NATURAL DRUGS
Morphologic and Taxonomic Consideration

NATURAL DRUGS

Morphologic and Taxonomic Consideration

— *2nd edn* —

by

Heber Wilkinson Youngken

Professor of Pharmacognosy and Materia Medica in the Massachusetts College of Pharmacy Boston; Member of the Committee of Revision of the Pharmacopoeia of the United States of America; Editor of the Section of Pharmacognosy and Pharmaceutical Botany of "Biological Abstracts;" Botanical Editor of The United States Dispensatory;" Author of Pharmaceutical Botany," etc.

2004

BIOTECH BOOKS

DELHI - 110035

Heber Wilkinson Youngken (1885–)
Original Title: A Textbook of Pharmacognosy
First Indian Impression 2003
Second Indian Impression 2004

ISBN 81-7622-090-6

Published by : **BIOTECH BOOKS**
1123/74, Tri Nagar,
Delhi - 110 035
Phone: 27382765
e-mail: biotechbooks@yahoo.co.in

Showroom : 4762-63/23, Ansari Road, Darya Ganj,
New Delhi - 110 002
Phone: 23245578, 23244987

Printed at : **Chawla Offset Printers**
New Delhi - 110 052

PRINTED IN INDIA

PREFACE TO THE SECOND EDITION

Since the publication of the first edition, the results of many investigations have been added to the literature of pharmacognosy. *The United States Pharmacopœia X* and *National Formulary V* have recently appeared with their many changes in the standards of official drugs. These, together with changes in the methods of production and in the commercial sources of drugs, have made it necessary to give the work a most thorough revision. As a result many parts had to be rewritten and new facts gleaned from the current literature, correspondence and personal observation, introduced.

The general plan of the text, which has proven acceptable, remains the same, save for the addition of a Chapter on Microanalytical Methods to Part II and the incorporation of the more important uses of drugs in their respective monographs.

One hundred and fifty-four pages of new subject matter and ninety-one figures have been added to the body of the work. The Index and the Bibliography, the latter containing many references which the author consulted, have been proportionately increased.

Part I has been augmented by the introduction of new data on the drying, sampling and examination of crude drugs. In Part II, the Chapter on "Crude Drugs of Vegetable Origin" has been increased by 133 pages, and several additional drugs have been treated therein. The classification of the drugs in the Chapter on "Crude Drugs of Animal Origin" has been altered to conform with the evolutionary system used in the preceding chapter, and several additional drugs have been added thereto.

The author wishes to express his appreciation to his former pupil and assistant, Prof. W. J. Stoneback, for his kindly aid in the preparation of a number of the photographs on crude drugs from which new cuts were made.

To Mr. L. J. Schwarz, Pharmacognosist of the United States Department of Agriculture at the port of New York, who extended much recent information on commercial sources of foreign drugs and to the authors and publishers of the other works from which cuts were borrowed or reproduced my thanks are due.

PREFACE TO THE FIRST EDITION

The primary aim of the author, in preparing this book, was to supply a systematic text which could be used by students of pharmacognosy in colleges and universities where the science of pharmacognosy is taught either from the morphologic or taxonomic viewpoint or from both. To this end the contents of this volume have been arranged in two parts. Part I embraces the "Morphologic Consideration of Crude Drugs" and Part II the "Taxonomic Consideration of Crude Drugs."

The secondary aim of the author was to provide a book which could also be used by the drug analyst, pharmacognosist, wholesale and retail pharmacist and collector of crude drugs. To meet these varied requirements, there has been included information not only dealing with the synonyms, titles, habitats, ash, limit of impurities, physical characteristics, microscopical structure, and constituents of crude drugs of the *United States Pharmacopœia IX and National Formulary IV*, but in addition, many of the more common unofficial crude materials such as unofficial drugs, condiments, spices, cereals, tea, chocolate, etc., the adulterants of drugs, drug production and commerce, and descriptions of medicinal plants.

The tables of comparison between commercial varieties of crude drugs as well as between drugs and their more common past adulterants, it is hoped will prove helpful.

The World War has wrought some marked changes in the geographical sources of supply of many foreign drugs. Through considerable correspondence, the perusal of recent Consular reports and from up-to-date information kindly extended by Professor C. J. Zufall, Assistant Pharmacognosist of the United States Department of Agriculture, at the port of New York, valuable modern data has been acquired on the commercial phase of the subject which has been introduced in the text. A growing demand exists for information bearing upon the cultivation of medicinal plants. Many of these which can be grown successfully in the United States are considered under "Production" in Part II. In the arrangement of the plant families appearing in Chapter I of Part II, the author has adopted the Evolutionary system. In respect to nomenclature of plants, he has mainly followed Engler and Prantl's "Die naturlichen Pflanzenfamilien and "Gray's New Manual of Botany," being careful to include, in respect to official vegetable drugs, those botanical names given in the latest editions of the "U.S.P." and "N.F.," so as to avoid confusion amongst students.

The names adopted for animals, appearing in Chapter II of Part II, are those appearing in the ninth edition of the U.S.P. and in the last edition of Maisch's "Organic Materia Medica."

In marshalling together the information contained within the covers of this volume, the author, in addition to his own research and study has consulted a wide range of foreign and domestic literature including books, bulletins of the United States Department of Agriculture, magazine articles and scientific papers. The titles and authors of many of these are given in the text and Bibliography and hereby acknowledged.

To Mr. Benjamin F. Hoffstein, Instructor in Pharmacognosy and Mr. Winfield F. Smith, Assistant in Botany, who aided in furnishing several of the drawings, and to Dr. Wm. R. Taylor of the University of Pennsylvania, who read the pages on the Algae, my thanks are due.

Grateful acknowledgment is made to Marin S. Dunn, A.M., Instructor in Botany and Pharmacognosy in the college, for material aid both on many of the drawings and in the compiling of the index. Finally, the writer desires to express his appreciation to Mr. I. A. Hagy of P. Blakiston's Son and Co. for the encouragement he has given during the publication of this book.

HEBER W. YOUNGKEN.

CONTENTS

PART I

MORPHOLOGIC CONSIDERATIONS OF DRUGS

CHAPTER I

FUNDAMENTAL CONSIDERATIONS

CHAPTER II

MORPHOLOGICAL CLASSIFICATION OF CRUDE VEGETABLE DRUGS

PART II

TAXONOMIC CONSIDERATION OF DRUGS

CHAPTER I

Crude Drugs of Vegetable Origin

CHAPTER III

MICROANALYTICAL METHODS

PART I

MORPHOLOGIC CONSIDERATION
OF
DRUGS

CHAPTER I

FUNDAMENTAL CONSIDERATIONS

Pharmacognosy is the science which treats of the history, commerce, collection, selection, identification, valuation and preservation of crude drugs, and other raw materials of vegetable and animal origin.

Crude Drugs occur in commerce either in the entire, nearly entire, or broken condition, as in most roots, rhizomes and roots, barks, fruits, seeds and some leaves, or in the matted together condition, as in Chondrus and many leaf and leaf and top drugs, in the form of transverse slices as in Colchicum Corm, Bryonia and Calumba, in longitudinal slices, as Veratrum Viride, etc., in the cut form, as some of the commercial Althæa and Licorice root, in the pressed condition, as in the pressed herbs, in the peeled condition, as Colocynth, or deprived of cork (periderm), as Jamaica Ginger, Althæa, Ulmus, etc., in the peeled and elongated cut form, as orris and rhubarb fingers, or in the ground or powdered condition, as most drugs, or finally, they may be first powdered and then molded into various shapes, as "compressed rhubarb."

There has always been a wide variance in the quality of crude drugs. This is generally due to one or more of the following causes: (1) Deficiency in knowledge or carelessness on the part of the collector; (2) want of care in preparing them for the market; (3) carelessness in garbling them; (4) carelessness in storing and preserving them; (5) accidental contamination with another drug; (6) adulteration; and (7) substitution.

Drugs are either official or unofficial. An official drug is one that is listed and described in a book recognized by the government as the legal authority for standards. In the United States all drugs are official, at present, which are listed in the United States Pharmacopœia X and National Formulary V. Every drug in either of these two standard books has a Latin official name and an English official name.

Some of the drugs in addition have one or more official common names or synonyms. The *Latin official* name is derived either from the name of the genus of the plant or animal yielding the drug, as Podophyllum and Cantharis, or from the specific name, as Ipecacuanha, or from the combined names of the genus and species, as Viburnum Opulus, or from a previous synonym, as Cascara Sagrada, or from other sources, as Pix Pini, Opium, etc.

The *botanical origin* represents the scientific name of the plant or scientific names of the plants yielding the drug. Thus, the botanical origin of Wild Cherry Bark is *Prunus serotina;* that of Burdock Root is *Arctium Lappa* and *Arctium minus;* that of American Wormseed is *Chenopodium ambrosioides anthelminticum.*

The *zoölogical origin* represents the scientific name of the animal or scientific names of the animals yielding the drug. Thus, the zoölogical origin of Cantharides is *Cantharis vesicatoria*, whilst that of Civet is *Viverra Civetta* and *Viverra Zibetha.*

The *habitat* is the original home of the plant or animal yielding the drug. Plants or animals found thriving in their original or native home are said to be *indigenous* thereto. When these organisms thrive in some locality other than that to which they are native, they are said to be *naturalized.* Thus, the Belladonna plant (*Atropa Belladonna*) is indigenous to central and southern Europe and naturalized in the United States.

The *commercial origin* of a drug represents its trade or commercial source. This may be the country or district in which the plant or the animal furnishing the drug is grown or the country or the port from which the drug is shipped. Thus, English Valerian is the product of plants grown in England; Shensi Rhubarb is the product of plants grown in the Shensi district of China; Bombay Mace is the product of plants grown in the interior of India but shipped from the port of Bombay; Alexandria Senna is the product of plants grown in El Hejaz but shipped in part to the markets of the world from Cairo, Egypt.

The *official definition* of a crude drug is found as the initial paragraph beneath the name or names of a drug in the pharmacopœia or national formulary. It consists of the part used, botanical or zoölogical origin, and family, and in some instances of the commercial varieties, habitat, preparation for the market, and purity rubric. The *official description* follows the official definition and generally comprises the occurrence, external and internal appearances, fracture, odor and taste. In some instances the microscopical characteristics of the crude drug and its powder are also included as well as tests for identity, purity, etc.

Collection of Drugs.—The best time for the collection of various drugs is considered in other parts of the text. It is the result of painstaking investigations in chemistry and pharmacodynamics. It may be said broadly, however, that the general rules for the collection of the greater number of vegetable crude drugs in each of the several classes are as follows: Autumn for roots, rhizomes, bulbs, tubers or barks; when fully expanded for flowers; just before expansion for leaf or flower buds; when the flowers of the plant are opening for leaves; when full grown for fruits; and when fully developed for seeds.

In the collection of fleshy subterranean plant organs such as Squill, Poke Root, American Hellebore, Calumba, etc., it is necessary to slice them before they are dried, in order to properly insure against mold attack. Mold spores germinate quickly in the presence of warmth and moisture and so these drugs should be dried rapidly and yet at a temperature not high enough to injure their active constituents.

It is well for the collector to know the plants yielding the drugs he seeks to collect; indeed he should be thoroughly acquainted with their most important gross features, but it is folly to expect him to be that sufficiently learned in morphology or taxonomy as to be able to distinguish between closely related varieties of a given species. This is a matter for the drug broker's or wholesaler's pharmacognosist to determine.

All crude drugs should be carefully garbled before being sold to the public or used in the manufacture of preparations. By *garbling* is meant the removal of extraneous matter from the drug, such as sand, dirt, or parts of plants which are at variance with the officially indicated portion. In many instances it is practically impossible to prevent some degree of harmless contamination. For this reason the pharmacopœia and national formulary give a limit of permissible impurities in many of the drug definitions.

It is well known that certain crude drugs must undergo a curing process in order that important active constituents may be developed. This generally involves a slow drying or sweating during which substances of biologic origin, known as ferments, initiate chemical changes which result in the alteration of their constituents. Among these might be mentioned Coca, Guarana, Gentiana, Belladonna, Hyoscyamus, Tonka, Sabal, Tobacco, and Vanilla.

In the cases of Cascara and Frangula barks it is necessary to destroy a contained irritant principle, before they can be used. This may be accomplished either by heating these barks at a temperature of 100°C. for 48 hours or by keeping them at least a year before using.

Drying of Drugs.—Crude drugs are dried in order that sufficient moisture may be removed from them to insure their good keeping qualities. Effective drying is best accomplished through the proper regulation of temperature, humidity and circulation of air. The loss of moisture should be gradual. Freshly gathered drugs are either air dried or dried by artificial heat.

In air drying, the drug is spread on trays, screens or floors or hung on wires in a room where the air can properly circulate. At the beginning, the fresh drug is spread out one layer thick and as drying progresses, it is often piled in thicker layers which are frequently turned. Drying in the shade under a roof, as on a barn floor, is recommended for most drugs, although many barks, rhizomes and roots can be adequately dried in the sun. In all cases the drying drug should be protected from rain and humid atmosphere.

In drying by artificial heat, a controlled heating and ventilating system is recommended. While small lots can be successfully dried in a heated room, special drying houses or drying apparatus equipped with tiers of trays or racks and a controlled heating and ventilating system is desirable (see Farmer's Bull. 1231, U. S. Dept. Agric.). For most barks, roots, rhizomes, leaves, herbs, seeds and some fruits, it has been found that a gradual raising of the temperature from 25°C. to 50°C. will give a satisfactory product; in the case of flowers and drugs containing volatile constituents, the temperature should not be raised over 35°C.

Valuation of Drugs.—This may be determined qualitatively by *organoleptic tests*, such as the application of sight, smell, taste and touch, and by *microscopical observation.* In some cases the organoleptic tests alone suffice. In others, as in the case of all powdered and ground drugs of vegetable or animal origin, the use of the compound microscope is essential.

In many instances a good idea of the quality of a drug can be ascertained by employing *microchemic methods.* These generally consist of examining mounts of sections or powdered drug in various reagents which either form salts of the contained active principles, that have constant characters, or show definite color reactions. It is often possible to determine whether a powdered drug has been exhausted by examining the crystals found in its sublimate. These have been found to be characteristic for many drugs.

Crude drugs are valued by *physical methods* when it is necessary to determine their specific gravity, optical rotation, melting point, or their degree of elasticity.

Chemical methods of valuation are employed when it is necessary to determine the percentage of active principle or principles, of oil, fat, carbohydrate, protein, ash, or crude fiber present in the sample (quantitative chemical methods) or when it is essential to determine by the use of reagents the color reactions or solubilities of drugs or their constituents (qualitative chemical methods).

Pharmacodynamic methods are employed in valuing a number of potent drugs or their preparations, such as Cannabis, Digitalis, Strophanthus-Aconite, Ergot, etc. These involve the study of the effect of a preparation or constituent of the crude drug on normal, healthy animals or plants.

Sampling of Crude Vegetable Drugs.—The problem of obtaining truly representative samples of a crude vegetable drug is one often requiring experience, judgment and skill. The samples are taken either by means of a specially devised tool called a trier or sampler or by hand.

The U.S.P. X and N.F. V recommend a schedule for sampling which is as follows:

No. of packages in shipment	No. of packages to be sampled
1 to 10	1 to 3
20 to 25	2 to 4
25 to 50	3 to 6
50 to 75	6 to 8
75 to 100	8 to 10
Over 100	Not less than 10

An excellent sampler has been developed by Mr. L. J. Schwarz of New York (see Fig. 1) which consists of a hollow drill spindle with provision for fitting a hollow drill on one end and a quick release and cap on the other. The drills used are made from tool steel and are of knife-edge or saw-tooth design. They can be used interchangeably depending upon the nature of the material which is to be sampled. The saw-toothed drill is better for tightly baled leaves, whereas the knife-edge drill is better for sarsaparilla and ipecac, etc. One end of the hollow spindle is threaded to accommodate the drill or an extension drill spindle. The other end is provided with pins for the attachment of the end cap. The

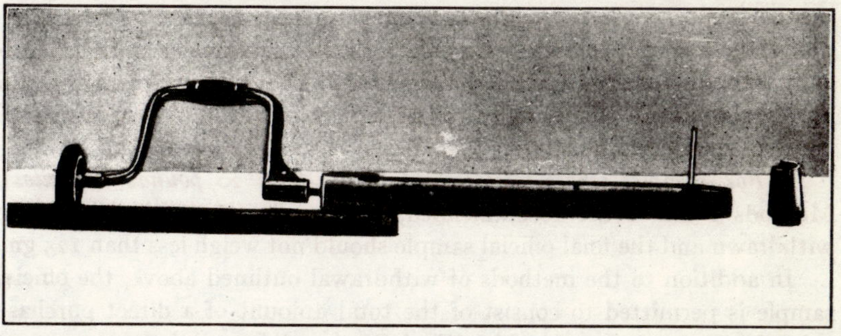

FIG. 1.—Sampler employed in taking samples of various kinds of crude vegetable drugs. (*Courtesy of L. J. Schwarz.*)

end cap is provided with a shank suited to a standard brace, an arrangement which will permit of hand drilling.

In using this sampler, the operator cuts out the desired number of cores of the drug to be sampled. As each core is cut, the end cap is released and the drug column in the sampler is forced into a suitable container by means of a wooden plunger.

While the sampler described is suited for the sampling of a large number of drugs, it is unsuited for material baled under hydraulic pressure, for heavy barks such as yohimbe or such roots as gentian, hydrangea, etc., or for some of the gum drugs.

The U.S.P. X. and N.F. V. give 3 methods for the withdrawal of official samples of vegetable drugs. They are essentially as follows:

1. *For gross samples whose component parts are 1 cm. or less in any dimension, and for all powdered or ground drugs.* It is recommended that a sampler be employed which removes a core from the top to the bottom of the container, not less than 2 cores being taken in opposite directions.

If the total weight of the drug to be sampled is less than 200 pounds (100 kilos), at least 250 gm. constitutes an official sample, when the total weight exceeds 200 pounds, repeated samples shall be taken by the above method according to the schedule recommended for sampling, mixed and quartered, 2 of the diagonal quarters being rejected, the remaining 2 quarters being combined and carefully mixed and again quartered in the same way until 2 of the quarters weigh at least 250 gm., which latter quarters shall constitute an official sample.

2. *For gross samples whose component parts are over 1 cm. in any dimension,* the sample is taken by hand. When the total weight of the drug sampled is less than 200 pounds (100 kilos), at least 500 gm. constitutes an official sample and this must be taken from different parts of the container or containers. When the total weight is in excess of 100 kilos, repeated samples must be taken by the above method and according to the schedule recommended for sampling, mixed and quartered, 2 of the diagonal quarters being rejected, the remaining 2 quarters carefully combined, mixed and again subjected to the quartering process until 2 of the quarters weigh not less than 500 gm. which latter quarters shall constitute an official sample.

3. *For samples whose total weight is less than* 20 *pounds* (10 *kilos*). Methods 1 and 2 are recommended, but smaller quantities should be withdrawn and the final official sample should not weigh less than 125 gm.

In addition to the methods of withdrawal outlined above, the official sample is permitted to consist of the total amount of a direct purchase made by Federal, State or Municipal Food and Drugs' Act enforcement officials.

Preservation of Drugs.—Insects, mites, molds, rusts, moisture and temperature are important factors which must be taken into consideration, if crude drugs are to be kept so as to be of salable appearance and therapeutically active.

Most of the crude drugs are subject to attacks by *insects* which render them unsightly and so unfit for sale. Chief among these pests, which ruin huge amounts of crude drugs yearly, are various species of beetles (*Coleoptera*) and moths (*Lepidoptera*). Both of these orders of insects have four stages in their life histories, viz.: egg, larva, pupa and imago. The eggs are frequently deposited on the drug by the adult (imago) female, before the drug reaches the dealer (at times before it is even collected). Under favorable conditions, such as are often prevalent in places where drugs are stored, these eggs hatch out into worm-like creatures called larvæ (sing. larva). The larvæ have biting mouth parts and feed on the drug making it unsightly. If not combatted, they may travel from one box, drawer, package or can to another and in time cause wholesale destruction. After a time each larva develops into a pupa and then into an imago or winged adult. All of these stages may be passed inside of one container and several generations or broods may be reared, until the drug is eventually reduced to debris.

Probably the most common drug infesting beetle is *Sitodrepa panicea*, a member of the *Ptinidæ* family. It possesses a brown colored, subcylindrical body, rounded at anterior and posterior ends, with head nearly concealed by prothorax and with striated wing covers (elytra). Its length is from 2 to 3 mm. The larva of this insect is characterized by a brown head with strong jaws (mandibles) and a white abdomen. It channels its way through the drug leaving evidences of its presence in the form of holes. In the course of a couple of weeks it changes to a pupa which soon develops into an adult beetle that also feeds upon the drug. I have found this insect in specimens of most of the spices, in black hellebore, aconite, belladonna, poke, angelica, marshmallow and parsley roots, in scopola and in wheat middlings.

Another drug ravaging beetle, *Lasioderma serricorne*, has a somewhat similar appearance to the preceding species but is larger and broader with smooth elytra. It has been found to attack spices and tobacco. Other beetles responsible for considerable damage are *Ptinus brunneus* and *Niptus hololeucus*.

The most prevalent drug attacking moth is the corn meal moth, *Tinea zea*. In its larva (caterpillar) stage it has been found in ergot, flaxseed, the *Compositæ* root drugs such as dandelion and burdock, in aconite, as well as many other drugs and cereals. A member of the fly and mosquito order (*Diptera*), namely, *Trypeta arnicivora* lays its eggs on the receptacles of Arnica flowers before they are gathered. These eggs frequently hatch out in the drug later and, feeding on it, do considerable damage.

A number of animal products and cereals are subject to attack by *mites*. Mites differ mainly from insects in not being differentiated, as to their bodies, into distinct head, thorax and abdomen, and in possessing in their fully developed condition eight legs instead of six. Several species of the mite genus, *Glyciphagus*, have been commonly found in Cantharides. Their presence is indicated when powder and fragments of the whole drug and minute, motile, white specks are observed in the container.

The most effective means of ridding crude drugs of eggs, larvæ and adult insects is to expose them to a temperature of 60°C. for a period varying from 15 minutes for small quantities to two or three days for supplies in large store rooms.

A practical means of combatting insects and mites in crude drugs kept on a small scale is to keep them in air-tight tin cans or jars into which a few drops or more (depending on the size of the container) of carbon tetrachloride or chloroform are introduced from time to time. At least two treatments of each new lot of drug with either of these insecticides is essential, if any degree of success is to be attained. The first treatment will kill any larvæ present in the container, but it should be known that the vapors of these insecticides will not penetrate the eggs. A second treatment in the course of about a week or two, after the remaining eggs have had time to hatch out, generally insures against the depredations of these pests. A third treatment in the course of another week or two will insure the effectiveness of the remedy with a certainty.

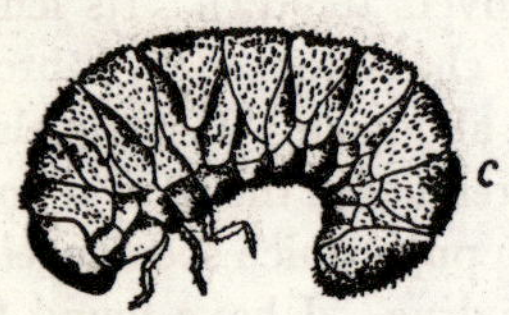

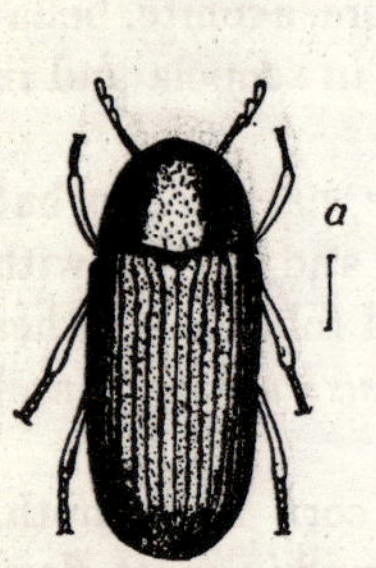

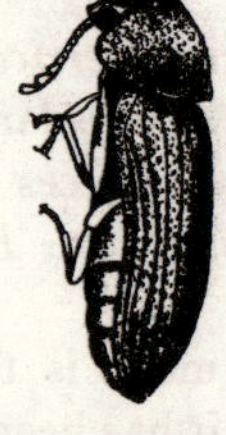

FIG. 2.

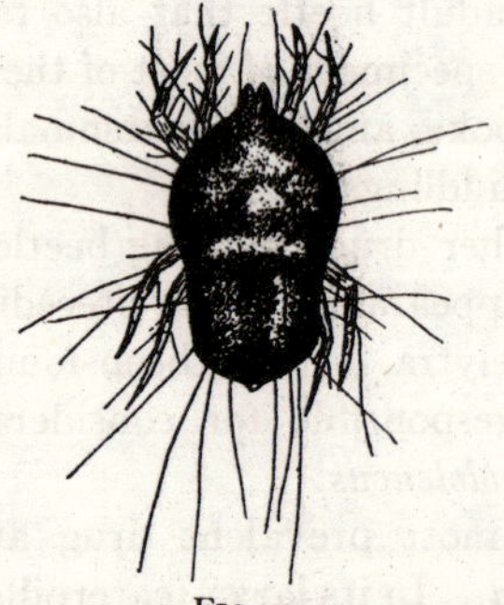

FIG. 3.

FIG. 2.—*Sitodrepa panicea* Linné. The common drug-eating insect. *a*, Dorsal view of adult bettle. *b*, Side view of adult beetle. *c*, Larva.—(*Sayre after Smith.*)

FIG. 3.—A Cantharid-eating Mite (*Glyciphagus spinipes*).—(*Sayre after Fum. and Rob.*)

Tar camphor may be used effectively in the preservation of Cantharis, Coccus and other dried animal drugs.

Molds are apt to attack fleshy rhizomes, roots, corms, and bulbs as well as various leaf and herb drugs. Their spores are constantly present in the atmosphere and only require the presence of moisture and warmth in order to germinate and grow into hyphæ. These hyphæ or mold filaments penetrate the drug and in time form a mycelium which appears as a whitish or colored intertangled mass of hyphal threads. The protoplasm of every mold secretes enzymes which not only digest and dissolve the cellular tissue of the drug but alter its constituents and make it in time worthless. To insure against mold attack all vegetable drugs should be carefully dried and stored in dry containers in a cool room.

Rusts occasionally attack leaves or herbs before they are collected. They are parasitic plants whose spores form hyphæ in the presence of moisture and warmth that ramify through the intercellular-air-spaces of the host and send branches into the cells. These secrete enzymes which alter the constituents present. The presence of rusts may often be detected by their brownish or reddish fruiting bodies which appear on the surface of the drug. Malvæ Folia N.F. is more apt to contain considerable rust infested material than any other official drug concerning which the writer is aware. In this case *Puccinia Malvacearum* is the fungus responsible, producing brownish fruiting bodies on many of the leaves. All rust infested material should be rejected before the drug is stored or used in any way.

Yeasts, bacteria and molds all secrete enzymes which destroy or alter constituents, and have the ability to develop in the presence of moisture, air and warmth. Vegetable drugs, therefore, should be kept in dry air-tight containers and in a cool room, if they are to be kept in good condition. All cellular vegetable drugs should be perfectly dry before they are stored.

Apart from the influence of temperature on the development of bacteria and fungi, it should be remembered that it bears a direct relation to the quality of many drugs. All drugs, for instance, containing volatile principles are deleteriously influenced by being dried or stored at the higher temperatures. Care should therefore be exercised in drying these slowly at moderate temperatures and in storing them in air-tight containers, in a room having a fairly uniform cool temperature.

Historical.—The word "Pharmacognosy" was introduced by Seydler in 1815 and literally translated means the science of drugs or medicines. If we consider that up to the last 50 or 75 years it was customary for pharmacists, physicians and others to collect drugs directly from plants in the field and so required of these more of a knowledge of the characteristics of living medicinal plants than of their products, we can well agree with Tschirch that the ancient herbalists were the first pharmacognosists.

The collection of herbs for medicinal use dates backward to remote antiquity. The papyri of the ancient Egyptians written as early as 1600 B.C. record the names of many drugs in use by the physicians of that period including acacia, myrrh, cannabis, coriander, opium, myrrh, aloe, frankincense, hemlock and cassia.

The ancient Greeks were familiar with a number of drugs in use to-day. Pythagoras (B.C. 582), a Greek philosopher, was acquainted with mustard and squill and Hippocrates (B.C. 466), a Greek physician, with absinthium, cinnamon, conium, gentian, hyoscyamus, rhubarb, acacia, myrrh, chamomile and many others. Theophrastus (B.C. 372), a pupil of Aristotle, wrote ten books "On the History of Plants" and eight "On the Causes of Plants." He was familiar with ergot, pepper, opium, aspidium and cinnamon.

Pedanios Dioscorides, a Greek physician, who lived in the first century B.C. was the first to write extensively on medicinal plants. His great work "De Materia Medica," written in 77 or 78 B.C., treats of all the medicinal substances then known and of their properties. During fifteen centuries his work was the authority in botany and materia medica and is even now held in high esteem among many of the Turks and Moors.

Pliny, the Elder (23–79 A.D.), a Roman soldier and writer, wrote 37 large volumes on natural history which contained information on about 1000 plants. While his works treat extensively with fabled monsters, they were, nevertheless, considered authoritative during the middle ages. Henna, cassia, piper, linum, anise, aspidium and other drugs still in use are mentioned in his writings. Galen (131–200 A. D.), a Greek physician, noted in his writings the adulteration of saffron, myrrh, cinnamon and rhubarb.

Very little of original work was produced by writers on medicinal plants from Dioscorides' time until the 13th century A.D., when Ibn Baitar (1197–1248 A.D.), a physician of Malaga, contributed an extensive treatise on materia medica entitled "Liber magnæ collectionis simplicium alimentorium et medicamentorum." This work contains much of value on the economic plants of the East. In 1530, 1531 and 1536, Otto Brunfels, a German botanist and physician, published three volumes entitled "Herbarum Vivæ Icones," which contained 229 woodcuts of plants and was famed for having been the first work to contain good botanical illustrations. Brunfels was also the first to write on local floras and to describe the native plants of Germany and as such is regarded by many as the "father of botany."

Valerius Cordus (1515–1544), Professor of materia medica at the University of Wittenburg, wrote several papers on medicinal plants which were published after his death by Conrad Gesner in 1561, at Strassburg. This publication is a large volume which not only contains the papers of Cordus (Historiæ stirpium, etc.) but also a treatise, "De Hortis Germaniæ" by Gesner himself.

In 1737, Carl von Linné (Linnæus) (1707–1778) a Swedish botanist, published his "Genera Plantarum" which was considered the starting point of systematic botany. Linnaeus published a number of works dealing with botany and zoology, but by far his most notable accomplishment was his "Species Plantarum." This work appeared in 1753 and includes a lengthy list of species of plants together with their descriptions and classification, according to a natural system, based upon a study of the resemblances and differences of their sexual organs. To Linnaeus belongs the credit of having brought order and system out of chaos, for his "Species Plantarum" is regarded by all modern botanists as the starting point of Systematic Botany, and this binomial system of nomenclature therein introduced is followed by all naturalists of note even to the present day.

In 1816, morphine was discovered in opium by Friederich Wilhelm Adam Setürner, an apothecary of Eimbeck, in Hanover, Germany, who demonstrated its poisonous character and prepared a number of its salts. This discovery led probably more than any other to changing the focus of scientists from drug plants to crude drugs and their contents.

In 1820, Guibourt, a Frenchman, of Paris issued a valuable treatise entitled "Historie Naturelle des Drogues Simples" which passed through several editions.

Modern Pharmacognosy may be said to begin with the work of Theodor W. C. Martius, an apothecary of Erlangen, Germany. Martius conducted a series of investigations on drugs, publishing some of his results in 1825 and all of them in 1832, in a book entitled, "Grundniss der Pharmakognosie des Pflanzenreiches. This was the first extensive treatise on Pharmacognosy written.

In 1838, Histological Pharmacognosy had its beginning with the announcement by Mathias Jacob Schleiden, a German botanist, that the cell is the fundamental unit of plant structure and that all tissues are combinations of cells.

The following year Jonathan Pereira published, in London, a valuable work entitled "Elements of Materia Medica and Therapeutics."

In 1842, M. J. Schleiden, then a professor of Botany at Jena, wrote his most important work, "Grundzüge der Wissentschaftliche Botanik." In this work he emphasized the inductive method of botanical research and sharply attacked the hazy, philosophical treatment of questions bearing on morphology. In 1857, he issued one of the early Pharmacognosies, entitled "Handbuch der Medicinisch-Pharmazeutischen Botanik und botanischen Pharmakognosie," which was published at Leipsic. He shows therein that drugs of different kinds must be determined by their cellular differences and he designated Pharmacognosy, on account of its exacting character, as "the mother of all scientific discipline."

In 1858, O. Berg, of Berlin, Germany, issued his "Pharmazeutischen Waarenkunde" and in 1865 his "Anatomischer Atlas zur Pharmazeutischen Waarenkunde."

From this time on Pharmacognosy developed rapidly in Europe, largely due to the researches and publications of such scholars as Vogl, Wiegand, Wittstein, Behrens, Tunmann, Oesterle, Hoffman, Flückiger,

Moeller, Hanausek, Meyer, Gilg and Dragendorff of Germany, Tschirch and Zörnig of Switzerland, Baillon and Collin of France, and Holmes, Hanbury, Greenish and Wallis of England.

Among the works of these scientists the following should be consulted by all who seek an intimate acquaintanceship with the cream of foreign pharmacognic classics:

"Pharmakognosie," by A. Vogl.
"Anatomischer Atlas zur Pharmakognosie," by A. E. Vogl.
"Lehrbuch der Pharmakognosie," by Albert Wiegand.
"Pharmakognosie des Pflanzenreichs," by G. C. Wittstein.
"Pharmakognosie des Pflanzenreiches," by F. A. Fluckiger.
"Pharmacographia," by F. A. Fluckiger and Daniel Hanbury.
"Pharmakognosi," by Hoffman.
"Microscopy of Technical Products," by T. F. Hanausek and A. Winton.
"Pharmakognostischer Atlas," by Joseph Moeller.
"Lehrbuch der Pharmakognosie," by Joseph Moeller.
"Mikroskopie der Nahrungs und Genussmittel," by Joseph Moeller.
"Microscopy of Vegetable Foods," by Winton and Moeller.
"Lehrbuch der Pharmakognosie," by Ernst Gilg.
"Anatomischer Atlas," by Tschirch and Oesterle.
"Handbuch der Pharmakognosie," by Alexander Tschirch.
"Arzneidrogen," by Heinrich Zörnig.
"Traite de Toxocologie Vegetale," by Eugene Collin.
"Anatomical Atlas of Vegetable Powders," by Henry G. Greenish and Eugene Collin.
"Microscopical Examination of Foods and Drugs," by Henry G. Greenish.
"A Text Book of Materia Medica" by Henry G. Greenish.
"Anleitung zur Microchemischen Analyse," by H. Behrens.
"Grundriss einer Histochemie der Pflanzlichen Genussmittel," by Hans Molisch.
"Pflanzenmikrochemie," by Otto Tunmann.
"Microchemie der Pflanze," by Hans Molisch.
"Wissenschaftliche Droguen Kunde," by Arthur Meyer.

In the United States, apart from work done on medicinal plants by Bartram, Carson, Millspaugh, and others, Pharmacognosy did not begin to develop to the standing of a distinct science until up to about 40 years ago.

Since that time it has advanced by leaps and bounds, largely due to the researches and publications of an increasing number of American investigators, until it is now recognized as a major study in the curriculum of nearly every pharmaceutical institution of this country. The pure food and drug act of 1906 and the adoption of microscopical descriptions for crude and powdered drugs in the subsequent revisions of the United States Pharmacopœia and National Formulary gave wonderful impetus to its growth.

Some of the books written by American authors which bear upon one or more phases of the science are as follows:

"Organic Materia Medica," by John M. Maisch.
"American Medicinal Plants," by Charles F. Millspaugh.
"College Botany," by Edson S. Bastin (revised by W. B. Day).
"Introduction to Pharmacognosy," by Smith E. Jeliffe.
"Scientific and Applied Pharmacognosy," by Henry Kraemer.
"Pharmacognosy," by Otto A. Wall.
"Materia Medica and Pharmacology," by D. M. R. Culbreth.
"Organic Materia Medica and Pharmacognosy," by Lucius E. Sayre.
"Histology of Medicinal Plants," by William Mansfield.
"Squibb's Atlas of The Official Drugs," by William Mansfield.
"Manual of Botany," by Henry H. Rusby.
"Microanalysis of Powdered Vegetable Drugs," by Albert Schneider.
"Pharmaceutical Botany," by Heber W. Youngken.
"Origin and History of Pharmacopoeial Vegetable Drugs, etc." by John Uri. Lloyd.
"A Text Book of Pharmacognosy" by Heber. W. Youngken.

CHAPTER II

MORPHOLOGICAL CLASSIFICATION OF CRUDE VEGETABLE DRUGS

ROOTS

These represent descending axes of plants which are devoid of leaves.

A. Those official in the U.S.P. x.

Title	Botanical Origin	Family
1. *Monocotyledonous:*		
Sarsaparilla	Smilax medica; Smilax ornata; Smilax officinalis (or undetermined sp.)	Liliaceæ
2. *Dicotyledonous:*		
Althæa	Althæa officinalis	Malvaceæ
Belladonnæ Radix	Atropa Belladonna	Solanaceæ
Calumba	Jateorrhiza palmata	Menispermaceæ
Ipomœa	Ipomœa orizabensis	Convolvulaceæ
Krameria	Krameria triandra; Krameria argentea	Leguminosæ
Senega	Polygala Senega	Polygalaceæ

B. Those official in the N.F. v. All dicotyledonous.

Title	Botanical Origin	Family
Asclepias	Asclepias tuberosa	Asclepiadaceæ
Baptisia	Baptisia tinctoria	Leguminosæ
Bryonia	Bryonia alba; Bryonia dioica	Cucurbitaceæ
Lappa	Arctium Lappa; Arctium minus	Compositæ
Manaca	Brunfelsia Hopeana	Solanaceæ
Pareira	Chondodendron tomentosum	Menispermaceæ
Phytolacca	Phytolacca decandra	Phytolaccaceæ
Rumex	Rumex crispus; Rumex obtusifolius	Polygonaceæ
Stillingia	Stillingia sylvatica	Euphorbiaceæ
Tonga	Epipremnum pinnatum	Araceæ

In the examination of root drugs the physical characteristics, including occurrence, size, shape, color, surface markings, fracture, internal appearance, odor, and taste are first taken into consideration.

Roots ***occur*** either in the entire or nearly entire condition, as Senega, Stillingia, Pyrethrum, or as longitudinal slices, in some specimens, as Althæa, Belladonna, and Lappa, or as transverse and oblique slices, as in Calumba and Bryonia, or in small cubical pieces, as in some specimens of Althæa, or as peeled, broken or longitudinally sliced roots, as in other specimens of Althæa, or as bales of rootlets, as in Sarsaparilla.

The *size* of the root includes a consideration of length and diameter, and is stated usually in terms of centimeters (cm.) and millimeters (mm).

In the consideration of *shape*, the general outline or form of the root is observed. This may be *conical*, as in Aconite; *fusiform*, as in Stillingia; *cylindrical*, as in Sarsaparilla; *disk-like*, as in Columba and Bryonia; *simple*, as in Pellitory; *branched*, as in Krameria and Senega; *twisted*, as in Scammoniæ Radix; etc.

The surface markings of roots may be of the nature of scars, furrows, wrinkles, annulations, nodules, fissures or abrasions. When roots exhibit more or less parallel well defined ridges and depressions, as in Mexican and Jamaica Sarsaparillas and Scammony root, they are *furrowed;* when the furrows are less defined, as in Baptisia, they are *wrinkled;* when transverse, ring-like outgrowths are evident, as in Ipecacuanha and Petroselini Radix, they are *annulated;* when openings occur running into the tissues, as in Ipecac and Savanilla Krameria, they are *fissured;* when more or less rounded outgrowths occur on the surface, as in Muira Puama, they are *nodulated;* when portions of the outer tissues are rubbed off, as in Belladonna Root, they are *abraded*.

Fracture has to do with the way a root or other plant part breaks when subjected to enough pressure. The fracture of most official roots is *complete*, since they break clean across. That of Sarsaparilla and Aralia is *incomplete*, since both of these break only part way across. The terms *short*, *brittle*, *fibrous*, *horny*, *strongly* or *slightly*, etc., are used to describe the nature of complete or incomplete fractures. To these are frequently added the terms *even*, *uneven*, *starchy*, *resinous*, *conchoidal*, etc., in order to describe the nature of the fractured surface.

Those roots which are too tough to be fractured are *breakable*, as Pareira, Ipomœa, and the thicker pieces of Krameria and Asclepias.

After the root has been broken or fractured, its *internal characteristics* should be observed. In respect to this, it is necessary to observe the color and other characters of cortex, wood, cambium, and, in the case of monocotyl roots, the nature of the endodermis and stele.

The ratio in diameter of bark to wood should be observed as well as the color and markings of each of these regions. In Monocotyl roots it is essential to note the ratio in diameter of cortex and central cylinder or *stele*.

Attention to odor and taste is particularly important in determining the quality of drugs.

The *odor* of a drug is either *distinct* or *indistinct*. It is distinct in the vast majority of root drugs. In such roots as Asclepias, Krameria, Phytolacca, and Sarsaparilla, it is indistinct. The distinctness of the odor of a drug bears a direct relation to the volatile constituents it possesses. The term "characteristic" is employed to qualify an odor or taste which has not been correlated with that of any other substance in nature.

The taste of a drug may be *simple*, when it has but one taste, as Krameria, which is astringent. Whenever, more than one taste sensation is imparted by a drug, as for example Aconite, which is successively sweet, acrid, tingling and benumbing, the taste is described as *complex*.

Following a study of the physical characteristics, an inquiry into the microscopic structure of the root drug is made. In many instances the examination of transverse sections suffices to identify the drug. But in no case is the inquiry complete without the examination of longitudinal-radial and longitudinal-tangential sections.

All roots of Monocotyledons used as drugs are characterized by showing primary root structure and a polyarch radial fibrovascular bundle. The Dicotyledonous root drugs all show secondary root structure and so possess secondary cortex, one or more circles of collateral bundles, but no pith, Aconite excepted.

The study of the powdered root is next taken up. Powdered roots are characterized by the absence of mesophyll, the presence of cork or epidermal tissue, fibrovascular elements and ordinary parenchyma.

TUBEROUS ROOTS

These are swollen roots which show anomalous structure. See part 2. Both Dicotyledonous, and official in the U.S.P. x.

Title	Botanical Origin	Family
Aconitum	Aconitum Napellus	Ranunculaceæ
Jalapa	Exogonium Jalapa	Convolvulaceæ

TUBERS

These are short, thick and solid underground stems borne usually at the end of slender creeping branches. There is but one official tuber, namely, that of Corydalis. See part 2.

RHIZOMES

Rhizomes are creeping underground stems of horizontal, vertical or oblique growth.

A. Those official in the U.S.P. x.

Title	Botanical Origin	Family
1. *Fern rhizome and stipes:*		
Aspidium	Dryopteris Filix-mas	Polypodiaceæ
2. *Monocotyledonous rhizome:*		
Zingiber	Zingiber officinale	Zingiberaceæ

B. Those official in the N.F. v.

Title	Botanical Origin	Family
1. *Monocotyledonous:*		
Dioscorea	Dioscorea villosa	Dioscoreaceæ
Galanga	Alpinia officinarum	Zingiberaceæ
Iris	Iris germanica Iris florentina Iris pallida	Iridaceæ
Iris Versicolor	Iris versicolor Iris caroliniana	Iridaceæ
Zedoaria	Curcuma Zedoaria	Zingiberaceæ
2. *Dicotyledonous:*		
Geranium	Geranium maculatum	Geraniaceæ

In the examination of rhizomes, the physical characteristics are first to be noted. These should include occurrence, size, shape, direction of growth, surface markings (including stem and leaf bases and scars), fracture, internal appearance, odor and taste.

Rhizomes occur either in the entire condition as Trillium or Geranium; or in broken pieces as in Dioscorea, Zingiber, Iris, Iris Versicolor and Galanga; or in transverse slices as Zedoaria; or in longitudinal slices as some specimens of Iris Versicolor. Iris and some varieties of Zingiber are peeled or partially peeled. All of the official rhizomes excepting Trillium tend to be branched. They all grow in a horizontal direction except Zedoaria which has vertical growth.

The surface markings of rhizomes include annulations from the bases of leaves which have withered, stem scars, root scars and wrinkles, the last due to the contraction of the tissues in the drying process. In addition to these, Aspidium shows numerous curved stipe bases.

The fracture of the official rhizomes varies from short, brittle and even in Zedoaria, and Aspidium to short, tough and even in Dioscorea, Iris and Geranium to strongly tough and uneven in Galanga to short, brittle and uneven in Iris Versicolor and Zingiber.

In the study of the internal appearance, width, and color of bark or of cortex and central cylinder, bundle markings, prominence of endodermis and relative diameter of pith are taken into consideration. All of the official rhizomes excepting Aspidium and Geranium show scattered bundle markings in the central cylinder or stele. There is something diagnostic in the microscopic appearance of the fractured or cut surface of each of the official rhizomes. Thus, Aspidium is green and shows an interrupted circle of bundles; Zingiber shows scattered resin cells with yellowish, brown or reddish contents and a pale yellow endodermis; Dioscorea has a whitish or pale brown appearance and shows numerous scattered yellow bundles; Zedoaria shows a thick grayish-yellow cortex, separated from the very broad, grayish-brown stele by a light colored endodermis; in both cortex and stele will be noted numerous scattered, small brown spots, representing the contents of resin cells; Galanga shows an orange-brown broken surface with endodermis indistinct; Iris is yellowish-white, shows a narrow cortex, prominent endodermis and broad stele; Iris Versicolor resembles Iris but its internal color is pale purplish-brown; Trillium has numerous brownish root scar markings in its thick cortex; Geranium has a thin bark, distinct cambium and broad pith, and its color is light purple-brown.

The odor of Iris Versicolor, Dioscorea, Aspidium and Geranium is indistinct; that of Iris resembles violets; that of Zedoaria is camphor-like; that of the remainder is aromatic and distinctively characteristic.

The taste varies from aromatic and pungent in Zingiber, to aromatic, pungent and pepper-like in Galanga, to acrid in Iris and Iris Versicolor, to starchy and acrid in Dioscorea; to strongly astringent in Geranium.

Following the study of the physical characteristics, a study of the microscopical features should be undertaken, in order to prepare one not only to detect adulterants but to know what to expect in the study of the powdered drugs. This is applicable in the case of every crude drug representing a plant organ.

All of the official rhizomes excepting Aspidium and Geranium exhibit Monocotyl stem structure. In the examination of Monocotyl rhizomes the following tissue regions are to be studied:

1. Epidermis
2. Cortex
3. Endodermis
4. Central Cylinder or Stele.

As in aerial stems of Monocotyledons, fibrovascular bundles of the closed collateral or concentric type will be noted scattered throughout central cylinder and cortex regions. Some of these, namely the main rhizome bundles, run nearly straight but others, which course out toward leaves and roots, run obliquely or transversely. In rhizomes, where the nodes are closely approximated, relatively few straight or nearly straight bundles are encountered.

Epidermis is usually the outermost tissue, but in rhizomes of the *Zingiberaceæ* including Zingiber, Zedoaria and Galanga, cork arises in the subjacent cortex and so, in older portions of these, may be seen entirely replacing epidermis.

The parenchyma of the cortex and central cylinder should be particularly examined in respect to the nature of cell walls and cell contents.

In many instances diagnostic starch grains or crystals will be found. Scattered through this tissue may often be found secretion sacs with suberized walls and oleoresin contents, as in the Gingers, Zedoary and Galangal.

The nature of the thickenings of the endodermal cells should be observed as should also the markings on the walls of tracheæ and sclerenchyma fibers.

Aspidium is characterized microscopically by exhibiting both in its rhizome and stipe portions an interrupted circle of concentric bundles, each of which shows a central xylem composed for the most part of tracheæ and tracheids of the scalariform type and a phloem which completely envelops the xylem. Surrounding the bundle, in each instance, is a brownish endodermis or bundle sheath of a single layer of cells. In this drug, also, internal glands containing a greenish oleoresin are to be noted, projecting into the intercellular-air-spaces.

Geranium exhibits dicotyl stem structure and so shows the following regions: (1) cork, (2) cork cambium, (3) cortex, (4) fibrovascular bundles of the open collateral type arranged in a circle, connected by interfascicular cambium and separated by medullary rays, and (5) pith. Particularly diagnostic of this drug are the numerous colored tannin masses in the parenchyma of the cortex and pith, the abnormal development of the interfascicular cambium, showing several patches of soft bast on its outer face in each medullary ray region, the presence of rosette aggregates in various cells of the cortex, and the absence of sclerenchyma fibers.

RHIZOME AND ROOTS

A. Those official in the U.S.P. x.

Title	Botanical Origin	Family
1. *Monocotyledonous:*		
Veratrum Viride	Veratrum viride	Liliaceæ
2. *Dicotyledonous:*		
Cimicifuga	Cimicifuga racemosa	Ranunculaceæ
Gentiana	Gentiana lutea	Gentianaceæ
Glycyrrhiza	Glycyrrhiza glabra var. typica, Glycyrrhiza glabra var. glandulifera and other var. of G. glabra	Leguminosæ
Hydrastis	Hydrastis canadensis	Ranunculaceæ
Ipecacuanba	Cephaëlis Ipecacuanba Cephaelis acuminata	Rubiaceæ
Podophyllum	Podophyllum peltatum	Berberidaceæ
Rheum	Rheum officinale, R. palmatum Other sp. of Rheum grown in China and Thibet.	Polygonaceæ
Serpentaria	Aristolochia Serpentaria Aristolochia reticulata	Aristolochiaceæ
Valeriana	Valeriana officinalis	Valerianaceæ

B. Those official in the N.F. v.

Title	Botanical Origin	Family
1. *Monocotyledonous:*		
Aletris	Aletris farinosa	Liliaceæ
Convallariæ Radix	Convallaria majalis	Liliaceæ
Cypripedium	Cypripedium hirsutum Cypripedium pubescens Cypripedium parviflorum	Orchidaceæ
Helonias	Chamælirium luteum	Liliaceæ
Trillium	Trillium erectum et al sp.	Liliaceæ
Triticum	Agropyron repens	Gramineæ
2. *Dicotyledonous:*		
Angelicæ Radix	Angelica Archangelica et al. sp. of Angelica	Umbelliferæ
Apocynum	Apocynum cannabinum	Apocynaceæ
Aralia	Aralia racemosa	Araliaceæ
Asarum	Asarum canadense	Aristolochiaceæ
Berberis	Sp. of Sect. Mahonia of genus Berberis	Berberidaceæ
Caulophyllum	Caulophyllum thalictroides	Berberidaceæ
Echinacea	Brauneria pallida Brauneria angustifolia	Compositæ
Gelsemium	Gelsemium sempervirens	Loganiaceæ
Taraxacum	Leontodon Taraxacum	Compositæ
Hydrangea	Hydrangea arborescens	Saxifragaceæ
Inula	Inula Helenium	Compositæ
Kava	Piper methysticum	Piperaceæ
Leptandra	Veronica virginica	Scrophulariaceæ
Sanguinaria	Sanguinaria canadensis	Papaveraceæ
Sumbul	Ferula Sumbul and closely related sp.	Umbelliferæ

The physical characteristics and microsopical features of rhizomes and roots should be studied as to the various points indicated under the heading of "Roots" and "Rhizomes."

Since there are instances among the dicotyledonous drugs of this group as in Gentiana, Apocynum and Echinacea, where the drug often consists of short separate pieces of rhizomes and of roots, it is often necessary to examine the cut surface to determine which of these organs one is dealing with. The presence of pith in the center of the piece examined always indicates rhizome and its absence, root.

Many of the drugs of this class have characteristic stem scars or stem bases as in Podophyllum, Cimicifuga, Caulophyllum. Others as Veratrum, Aletris and Helonias have characteristic leaf bases. Taraxacum shows a multiple crown. In Serpentaria leaves frequently occur with the rhizomes and roots.

As to the direction of growth, the majority are horizontal; a few as Veratrum Viride, Taraxacum, Angelica, Valeriana and Gentiana are vertical; Aralia and Helonias are oblique. The vertical rhizome and root drugs show characteristic annulated outer surfaces in respect to their rhizomes.

BULBS

Bulbs are short, vertical, subterranean stems covered with numerous scales, the latter comprising their greater bulk.

A. Official in the U.S.P. x.

Title	Botanical Origin	Family
Scilla	Urginea maritima	Liliaceæ

B. Official in the N.F. v.

Allium	Allium sativum	Liliaceæ

Scilla consists of grayish to yellowish-white, entire or broken, transverse slices of fleshy scales, which are frequently curved or arranged in concentric fashion. These have a weak fracture and mucilaginous, bitter taste. The diagnostic microscopical features are numerous mucilage sacs, long raphides and spiral ducts.

Allium occurs as entire, compound, fresh bulbs of a white or pink color with smooth stems. Each compound bulb consists of 8 to 15 ovoid bulbels surrounded by whitish membranous scales and showing numerous yellowish-white rootlets arising from a circular base. The odor is strongly and characteristically aromatic, and the taste is strongly pungent.

CORM

A corm is an excessively thickened, solid and erect subterranean stem.

Title	Botanical Origin	Family
Colchici Cormus U.S.P.	Colchicum autumnale	Liliaceæ

Colchicum Corm consists of transverse, reniform, or longitudinal, somewhat ovate slices of the corm, the cut surfaces of which are grayish-white, dotted with resin. They have a starchy, bitter and acrid taste.

BARKS

Bark is all that portion of a woody exogenous plant axis found outside of the cambium.

A. Those official in the U.S.P. x.

Title	Botanical Origin	Family
Cascara Sagrada	Rhamnus Purshiana	Rhamnaceæ
Cinchona	Cinchona Ledgeriana, C. Calisaya, Cinchona succirubra and hybrids	Rubiaceæ
Cinnamomum	Cinnamomum Loureirii	Lauraceæ
Granatum	Punica Granatum	Punicaceæ
Prunus Virginiana	Prunus serotina	Rosaceæ
Ulmus	Ulmus fulva	Ulmaceæ

B. Those official in the N.F. v.

TITLE	BOTANICAL ORIGIN	FAMILY
Canella	Canella Winterana	Canellaceæ
Cascara Amarga	Picramnia sp.	Simarubaceæ
Chionanthus	Chionanthus virginica	Oleaceæ
Cocillana	Guarea Rusbyi	Meliaceæ
Condurango	Marsdenia Condurango	Asclepiadaceæ
Cornus	Cornus florida	Cornaceæ
Euonymus	Evonymus atropurpureus	Celastraceæ
Frangula	Rhamnus Frangula	Rhamnaceæ
Gossypii Cortex	Gossypium herbaceum, G. Barbadense and G. hirsutum	Malvaceæ
Juglans	Juglans cinerea	Juglandaceæ
Mezereum	Daphne Mezereum Daphne Gnidium Daphne Laureola	Thymelæaceæ
Myrica	Myrica cerifera and M. carolinensis	Myricaceæ
Pinus Alba	Pinus strobus	Pinaceæ
Quercus	Quercus alba	Fagaceæ
Quillaja	Quillaja Saponaria	Rosaceæ
Rubus	The Section Eubatus of the genus Rubus	Rosaceæ
Sassafras	Sassafras variifolium	Lauraceæ
Tonga	Bark of Premna arborea Root of Epipremnum pinnatum	Verbenaceæ Araceæ
Viburnum Opulus	Viburnum Opulus var. americanum	Caprifoliaceæ
Viburnum Prunifolium	Viburnum Prunifolium	Caprifoliaceæ
Xanthoxylum	Zanthoxylum americanum Zanthoxylum Clava-Herculis	Rutaceæ

Barks are considered as to their physical characteristics, histology and microscopical features of their elements, as examined in the form of a powder.

The study of their physical characteristics should include occurrence, nature of outer surface, inner surface, fracture, internal appearance, odor and taste.

Most of the official barks have periderm (cork) present. The exceptions to this rule are Cinnamomum Zeylanicum, Sassafras, Ulmus, Canella, Fraxinus, Juglans, Pinus Alba, Quercus, rossed Prunus Virginiana and Quillaja.

When the term bark without limitation is employed in pharmacognic and materia medica texts, the stem bark is usually to be inferred. Either the stem or root bark of Granatum and Cinchona is recognized.

Several of the official barks are directed by the official standards to be obtained only from the root. These are Sassafras, Cornus, Euonymus, Chionanthus, Gossypii Cortex, Myrica and Juglans. Rubus consists of the bark of the rhizome and root. Myrica of commerce sometimes consists of the bark of the aerial stem, rhizome and root.

Barks occur either in the form of single quills as Cinnamomum Saigonicum and the Cinchonas, or in double quills as Cinnamomum Zeylanicum where several quills are inside of each other, or in transversely curved pieces as Condurango and Xanthoxylum, or in flat pieces as Cornus, or in flat, slab like pieces as in Quillaja and Ulmus, or as a mixture of partially quilled and quilled pieces as Gossypii Cortex and Rubus.

In the examination of the outer surface of a bark, it is important to note the presence or absence and character of prickles, lenticels, lichens and their apothecia, fissures, as well as its color.

The examination of the inner surface should embody color, markings, the tendency of the inner fibers to separate, as in Gossypii Cortex, Mezereum, Condurango, Quercus and Ulmus.

The fracture may be short and very weak as in Viburnum Opulus, Cinnamomum Zeylanicum and Cascarilla, short and brittle as in Cascara Amarga, Prunus Virginiana, Sassafras, Cascara, etc., tough fibrous as in Cinchona, Chionanthus, Condurango, etc., or very tough fibrous as in the unofficial Aspidosperma and Paracoto. The examination of fractured surface should include color and the presence or absence of projecting fibers or stone cells.

The microscopical study of barks should embrace their study in transverse, longitudinal-radial and longitudinal-tangential sections as well as their appearance in powdered form. In some instances it is advisable to digest small pieces or shavings of the bark in Schulze's maceration fluid, wash in water and tease apart the lignified elements, in order to best observe them in their entire condition. Scrapings of the bark surfaces have been found very helpful in studying the characteristics of their histological elements.

Stem barks in their entire condition show the following tissue regions, passing from outer to inner surface:

1. Cork (periderm).
2. Cork cambium (phellogen).
3. Cortex { a. secondary—usually (phelloderm). b. primary—constant.
4. Pericycle.
5. Phloem, traversed by phloem medullary-rays.

Root barks in their entire condition exhibit the following regions of tissues, passing from outer to inner surface:

1. Cork (periderm).
2. Cork cambium (phellogen).
3. Secondary cortex.
4. Phloem, traversed by phloem medullary-rays.

Whenever no sclerenchyma elements occur in the pericycle, for all practical purposes the pericycle is included with the cortex and the two regions collectively termed "cortex."

The three most important regions in the average bark upon which detailed histological studies should be made are (1) outer bark or cork, (2) middle bark or cortex and (3) inner bark or phloem.

The cork tissue varies in different barks as to the size and nature of its cells as well as to their arrangement. The cell walls in particular should be observed to determine first whether any lignification is present or whether they are entirely suberised and second, whether they differ as to thickening. The character of the cell contents should likewise be noted.

In most barks cork is found only on the outer face as a product of the secondary meristem known as cork cambium, but in others, as Quercus, zones of cork may occur at varying levels in the cortex, pericycle and phloem, due to the appearance in these regions of tertiary meristems.

WOODS

A. Those official in the U.S.P. x.

Title	Botanical Origin	Family
Carbo Ligni	Salix, Populus, Acer, etc.	Salicaceæ, Aceraceæ, etc.
Quassia	Picrasma excelsa Quassia amara	Simarubaceæ
Santalum Rubrum	Pterocarpus santalinus	Leguminosæ

B. Those official in the N.F. v.

Title	Botanical Origin	Family
Hæmatoxylon	Hæmatoxylon campechianum	Leguminosæ
Santalum Album	Santalum album	Santalaceæ

PITH

Official in the N.F. v

Title	Botanical Origin	Family
Sassafras Medulla	Sassafras variifolium	Lauraceæ

The wood drugs include those portions of woody exogenous plant axes lying inside of the cambium line. Those official represent the wood of Dicotyl stems. The outer whitish layers of wood which contain living cells, functioning in the vegetative processes of the plant, make up what is termed *sapwood* or *alburnum.* Quassia is the only official example of a sapwood. The inner dead layers of wood which have been more or less infiltrated with extractive and coloring matter and which have ceased to function as sap-transporting elements constitute what is called *heartwood* or *duramen.* The official representative of this class are Santalum Rubrum, Hæmatoxylon and Santalum Album.

Carbo Ligni represents a black powder obtained from soft wood.

In the macroscopic examination of woods cognizance is taken of their manner of occurrence, color, markings, fracture, odor and taste.

In the microscopic examination of woods, the following points should be considered:

1. The distribution and arrangement of the tissues particularly the tracheæ, wood parenchyma and medullary-rays.

2. The range in width of the medullary rays as observed in tangential sections.

3. The character of the tracheæ, tracheids and wood fibers in respect to relative width, thickness of walls, markings on walls, etc.

4. The presence or absence of starch and crystals. If these be present, their shape and size should be acertained.

5. The presence or absence of secretion sacs or reservoirs and the nature of their contents.

6. The presence of an abnormal structure or absence of one known to occur in the authentic article.

LEAVES

A. Those official in the U.S.P. x.

Title	Botanical Origin	Family
Buchu	Barosma betulina, B. crenulata, and B. serratifolia	Rutaceæ
Digitalis	Digitalis purpurea	Scrophulariaceæ
Eucalyptus	Eucalyptus globulus	Myrtaceæ
Eriodictyon	Eriodictyon californicum	Hydrophyllaceæ
Hyoscyamus	Hyoscyamus niger	Solanaceæ
Uva Ursi	Arctostaphylos Uva Ursi	Ericaceæ

B. Those official in the N.F. v.

Althææ Folia	Althæa officinalis	Malvaceæ
Boldus	Boldu Boldus	Monimiaceæ
Castanea	Castanea dentata	Fagaceæ
Chimaphila	Chimaphila umbellata	Ericaceæ
Damiana	Turnera diffusa; Turnera aphrodisiaca	Turneraceæ
Farfara	Tussilago Farfara	Compositæ
Hamamelidis Folia	Hamamelis virginiana	Hamamelidaceæ
Malvæ Folia	Malva rotundifolia; Malva sylvestris	Malvaceæ
Matico	Piper angustifolium	Piperaceæ
Verbasci Folia	Verbascum Thapsus	Scrophulariaceæ

LEAFLETS

Official in U.S.P. x.

Senna	Cassia Senna; Cassia angustifolia	Leguminosæ

LEAF BUDS

Official in N.F. v.

Title	Botanical Origin	Family
Populi Gemmæ	Populus nigra Populus balsamifera Populus candicans	Salicaceæ

Leaves are generally flattened, rarely semi-centric, or centric-lateral expansions developed by the stem or by branches and in whose axils one or more branches arise.

In the study of the physical characteristics of leaves and leaflets it is important to note the general outline, apex, base, margin, nature of petiole if present, length and breadth of lamina, surfaces, texture, color of both surfaces and venation, odor and taste. Very frequently, as in Hamamelidis Folia, Digitalis, Stramonium, Castanea and Matico, the leaves are more or less crumpled and broken. Such specimens should be spread out, after first macerating in water, in order to properly study the nature of the margin.

The microscopic examination should include the study of surface sections of both upper and lower epidermis as well as transverse sections. In this connection it is well to state that dried leaves are best prepared for sectioning by exposure to the atmosphere of a moist chamber for 24 hours or longer until sufficiently supple. Transverse sections can then be had by imbedding between the halves of elder pith preparatory to cutting. Surface sections may be prepared for cutting by bending the leaf over the index finger and holding it firmly between the index finger and the third finger on the one end and with the thumb on the other. Another method of preparing surface sections is as follows: Place a representative portion of the leaf not over ¼ inch square in a watch crystal with chloral hydrate solution, warm gently for several minutes, according to the texture of the leaf, transfer to clean slide, add a drop or two of chloral solution, cover with cover slip and exert pressure on the slip with a rotary movement. The epidermis will thereby readily be separated from the leaf parenchyma and fibrovascular tissue.

In case good sized portions of leathery leaves are available and the task is that of studying large areas of epidermis, these may be prepared by boiling the leaf material in 10 to 20 per cent. solutions of sodium or potassium hydroxide until the epidermis puckers up in the form of blisters, when they should be removed to a slide and the epidermis lifted off by means of fine forceps or dissecting needles.

It is frequently necessary to clear leaf material before examination. This may be accomplished by allowing it to macerate in saturated solution of chloral hydrate for a day or longer or by the use of Labarraque's solution or Javelle Water in case hasty examination is urgent. The main disadvantages in the use of Labarraque's and Javelle Water are first—the appearance of numerous bubbles in material which frequently obscure the field and second—the danger of over bleaching, when conducted by an inexperienced individual. In all cases the material should be washed in water before examination.

The microscopic structures to be observed in leaves are as follows:

1. Upper and lower epidermis—thickness and color of cuticle; outline of epidermal cells as seen in transverse and vertical view; nature of vertical walls, whether rectilinear (straight) or curvilinear (wavy); presence or absence of stomata with accompanying guard cells or of water stomata; the number and arrangement of the neighboring-cells, if present; presence or absence of hairs and their character, whether non-glandular or glandular; if non-glandular, whether simple or branched, unicellular or multicellular, uniseriate or multiseriate, non-papillated or papillated, whether certain cells are collapsed in the course of the hair as in Digitalis, and whether the hair is inserted between epidermal cells or occurs as an outgrowth of them; if glandular, whether stalked or sessile, whether stalk, if present, is uniseriate or multiseriate and the number of cells in length or rows of cells (in the case of multiseriate hairs) comprising the stalk, the number of cells comprising the head and the shape of the head. In certain instances it is necessary to measure the length of the hairs and their breadth at the base. The nature of the distal cell of the non-glandular hair is also to be observed.

2. Mesophyll—including arrangement of the palisade and spongy parenchyma regions, presence or absence of crystals, their nature, size and position, presence or absence of stone cells or idioblasts, size of cells and intercellular-air-spaces, presence or absence of secretion sacs or internal glands and the character of their contents, nature of fibrovascular elements.

3. Midrib and Petiole—outline in cross section, arrangement and character of bundles, nature of endodermis, presence or absence of sclerenchyma elements in the pericycle adjacent to the bundles, presence or absence of crystals, their nature and size, presence or absence of collenchyma and its position.

STEMS

Stems are those parts of plant axes which bear leaves or leaf modifications.

Official in the N.F. v.

Title	Botanical Origin	Family
Cactus Grandiflorus	Selenicereus grandiflorus	Cactaceæ
Dulcamara	Solanum Dulcamara	Solanaceæ
Scoparius	Cytisus scoparius	Leguminosæ
Thuja	Thuja occidentalis	Pinaceæ

The official aerial stems are all derived from Dicotyledons, and therefore exhibit dicotyl stem structure. In the study of the physical characteristics of stems, attention should be paid to the following points: occurrence, range in diameter, outline, whether simple or branched, surface, color, fracture, internal appearance, odor, and taste.

Cactus occurs as fresh stems and Dulcamara as dried stems. The former is cut into long segments, the latter into very short segments with a hollow center. Scoparius occurs in cut and broken branches, Thuja in broken branches. The range in diameter of Cactus if from 1.5 cm. to 4 cm.: of Dulcamara, 4 mm. to 7 mm., of Scoparius, 1 mm. to 3 mm., and Thuja, from 2 mm. to 4 mm. The outline of Cactus is wavy and angular; of Dulcamara cylindrical; of Scoparius five angled; and of Thuja irregular. Scoparius and Thuja alone show branching. Cactus has a succulent texture, the others are fibrous. The surface of Cactus is deeply longitudinally channeled and marked by tufts of spines, and at irregular intervals shows nodes, some with branched rootlets; of Dulcamara striated; of Scoparius five angled; of Thuja, covered with four rows of appressed leaves. The color of Cactus is dark green; of Dulcamara greenish-brown; of Scoparius greenish-brown to greenish-black; of Thuja dark green to reddish brown.

The fracture of all these stems (except Cactus, which bends) is uneven. The fracture of Scoparius is tough and uneven; of Dulcamara, brittle and uneven; of Thuja, fibrous.

Internally, Cactus shows a broad mucilaginous cortex and a small fibrous pith; Dulcamara shows a thin greenish-brown cortex, a narrow brownish wood and usually a hollow pith; Scoparius has a thin cortex, broad yellow wood and narrow pith; Thuja a thin cortex and fibrous wood.

The odor of Cactus is slightly aromatic; of Dulcamara and Scoparius indistinct; of Thuja characteristically aromatic.

The taste of Cactus is acidulous and mucilaginous; of Dulcamara bitter, then sweet; of Scoparius bitter; of Thuja terebinthinate and bitter.

The histological study of the stem drug should include an inquiry into its appearance in transverse, radial-longitudinal, and tangential-longitudinal sections, as well as the examination of its cellular elements, when isolated. While transverse sections through the internodal portions of the official stems are frequently diagnostic for the whole stem drugs, it is, nevertheless, important to study longitudinal sections in order to learn the lengthwise appearance of the cellular elements, which usually are so cut in the grinding of drugs. The range in width and the depth of the medullary rays can be best ascertained through the examination of the stem in tangential-longitudinal sections, and types of crystals as well as the lengthwise characteristics of the cellular elements from radial-longitudinal sections. The latter type of section is most helpful in preparation for the study of the powdered drug.

Every dicotyl or gymnosperm stem exhibits internally a central pith which is immediately surrounded by a circular zone of wood; outside of the wood is a delicate growing layer of cambium which separates the internal wood from the external ring of bark. If the aerial stem be that of less than one year's growth, the following regions will be observed, passing in order from outer surface to center: Epidermis, primary cortex, endodermis, pericycle, protophloem, cambium, protoxylem, and pith. If it be of more than one year's growth, as in the aerial stems of perennials below the distal node, the following regions will be observed: (1) Epidermis, in the process of peeling off, or entirely absent; (2) Cork; (3) Cork cambium (generally shrunken in dried stems); (4) Secondary cortex; (5) Primary cortex; (6) Endodermis; (7) Pericycle; (8) Protophloem (primary phloem); (9) Secondary phloem (Metaphloem); (10) Cambium (usually with cells more or less collapsed in dried stems); (11) Secondary Xylem; (12) Protoxylem; (13) Pith.

The phloem, cambium, and xylem regions are separated into a number of wedges by means of strands of parenchymatous cells, known as medullary rays, that course like the spokes of a wheel through these regions. The primary medullary rays (coursing from pith to cortex) separate the fibro-vascular bundles one from the other. It is this type of medullary ray which, if followed outward to its termination, marks the outer limit of the phloem, and so is helpful in the study of transverse sections of stems whose phloem shows few or no bast fibres in determining the boundary line between phloem and pericycle.

The epidermis consists of a single row of epidermal cells, that are usually tangentially elongated in transverse sections, and axially elongated in the longitudinal sections. In drug stems, it is always covered with a cuticle and usually shows stomata. Hairs (trichomes) are sometimes found which are outgrowths of epidermal cells. They may be non-glandular or glandular in character.

The cortex is commonly composed of cortical parenchyma tissue, the cells of which are frequently collenchymatic, in the outer part abutting the epidermis. (Their walls are thickened with a colloidal substance, particularly at the angles.) Moreover, outer rows of cells are generally tangentially elongated, and usually contain chloroplasts. In passing toward the inner margin of the cortex, the cells generally become rounded off and isodiametric. In the examination of this region, it is important to note any variation from the structure outlined, for such aids in the diagnosis of the drug.

The following kinds of cellular elements are to be looked for: stone cells; sclerenchyma fibres; secretion sacs; internal glands; laticiferous cells or vessels; and internal hairs.

The character of the cell contents should also be noted. Among those apt to occur are the following: starch; calcium oxalate crystals; cystoliths; resin; tannin; oil; sugars; alkaloids; glucosides; etc.

The endodermis, or innermost layer of cells of the cortex, is generally indistinguishable from the other layers of the cortex, but in some stems, especially in their early growth, can be recognized by the following characteristics: 1. The rectangular form of the cells in cross section; and the absence of intercellular air spaces; 2, the presence of abundant starch, and 3, the appearance of suberized or lignified walls, especially the radial walls of the cells of this layer.

The pericycle, in many stems, is also indistinguishable from the cortex but in many others, especially stems of climbing plants, can be made out by the presence of sclerenchyma fibres or stone cells or both, which may either be isolated, occur in small groups, or form a continuous or discontinuous ring. This region may consist of one or more rows of parenchymatous cells.

The phloem, which follows the pericycle, tends to be narrow in herbaceous stems, broader in stems of shrubs and trees. It always contains sieve tubes and phloem parenchyma, and phloem medullary rays. In addition, bast fibres and stone cells as well as laticiferous tissue, oil glands, and calcium oxalate cells are apt to be found, either of which is helpful in diagnosis, and should be noted. The absence of bast fibres, etc., in the phloem is also frequently diagnostic.

The xylem or wood region, found directly within the cambium, shows variation in structure depending upon the group of plants in which it occurs. In stems of conifers it is composed wholly or chiefly of tracheids with a single row of bordered pores and xylem medullary rays. In stems of Dicotyledons, it varies often with tracheids with bordered pores and xylem medullary rays, but the pitted tracheids are marked on their longitudinal walls by more than one layer of bordered pores. Moreover, in addition to these elements, wood parenchyma is almost always present, and tracheæ and wood fibres are very common.

In the stems of some dicotyledons isolated patches of sieve tissue will be found scattered here and there in the xylem region. This is called "*interxylary phloem*" and has been observed in the following families: *Loganiaceæ*, *Gentianaceæ*, *Convolvulaceæ*, *Cucurbitaceæ*, *Combretaceæ*, *Myrtaceæ*, *Punicaceæ*, *Apocynaceæ*, *Asclepiadaceæ*, *Acanthaceæ*, *Euphorbiaceæ*, *Melastomaceæ*, etc. *Intraxylary phloem* in the form of sieve tissue with or without accompanying bast fibres may be found on the inner face of the xylem and, when present, should be noted. It has been observed in the stems of members of the following drug-yielding families: *Loganiaceæ, Gentianaceæ, Papilionaceæ, Oleaceæ, Combretaceæ, Solanaceæ, Cucurbitaceæ, Convolvulaceæ, Melastomaceæ, Apocynaceæ, Asclepiadaceæ, Thymeleaceæ, Acanthaceæ, Euphorbiaceæ, Malphigiaceæ,* and *Polygonaceæ.*

Such microscopic features as enumerated under the captions of Wood and Xylem of roots should be noted in addition to those here presented.

The pith consists of parenchyma cells which are frequently pitted. In some instances, during the development of this region, modifications of the walls and contents of the cells occur. The presence of lignified walls, stone cells, sclerenchyma fibres, laticiferous elements, crystals of calcium oxalate, cystoliths, secretion sacs, internal glands, hairs, starch grains, mucilage sacs, tannin cells, etc., should always be noted.

Fibrovascular bundles occur in the pith region of certain stems belonging to the *Polygonaceæ, Piperaceæ,* etc., and when present are valuable aids in diagnosis. The stems of several genera, including *Phytolacca, Ipomoea, Exogonium, Amaranthus, Cucurbita,* etc., show more than one circle of bundles outside the pith region.

LEAVES AND FLOWERING OR FRUITING TOPS

A. Those official in the U.S.P. x.

Title	Botanical Origin	Family
Belladonnæ Folia	Atropa Belladonna	Solanaceæ
Cannabis	Cannabis sativa	Moraceæ
Hyoscyamus	Hyoscyamus niger	Solanaceæ
Lobelia	Lobelia inflata	Lobeliaceæ
Mentha Piperita	Mentha piperita	Labiatæ
Mentha Viridis	Mentha spicata	Labiatæ
Stramonium	Datura Stramonium	Solanaceæ

B. Those official in the N.F. v.

Title	Botanical Origin	Family
Cataria	Nepeta Cataria	Labiatæ
Eupatorium	Eupatorium perfoliatum	Compositæ
Grindelia	Grindelia camporum Grindelia cuneifolia Grindelia squarrosa	Compositæ
Melilotus	Melilotus officinalis	Leguminosæ
Thymus	Thymus vulgaris	Labiatæ

ENTIRE PLANT DRUGS

Those official in the N.F. v.

Title	Botanical Origin	Family
Centaurium	Erythræa Centaurium	Gentianaceæ
Chirata	Swertia Chirayita	Gentianaceæ
Chondrus	Chondrus crispus Gigartina mamillosa	Gigartinaceæ

Title	Botanical Origin	Family
Coptis	Coptis trifolia	Ranunculaceæ
Drosera	Drosera rotundifolia Drosera anglica Drosera longifolia	Droseraceæ
Euphorbia	Euphorbia hirta	Euphorbiaceæ
Fucus (dried thallus)	Fucus vesiculosus	Fucaceæ
Mitchella	Mitchella repens	Rubiaceæ
Senecio	Senecio aureus	Compositæ

OVERGROUND PORTIONS OF PLANTS ("HERBS")

Official in the N.F. v.

Title	Botanical Origin	Family
Adonis	Adonis vernalis	Ranunculaceæ
Galega	Galega officinalis	Leguminosæ
Passiflora	Passiflora incarnata	Passifloraceæ
Pulsatilla	Pulsatilla vulgaris Pulsatilla pratensis Pulsatilla patens	Ranunculaceæ
Scutellaria	Scutellaria lateriflora	Labiatæ

FLOWERS AND FLORAL PARTS

Flowers are shoots which have undergone modifications so as to serve as a means for the propagation of the individual.

A. Those official in the U.S.P. x.

Title	Botanical Origin	Family
1. Unexpanded Bud		
Caryophyllus	Caryophyllus aromaticus	Myrtaceæ
2. Petals		
Rosa	Rosa gallica	Rosaceæ

B. Those official in the N.F. v.

Title	Botanical Origin	Family
1. Flowers		
Sambucus	Sambucus canadensis Sambucus nigra	Caprifoliaceæ
2. Corollas (with adhering stamens)		
Verbasci Flores	Verbascum phlomoides Verbascum thapsiforme	Scrophulariaceæ
3. Stigmas		
Crocus	Crocus sativus	Iridaceæ
4. Fresh Styles and Stigmas		
Zea	Zea Mays	Gramineæ
5. Ligulate Floret		
Calendula	Calendula officinalis	Compositæ
6. Inflorescences		
Brayera (panicle)	Hagenia abyssinica	Rosaceæ
7. Flower Heads		
Arnica	Arnica montana	Compositæ
Matricaria	Matricaria Chamomilla	Compositæ
Trifolium	Trifolium pratense	Leguminosæ

The official flower drugs have all been derived from Angiosperms. A typical angiospermous flower consists of four whorls of floral leaves arranged upon the swollen summit of the flower stalk known as the *Receptacle*. These, from without inward, are the *Calyx*, *Corolla*, *Andrœcium* and *Gynœcium*. The arrangement of the flowers upon the stem is termed *Inflorescence* or *Anthotaxy*. The flowers may occur singly on the stem or in clusters. In a flower cluster, the stalk bearing the cluster is termed the *Peduncle;* the continuation of the peduncle as an axis along which the flowers are arranged, the *Rachis*. The stalks which arise either from the summit of the peduncle or the rachis are termed *Pedicels*. The modified leaves occurring along the peduncle or rachis are known as *Bracts*, while those occurring on the pedicels are known as the *Bracteoles*. The *Involucre* represents one or more whorls of bracts.

The types of inflorescences represented among the flower drugs are the *Raceme*, *Panicle*, and *Capitulum* (Flower head). The raceme, illustrated by Convallariæ Flores (unofficial) consists of a peduncle with its elongated rachis, the latter bearing alternate bracts in the axils of which pedicels arise, each of which terminates in a single flower. The flowers open in order from the base toward the summit.

The *Panicle*, illustrated by the drug Brayera, is a compound raceme, which differs from a raceme in showing branched pedicles, the secondary pedicels terminated by flowers.

The *Capitulum*, or flower head, is the common type of inflorescence for all the *Compositæ*, as well as for some of the *Campanulaceæ* and the *Leguminosæ*. It consists of a number of small flowers called *Florets* inserted on a compound receptacle that terminates the flower stalk. The common receptacle is usually surrounded on its exterior by one or more circles of bracts, often arranged in imbricate fashion. The florets which are imbedded in the receptacle may be all tubular, as in the flower heads of Santonica, Eupatorium, and Absinthium, or they may be all ligulate, as in Dandelion, Chicory, the Hawkweeds, and cultivated *Anthemis nobilis*. Sometime the florets may be partly tubular (disk florets) and partly ligulate (ray florets) as in Matricaria, wild Anthemis, Pyrethri Flores, Arnica, or they may be all papilionaceous as in Trifolium.

In the study of flowers, the physical characteristics of the peduncle and the various whorls should be first considered. In this work, a hand lens or dissecting microscope, needles and penknife will be found advantageous during dissection. The presence or absence of nectaries and their position should be ascertained. Following this, examination with the aid of the compound microscope can be made of the various parts, and finally, the powdered drug can be examined.

In the examination of the calyx, the methods employed in leaf examination obtain. Often, diagnostic structures may be found in the nature of hairs, stomatal apparatus, internal glands and crystals.

In the examination of the corolla, which is usually thinner and more delicate in structure than the calyx, mounts of petals should be made, and the characteristics of the epidermis ascertained, particularly as to the presence or absence of papillæ and cell contents. The mesophyll may then be examined for crystals, secretion sacs, and other diagnostic features.

In the examination of the stamens, attention should be particularly focused upon the pollen grains and the endothecium of the anther. Pollen grains are very frequently diagnostic for families, genera, and even species of plants. The shape and character of the outer wall of these should always be observed. The character of the thickenings of the endothecium of the anther, which may be annular, spiral, or reticulate, may be determined.

In the study of the pistil, attention should be directed toward ascertaining the number of chambers in the ovary, the presence or absence of epidermal hairs and secretory tissue, size and character of papillæ, shape of the stigma, and the characteristics of the stigmatic papillæ.

It frequently happens that floral parts are densely colored, as in numerous petals, anthers, and stigmas. These can be decolorized, preparatory to microscopic examination, by maceration in water, or in very dilute ammonia water.

FRUITS

Fruits consist of matured pistils or ovarian portions thereof, or in some instances matured flowers or flower clusters. See part 2.

A. Those official in the U.S.P. x.

Title	Botanical Origin	Family
1. Berries		
Capsicum	Capsicum frutescens	Solanaceæ
Colocynthis (pulp)	Citrullus Colocynthis	Cucurbitaceæ
2. Drupes		
Cubeba	Piper Cubeba	Piperaceæ
Rhus Glabra	Rhus glabra	Anacardiaceæ
3. Caryopsis		
Maltum	Hordeum vulgare varieties	Gramineæ
4. Cremocarps		
Carum	Carum Carvi	Umbelliferæ
5. Rinds of Fruits		
Aurantii Amari Cortex	Citrus Aurantium	Rutaceæ
Aurantii Dulcis Cortex	Citrus Aurantium sinensis	Rutaceæ
Limonis Cortex	Citrus medica Limonum	Rutaceæ

B. Those official in the N.F. v.

Title	Botanical Origin	Family
1. Berries		
Cocculus	Anamirta Cocculus	Menispermaceæ
Rhamnus Cathartica	Rhamnus Cathartica	Rhamnaceæ
Solanum	Solanum carolinense	Solanaceæ
Pimenta	Pimenta officinalis	Myrtaceæ
2. Drupes		
Piper	Piper nigrum	Piperaceæ
Sabal	Serenoa serrulata	Palmæ
Prunum	Prunus domestica	Rosaceæ
3. Caryopsis (grain)		
Avena Sativa	Avena sativa	Gramineæ
4. Cremocarps		
Anisum	Pimpinella Anisum	Umbelliferæ
Angelicæ Fructus	Angelica Archangelica and other sp. of Angelica	Umbelliferæ
Apii Fructus	Apium graveolens	Umbelliferæ
Conium	Conium maculatum	Umbelliferæ
Coriandrum	Coriandrum sativum	Umbelliferæ
Fœniculum	Fœniculum vulgare	Umbelliferæ
5. Capsules		
Vanilla	Vanilla planifolia	Orchidaceæ
6. Follicles		
Xanthoxyli Fructus	Zanthoxylum americanum Zanthoxylum Clava-Herculis	Rutaceæ
7. Galbulus		
Juniperus	Juniperus communis	Pinaceæ
8. Syconium		
Ficus	Ficus Carica	Moraceæ
9. Aggregate Fruit		
Rubi Idæi Fructus	Rubus Idæus Rubus strigosus	Rosaceæ
10. Preserved Pulp		
Tamarindus	Tamarindus indica	Leguminosæ
11. Loment		
Cassia Fistula	Cathartocarpus Fistula	Leguminosæ
12. Strobile		
Humulus	Humulus Lupulus	Moraceæ

SEEDS AND SEED PARTS

A seed is a fertilized and ripened ovule containing an embryo.

A. Those official in the U.S.P. x. See part 2.

Title	Botanical Origin	Family
1. Exalbuminous Seeds		
Pepo	Cult. var. of Cucurbita Pepo	Cucurbitaceæ
Sinapis Nigra	Brassica nigra	Cruciferæ
2. Albuminous Seeds		
Cardamomi Semen	Elettaria Cardamomum	Zingiberaceæ
Colchici Semen	Colchicum autumnale	Liliaceæ
Linum	Linum usitatissimum	Linaceæ
Myristica	Myristica fragrans	Myristicaceæ
Nux Vomica	Strychnos Nux-Vomica	Loganiaceæ
Strophanthus	Strophanthus Kombé and S. hispidus	Apocynaceæ

B. Those official in the N.F. v.

Title	Botanical Origin	Family
1. Albuminous Seeds		
Delphinium	Delphinium Ajacis	Ranunculaceæ
Coffea Tosta	Coffea arabica Coffea liberica	Rubiaceæ
Ignatia	Strychnos Ignatii	Loganiaceæ
2. Cotyledons		
Kola	Cola nitida and other sp. of Cola	Sterculiaceæ
3. Powder prepared from Kernels		
Cacao Præparatum	Theobroma Cacao	Sterculiaceæ
4. Paste chiefly consisting of crushed seeds.		
Guarana	Paullinia Cupana	Sapindaceæ

TRICHOMES (PLANT HAIRS)

Trichomes are outgrowths of epidermal cells. See part 2.

A. Official in the U.S.P. x.

Title	Botanical Origin	Family
1. Non-glandular		
Gossypium Purificatum	Cultivated varieties of Gossypium herbaceum and other sp. of Gossypium	Malvaceæ

B. Official in the N.F. v.

Title	Botanical Origin	Family
1. Glandular		
Lupulinum	Humulus Lupulus	Moraceæ

GUMS, MUCILAGE, RESINS, GUM RESINS, OLEORESINS AND BALSAMS

A. Those official in the U.S.P. x.

Title	Botanical Origin	Family
1. Gums		
Acacia	Acacia Senegal or other sp. of Acacia	Leguminosæ
Tragacantha	Astragalus gummifer and other Asiatic sp. of Astragalus	Leguminosæ
2. Dried mucilaginous substance		
Agar	Gelidium corneum, other sp. of Gelidium and related algæ.	Florideæ
3. Resins		
Resina	Pinus palustris and other Pinus species	Pinaceæ
4. Gum Resins		
Asafœtida	Ferula Asafœtida Ferula fœtida and some other sp. of Ferula	Umbelliferæ
Cambogia	Garcinia Hanburyi	Guttiferæ
Myrrha	Commiphora Myrrha and other sp. of Commiphora	Burseraceæ
5. Oleoresin		
Copaiba	So. Amer. species of Copaiba	Leguminosæ

GUMS, RESINS, INSPISSATED JUICES, ETC.

Title	Botanical Origin	Family
6. Balsams		
Balsamum Peruvianum	Toluifera Pereiræ	Leguminosæ
Tolu	Toluifera Balsamum	Leguminosæ
Benzoinum (balsamic resin)	Styrax Benzoin and other sp. of Styrax	Styracaceæ
Styrax	Liquidambar orientalis Liquidambar Styraciflua	Hamamelidaceæ

B. Those official in the N.F. v.

Title	Botanical Origin	Family
1. Gum: Eucalypti Gummi	Eucalyptus rostrata et al. Eucalyptus sp.	Myrtaceæ
2. Resin		
Guaiacum	Guajacum officinale Guajacum sanctum	Zygophyllaceæ
Mastiche	Pistacia Lentiscus	Anacardiaceæ
3. Oleoresins		
Terebinthina (concrete)	Pinus palustris and other sp. of Pinus	Pinaceæ

INSPISSATED JUICES, LATEX, TAR AND EXTRACTS

A. Those official in the U.S.P. x.

Title	Botanical Origin	Family
1. Inspissated Juices		
Aloe	Aloe vera, A. Perryi and A. ferox	Liliaceæ
Kino	Pterocarpus Marsupium	Leguminosæ
2. Latex		
Opium	Papaver somniferum and its var. album	Papaveraceæ]
3. Tar		
Pix Pini	Pinus palustris, or other sp. of Pinus	Pinaceæ
4. Extract		
Gambir	Ourouparia Gambir	Rubiaceæ

MISCELLANEOUS DRUGS OF VEGETABLE ORIGIN

A. Those official in the U.S.P. x.

Title	Botanical Origin	Family
1. Starch		
Amylum	Zea Mays	Gramineæ
2. Saccharine exudate		
Manna	Fraxinus Ornus	Oleaceæ
3. Camphor		
Camphora	Cinnamomum Camphora	Lauraceæ
4. Excrescence		
Galla	Quercus infectoria and other sp.	Fagaceæ
5. Sclerotium		
Ergota	Claviceps purpurea	Hypocreaceæ
6. Spores		
Lycopodium	Lycopodium clavatum	Lycopodiaceæ
7. Diatom frustules		
Terra Silicea Purificata	Bacillarieæ sp.	

B. Those official in the N.F. v.

Title	Botanical Origin	Family
1. **Yeast**		
Cerevisiæ Fermentum Compressum	Saccharomyces sp.	Saccharomycetaceæ
2. Sporophore (fruit body)		
Agaricus	Polyporus officinalis	Polyporaceæ
3. Purplish-red Powder		
Persio	Sp. of Rocella, Lecanora and other Lichens	Parmeliaceæ

PART II

TAXONOMIC CONSIDERATION OF DRUGS

CHAPTER I

CRUDE DRUGS OF VEGETABLE ORIGIN

DIVISION I—THALLOPHYTA (THALLOPHYTES)

Plants, the greater number of which, consist of a *thallus*, a body undifferentiated into root, stem or leaf. This group, nearest to the beginning of the plant kingdom, presents forms showing rudimentary structures which are modified through division of labor, differentiation, etc., in higher groups. Under the microscope the thallus shows neither tracheæ nor wood fibers. To this assemblage belong the bacteria, slime-molds, blue-green algæ, green, brown and red algæ, fungi and lichens.

SUBDIVISION—ALGÆ

Low forms of thallophytes of terrestrial and aquatic distribution consisting for the most part of single cells or rows of single cells joined end to end to form filaments. The higher forms, however, possess structures, which might be compared to stems and leaves of higher plants, although more rudimentary in structure. All excepting the saprophytic forms contain chlorophyll, with the addition in blue-green, brown and red algæ of other pigments. Many of the blue-green and green algæ as well as the diatoms have been responsible for disagreeable tastes and odors in water supplies during certain periods of the year. The commercially important algæ are limited to the diatoms and marine forms of the brown and red groups. A number of the brown algæ such as the kelps and rockweeds represent the most important source of iodine and have also been harvested for their potash content, as fertilizer. Because of their abundant mucilage content, some of the red algæ, as Irish Dulse and Chondrus. have long been used as demulcents and nutritives.

CLASS—BACILLARIEÆ OR DIATOMS

This class comprises several thousand species of unicellular plants called *Diatoms* which are found in fresh, brackish and salt water, forming much of the diet of small animals. While unicellular, they frequently are united in colonies. They all possess chromatophores containing chlorophyll but this green pigment is often obscured by the presence also of a brown pigment.

The most striking peculiarity of the group is the structure of the enclosing cell wall. This is in the form of a siliceous case consisting of two *valves* which fit into each other like the halves of a pill box. The valves, which are beautifully sculptured, are similar except that one is slightly larger than the other so as to fit over it. Diatoms vary in form being either circular, linear, elliptical, cylindrical, rhomboidal, triangular or fan-shaped, etc. Some are borne on the ends of stalks, while others are held in gelatinous masses. Their siliceous skeleta are deposited constantly on the floor of ponds, rivers, lakes and seas, often in such abundance as to form Diatomaceous earths or Kieselguhrs (Siliceous Earths). Huge geological deposits of this material have been found in various parts of the world.

One of the largest of these is that at Richmond, Virginia. Many of the diatomaceous earths are useful as polishing powders and as absorbents for nitroglycerin in producing the explosive, dynamite. When purified they have been found valuable in pharmacy as filtering media for elixirs and aromatic waters.

TERRA SILICEA PURIFICATA U.S.P. (PURIFIED SILICEOUS EARTH)

Synonyms.—Purified Kieselguhr, Purified Infusorial Earth.

Definition.—A form of silica (SiO_2) consisting of the frustules and fragments of diatoms, purified by boiling with dilute hydrochloric acid, washing and calcining.

Commercial.—Crude siliceous earth (Kieselguhr) occurs in the form of rock masses in this country in the states of Virginia, Maryland, California, Oregon and Nevada. These are mined and the official (purified) article is calcined to destroy organic matter, washed, boiled with diluted hydrochloric acid, washed again and calcined.

Description.—A bulky and very fine, white or light gray to pale buff powder without odor or taste, readily absorbing moisture and retaining about four times its weight of water without the mixture becoming fluid. It is insoluble in water, dilute alkali, or in acids.

Impurities.—Samples of purified siliceous earth have been found which contained organic impurities, excess of moisture, iron, sulphates and carbonates. If organic impurities be present, it is darkened upon ignition. More than 10 per cent. loss by weight, upon ignition, would signify excess moisture.

If effervescence occurs after 1 Gm. of sample is added to 25 cc. of diluted hydrochloric acid, carbonates are present; if this mixture be boiled and filtered and barium chloride test solution added, a precipitate would indicate sulphate; if to the filtrate potassium ferrocyanide test solution be added and a blue color develop, soluble iron is present.

Microscopical Characteristics.—Temporary mounts made in water or chloral hydrate solution show upon examination a variety of forms of frustules of diatoms. In some instances these are for the most part in the entire condition whilst in others they are more or less broken up.

Uses.—As a filtering medium and in the preparation of dermatologic pastes.

CLASS—PHÆOPHYCEÆ, THE BROWN ALGÆ

Mostly marine forms showing great diversity in the form of their vegetative bodies. They occur for the most part in salt water between the high and low tide marks. Their bodies are usually fixed to some support in the water by means of a holdfast, and are often highly differentiated as to form and tissues. Some reach hundreds of feet in length as, for example, *Macrocystis,* which grows in the Pacific Ocean off the coast of California. Several, like *Fucus* and *Sargassum* (Gulf Weed), possess floating bladders containing oxygen. They all contain the brown pigment called *phycophœin* and the green pigment, *chlorophyll*, both of which are present in their chromatophores. A yellowish pigment called *phycoxanthin* has also been isolated from some of the species. Many of the kelps and rockweeds belonging to this class have long been sources of iodine, potash and sodium.

FUCACEÆ OR ROCKWEED FAMILY

The highest evolved group of brown algæ in which the male sexual organs (antheridia) and female sexual organs (oögonia) are lodged in conceptacles.

FUCUS N.F. (FUCUS)

Synonym.—Bladderwrack, Bladder Fucus, Sea-wrack, Black-tang; *Ger.* Blasentang, Meeriche; *Fr.* Fucus vesiculeux.

Botanical Origin.—*Fucus vesiculosus* Linné (and probably other species of *Fucus*).

Part Used.—The dried thallus.

Habitat.—Along coasts and borders of inlets of the North Atlantic Ocean between low and high tide marks.

Purity Rubric.—Fucus contains not more than 3 per cent. of foreign organic matter and yields not more than 4 per cent. of acid-insoluble ash.

Plant.—*Fucus vesiculosus* occurs as a flat, mucilaginous, olive-brown thallus, which forks repeatedly, - type of branching called dichotomous. It grows near the surface of sea water, attached to rocks or to mussels along banks by means of a basal *disc-shaped holdfast.* In the upper branches of the thallus are to be found *air bladders* which are more or less spherical and usually in pairs. The tips of old branches become swollen and are termed *receptacles*. They are dotted over with minute orifices which communicate with cavities called *conceptacles.* Within these conceptacles of some of the plants the *antheridia*, or male sexual organs are produced, while in conceptacles of other plants *oögonia*, or female sexual organs, arise. The conceptacles also contain numerous branching filaments called *paraphyses*, which arise from the cells lining the cavities. The antheridia are found as outgrowths of antheridiophores which arise from the wall of the conceptacle. They produce *sperms* or male sexual cells. The *oögonium* is a large, ovoid, stalked cell and produces eight *eggs*, each of which is a female sexual cell. The eggs and sperm escape into the sea water. The eggs sink gradually and are surrounded by myriads by sperms. One sperm, only, gains an entrance, after which its nucleus fuses with that of the egg to form an oöspore. The oöspore at once develops into a new Fucus plant.

Commercial.—The several varieties of *Fucus vesiculosus* are gathered when in the fruiting condition, which occurs throughout the year but mostly during late summer and autumn. They are spread out on the shore to dry and then packed in barrels for shipment. Considerable is employed as fertilizer and for the production of iodine.

Description.—The dried article constituting the drug occurs in the entire condition or in segments thereof. The thallus is flattened, dichotomously-branched, brownish-black to slightly reddish, usually with a slight, whitish incrustation and attains a length of up to 1 meter. Two kinds of plants occur, one bearing male receptacles, the other female. Both show forked branching and a stcut midrib. On either side of the midrib occur spherical to ellipsoidal shaped bladders which contain oxygen and other gases. The receptacles occur as swollen, ovate to ellipsoidal, often forked structures on the ends of some of the branches. The color is blackish-brown; the odor seaweed-like; the taste, saline, mucilaginous and nauseous. If sections of the thallus are placed on a slide with starch, and nitric acid be added, the starch grains will be stained blue, due to liberated iodine.

Histology.—Sections of the plant cut outside of the receptacles exhibit a layer of colorless, epidermal cells polygonal in surface view, a hypodermis of about 4 rows of longitudinally elongated mucilaginous cells, the remaining central tissue consisting of loosely arranged pseudo-parenchyma with large intercellular air-spaces.

Sections through the receptacles exhibit spherical conceptacles containing either antheridiophores bearing pyriform antheridia and sterile cells or rounded oögonia separated by paraphyses.

Powdered Drug.—Reddish-brown; numerous fragments of epidermis with polygonal cells, elongated hypodermal cells and irregular fragments of pseudo-parenchyma with thick mucilaginous walls.

Constituents.—A gelatinous substance termed algin, iodine (0.21 per cent.), bromine, chlorides, mannite and about 0.1 per cent. volatile oil.

Adulterants.—*Fucus serratus*, distinguished by its absence of air-bladders and serrated margin and *Fucus nodosus* L. which has single air-bladders.

Uses.—Bladderwrack is used in obesity because of its iodine content.

CLASS—RHODOPHYCEÆ, THE RED ALGÆ

A greatly diversified group comprising marine algæ but represented also by some fresh-water forms. The marine red algæ are generally

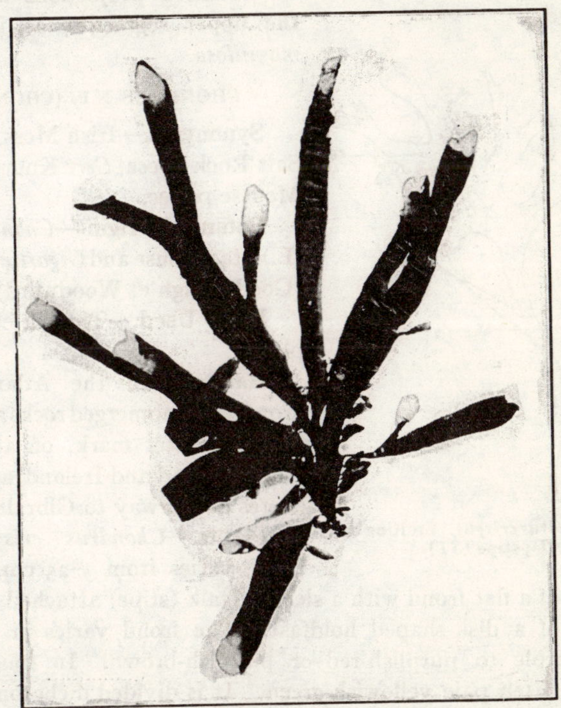

FIG. 4.—Irish Dulse (*Rhodymenia palmata*), a purplish-red, flat, membranous, dichotomously branched, red alga found along the northern shores of Atlantic ocean between low and high tide marks.

found below the low water mark. Their vegetative bodies vary from simple branching filaments through all gradations to forms differentiated into branching stems, holdfasts and leaf-like organs. It has been observed that many of the higher types are composed of numerous filaments which are arranged so closely and connected so intimately by protoplasmic processes as to resemble the tissues of higher plants. Their color may be red, purple, violet, or reddish-brown or even green and is due to the presence of phycoerythrin, a red pigment, which is found in the chromatophores with but frequently masking the chlorophyll.

GIGARTINACEÆ FAMILY

A family of red, purple or violet colored Rhodophyceæ with a more or less fleshy thallus, irregularly or dichotomously lobed. They are usually gelatinous forms with flattened, furcate bodies. The cystocarps or spore-bearing organs are either imbedded in the flat portions of the thallus, as in *Chondrus crispus*, or borne on short tuberculated projections arising from the upper segments, as in *Gigartina mamillosa*.

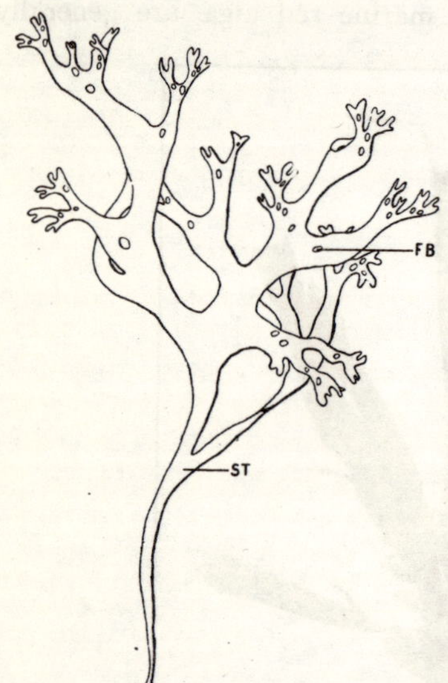

FIG. 5.—*Chondrus crispus.* Fruiting body (*FB*); stipe (*ST*).

CHONDRUS N.F. (CHONDRUS)

Synonyms.—Irish Moss, Carrageen, Salt Rock Moss; *Ger.* Knorpeltang; *Fr.* Mousse perlee.

Botanical Origin.—*Chondrus crispus* (L.) Stackhouse and *Gigartina mamillosa* (Goodenough et Woodward) J. Agardh.

Part Used.—The dried bleached plant.

Habitat.—In the Atlantic Ocean growing on submerged rocks at or beyond the low water mark, off the coast of New England and Ireland, and from the shores of Norway to Gibraltar.

Plants.—*Chondrus crispus*, when fresh, varies from 3–25 cm. in length. It consists of a flat frond with a slender stalk (stipe) attached to the rock by means of a disk-shaped holdfast. The frond varies in color from greenish-purple to purplish-red or purplish-brown. In rough shallow water it is often pale yellowish-green. It is divided dichotomously into several wedge shaped segments. These are repeatedly forked and terminate in a number of notched or 2-lobed segments. The fruiting bodies are ovate cystocarps.

Gigartina mamillosa, when fresh, somewhat resembles *Chondrus crispus*. It is purplish with a tinge of green. Its frond is irregularly branched in dichotomous fashion, the branches being forked at the apex. Its fructifications consist of small, more or less spherical, slightly elongated, sessile, bright red sporangia, borne on tuberculated stalks, which are scattered over the primary and secondary branches.

Commercial.—Most of the *Chondrus crispus* used in the United States is gathered along the coast of Massachusetts from 15 to 25 miles south of Boston, while most the *Gigartina mamillosa* is collected along the coast north of Boston. Both plants are collected from the latter part of May until September, although the greatest harvest is reaped in June and July. The collectors go out in boats with long rakes and scrape the algæ off the rocks. They bring large quantities of it ashore and spread it out on the higher parts of the beach. Here it is exposed to the action of the sun and dews for a week or more and partially bleached. At the end of a week, after it has been turned over two or three times, it has assumed a pale purplish-yellow color. It is then placed in barrels which are filled with salt water and covered with canvas. These barrels are rolled to the beach and the alga again spread out to be further bleached. It is then raked over until dry and until the alga is of a pale yellowish color. It is stored in barns and later packed in barrels holding about 100 pounds, for shipment into the market. The article is also imported from Dublin, Ireland, and Nimes, France.

Description.—Entire plants more or less matted together, consisting of a slender stalk from which arises a series of dichotomously branching, somewhat flattened segments, notched or deeply cleft at the tips; from 5 to 15 cm. in length, and 1 to 10 mm. in width; yellowish-white, occasionally with a tinge of purple, or red, translucent, often coated with a calcareous deposit; sometimes with fruit bodies (sporangia) embedded near the apex of the segments (*Chondrus crispus*), or, with sporangia borne on short tuberculated projections, scattered over the upper portion of the segments (*Gigartina mamillosa*); cartilaginous; odor seaweed-like; taste mucilaginous, saline.

When one part of Chondrus is boiled with 30 parts of water for ten minutes (the water lost by evaporation being replaced), the strained liquid forms a thick jelly upon cooling. When softened in cold water, Chondrus becomes gelatinous and transparent, the thallus only showing slight swelling at its tips.

Constituents.—Carrageenin (a mucilaginous principle), compounds of sodium, magnesium, potassium and calcium with chlorine, iodine and bromine; proteins, etc

Uses.—Demulcent and nutrient.

FLORIDEÆ FAMILY

Marine or very rarely fresh water algæ (*Batrachospermum*, etc.) in color either rose, violet, purple, reddish-brown or rarely green, frequently mucilaginous, consisting of simple or branched filaments (*Callithamnion*) or of rows of cells called *siphons* that are connected with one another by strands of protoplasm (*Polysiphonia*), or of membranous or cartilaginous forms. Monœcious or diœcious. The most striking feature of their reproductive system is seen in the nature of the male sexual cells or antherozoids which are devoid of cilia.

AGAR. U.S.P (AGAR)

Synonyms.—Agar-agar, Vegetable Gelatin, Japanese or Chinese Gelatin, Japanese Isinglass. *Fr.* Mousse de Chine; *Ger.* Thav.

Botanical Origin.—*Gelidium corneum*, other species of *Gelidium* and closely related algæ.

Part Used.—Dried mucilaginous substance.

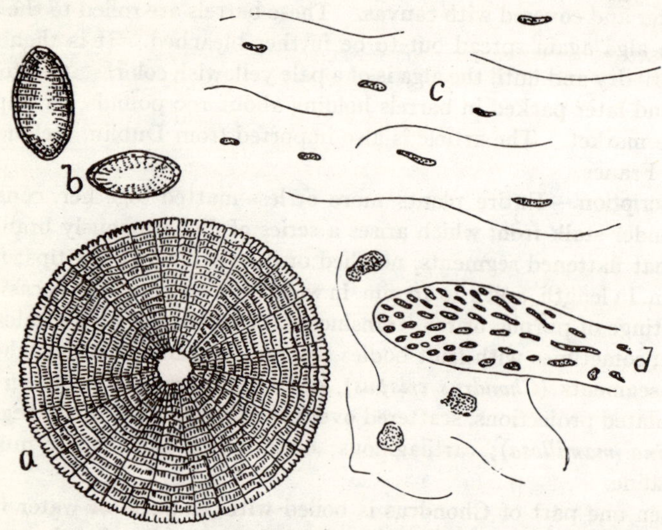

FIG. 6.—Agar. *a* and *b*, two species of diatoms which are constantly present in agar. The larger species is *Arachnoidiscus Ehrenbergii* Bail. *c* and *d*, mucilaginous tissue elements of agar as they appear in the commercial article. (*Schneider.*)

Purity Rubric.—Agar contains not more than 1 per cent. of foreign organic matter, and yields not more than 1 per cent. of acid-insoluble ash and not more than 16 per cent. of moisture.

Habitat.—In Japan, Yellow and China seas, along the eastern coast of Asia, and in the Pacific ocean, along the coast of California.

Production and Commerce.—The algæ are collected in summer and autumn along the coast of Eastern and Southern Asia, spread out on the beach until bleached and dried. During the winter months, they are then boiled with water and the mucilaginous liquid separated by straining through a cloth. The strained liquid is then cooled, the jelly cut into strips and dried by exposure to the air and sun, in the cold, to prevent growth of bacteria and molds. Most of the agar used in the United States comes from Japan. Agar is also being manufactured at San Diego, California, from red algæ growing along the coast of lower California. California now supplies about 35 per cent of the agar used in this country.

Description.—Agar occurs mostly in bundles 4–6 dm. in length which consist of thin, translucent, membranous, agglutinated pieces from 4–10 mm. in width; externally yellowish-white or brownish-white, tough when damp, brittle when dry; odor not distinct; taste mucilaginous. Insoluble in cold water but slowly soluble in hot water. When 1 part of Agar is boiled for 10 minutes with 100 parts of water and the product cooled, a stiff jelly results.

Microscopical Characteristics.—A fragment mounted in water gradually becomes more transparent, showing a granular structure and a few diatoms. The most diagnostic diatom is *Arachnoidiscus Ehrenbergii* which is disk-shaped and from 100 to 300μ in diameter. Spicules of sponges or fragments thereof and starch grains of algæ are also evident in some fragments of the drug.

Constituents.—About 65 per cent. of gelose (a mucilaginous substance, which, according to Takao, yields galactose with small quantities of fructose and arabinose, on hydrolysis and mucic acid on oxidation), nitrogenous substances, etc.

Uses.—As a laxative and in the preparation of culture media for bacteriologic and mycologic work.

SUBDIVISION—FUNGI

This great assemblage of thallophytes is characterized by the total absence of chlorophyll and so its members possess no independent power of manufacturing food materials such as starches, sugars, etc., from CO_2 and H_2O. Consequently they are either *parasites*, depending for their nourishment upon other living plants or animals, called *hosts;* or *saprophytes*, depending upon decaying animal or vegetable matter in solution. Some forms are able to live either as saprophytes or parasites, while others are restricted to either the parasitic or saprophytic habit. The vegetative body of a fungus is known as a *mycelium.* It consists of interlacing and branching filaments called *hyphæ*, which ramify through decaying matter or invade the tissues of living organisms and derive nourishment therefrom. In the cases of parasites, the absorbing connections which are more or less specialized and definite are called *haustoria.* In the higher forms the hyphæ become consolidated into false tissues, and assume definite shapes according to the species. Of this character are the fructifying organs which constitute the above ground parts of Puff Balls, Morels,

Ergot, Cup Fungi, Mushrooms, etc. There are four classes of Fungi, viz.: Phycomycetes, Ascomycetes, Basidiomycetes and Fungi Imperfecti. Of these only the Ascomycetes and Basidiomycetes yield official drugs.

CLASS—ASCOMYCETES OR SAC FUNGI

This is the largest class of fungi, containing thousands of species which vary from unicellular organisms such as the yeasts to multicellular forms like *Penicillium*, *Aspergillus*, *Claviceps*, *Peziza*, etc. In all, the life history is characterized by the appearance of a sac called an *ascus* in which *ascospores* are formed. The mycelium is composed of septated filaments (*hyphæ*).

SACCHAROMYCETACEÆ OR YEAST FAMILY

Unicellular plants of spheroidal, oval, ellipsoidal or pyriform shape, in whose life history a mycelium is wanting. They occur either in the wild or cultivated condition and are of considerable economic value on account of their ability to break down some form of carbohydrate substance into carbon dioxide and alcohol. Reproduction is by gemmation (budding) and through the formation of ascospores.

CEREVISIÆ FERMENTUM COMPRESSUM N.F. (COMPRESSED YEAST)

Synonym.—Fæx Compressa, *Ger.* Hefe; *Fr.* Levure.

Botanical Origin.—*Saccharomyces cerevisiæ* Meyen, or other species of *Saccharomyces*.

Part Used.—The moist living cells, combined with a starchy or absorbent base.

Habitat.—In dilute saccharine solutions which are exposed to the air.

Saccharomyces cerevisiæ, commonly called Brewer's Yeast, is a cultivated species with many strains. It is used extensively in the brewing and baking industries and in recent years has met with considerable esteem by the medical profession in the treatment of certain skin diseases.

When examined under the microscope it is found to be somewhat spheroidal to ellipsoidal in outline, 8 to 12μ long, and 8 to 10μ broad. It consists of an outer cell wall of *fungous cellulose* enclosing cytoplasm and a nucleus, the latter invisible without special staining. The cytoplasm is differentiated into a clear outer membrane lying directly within the cell wall and termed the *ectoplasm* and an inner granular region, the *endoplasm*. In the young condition of the yeast cell numerous glycogen vacuoles are found scattered more or less uniformly throughout this region, but, as the cell matures, these coalesce, until, in a very old cell, a huge glycogen vacuole may be seen occupying most of the interior, with the cytoplasm and nucleus pushed up against the cell wall and forming there a very narrow layer.

Yeast plants grow in dilute saccharine solutions containing dissolved nitrogenous substances such as beerwort, Pasteur's solution, grape juice, etc. Here they are constantly wasting away and as constantly being built up. The question may well arise: "How do they obtain the material necessary for growth and repair?" The answer, in a general way, is not difficult. The fluid in which they live is a solution of sugars and of nitrogenous and other matters. The cell walls are readily permeable. Food substances diffuse through it into the cell, and by a series of changes are converted into new living substance. The waste products likewise diffuse readily outward. This method of nutrition is called saprophytic, and the yeast plant is said to be a saprophyte.

A striking fact must be briefly mentioned in connection with the metabolism of yeast. Many organisms exercise a profound effect on the medium in which they live. Yeast causes a wholesale destruction of sugar in the surrounding fluid. The fermentative ability of the plant is due to two enzymes, *invertase* and *zymase*. *Invertase*, an extracellular enzyme, diffuses out of the cell into the solution in which the yeast is growing and hydrolyzes cane sugar into dextrose and levulose; *Zymase*, an endocellular ferment, remains within the cell, being incapable of osmosis, and there ferments the dextrose and levulose to form carbon dioxide and alcohol. The alcohol of commerce is produced by the activity of this plant.

Saccharomyces has its times of danger and stress when the cells perish in great numbers from cold, starvation, poisons, etc. If not too suddenly exposed, however, they are able to meet adverse conditions by eliminating most of their water, suspending physiological processes, and becoming dormant. Sometimes they enter the resting condition after a process of division, when each cell divides into four parts, each of which becomes nearly dry and is surrounded by a thick wall. Such cells are called *ascospores*, and their production serves both as a method of multiplying the plant and of tiding over adverse conditions. They can survive for a long time without food or water, and can endure higher temperatures than the active cells and almost any degree of cold.

The dried cells and spores float in the air as dust and so accomplish a dispersal of the organism. Doubtless most of them never again meet suitable environment and so sooner or later perish. But some will fall into favorable conditions and be able to multiply enormously again, and so the species is continued.

The vegetative method of reproduction in *Saccharomyces* is that of *gemmation* or *budding*. A small protuberance of the cell wall commences to form on the parent-cell. This grows larger and a portion of the cytoplasm and nuclear material pass into it. Eventually a daughter-bud, which may assume the size of the parent-cell, is formed. This generally adheres to the parent-cell and produces one or more granddaughter-buds which in turn may produce great-granddaughter-buds before separation from the parent-cell takes place.

There are two-well known varieties of brewer's yeast, viz.: Top yeasts and Bottom yeasts. Top yeasts grow on or near the surface of the liquid and produce rapid fermentation at summer temperatures, causing great quantities of carbon dioxide to arise to the surface and thus forming the froth which is characteristic of ale, stout and porter.

Bottom yeasts grow at about 4°C. at or near the bottom of the vat. They are used in the manufacture of larger beers.

Description.—Compressed yeast is found on the market in the form of white or yellowish-white masses or cakes of variable size. It is soft and easily broken, has a characteristic slightly sour odor and taste. Its reaction to litmus is faintly acid. When examined under the microscope, it exhibits, besides the yeast cells described above, numerous starch grains and oidium and mycoderma cells. It should be free from molds and mildews.

Constituents.—The enzymes zymase, invertase and endotryptase; the water-soluble vitamin-B or accessory growth promoting substance; fat, nucleins, nucleoproteins and carbohydrates.

Uses.—Apart from its use in the brewing industry, yeast is used to raise dough. It is employed medicinally as a laxative and in the treatment of boils, unhealthy wounds and various skin eruptions.

HYPOCREACEÆ FAMILY

This family includes about 57 genera of parasites found on fungi, grasses and cereals, trees and insects. It is characterized by the perithecia being more or less spherical and opening by means of an apical pore. Arising from the base of each perithecium are to be noted a cluster of eight-spored asci.

ERGOTA U.S.P. (ERGOT)

Synonyms.—Ergot of Rye, Spurred Rye, Secale Cornutum, Horn-seed; *Ger.* Mutterkorn; *Fr.* Ergot de Seigle.

Botanical Origin.—*Claviceps purpurea* (Fries) Tulasne.

Part Used.—The dried sclerotium, replacing the grain of the rye (*Secale cereale*).

Standard of Assay.—Ergot in the form of the fluidextract, administered by intramuscular injection to single-comb, white Leghorn cocks, in doses not exceeding 0.5 cc. for each kilogram of body weight of cock, produces a darkening of the comb, corresponding in intensity to that caused by the same dose of a standard fluidextract of ergot prepared in accordance with U.S.P. x.

Limit of Impurities.—5 per cent. of seeds, fruits, or other foreign organic matter.

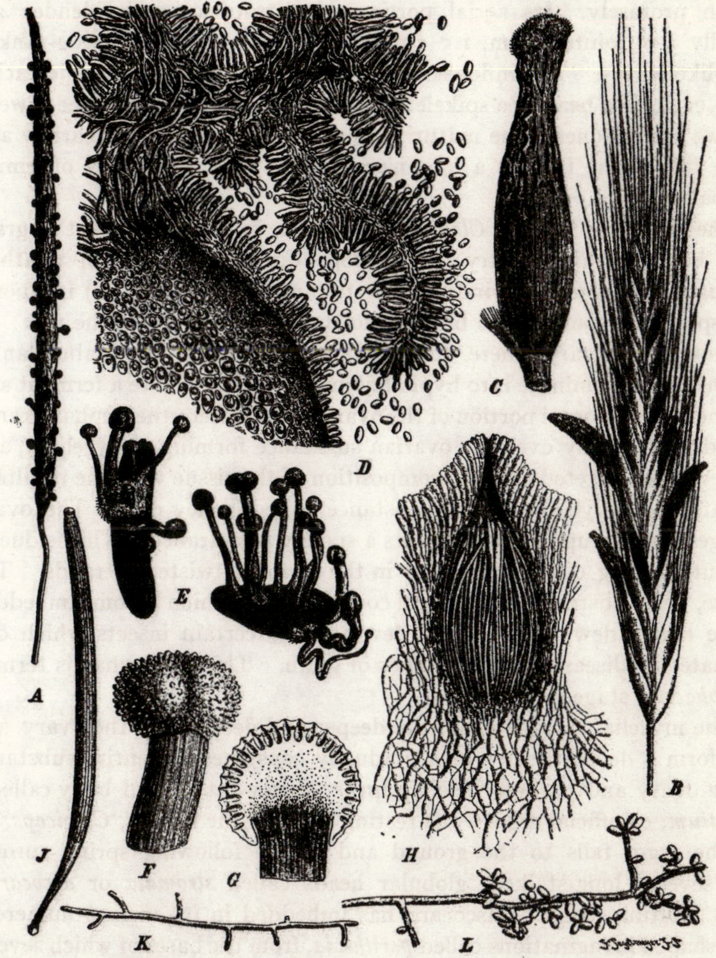

FIG. 7.—*A*, *Balansia claviceps* on ear of *Paspalum; B–L, Claviceps purpurea; E*, sclerotium; *C*, sclerotium with *Sphacelia; D*, cross-section of sphacelial layer; *E*, sprouting sclerotium; *F*, stalked ascocarp (*stroma*) from sclerotium; *G*, section of same; *H*, section of perithecium; *J*, ascus; *K*, germinating ascospore; *L*, conidiospores produced on mycelium. (*See Die natürlichen Pflanzenfamilien* I, I, p. 371.)

Habitat.—Russia, Spain and other eastern countries, infesting the ovaries of various cereals and grasses.

Plants.—Two plants are concerned in the formation of Ergot, namely, *Secale cereale*, the common rye, which is the host and *Claviceps purpurea*, the parasite. *Secale cereale* is an annual member of the grass family. Its underground portion consists of a whorl of four primary roots which branch profusely. Its aerial portion consists of a tough, slender 4–7 (usually 5–6) jointed stem, 1.5–2 m. high, which bears alternate, 2-ranked grass-like leaves. The inflorescence is a 4-rowed spike with 20–30 rachis joints, each joint bearing a spikelet. Each spikelet consists of three flowers, the two lateral ones alone maturing grains. The glumes are narrow and bristle-like. The fruit is a long narrow grain that is destitute of lemma and palet.

The parasitic fungus, *Claviceps purpurea*, is very prevalent in grain fields both in this country and Europe during moist warm weather. Through the agency of winds or insects (ants, flies, or beetles) its spores (ascospores or conidia) are brought to the young ovaries of the rye. At the base of the ovary, where, during damp weather moisture is abundantly present, they germinate into hyphal filaments which secrete a ferment and so penetrate the basal portion of the ovary. From here the hyphal strands extend superficially over the ovarian substance forming a mycelium, and the ferments secreted cause decomposition of the tissue with the resultant formation of a yellow-mucus substance called honey dew. The ovary enlarges and its upper end presents a spongy appearance. This is due to the outcropping of the mycelium in the form of twisted strands. The hyphæ, here, abstrict off chains of conidiospores, which become imbedded in the honey dew. The honey dew attracts certain insects which disseminate the disease to other spikes of grain. This ends what is termed the *sphacelia* stage.

The mycelial threads penetrate deeper and deeper into the ovary and soon form a dense tissue which gradually consumes the entire substance of the ovary and hardens into a purple, somewhat curved body called a *sclerotium*, or official ergot—the resting stage of the fungus, *Claviceps*.

The ergot falls to the ground and in the following spring sprouts into several long-stalked, globular heads called *stromata* or *ascocarps*. Each (fruiting) head or ascocarp has imbedded in its surface numerous flask-shaped invaginations called *perithecia*, from the bases of which several sacs or *asci* develop. Within each ascus are developed eight filiform spores (*ascospores*) which, when the ascus ruptures, are discharged and are carried by the wind to other fields of grain, there to begin over a new life cycle.

Production and Commerce.—Ergot is gathered chiefly in Spain, Russia, Germany, Galicia and Austria being usually separated from the rye after it has been thrashed by special machinery, although also picked by hand. It is dried at a low temperature. The supplies imported into the United States come chiefly from ports of Spain in cases or bags. Some supplies also come from Portugal, Holland, Germany, Trieste and from Russia.

Description.—The sclerotium is somewhat cylinder-like, obscurely 3-angled, tapering toward both ends, obtuse, somewhat curved, from 1 to 4.5 cm. in length and from 3 to 5 mm. in thickness; externally purplish-black, or brownish-black, longitudinally furrowed; fracture short, pinkish or reddish white, sometimes grayish-white; odor peculiar, disagreeable, free from mustiness; taste oily and disagreeable. No ammoniacal or rancid odor should develop when hot water is poured on bruised Ergot.

Histology.—Transverse sections exhibit under the microscope a thin outer zone of small compact cells of a purplish or violet color, turning red with 50 per cent. H_2SO_4 or with chloral hydrate solution and a broad inner zone of pseudoparenchyma composed of colorless, thin-walled cells, each less than 15μ in width, which contain globules of fixed oil.

Powdered Drug.—Grayish-brown to purplish brown. It shows for the most part whitish fragments composed of false parenchyma (compacted hyphæ) and a few purplish fragments of the outer region of the sclerotium. Upon mounting a small portion in chloral hydrate T.S. or in 50 per cent. sulphuric acid, numerous globules of fixed oil separate and many of the fragments are colored yellow, red, or rose-purple.

Constituents.—Ergotoxine (an amorphous alkaloid yielding crystalline salts), ergotamine (a crystalline alkaloid), histamine, tyramine, acetylcholine, etc.

Uses.—As a parturient (in labor) and hemostatic (in uterine hemorrhage).

POLYPORACEÆ (PORE FUNGI)

The sporophores or fruiting bodies of these fungi are various. They may be entirely supinate with pores or shallow depressions on their upper surfaces (*Merulius*), or mushroom-like (*Boletus*), or of the nature of woody (*Polyporus* and *Fomes*) or fleshy (*Fistulina*) brackets. In all cases the hymenium or basidial layer lines the inner surface of pores.

AGARICUS N.F. (AGARIC)

Synonyms.—Larch Agaric, White Agaric, Surgeon's Agaric; *Fr.* Polypore du Méleze; *Ger.* Larchenschwamm.

Botanical Origin.—*Polyporus officinalis* Fries.

Part Used.—The dried fruit body, deprived of its outer rind.

Limit of Impurities.—5 per cent. of foreign organic matter.

Standard of Assay.—It yields to boiling alcohol not less than 50 per cent. of a non-volatile resinous extract.

Habitat.—On species of *Pinus*, *Larix* and *Picea* (Pines, Larches and Spruces) of the eastern and western hemispheres.

Description.—This drug is found as irregular, light, fibrous and somewhat spongy pieces of the sporophore; externally grayish-white to pale brown; internally pale yellow and resinous; fracture tough, fibrous; odor indistinct; taste sweet, acrid and bitter.

Constituents.—Resin, agaricinic acid, tannin, phosphoric acid, tartaric acid, oxalic acid, malic acid, fat, protein, etc.

Use.—Surgeon's agaric is used as a styptic in hemorrhage.

SUBDIVISION—LICHENS

Lichens are variously colored, usually dry leathery plants consisting of symbioses of algæ and fungi. Blue-green and Protococcus forms of Green Algæ and Ascomycete Fungi represent the main forms concerned in lichen formation. The body of a lichen, when examined microscopically, shows differentiation into 2 regions: (1) a more or less compact row of cells on both surfaces called the epidermis and (2) an inner portion composed of fungal hyphæ in close association with algal cells. Lichens reproduce by spores which are borne in asci. The latter are borne in open or closed fruiting bodies called apothecia. Many of the lichens, like *Cetraria islandica* or *Iceland Moss* have been valued because of their demuicent properties while others, as species of *Rocella* and *Lecanora*, yield upon fermentation valuable coloring principles.

PERSIO N.F. (PERSIO)

Synonyms.—Cudbear; *Fr.* Orseille de terre.

Botanical Origin.—Species of *Rocella* DC., *Lecanora* Ach. and other lichens.

Part Used.—A purplish-red powder.

Purity Rubric.—Not more than 12 per cent. of total ash.

Habital.—Eastern and Western Hemispheres.

Production and Commerce.—The lichens used in the preparation of cudbear belong to several genera. Chief among those identified are *Rocella tinctoria* Ach. or Orchilla Weed, from the Mediterranean coasts, Canary and Cape Verde Islands, *Lecanora tartărea* Ach. or Tartarean Moss from Northern Europe, *Rocella Montagnei* Bel. from Mozambique and Madagascar and *Dendrographa leucophœa* Darb. from California. The substances or mother principles in these plants which yield cudbear are themselves colorless and are said to be acids or acid anhydrides as lecanoric acid, orsellic acid, etc. The lichens are gathered from rocks, cleaned, dried and ground. They are then macerated in an ammoniacal liquid of urine, lime, and potash or soda for nearly a week during which time a purplish-red color develops. The resultant paste is dried and reduced to a powder.

Description.—A purplish red powder which imparts to aqueous or alcoholic preparations a deep red color. This color is rendered lighter in tint by the addition of acids, and is changed to purplish red by the addition of alkalies.

Uses.—Coloring agent for various pharmaceutical preparations and as a dye in the arts.

DIVISION II—BRYOPHYTA (BRYOPHYTES)

Plants showing a beginning of definite alternation of generations, *i.e.*, gametophyte (sexual phase) alternating with sporophyte (asexual phase of development) in their life history, the two phases being combined in one plant. The female sexual cell is always lodged in an *archegonium* (a multicellular female sexual organ).

SPHAGNUM

Synonyms.—Peat Moss, Bog Moss.

Botanical Origin.—*Sphagnum imbricatum*, *S. palustre*, *S. papillosum*, *S. magellanicum* and probably other species of *Sphagnum*.

Part Used.—The entire plant.

Habitat.—In bogs of the eastern and western hemispheres.

Plants.—**Sphagnum imbricatum** belongs to the Cymbifolia group. The imbricated leaves are borne on the crowded fascicles of tapering and short branches. Plant brown in color and grows in thick tufts. **S. palustre,** belonging to group Cuspidata, is pale green, and appears in loose tufts. The stem leaves are at the apex, 5-toothed, and in outline ovate. The branches are in 3's to 5's per fascicle with ovate-lanceolate leaves. Monœcious or diœcious. **S. papillosum,** of the group Cymbifolia, is robust with turgid branches. In the stem are four layers of cuticular cells. The branch leaves, in contrast to the rounded, serrulate stem leaves, are closely imbricated and somewhat concave. Plants are diœcious.

Production and Commerce.—The richest areas for Sphagnum in North America are from Nova Scotia to southern New Jersey, Alaska to lower Oregon and in the vicinity of the Great Lakes. A particularly fine zone for the collection of those species which can be employed as a substitute for cotton is around Ilwaco, Washington. That moss is best which has the highest capacity for absorbing liquids. It should be soft, pliable and fairly strong. These requirements are possessed to an excellent degree by *Sphagnum imbricatum*, *S. palustre*, *S. papillosum* and *S. magellanicum*.

The moss may be collected during any season. It is pulled up in chunks and partially dried, packed in gunny sacks and sent to railroad centers for cleaning. Here it is freed from all sticks, foreign leaves and wiry stems and baled or boxed for shipment to various points.

Histology.—Under the microscope, sphagnum leaves show bread areas of colorless, porous cells with oblique septa, capable of absorbing and holding quantities of liquid. It is these cells which give sponginess to even partially dried and dead specimens. Elongated and slender chlorophylloid cells are present surrounding the colorless cell areas.

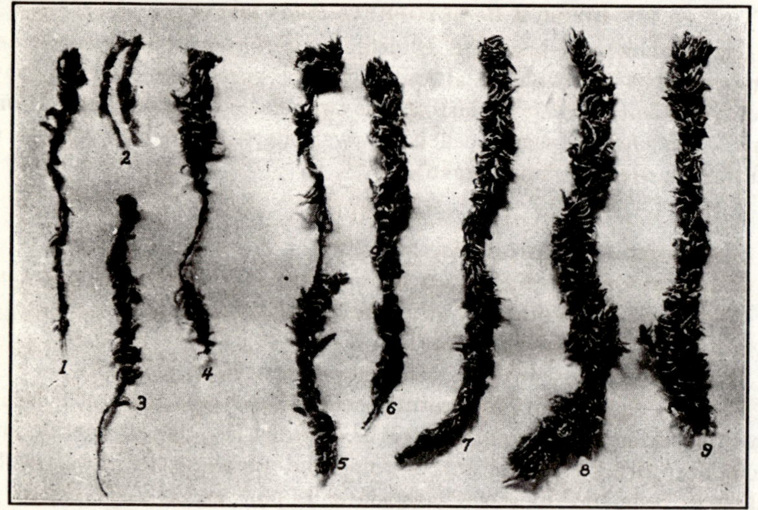

FIG. 8.—Sphagnum (*Peat Moss*).

Uses.—Sphagnum has proven a more excellent absorbent than cotton and as such has been extensively employed in surgery in the form of pads. It is also used in the manufacture of sanitary napkins. Its saturation time is but 1/3 to 1/2 that of absorbent cotton and it possesses the additional advantages of being antiseptic because of its iodine content, and less expensive.

DIVISION III.—PTERIDOPHYTA (PTERIDOPHYTES)

This division includes the club mosses, scouring rushes and ferns. All of these show a distinct alternation of generations in their life history. The sporophyte is characterized by separating very early from the gametophyte (prothallus) and living thereafter an independent existence. It is furthermore leafy, vascular and root bearing.

SUBDIVISION—LYCOPODINEÆ OR CLUB MOSSES

Small, perennial, vascular, dichotomously branched herbs with stems thickly covered with awl-shaped leaves. The earliest forms of vascular plants, differing from ferns in being comparatively simple in structure, of small size, leaves sessile and usually possessing a single vein. Except in a few instances the sporangia are borne on leaves, crowded together and forming cones or spikes at the ends of the branches—homosporous (spores of one kind).

LYCOPODIACEÆ (CLUB MOSS FAMILY)

A family of trailing or upright, moss-like herbs with many small, usually subulate or lanceolate leaves and elongated stems. The prothallus is subterranean.

LYCOPODIUM U.S.P. (LYCOPODIUM)

Synonyms.—Vegetable Sulphur, Common Club Moss, Wolf's Claws, Lamb's or Fox Tail; *Fr.* Saufre végétale; *Ger.* Streupulver, Bärlappsamen.

Botanical Origin.—*Lycopodium clavatum* Linné.

Part Used.—The spores.

Habitat.—Europe and Asia.

Plant.—A creeping, prostrate, horizontally branching, perennial club moss. From the main prostrate stems arise aerial stems. The leaves are crowded, many ranked, linear-awl-shaped and bristle tipped. The peduncles are stout, often forked near the summit, with slender bristle-tipped bracts. The spikes are elongated, the sporophylls deltoid, ovate, acuminate and bristle-tipped.

Production and Commerce.—The plant grows in Europe, Asia, North America and Central America. When the sporophylls are mature, the tops are shaken and the spores collected with foreign matter. The latter is separated by sieving. Considerable of the drug is produced in Poland and Ukraine. Switzerland and Germany also produce it. The commercial supplies used in this country come in bags within cases and are chiefly imported from Danzig, Hamburg and London. Much of it is consumed by manufacturers of fireworks.

Description.—A mobile powder of light yellow color and devoid of odor and taste. It floats on water, and, when boiled with it, sinks. It burns with a quick flash when thrown into a flame.

Microscopical Characteristics.—Chloral or water mounts exhibit the spores as spheroidal tetrahedrons from 25μ to 40μ in diameter. The exosporium or outer wall is marked by a reticulated surface, the meshes being surrounded by polygonal ridges with straight sides. When observed with the rounded surface facing downward, the upper surface is characterized by a triangular marking which represents the intersection of the 3 plane surfaces.

Constituents.—Fixed oil (about 50 per cent.) consisting chiefly of lycopodium-oleic acid; sugar, phytosterin, protein, etc.

Uses.—As a dusting powder for abraded surfaces and for preventing the adhesion of pills.

Adulterants.—(1) Pine pollen, which consists of dumb-bell shaped pollen grains, each having a central convex generative cell and 2 spherical wing cells, one on either side of the generative cell. (2) Altered corn starch colored with methyl-orange. (3) Sulphur, detected by its solubility in carbon disulphide.

SUBDIVISION—FILICINEÆ

The group Filicineæ is the largest among the vascular cryptogams and includes all the plants commonly known as Ferns. The main axis of a typical fern is a creeping underground stem or *rhizome* which at its various nodes bears *rootlets* below and *fronds* above. These fronds are highly developed, each being provided with a petiole-like portion called a *stipe* which is extended into a *lamina* usually showing a forked venation. Some ferns possess laminæ which are lobed, each lobe being called a *pinna*. If a pinna be further divided, its divisions are called *pinnules*. The unfolding of a frond is circinate and it increases in length by apical growth. On the under surface of the laminæ, pinnæ, or pinnules may be seen small brown patches, each of which is called a *sorus*, and usually covered by a membrane called the *indusium*. Each sorus consists of a number of *sporangia* (spore cases) developed from epidermal cells. In some ferns the entire leaf becomes a spore-bearing organ (sporophyll). Most sporangia have a row of cells around the margin, the whole beng called the *annulus*. Each cell of the annulus has a U-shaped, thickened cell-wall. Water is present within these cells and when it evaporates it pulls the cell walls together, straightening the ring and tearing the weak side. The annulus then recoils and hurls the spores out of the sporangium. Upon coming into contact with damp earth each spore germinates, producing a green septate filament called a *protonema*. This later becomes a green heart-shaped body called a *prothallus*. It develops on its under surface *antheridia* or male organs and *archegonia* or female organs, as well as numerous *rhizoids*. Within the antheridia are developed motile *sperms*, while *ova* are produced within the archegonia. The many ciliate sperms escape from the antheridia of one prothallus during a wet season, and, moving through the water, are drawn by a chemotactic influence to the archegonia of another prothallus, pass down the neck canals of these and fuse with the ova, fertilizing them. The fertilized egg or oöspore divides and redivides and soon becomes differentiated into stem-bud, first leaf, root, and *foot.* The foot obtains nourishment from the prothallus until the root grows into the soil, when it atrophies, and the sporophyte becomes independent. Unequal growth and division of labor continue until a highly differentiated sporophyte results, the mature "fern plant."

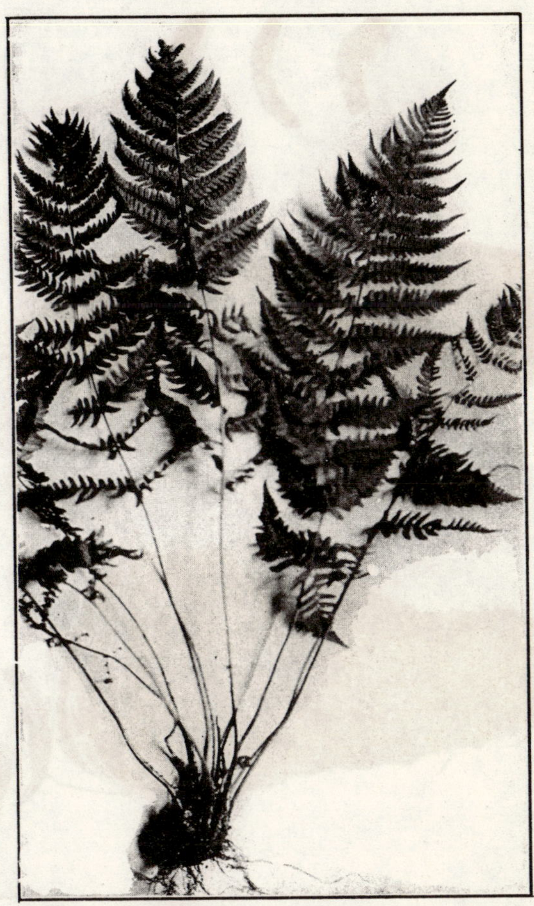

FIG. 9.—*Dryopteris marginalis*, a fern whose rhizome and stipes yields the drug, known as American Aspidium.

To this subdivision belong the true ferns or Filicales, which bear spores only of one kind, and the water ferns or Hydropterales, which bear spores of two kinds. The ferns used in medicine belong to the former of these.

POLYPODIACEÆ (POLYPODIUM FAMILY)

Ferns characterized by possessing creeping rhizomes and leafy aerial fronds. The spores are formed in sporangia which are associated in

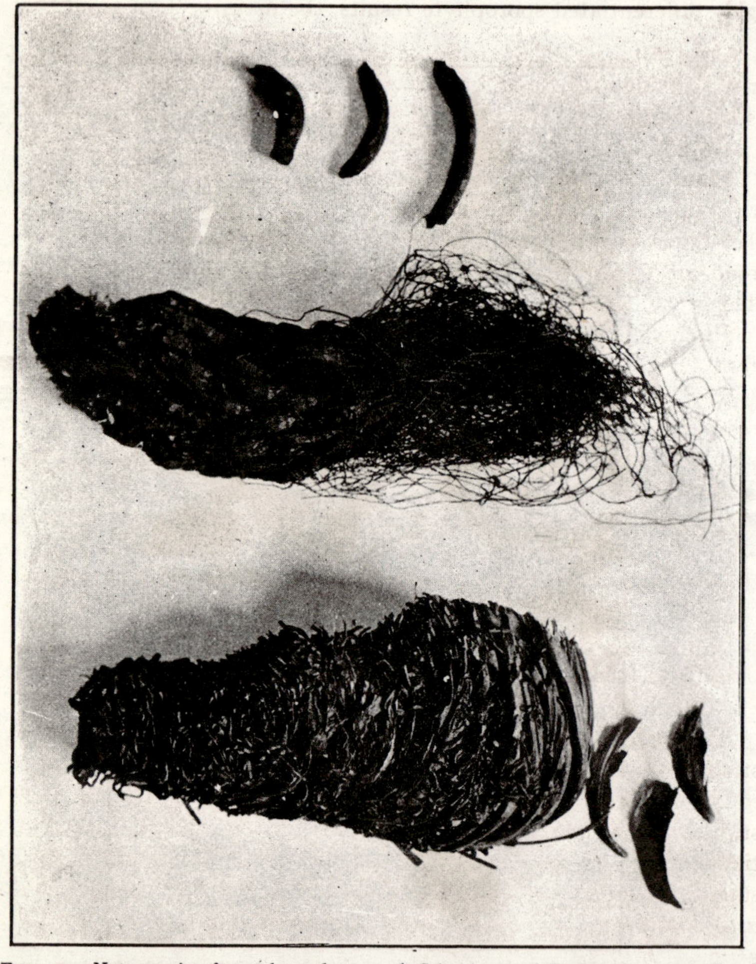

FIG. 10.—Note passing from above downward: Stipe bases of *Dryopteris marginalis;* rhizome and roots of *Dryopteris marginalis*, the rhizome covered with stipe bases; rhizome of *Osmunda Claytoniana* covered with stipe bases and 3 separated stipe bases at its right.

dot or line-like clusters (sori) on the dorsal surface or margins of the frond or its divisions. Each spore case has an annulus. The sori are often covered by an indusium.

ASPIDIUM U.S.P. (ASPIDIUM)

Synonyms.—Male Fern, European Aspidium; *Fr.* Fougère mâle; *Ger.* Wurmfarn.

Botanical Origin.—*Dryopteris Filix-mas* (Linné) Schott.

Part Used.—The rhizomes and stipes.

Purity Rubric.—Aspidium yields not less than 6.5 per cent. of oleoresin, and not more than 3 per cent. of acid-insoluble ash. Only such portions as have retained their green color should be used.

Habitat.—Europe, Asia and northern North America.

Plant.—A perennial fern with an oblique rhizome which is covered with stipe bases. From the anterior region of each arises a circle of lanceolate, bipinnate fronds. The pinnæ or first divisions of the lamina of the frond are linear-lanceolate and the pinnules or divisions of the pinnæ, oblong. The sori are nearer the midvein than the margin.

Production and Commerce.—The ferns are uprooted in autumn, freed from roots, dead portions of rhizomes and stipes and dried at a temperature of 70°C. Many of the rhizomes are cut longitudinally to facilitate drying. The drug is gathered in various parts of Europe, particularly in the Harz and Thuringian mountains. It is imported into the U.S.A. chiefly from Germany and Holland.

The European article is characterized by occurring in the form of partially peeled stipes and longitudinally cut rhizomes. About 1000 pounds were imported in 1924 chiefly through Rotterdam, Holland.

American Aspidium is yielded by *Dryopteris marginalis* (L.) A. Gray. It occurs as entire rhizomes and stipe bases or as stipe bases only. It is collected sparingly in scattered parts of the eastern and central United States.

Description.—Rhizome cylindraceous, 1 to 3 cm. in thickness, nearly straight or curved and tapering toward one end, often split longitudinally, roughly scarred with stipe base remains, or with stipe bases attached; stipes subcylindrical, somewhat curved, tapering toward one end, partially peeled or unpeeled; fracture short; texture spongy; fractured surface pale green and exhibiting 6 to 12 small vascular bundles, arranged in an interrupted circle; odor slight; taste sweetish, astringent, bitter and acrid.

Rhizomes and stipes devoid of a green color internally should be rejected.

Histology of Rhizome.—Passing from periphery toward the center the following structures are to be observed:

1. **Epidermis,** a protective outer covering tissue, composed of a single layer of brownish polyhedral cells from which are given off scaly hairs.

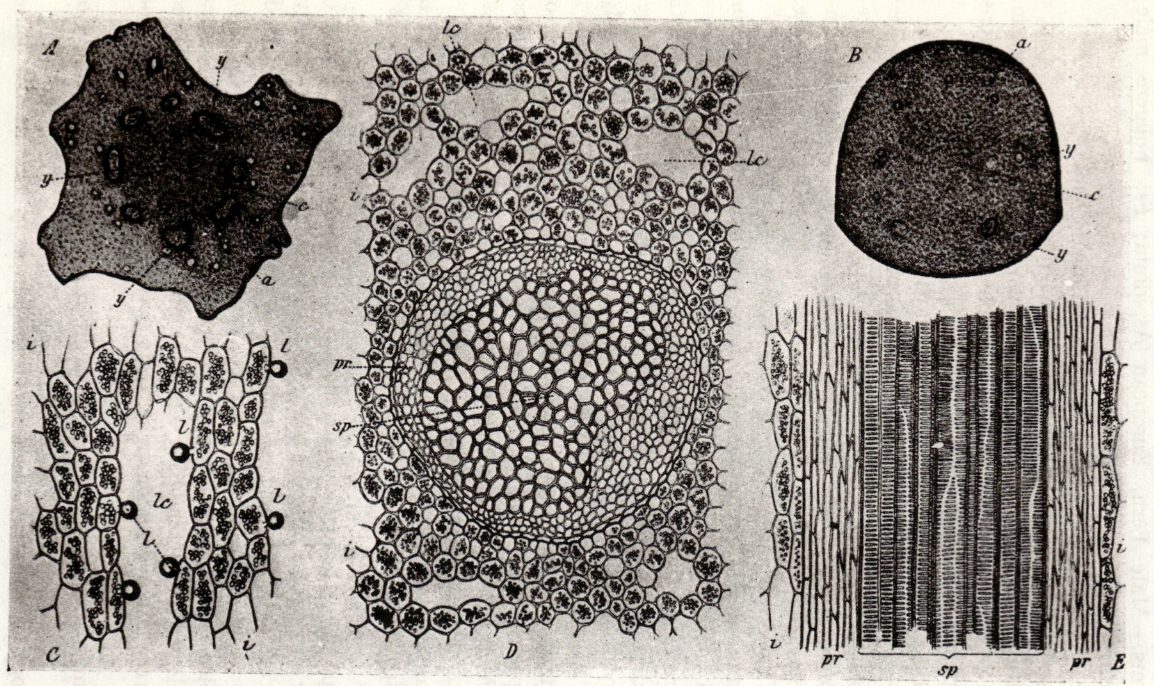

FIG. 11.—*Aspidium Filix-mas.* *A.* Transverse section of the rhizome, × 3. *B.* Transverse section of the stipe base × 5. *C.* Longitudinal section through a portion of the parenchyma region showing intercellular-air-spaces into which oleoresin-containing glandular hairs (*l*) project, × 65. *D.* Transverse section through a concentric bundle and adjacent parenchyma, × 65. *E.* Longitudinal section through the same, × 65. *a*, cortex; *c*, pith; *i*, parenchyma; *y*, concentric bundles; *lc*, intercellular-air-spaces; *l*, internal glandular hairs; *pr*, phloem; *sp*, scalariform tracheae. (*After Berg.*)

The latter show 2 small glands at their bases and the margins have 2-celled projections.

2. **Outer cortex** (hypodermis), a zone of several layers of thick-walled lignified cells separating the epidermis from the inner cortex beneath.

3. **Inner cortex** of several layers of more or less isodiametric cells (cells of nearly the same length, breadth and thickness) with thin cellu-

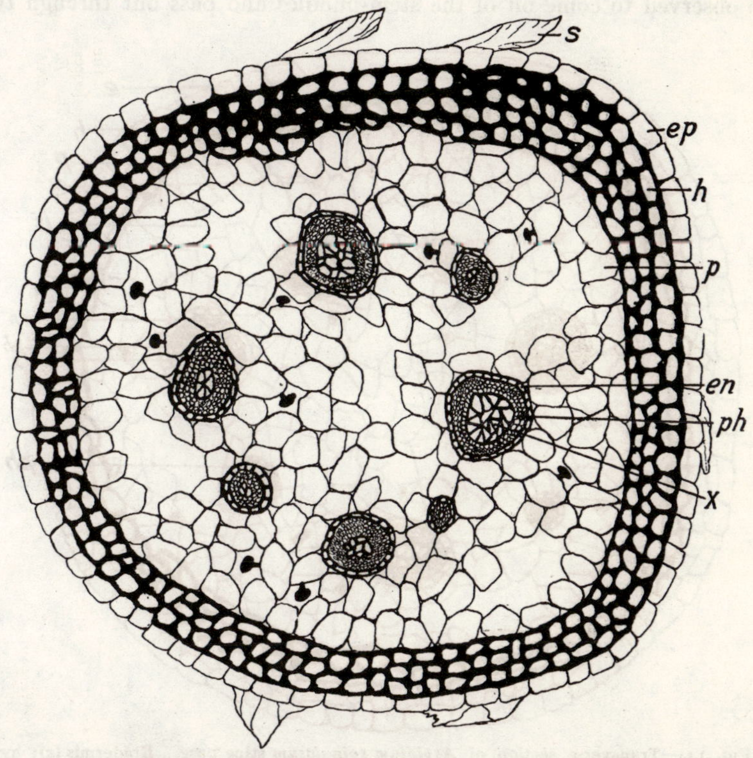

FIG. 12.—Transverse section of *Dryopteris marginalis* (American Aspidium) stipe base. Epidermis (*e*); hypodermis (*h*); parenchyma (*p*); internal gland (*g*); xylem composed mainly of scalariform tracheids (*x*); surrounded by phlœm (*ph*) and forming a concentric fibro-vascular bundle; endodermis or bundle sheath (*en*); scales (*s*). Magnified.

lose walls and containing stored starch surrounded by a protoplasmic investment. Between the cells are to be noted intercellular-air-spaces, many of which contain internal glandular hairs.

4. **Fundamental tissue,** resembling the last in aspect and function.

5. **Vascular Bundles.**—These are of two kinds, viz.: stem bundles and leaf-trace bundles. Both are of elliptical outline and of concentric

type as seen in cross section, and are embedded in the parenchyma forming the broad central matrix. The stem bundles are comparatively broad and, as viewed in longitudinal sections, form a continuous network with good-sized meshes, each mesh being opposite the point of insertion of one of the leaves. In transverse section these bundles are seen to be 6 to 12 in number and arranged in an interrupted circle within the fundamental tissue. The leaf-trace bundles are comparatively narrow and are observed to come off of the stem-bundles and pass out through the

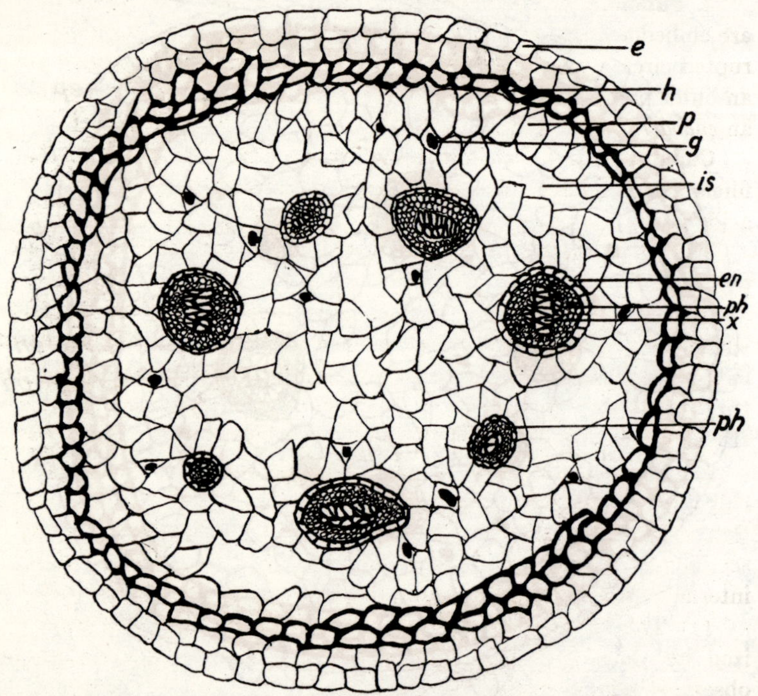

FIG. 13.—Transverse section of *Aspidium spinulosum* stipe base. Epidermis (*e*); hypodermis (*h*); parenchyma (*p*); intercellular-space (*is*); internal gland (*g*); xylem (*x*); phlœm (*ph*); endodermis (*en*). Magnified.

cortex into the leaves (fronds). When each bundle is examined under a high-power magnification it is seen to consist of a central xylem, composed of scalariform tracheids and xylem cells, which is completely surrounded by a phloem composed of rounded, thin-walled phloem cells and sieve tubes. Surrounding the bundle is a 1 to 3-layered pericambium and around this an endodermis or bundle sheath composed of a single layer of cells with yellowish walls and granular contents.

Histology of Stipe (Petiole).—This, in transverse section, passing from periphery toward the center, presents the following structural characteristics:

1. **Epidermis,** a single layer of epidermal cells with dark brown outer walls.

2. **Outer cortex** (hypodermis), a wide band of small cells with lignified walls.

3. **Inner cortex,** similar to inner cortex of rhizome but devoid of leaf-trace bundle.

4. **Fundamental parenchyma,** similar to same region of stem, in which are embedded 6 to 10 *concentric fibrovascular bundles* arranged in an interrupted circle. Each of these shows a central xylem mass surrounded by an outer phloem mass. Each bundle is enveloped by a *pericambium* and an *endodermis* or bundle sheath.

Constituents.—A yellowish amorphous substance called filmarone, filicic acid, aspidinol, flavaspidic acid, flavaspidinol, fixed oil, filicitannic acid, resins, starch, etc.

Use.—Aspidium is employed in the form of its official oleoresin as a tænifuge.

Adulterants.—(1) The rhizomes and stipes of *Osmunda Claytoniana* L., which may be detected by the presence of flattened stipe bases that show in transverse section one large central, more or less crescent-shaped, concentric bundle that is flanked on either side by brownish masses of sclerenchyma fibers. Moreover, the rootlets are thicker and wiry.

(2) The rhizomes and stipes of *Aspidium spinulosum* Sw., which are difficult to distinguish from the genuine drug without microscopical examination. They may, however, be detected by the examination of cross sections of the stipes. These show 6 to 8 concentric bundles, fewer internal glands, and a less indurated hypodermis (see Fig. 13).

(3) The rhizomes of *Athyrium Filix-fœmina* L., which are characterized by showing 2 large dumb-bell shaped fibrovascular bundles, as observed in cross-section.

(4) The old, inert, brownish, powdered drug has been admixed with powdered marshmallow leaves in order to give it the light green appearance of the recent article.

DIVISION IV.—SPERMATOPHYTA (PHANEROGAMIA)

Plants producing real flowers and seeds. The highest evolved division of the vegetable kingdom.

SUBDIVISION I.—GYMNOSPERMÆ—THE GYMNOSPERMS

The Gymnosperms comprise an ancient and historic group of seed plants which were more numerous in the Triassic and Carboniferous periods than now. They differ from the Angiosperms in several respects, viz.: they bear naked ovules on the edges or flat surfaces of leaves called carpels, while Angiosperms bear covered ones; each megaspore or embryo-sac produces within itself a bulky prothallus, in the upper portion of which originate one or more archegonia, while in Angiosperms no recognizable prothallus has been proven to exist; the stored food tissue within their seeds is prothallial tissue loaded with starch, etc., while that in Angiosperm seeds (endosperm) is developed from the endosperm nucleus; the mode of growth of their stems is always indefinite while that of Angiosperms is either indefinite or definite.

The groups still extant are the Cycads or Fern Palms, the Gnetums, the Ephedras, the Ginkgos and the Conifers. Of these the Conifers comprising over 300 species are the most numerous. Many of them yield valuable products to pharmacy and the arts.

The Conifers include the pines, spruces, hemlocks, cedars, firs, arbor vitæ, chamæcyparis, and larches. All of their number are evergreen except some of the larches, which drop their foliage upon the advent of winter.

PINACEÆ (CONIFERÆ) (PINE FAMILY)

Trees or shrubs with resinous juice whose wood is characterized by being composed largely of tracheids with bordered pits. Leaves entire, awl- or needle-shaped, frequently fascicled, exstipulate, usually evergreen. Flowers, monœcious or rarely diœcious, achlamydeous, in cones. Staminate cone of a large number of microsporophylls (stamens) closely packed together and arranged spirally around a central axis, each stamen bearing usually two pollen sacs. Carpellate cone composed of spirally arranged scales, each of which bears a pair of naked ovules (megasori) near the base of its upper face, or a single ovule springing from a cupuliform disc (*Taxus*). Fruit a cone with woody or fleshy scales (*Pinus*, *Thuja*, *Abies*, *Picea*, etc.), a galbulus (*Juniperus*), or a drupe composed of the thickened and fleshy disc surrounding an erect seed (*Taxus*). Seeds albuminous. Embryo with two or more cotyledons.

TEREBINTHINA N.F. (TURPENTINE)

Synonyms.—Crude Turpentine, Lump Turpentine, Gum Thus; *Ger.* Terpentin; *Fr.* Térébenthine commune.

Botanical Origin.—*Pinus palustris* Miller and other species of *Pinus*.

Part Used.—The concrete oleoresin.

Limit of Impurities.—2 per cent. of foreign matter.

Habitat.—From Virginia to Florida and Texas.

Plant.—*Pinus palustris* or "long leaf pine" is a large evergreen tree with thin scaly cork and hard resinous wood, growing in sandy soil in the southern states, mainly within 100 miles of the coast. Its leaves are in fascicles of 3 which range from 5 to 10 in. in length. Its cone scales are long, flattened, with short, sharp recurved spines. *Pinus Tæda* L. (Loblolly pine), *P. cubensis* Grisebach (Cuban pine) and *P. echinata* Miller (Short-leaf pine) also yield some of the drug.

Production and Commerce.—The oleoresin is formed in resin reservoirs contained in the wood and exudes spontaneously but not in sufficient

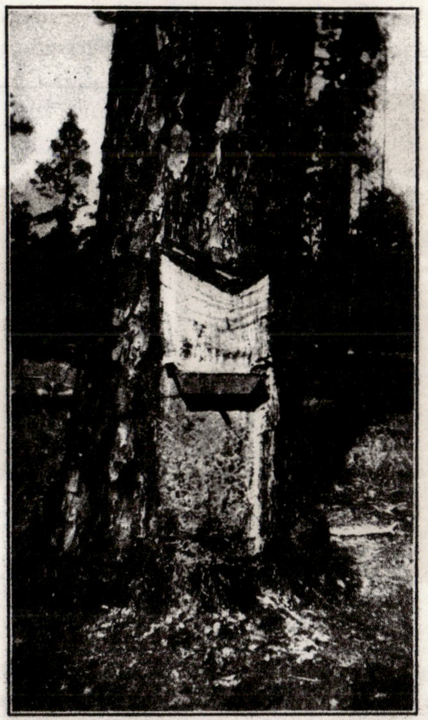

FIG. 14.—Trunk of a *Pinus palustris* tree growing in a Texas forest showing a common method of turpentining. Note the hacked wood and the affixed aluminum cup, the latter used to collect the flow of crude turpentine. (*Photograph by Ohmart.*)

quantities to make it worth while collecting on a commercial basis. It is obtained commercially by two methods. The first of these consists of cutting a series of downward and inward sloping V-shaped incisions into the trunk of the tree for a distance of about a foot, the bark and young wood being removed. This is usually done early in the year. At the base of these incisions an aluminum cup is affixed to the trunk and two aluminum strips ("aprons") are inserted above to deflect the flow of the oleoresin into the cup. The oleoresin soon begins to run and collects in the cup. As the cups become filled their contents are emptied into wooden barrels and others affixed to the trees. In about a week or ten days the flow of oleoresin diminishes and another series of incisions is started above the first excavation. Production continues until autumn.

The second method is known as "the cup and gutter system." This consists of making a small incision in the bark and inserting a strip of galvanized iron or aluminum. The oleoresin flows along this strip into an earthenware receptacle.

Turpentine is largely a pathological product formed in the wood of the trees due to the stimulation of the cambium, through injury, to form new

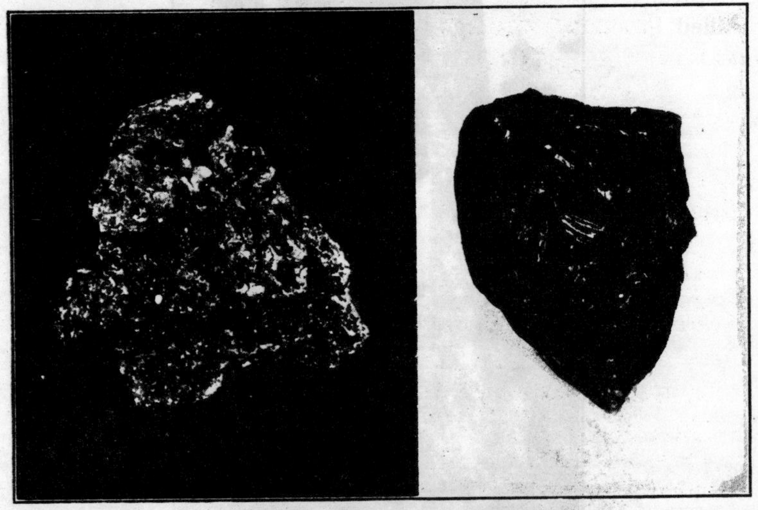

A B

FIG. 15.—*A*, Turpentine; *B*, rosin. × ⅛. (*Photograph by Stoneback.*)

wood containing large numbers of oleoresin reservoirs. "Scraps," "gum thus" or "American Frankincense" are terms applied to the white incrustation on the surface of the hacked wood of the excavations, consisting of the turpentine which has dried thereon without reaching the cup. This is scraped off and marketed as a distinct article. The turpentine collected from the first year's tapping is known as "virgin" turpentine and yields from 15 to 30 per cent. of volatile oil and an amber-colored rosin. That collected during subsequent years supplies the so-called "yellow dip" turpentine which is somewhat darker in color, contains less volatile oil and yields upon distillation a yellowish-brown or yellowish-red rosin.

The commercial supplies of turpentine are obtained chiefly from Florida, Mississippi, Louisiana, Texas, North Carolina, South Carolina and Georgia. Florida leads the country in turpentine and rosin production.

Description.—In yellowish, irregular, opaque masses, yellowish-white internally, sticky, more or less glossy, brittle in the cold; odor aromatic; taste characteristically pungent.

Constituents.—Volatile oil (10 to 30 per cent.) consisting of a mixture of several terpenes, chief among which are pinene, phellandrene, limonene and dipentene (all of them have the formula of $C_{10}H_{16}$); resin (70 to 90 per cent.), bitter principle, etc.

Oleum Terebinthinæ U.S.P., commonly known as Spirits of Turpentine or Turpentine Oil, is the volatile oil distilled from this drug. It is used as a solvent in the arts. The rectified article (Oleum Terebinthinæ Rectificatum U.S.P.) is employed as a counter irritant and diuretic.

Allied Product.—Bordeaux turpentine is an oleoresin obtained from *Pinus maritima* Poiret and other species of *Pinus* growing in southwestern France. It contains a strongly lævorotatory volatile oil, and a resin consisting of pimaric, pimarinic and pimarolic acids.

Uses.—Lump turpentine is used as an ingredient in preparing Compound Rosin Cerate N.F. or Deshler's Salve. Most of the crude article is distilled for oil of turpentine and rosin.

RESINA U.S.P. (ROSIN)

Synonym.—Colophony, *Ger.* Geigenharz, Fichtenharz; *Fr.* Colophone ou Arcanson.

Botanical Origin.—*Pinus palustris* Miller and other species of *Pinus*.

Part Used.—The residue left after distilling the volatile oil from Lump Turpentine.

Ash.—Not more than 0.05 per cent.

Description.—It occurs in irregular, more or less angular, light or dark amber-colored masses or sharp fragments, frequently covered with a yellowish dust, brittle at ordinary room temperature, translucent; fracture conchoidal; odor and taste slightly terebinthinate. It is soluble in alcohol, ether, benzene, fixed and volatile oils, glacial acetic acid and is dissolved by dilute solutions of fixed alkaline hydroxides. Its specific gravity is 1.07 to 1.09 at 25°C.

Constituents.—Chiefly abietic anhydride ($C_{44}H_{64}O_5$).

Uses.—Rosin is used because of its stimulating properties as an ingredient in Rosin Cerate, Deshler's Salve, as well as in some plasters and ointments. It is also employed an ingredient of some varnishes, and as a size for paper, etc.

TEREBINTHINA LARICIS (VENICE TURPENTINE)

Synonym.—Larch Turpentine, *Ger.* Venetianischer Terpentin; *Fr.* Térébenthine de Venise.

Botanical Origin.—*Larix europœa* De Candolle.

Part Used.—The viscid oleoresin.

Habitat.—Alps and Carpathian mountains of Europe.

Plant.—A deciduous conifer.

Production and Commerce.—The European Larch is cultivated extensively in the Alps and Carpathians for its oleoresin. This is procured by boring holes into the wood in the spring and conducting the exuded oleoresin by gutters into tubs. It is then filtered through sieves. The commercial supplies are obtained from France, Italy and southern Europe.

Description.—A yellowish-green, thick, heavy liquid, having an aromatic odor and a bitter, pungent taste. It is soluble in alcohol, chloroform, acetone or glacial acetic acid.

Constituents.—Volatile oil, resin, laricinolic acid, bitter principle, etc.

Use.—As an antiseptic protective in veterinary practice.

Adulterant.—Rosin oil. This may be detected by the use of reflected light. Rosin oil, in a sample thus examined, exhibits a violet or purple fluorescence whereas Venice Turpentine shows a slight greenish fluorescence.

TEREBINTHINA CANADENSIS (CANADA TURPENTINE)

Synonyms.—Balsam of Fir, Canada Balsam; *Fr.* Baume du Canada; *Ger.* Canadischer Balsam.

Botanical Origin.—*Abies balsamea* Miller.

Part Used.—The oleoresin.

Habital.—Northern United States and Canada.

Plant.—The Balsam Fir is a handsome evergreen tree attaining a height of 50 to 80 ft. and a trunk diameter of 15 to 30 in. Its leaves (needles) are ⅓ to 1¼ in. long, linear, obtusely pointed or emarginate, shiny dark green above, paler below. Its carpellate cones are at first purplish later becoming yellowish-brown, up to 4 in. long and erect on the upper side of spreading branches. Each of these cones shows a series of spirals of thin obovate serrulate scales (bracts) which are tipped with a short, slender point. The bark contains numerous oleoresin vesicles.

Production and Commerce.—The oleoresin commonly known as Balsam of Fir is secreted in oleoresin reservoirs in the bark of the tree but also collects in cavities which appear like blisters on the exterior of the trunk and branches. The blisters are punctured by collectors with the pointed spout of a collecting can and the oleoresin allowed to run into the can. The greater bulk of the commercial supply is produced in lower Canada, particularly in Quebec, although some is also collected in Maine.

Description.—A pale yellow, viscid, transparent liquid often exhibiting a slight greenish fluorescence, soluble in all proportions of ether, chloroform, oil of turpentine or benzene, but only partially soluble in alcohol; odor agreeable, terebinthinate; taste bitter and acrid. It dries to a solid, transparent film on evaporation.

Constituents.—Volatile oil composed chiefly of *l*-pinene (16 to 24 per cent.); resin (70 to 80 per cent.) and bitter principle. About 20 per cent. of the resin is canado-resene which is insoluble in alcohol, the remainder being composed of two amorphous resin acids (α- and β-canadinolic acids) and about 0.5 per cent. of crystalline canadolic acid.

Uses.—Canada Balsam is chiefly used as a microscopic mounting medium and as a cement for optical lenses, for which purposes it is dissolved in xylol, after warming. It is also employed in the preparation of flexible collodion and printing inks.

Allied Drug.—Oregon Balsam, yielded by *Pseudotsuga taxifolia* Brit. (*P. Douglasii* Carr), an evergreen conifer found in Western N. A. from British Columbia to Mexico, dries to a sticky film upon evaporation.

PIX PINI U.S.P. (TAR)

Synonyms.—Pine Tar, Pix Liquida, Wood Tar, *Ger.* Theer; *Fr.* Goudron végétal.

Botanical Origin.—*Pinus palustris* Mill. and other species of *Pinus*.

Part Used.—A product obtained by the destructive distillation of the wood.

Habitat.—Southern United States.

Plant.—*See under Terebinthina.*

Production.—The wood of several of the pines indigenous to the Southern United States, notably *Pinus sylvestris*, *P. Tæda* and *P. rigida*, is cut into billets which are distilled without access of air. The tarry liquid is then separated from the liquid consisting of pyroligneous acid, wood naphtha, etc., and poured into barrels for shipment.

Description.—It occurs as a viscid, blackish-brown, non-crystalline liquid, translucent in thin layers, becoming granular and opaque upon ageing; odor empyreumatic, terebinthinate; tàste pungent and empyrematic.

Upon distillation, tar gives off oil of tar and pyroligneous acid, the residue left in the retort being pitch.

Constituents.—Resins, turpentine, creosote, guaiacol, acetic acid, acetone, xylol, toluol, methyl-alcohol and empyreumatic substances.

Uses.—As a local irritant and antiseptic in certain skin diseases; internally as a stimulating expectorant and diuretic.

Allied Product.—*Pix Carbonis* also known as *Pix Lithanthracis* or Coal Tar is a nearly black, thick liquid or semi-solid obtained as a by-product in the destructive distillation of coal in the manufacture of illuminating gas. It is employed to combat inflammations in certain skin diseases.

PIX BURGUNDICA (BURGUNDY PITCH)

Synonyms.—*Ger.* Burgunder Harz, Burgundisches Pech; *Fr.* Poix de Bourgogne.

Botanical Origin.—*Picea excelsa* Link. [*Picea abies* (L.) Karst.; *Abies excelsa* Poiret].

Part Used.—A resinous exudation obtained from the stem.

Habitat.—Europe, in mountainous districts.

Plant.—The *Picea excelsa* or Norway Spruce is a handsome evergreen tree attaining a height of up to 150 ft. with spreading branches, reddish-brown bark and dense dark green foliage. Its leaves are quadrangular, acute, glossy and from ½ to 1 in. in length. It bears staminate and carpellate cones, the carpellate being conical, purplish when young, at length becoming cylindric-oblong, light brown and up to 7 in. long, the scales being obovate with erose denticulate margins.

Production and Commerce.—The Norway Spruce grows abundantly in the Black Forest, Jura mountains and in Finland where the drug is obtained by making deep incisions in the bark, extending into the wood. The oleoresin, naturally occurring in the secretion reservoirs therein, is thus induced to flow and collects in the incisions and solidifies. In due course of time it is scraped out, melted in boilers under water and finally strained through cloths.

The commercial supplies come chiefly from Finland and Germany, although little of the genuine article has been imported into this country within recent years.

Description.—An opaque or translucent, yellowish-brown to reddish-brown, hard substance, taking on the form of the container in which it is kept; brittle, breaking with a conchoidal fracture: soluble in strong alcohol and glacial acetic acid: odor aromatic; taste sweet and aromatic.

Constituents.—Chiefly resin consisting of α- and β-picea-pimarolic acids with smaller quantities of picea-pimarinic and picea-pimaric acids and juro-resene; volatile oil.

Use.—Counter-irritant in plasters.

Substitute.—Factitious Burgundy Pitch composed of a mixture of rosin, turpentine and palm oil. This article differs from the authentic drug in being incompletely insoluble in twice its weight of glacial acetic acid.

PINUS ALBA N.F. (WHITE PINE BARK)

Synonyms.—Pine Bark, Weymouth Pine.

Botanical Origin.—*Pinus Strobus* Linné.

Part Used.—The dried inner bark.

Purity Rubric.—Not more than 2 per cent. of outer bark and not more than 2 per cent. of foreign organic matter.

Habitat.—In forests of eastern and central North America.

Plant.—An evergreen timber tree having a trunk 1½ to 3 feet in diameter and attaining a height of 90 to 125 feet. At varying distances

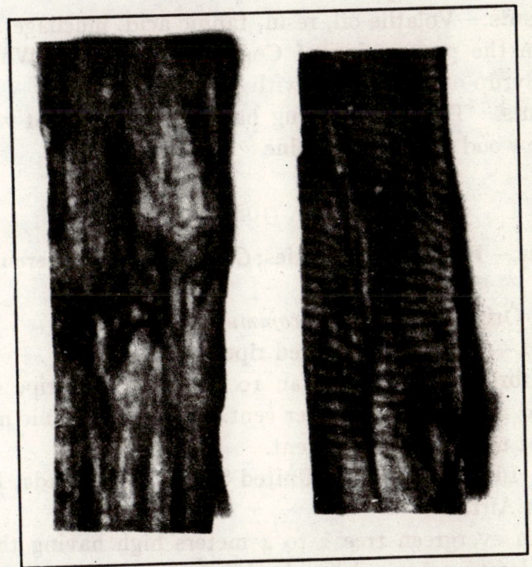

FIG. 16.—White Pine bark. Outer surface at left; inner corrugated surface at right. × ⅜

above the soil there arise whorls of lateral branches (3 to 7 in a whorl) at various levels becoming increasingly shorter up to the apex. These branches and their secondary branches end in terminal scaly buds. The spur shoots bear soft, flexible, bluish-green needles which are up to 5 in. in length, when mature, and occur in clusters of 5, each cluster being surrounded at its base by a deciduous sheath. The staminate cones are yellow and ovate and appear clustered at the base of the new growth about May. The young carpellate cones are pinkish-purple and occur in solitary fashion or in small groups, lateral along the new growth in early summer. The fruit is a slightly curved cone, 5 to 10 in. in length, having thin unarmed scales.

Production and Commerce.—The bark is stripped from the trunk and branches in long sheets and the cork and some of the cortex removed. It is then carefully dried. The commercial supplies are obtained from the northwestern and southeastern parts of the United States.

Description.—In flat, cut and broken pieces of variable size and from 1 to 3 mm. in thickness; sometimes folded, outer surface pinkish-yellow to yellowish-brown, coarsely striated, occasionally with small patches of brown to gray-brown periderm adhering and frequently showing small scattered pits; inner surface yellowish-brown, finely striated and corrugated; fracture tough, fibrous; fractured surface showing a yellowish fibrous surface; odor slightly terebinthinate; taste slightly mucilaginous, bitter, sweet and astringent.

Constituents.—Volatile oil, resin, tannic acid, mucilage, etc.

Uses.—In the preparation of Compound Syrup of White Pine and Compound Syrup of White Pine with Morphine.

Adulterants.—The ground drug has been adulterated with elm bark and with the wood of the white pine.

JUNIPERUS N.F. (JUNIPER BERRIES)

Synonyms.—Horse Savin Berries; *Ger.* Wachholderbeeren; *Fr.* Baies de Genièvre.

Botanical Origin.—*Juniperus communis* Linné.

Part Used.—The carefully dried ripe fruit.

Purity Rubric.—Not more than 10 per cent. of unripe or discolored "berries" and not more than 3 per cent. of foreign organic matter.

Ash.—Not more than 5 per cent.

Habitat.—In dry woods of United States and Canada, Europe, Asia and Northern Africa.

Plant.—An evergreen tree 2 to 4 meters high having thin, straight, long, acerose leaves arranged in whorls of 3 and diœcious flowers. The carpellate cones are ovoid and consist of 3 fleshy scales, each one ovuled. The fruit is a subglobose galbulus which contains 3 seeds.

Production and Commerce.—The fruits are collected when ripe and carefully dried. They are imported from Leghorn, Italy.

Description.—Subglobular, 5 to 10 mm. in diameter; externally smooth, shining purplish-black to dark brown with a blue-gray bloom; at the summit a 3-rayed furrow marks the cohesion of the three fleshy bracts forming the pericarp; internally exhibiting a greenish-brown pulp containing three triangular ovate, hard brown seeds, adhering to which are large uneven oil glands; odor aromatic; taste sweet, terebinthinate and pungent.

Powdered Drug.—Dark brown; numerous fragments of somewhat polygonal epicarp cells containing a brownish granular substance; fragments of brownish-red collenchyma cells from hypodermis; fragments of groups of sclerenchyma cells, some containing monoclinic prisms; fragments of endosperm containing aleurone and oil globules; fragments of loose parenchyma containing a brownish substance; fragments of oil glands and resin masses.

Constituents.—Volatile oil (U.S.P.) containing juniper camphor, pinene and cadinine; resin, fixed oil, etc.

Uses.—As a diuretic.

SABINA (SAVIN)

Synonyms.—Savin Tops, Cacumina Sabinæ; *Ger.* Sadebaumspitzen; *Fr.* Sabine.

Botanical Orign.—*Juniperus Sabina* L.

Part Used.—The young green tops of the twigs.

Habitat.—Mountainous regions of Central and Southern Europe to Siberia.

Plant.—A small evergreen shrub of more or less erect habit, attaining a height of 10 ft. or procumbent. It possesses slender branchlets bearing small, 4-ranked, overlapping, rhombic-lanceolate, obtuse or subacute green leaves and small globular 1 to 3-seeded fruits (galbuli) borne on curved peduncles.

Production and Commerce.—The young tender twigs are gathered in the spring, chiefly in the Alps and Great Britain. They are either distilled in the recent condition for the volatile oil or dried and later used in the manufacture of fluid extract and tincture.

Description.—Twigs, thin, averagely from 1 to 3 cm. long and 1 to 2 mm. thick, densely covered with 4 rows of appressed, scale-like, imbricated rhomboid leaves, each about 2 mm. long and with an oil gland directly under its dorsal surface; odor terebinthinate; taste bitter, resinous and acrid.

Histology.—Transverse sections of the leafy twigs may be such as to include the stem and the adnate bases of 2 opposite leaves or leaves separate from stem. The first type of section presents an elliptical outline interrupted by 2 notches, marking the places of separation of the leaf bases. It is characterized further by showing an epidermis with sunken stomata and thick cuticle, a slightly lignified hypodermis composed of small-lumened and thick-walled cells, a mesophyll with outer palisade and inner spongy parenchyma, imbedded in which are 2 oil glands, one at either pole directly beneath the hypodermis, while in the center of the section there will be observed coniferous stem tissues. On either side of each notch and imbedded in the mesophyll is a small group of irregularly lignified cells called transfusion tracheids.

The cross section of the leaf is almost semicircular in outline. The leaf is of the centric type. It shows an epidermis similar to that of the preceeding section, a hypodermis of interrupted groups of fibrous cells which tend to be missing beneath the middle portion of the upper epidermis, a mesophyll with an outer layer of palisade cells, the remainder becoming shorter toward the center. Imbedded in the center of this region is a meristele composed of a mass of tracheids facing toward the upper surface and a mass of phloem tissue facing toward the lower. Two groups of transfusion tracheids occur, one on each side of the meristele. A single large oil gland lies imbedded in the mesophyll just below the meristele and above the lower epidermis.

Constituents.—Volatile oil (Oil of savin) 2 to 4 per cent., tannin and resin.

Uses.—Uterine stimulant, emmenagogue, local irritant.

Adulterant.—The tops of *Juniperus Phœnicea* which may be distinguished both by the presence of large stone cells in the mesophyll and by the spiral arrangement of the leaves.

THUJA N.F. (THUJA)

Synonyms.—Arbor Vitæ, American Arbor Vitæ.

Botanical Origin.—*Thuja occidentalis* Linné.

Part Used.—The recently dried leafy young twigs.

Limit of Impurities.—Not more than 2 per cent. of its stems over 4 mm. in diameter or other foreign organic matter.

Habitat.—In low swampy localities and along streams from Southern Labrador west to Manitoba, south to North Carolina and Tennessee.

Commerce.—The commercial supplies are collected chiefly in North Carolina, Virginia and Michigan.

Plant.—A medium sized evergreen tree usually growing to the height of 20 to 50 feet with a tapering, furrowed and buttressed trunk and a dense, conical crown of branches bearing more or less 4-sided twigs that are completely covered by scale-like and closely overlapping leaves. The staminate and pistillate cones occur on different twigs in April and May, the staminate being small, rounded, and yellow, the pistillate small, ovoid and purplish. The fruit is a short, oblong, reddish-brown cone with from 6 to 12 thin, oblong and obtuse scales.

Description.—Twigs entire or broken, fan-shaped, flattened, bearing 4 rows of appressed, scale-like leaves, all bearing glands on back; odor balsamic, aromatic; taste camphoraceous, turpentine-like and bitter.

Powdered Drug.—Greenish to brownish-green. Fragments of chlorenchyma; fragments of epidermis with broadly elliptical stomata from 25 to 40μ in length, the guard cells having lignified walls; numerous thick walled lignified fibers with simple oblique pores.

Constituents.—Volatile oil containing pinene, fenchone and thujone; a bitter principle termed pinipicrin, a crystallizable coloring principle called thujin, tannin, etc.

Uses.—Uterine stimulant, emmenagogue, vermifuge and local irritant.

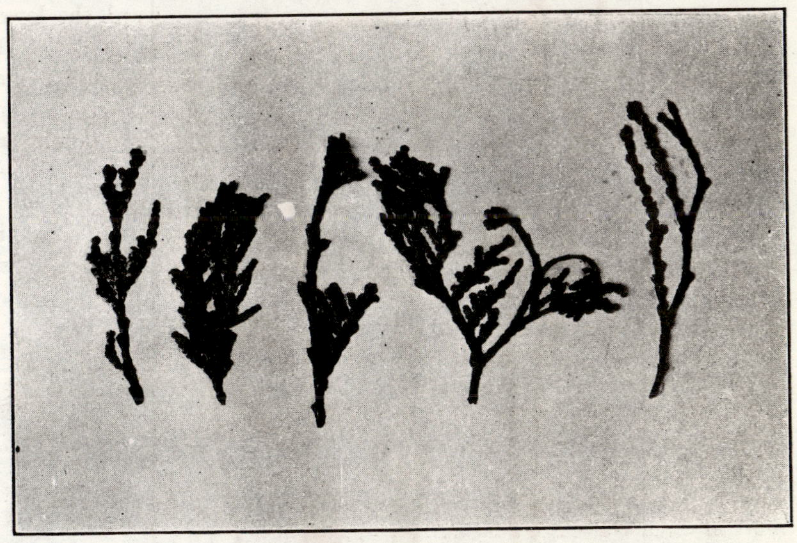

FIG. 17.—Leafy twigs of the Arbor Vitæ, *Thuja occidentalis* × ½. (*Photograph by Stoneback.*

SUBDIVISION II.—ANGIOSPERMÆ OR ANGIOSPERMS

(Plants with covered seeds)

CLASS A.—MONOCOTYLEDONEÆ

A class of Angiosperms characterized by the following peculiarities:

One cotyledon or seed leaf in the embryo.

Stems endogenous with closed collateral or concentric fibro-vascular bundles, which are scattered.

Leaves generally parallel veined.

Flowers trimerous (having the parts of each whorl in threes or multiple thereof).

Secondary growth in roots generally absent.

Medullary rays generally absent.

GRAMINEÆ (GRASS FAMILY)

Mostly herbs with cylindric, hollow, jointed stems whose nodes are swollen. The leaves are alternate, with long split sheaths and a ligule. Flowers generally hermaphroditic and borne in spikelets, making up a

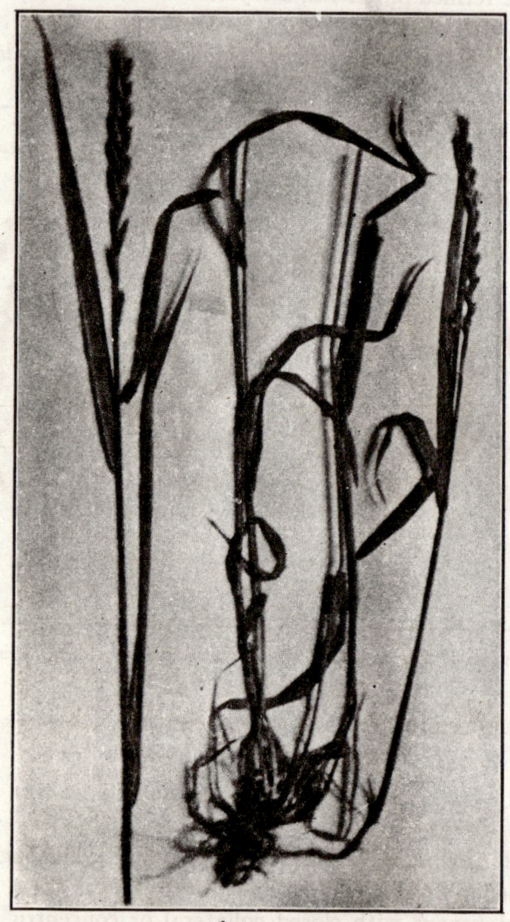

FIG. 18.—*Agropyron repens* (Couch Grass). Plant.

spicate inflorescence. Lowest floral leaves of each spikelet are called glumes, which are empty and paired. Fruit, a caryopsis or grain. Embryo with scutellum. Seeds, albuminous. Seed coat fused with fruit coat to form one layer.

TRITICUM N.F. (TRITICUM)

Synonyms.—Couch Grass, Dog Grass, Quack Grass, Witch Grass, Twitch Grass; *Ger.* Queckenwurzel; *Fr.* Chiendent officinal.

Botanical Origin.—*Agropyron repens* (Linné) Beauvois.

Parts Used.—The dried rhizome and roots, gathered in the spring.

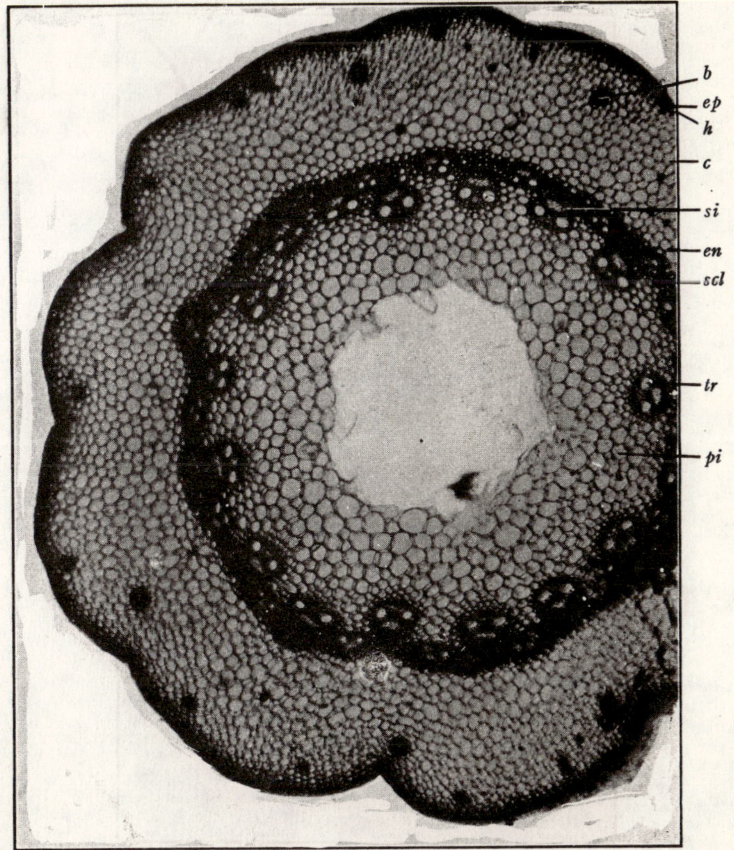

FIG. 19.—Transverse section through rhizome of *Agropyron repens* (Triticum). Epidermis (*ep*); hypodermis (*h*); cortex (*c*); sclerenchymatous ring (*scl*); pith (*pi*); endodermis (*en*); sieve tubes of a closed collateral bundle (*si*); trachea of a closed collateral bundle (*tr*); a concentric bundle of the cortex (*b*). Note bundles of pith attached to sclerenchymatous ring.

Purity Rubric.—Not more than 2 per cent. of foreign organic matter and not more than 3 per cent. of acid-insoluble ash.

Habitat.—In fields and along roadsides of Europe and Asia. Naturalized in North America.

Plant.—A perennial weed, the underground portion of which consists of a very long, slender, many-jointed rhizome from which numerous fibrous rootlets emanate from the nodes and by means of which the plant is extensively propagated. The aerial portion consists of a leafy simple culm attaining the height of 1 m. and bearing a terminal spike of numerous spikelets. Each spikelet is 3–7, usually 5-flowered, the glumes being

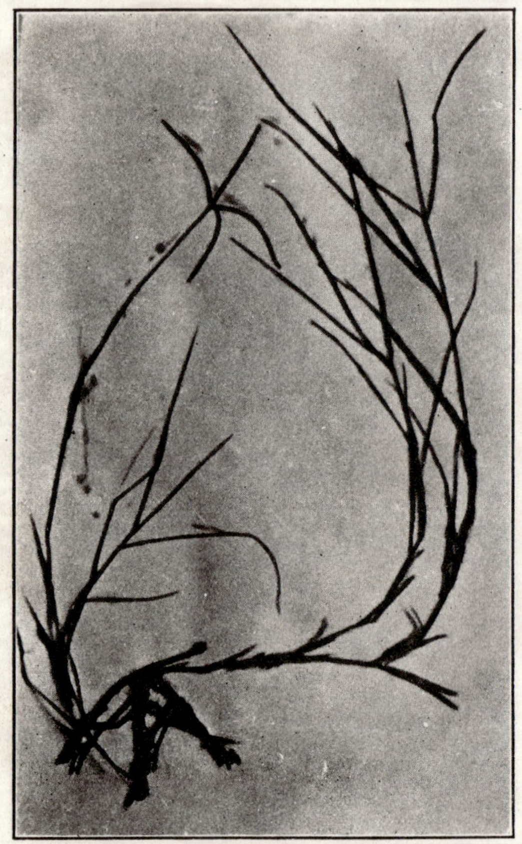

Fig. 20.—*Cynodon Dactylon* (Bermuda Grass). Plant.

8–10 mm. long, 5–7 nerved, acuminate or awn-pointed, the lemmas, about 1 cm. long, strongly nerved, acute or terminating in an awn.

Commercial.—Most of the drug is collected in Central Europe. The rhizomes and roots are gathered in the spring, usually cut into segments varying from 4–12 cm. in length and carefully dried. Samples, recently examined, which were shipped from Europe consisted entirely of the rhizome of *Cynodon Dactylon*, another grass, which somewhat resembles the genuine article. The commercial supplies of Triticum come from Hamburg, Germany, and London, England.

Description.—The drug occurs on the market either in bundles of folded entire and broken pieces attaining a length of 40 cm. or, more generally, in segments 4–12 mm. long and 1–3, seldom more than 2 mm. in diameter, straw-colored externally, smooth and lustrous, showing longitudinal furrows and nodes having circular scars from aerial stems that have fallen off, and root scars as well as occasional filiform rootlets.

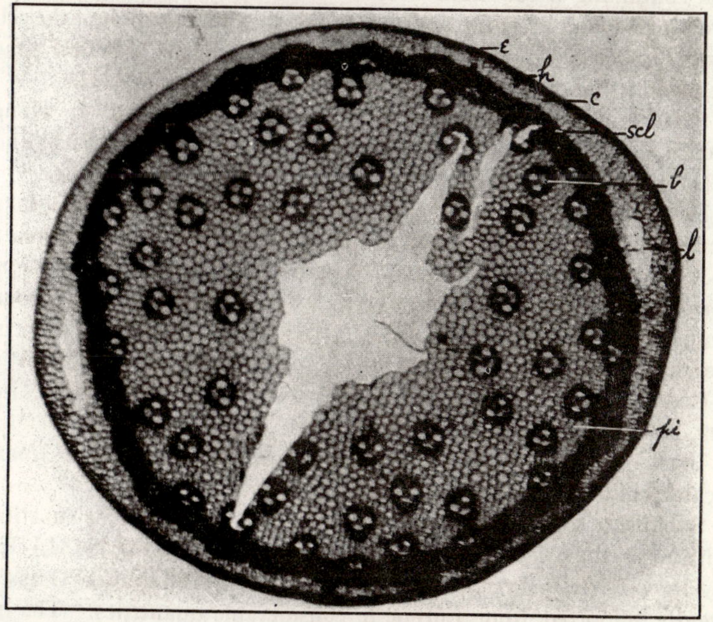

FIG. 21.—Transverse section of Bermuda Grass (*Cynodon Dactylon*) rhizome showing epidermis (*e*); hypodermis (*h*); cortex (*c*); sclerenchyma sheath (*scl*); fibrovascular bundle (*b*); pith parenchyma (*pi*) and lacuna (*l*).

The fracture is tough, irregular and fibrous. The cut ends exhibit a lemon-yellow color and hollow pith. Odor indistinct. Taste sweet.

Microscopical Characteristics.—Cross sections of the rhizome present the following characteristics:

1. Epidermis of a single layer of cells having lignified walls.
2. Hypodermis consisting of 3 to 4 layers of more or less polygonal cells with lignified walls.
3. Cortex of up to 16 layers of thin-walled parenchyma cells with carbohydrate contents either in irregular masses, or, rarely, small spheroidal

starch grains. A number of small concentric fibrovascular bundles occur in the region near the hypodermis. Each is surrounded by a closed sheath of sclerenchyma fibers.

4. Endodermis, a layer of endodermal cells whose radial and inner walls are porous, thick and strongly lignified.

5. A Sclerenchymatous Ring of several rows of sclerenchyma fibers in which are imbedded an irregular, interrupted circle of fibrovascular bundles.

6. Pith, composed of about 8 or 10 rows of thin-walled parenchyma cells containing a few fibrovascular bundles, most of which are found bordering on and partially surrounded by the inner portion of the sclerenchymatous ring. In the center of the pith region is a hollow space of irregular outline, due to a disintegration of the medullary cells.

Surface sections of the epidermis show sinuous-walled, elongated epidermal cells and small twin-cells having strongly silicified walls and of a ball and socket appearance.

Powdered Drug.—Light yellow and consisting of irregular fragments of tissues including fragments of thin-walled, lignified, sclerenchyma fibers associated with portions of annular, spiral or porous tracheæ, fragments of rectangular shaped, epidermal cells whose longer walls are porous and lignified, fragments of thin-walled parenchyma cells and of masses of sclerenchyma fibers.

Constituents.—Triticin, a carbohydrate; glucose, mannite, inosite, gum, malates, etc.

Uses.—Triticum is employed as a demulcent diuretic in the treatment of catarrhal diseases of the genito-urinary tract.

Substitute and Adulterant.—The common adulterant or substitute of Triticum is the dried rhizome and roots of *Capriola Dactylon* (L) Kuntze (*Cynodon Dactylon* Pers.), known to the trade as "Bermuda Grass" and recently imported from Europe in considerable quantities. The important gross and microscopic differences between the official and spurious rhizomes may be tabulated as follows:

Triticum Rhizome	Bermuda Grass Rhizome
Seldom more than 2 mm. in diameter.	Usually 3 mm. or more in diameter, seldom less than 2 mm.
Soft and pliable.	Hard and brittle.
Sweetish taste.	Somewhat starchy taste.
Outline of cross section—irregularly rounded.	Outline of cross section—somewhat oval.
Cortex comparatively broad and containing 6 to 7 or more fibrovascular bundles.	Cortex only about one-fourth as broad as Triticum and containing 1 or 2 fibrovascular bundles.
Endodermis with inner and radial cell walls considerably thickened.	No characteristic endodermis.

Triticum Rhizome	Bermuda Grass Rhizome
Parenchyma cells of cortex and pith with comparatively thin walls and usually containing no starch.	Parenchyma cells of cortex and pith with comparatively thick walls and containing numerous starch grains.
Pith comparatively narrow and containing only about 10 to 19 fibrovascular bundles, most of which are attached to the sclerenchymatous ring.	Pith comparatively broad and containing 30 to 35 fibrovascular bundles.

MALTUM U.S.P. (MALT)

Synonyms.—Barley Malt; *Ger.* Malz, Perlgerste; *Fr.* Orge Perlé, Dreche.

Botanical Origin.—One or more varieties of *Hordeum vulgare* Linné.

Part Used.—The grain, partially germinated artificially, and containing amylolytic enzymes.

Habitat.—Western Asia, Egypt; extensively cultivated.

Plant.—Barley is an annual grain attaining a height of from 0.6 to 1 m. The stem is a 5- to 7- (occasionally 8-) jointed culm bearing alternate leaves with pronounced auricles. The inflorescence is a cylindrical spike up to 10 cm. in length which consists of a compressed rachis bearing two rows of spikelet groups, 3 spikelets appearing at each joint. Each spikelet is one-flowered. The narrow, awn-like glumes form an investment about the spikelets. The lemma is broad, 5 nerved, and bears a long awn with barbed edges. The palet shows two ridges. The fruit is a caryopsis or grain containing an albuminous seed.

Production and Preparation.—The countries yielding the greatest supply of barley are Russia, United States, Germany and the Austrian States. Various types exist, some with two rows, others with four or six rows of spikelet groups. The two-rowed barleys are preferred for the preparation of malt since they have the largest and softest grains. The grain is separated from the straw by threshing. In the preparation of malt, barley grains are steeped for about forty-eight hours in water and then spread out on the floor of a malting room, the temperature of which is from 50 to 60°F. Germination is so regulated that when the young shoot begins to make its appearance the grain is quickly dried in kilns at a temperature not exceeding 55°C. During the process of germination the ferment, diastase, from the epithelial layer of the scutellum, is secreted, which converts starch into maltose (a sugar). It should be kept protected from moisture and heat.

Description.—Barley Malt occurs in entire, yellowish or amber colored grains, rounded at the base, grooved on one side and acuminate at the apex. The fracture is brittle, exhibiting a nearly white internal surface. The odor is characteristic and the taste sweet.

Uses.—Malt is employed medicinally chiefly in the form of its extract for its nutritive properties and as a vehicle for the administration of cod-liver oil, hæmoglobin, cascara sagrada and various salts.

Constituents.—Diastase, soluble starch, maltose, proteids, phosphoric and lactic acids.

ZEA N.F. (ZEA)

Synonyms.—Corn Silk, Stigmata Maydis; *Ger.* Maispistille; *Fr.* Filament de Mais.

Botanical Origin.—*Zea Mays* Linné.

Part Used.—Fresh styles and stigmas.

Habitat.—Tropical America; extensively cultivated.

Plant.—An annual herb.

Description.—It occurs in masses consisting of more or less tangled slender filaments of a light green, yellow, light brown or purplish-red color. Each entire filament consists of a long style (up to 30 cm.) and a bifid stigma. The odor is slight. The taste is slightly sweet.

Microscopical Characteristics.—The styles consist of an epidermis surrounding a matrix of parenchyma through which course two parallel bundles, possessing slender annular and spiral tracheæ. Many of the epidermal cells, particularly of the distal region, show outgrowths in the form of multicellular hairs from 200 to 800μ long. The basal portion of each of these hairs comprises two to five united cells, the distal portion usually one cell. Numerous spinose pollen grains are also evident either adhering to the style or upon the stigmatic surfaces.

Constituents.—Resin, fixed oil, volatile alkaloid, maizenic acid, sugar, etc. A pale purplish-red solution is produced by digesting a small portion of the fresh drug in diluted alcohol and filtering, separate portions of which, on the addition of acids, become yellowish-red; on the addition of alkalies, green; on the addition of ferric chloride T.S., olive green changing to greenish-brown; and on the addition of an aqueous solution of potassium alum, bluish or purplish.

Uses.—Diuretic.

AMYLUM U.S.P. (STARCH)

Synonyms.—Corn Starch; *Ger.* Maisstärke; *Fr.* Fécule de Maize.

Botanical Origin.—*Zea Mays* Linné.

Part Used.—Starch granules separated from the grain.

Purity Rubric.—It contains but a trace of foreign organic matter and yields not more than 0.5 per cent. of ash, and not over 14 per cent. of moisture.

Habitat and Plant.—See *Zea.*

Description.—A fine white powder which may contain irregular white masses. The odor is not distinct. The taste is starchy at first but subsequently sweet. Upon triturating about 0.5 Gm. of starch with 5 cc. of distilled water, the mixture is neutral to litmus. The presence of any iron in starch may be detected by adding 10 cc. of distilled water to 1 Gm. of starch, acidifying with 0.5 cc. HCl and adding 3 drops of potassium ferrocyanide solution, when the mixture will exhibit a blue color within 5 minutes, if iron is present.

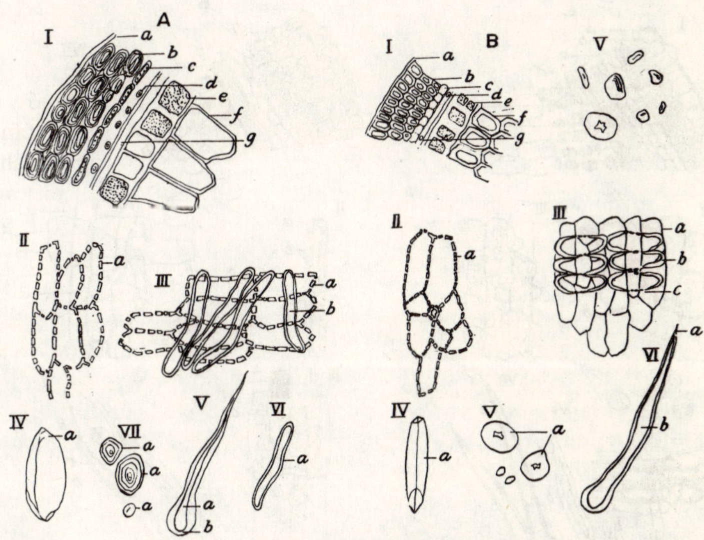

FIG. 22.—A, *Wheat*. I. Transverse section through outer part of fruit. Cuticle (*a*); epicarp (*b*); cross cells (*c*); tube cells (*d*); aleurone layer of endosperm (*e*); perisperm (*g*); starchy endosperm (*f*). II. Epicarp in surface view; cell wall (*a*). III. Surface view of cross cells (*a*) and tube cells (*b*). IV. Whole grain. V. Hair from beard of grain; wall (*b*); lumen (*a*). VI. Tube cell. VII. Wheat starch. B, *Rye*. I. Transverse section through outer portion of grain. Cuticle (*a*); epicarp (*b*); mesocarp (*c*); spermoderm (*d*); aleurone layer of endosperm (*e*); starchy endosperm (*f*); tube cells (*g*). II. Epicarp in surface view. III. Surface section of epicarp (*a*) and cross cells (*b*). IV. Whole grain. V. Rye starch; typical grains (*a*). VI. Hair apex; (*a*); lumen (*b*).

Microscopical Characteristics.—Corn starch grains are simple, polygonal or rounded, 10 to 35μ in diameter; hilum circular or a 2–5 rayed cleft; lamellæ indistinct; polarization cross distinct; no marked play of colors with selenite plate. Iodine T.S. colors starch grains a deep blue.

Preparation.—The dent or flint corn fruits are soaked in running water kept at a temperature of about 60°C. for several days. They are then crushed between burr-stones and the paste conveyed to sieves by means of water and strained. The strained mass is then ground and carried to bolting cloth sieves. The white fluid containing the starch is then run into vats where the starch settles out. A caustic soda solution is then employed to rid the starch of proteins and oil. The supernatant fluid is then decanted and the starch washed with water to remove alkali. Upon standing the starch separates out and is then dried.

Uses.—Starch is a nutrient and demulcent. It is employed pharmaceutically as a base for dusting powders and insufflatious, as a dusting

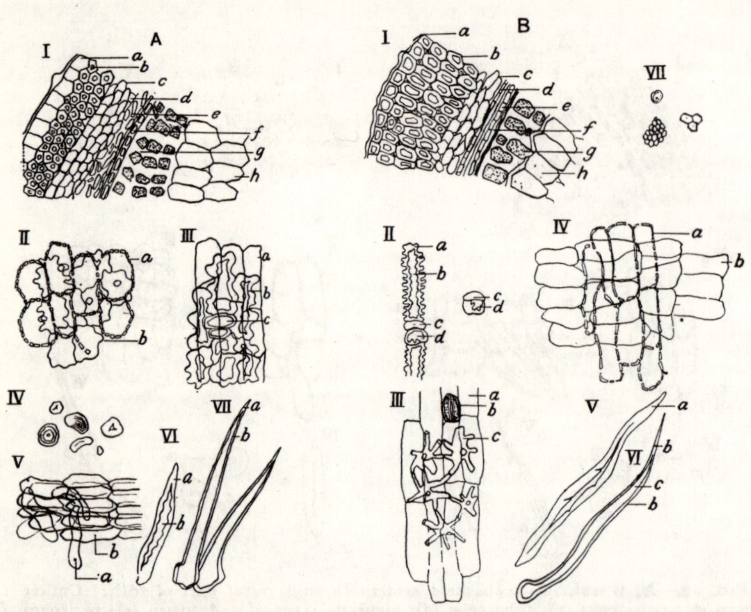

FIG. 23.—A, *Barley*. I. Transverse section through outer portion of grain. Palet (*a*, *b*, *c*); pericarp (*d*, *e*); spermoderm (*f*); aleurone layers of endosperm (*g*); starchy endosperm (*h*). II. Surface view of epicarp (*a*) and parenchyma of palet (*b*). III. Surface view of palet; inner epidermis (*a*), outer epidermis (*b*), and twin cells (*c*). IV. Barley starch. V. Surface section showing 2 layers of cross cells (*b*) and tube cells (*a*). VI. Hypodermal fiber. VII. Hairs fromepi carp; apex (*a*) and lumen (*b*). B, *Oats*. I. Transverse section through outer portion of glume and grain. Glume (*a*, *b*, *c*); pericarp and spermoderm (*d*, *e*, *f*); aleurone layer of endosperm (*g*); starchy endosperm (*h*). II. Elements of flowering glumes and palets. Cells of outer epidermis in surface view; elongated cells (*a* and *b*); crescent shaped cell (*c*); silica containing cell (*d*). III. Surface view of flowering glume and palet. Inner epidermis (*a*); stoma (*b*); spongy parenchyma (*c*). IV. Surface view of bran coats. Epicarp (*a*); cross cells (*b*). V. Hypodermal fiber of glume. VI. Hair from epicarp. Wall (*b*); lumen (*c*). VII. Oat starch.

powder for uncoated pills to prevent them adhering to each other and, in the form of glycorite as an emollient and base for suppositories. It is also an antidote for iodine and bromine poisoning.

AVENA SATIVA N.F. (OAT)

Synonyms.—Common Oats, Cultivated Oats, Panicle Oats.

Botanical Origin.—*Avena sativa* Linné.

Part Used.—The grain.

Limit of Impurities.—5 per cent. of other seeds or of foreign organic matter.

Habitat.—Eurasia. Cultivated extensively in temperate zones of both hemispheres.

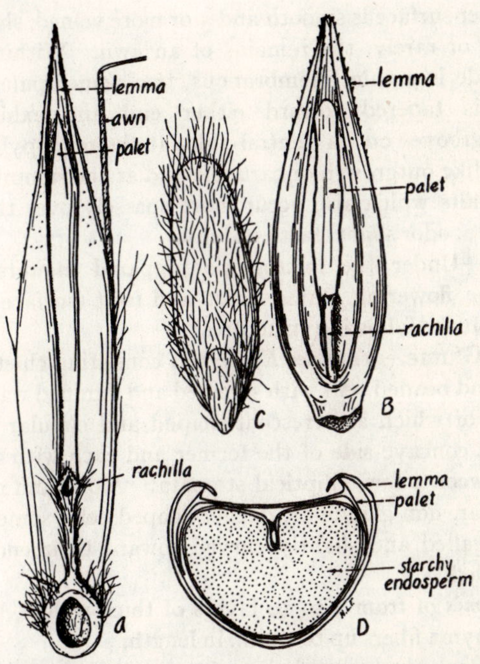

FIG. 24.—Oats. *A*, mature grain of wild oats (*Avena fatua*); *B*, mature grain of cultivated oats (*Avena sativa*); *C*, grain of same with "hull" removed; *D*, cross section of grain with the "hull." *A*, *B*, and *C*, × 5; *D*, × 10. (*After Robbins.*)

Plant.—An annual herb with a terminal spreading panicle of spikelets. The individual spikelets usually possessing 3 flowers. Subtending each spikelet are two large, membranous, empty glumes. The fruit is an elongated caryopsis (grain) tapered toward both ends.

Production and Commerce.—Oat thrives best in wet soil and a moderately cool, humid climate. It is extensively cultivated in the United States which for years has led the world in the production of this cereal. Russia, Germany, Canada, France, Austria, Great Britain, Sweeden and Argentina also produce large annual yields. The mature oat plants are mowed down and carried to the threshing floor where the grains are thrashed out, the stems with adhering glumes being separated as straw. The grains are dried on the floors of barns, cleaned and marketed in bags.

Description.—Whole oat occurs as a somewhat spindle-shaped grain up to 1.5 cm. in length and about 3 mm. broad, enveloped by chaff consisting of a larger scale or flowering glume (*lemma*) and a palet. The flowering glume surrounds the grain except on the ventral side where there is a distinct longitudinal groove showing usually a minute stalk at its base. Its outer surface is smooth and 5 or more veined, showing above the center a scar, or rarely, the remains of an awn. Within the groove on the ventral side is a thin, membranous, two veined palet. The fruit or naked grain is tapered toward either end and exhibits a distinct longitudinal groove on its ventral side, at the micropylar end of which occurs a wart-like outgrowth or caruncle and at the summit, a "beard" of long slender hairs which also occur more sparsely over the remainder of the fruit surface; odor slight; taste starchy.

Histology.—Under the microscope prepared mounts of macerated material of the flowering glume, palet and fruit (surface and transverse sections) exhibit the following structures:

Flowering Glume.—1. *Outer Epidermis* consisting chiefly of elongated wavy-walled and beaded cells with silicified and lignified walls, between the ends of many of which are crescent shaped and circular cells, the latter fitting into the concave side of the former and each with greatly silicified walls, and between a few, elliptical stomata. Along and near the margin occur unicellular, non-glandular, dagger-shaped cells, some being comparatively thick-walled and slightly curved toward their ends, others rigid and thick-walled.

2. *Hypodermis* of from 4 to 10 layers of thick-walled, lignified, taper-ended sclerenchyma fibers up to 1 mm. in length.

3. *Spongy Parenchyma* consisting of a narrow zone of somewhat star-shaped cells and large intercellular spaces.

4. *Inner Epidermis* composed of elongated, thin-walled cells and elliptical stomata.

Palet.—This portion of oat simulates closely the structure of the glume in its middle region except that the hypodermis is thinner. This region tapers off into membranous wings, in parts of which the hypodermal fibers become entirely wanting and the epidermis with entirely thin walls. Along the margins and keels of the palet are numerous stiff, sharp-pointed, straight or curved, unicellular, non-glandular hairs, while parallel to the keels are rows of elliptical stomata.

Fruit.—1. *Epicarp* of longitudinally elongated, thin-walled cells, except at apex and base where they are more or less isodiametric. From a number of these arise slender pointed, unicellular, non-glandular hairs, up to 200μ or more in length. Other layers of pericarp and the spermoderm and perisperm of collapsed or poorly defined cells.

2. *Endosperm* consisting of a outer layer of aleurone cells with thin walls, the remainder of the tissue composed of large, thin-walled, parenchyma cells filled with polygonal and spindle-shaped starch grains, the starch grains being gathered in ellipsoidal or rounded aggregates.

3. *Embryo*, forming a broad, spindle-shaped region about 2 mm. in length and found embedded in the endosperm near the micropylar end.

Powdered Drug.—Whitish. Fragments of flowering-glume and palet with characteristic tissues; fragments of epicarp with elongated, thin walled cells from a number of which arise slender pointed hairs, 200μ or more in length, about 20μ in diameter at the base, larger in the middle and with lumina up to 9μ in diameter and walls up to 8μ in thickness; fragments of endosperm with cells containing ellipsoidal or rounded, many-compound starch grains, the compound grains up to 60μ in diameter with individual grains polygonal or spindle shaped and rarely over 10μ in diameter.

Constituents.—Oats is composed of about 70 per cent. kernel and 30 per cent. chaff (husk); the kernel contains carbohydrates (67.09 per cent.), albuminoids (14.31 per cent.); fixed oil (8.14 per cent.), fiber (1.38 per cent.), ash (2.15 per cent.), water (6.93 per cent.).

Uses.—Nutrient and demulcent.

CEREALS

A number of cereals have been used in the ground condition to adulterate ground drugs and spices. The chief diagnostic peculiarities of these are indicated in the following table. See p. 94, also figs. 22 and 23.

PALMÆ (PALM FAMILY)

Tropical or sub-tropical shrubs, rarely trees, having unbranched trunks which are terminated by a crown of leaves, in the axils of which the flowers are produced. The leaves are well developed with pinnate (feather palms) or palmate blades (fan palms) and a fibrous sheathed, clasping petiole. The flowers are small, of one or two sexes, and crowded on a spike or spadix, which is subtended by a large bract or spathe which may become woody, as in the Cocoanut Palm. The perianth consists of 6 parts in 2 whorls (3 sepals and 3 petals) or it may be inconspicuous or absent. The stamens are 6 in number, rarely 3, inserted below the ovary. The ovary is superior, of 3 cells, with central placenta. The fruit is either a nut, with leathery epicarp, fibrous or cellular mesocarp and thin membranous endocarp, or a drupe (Cocoanut) with leathery epicarp, broadly fibrous mesocarp and stony endocarp, or a berry as in the Date Palm, *Phoenix*, with

	Wheat Triticum sativum	Rye Secale cereale	Barley Hordeum vulgare	Oats Avena sativa	Corn Zea mays	Rice Oryza sativa
Glumes and paleæ in whole product	Absent	Absent	Present	Present	Absent	Absent
Hairs	Up to 1 mm. long with walls thicker than the lumen.	Lumen of hairs thicker than the walls.	Conical hairs; lumen may be thicker than walls or vice versa. Less than 150μ long.	On glume, hairs are dagger-shaped, some hooked, broad base. May exceed 200μ in length on epicarp. Usually broadest in the middle.	Walls thinner than lumen. Unicellular or multicellular.	Dagger-shaped, up to 500μ in length. Hairs 40μ broad at base.
Cross cells	Cross cells with porous, radial walls. End walls are not swollen. Intercellular spaces rare.	Side walls thinner and less distinctly porous than wheat. End walls swollen or rounded. Pronounced intercellular spaces.	Two rows with non-porous walls. Inter-cellular-air-spaces between side walls and angles.	Cross cells are very thin-walled.	Spongy parenchyma takes the place of cross cells.	Either united or detached.
Aleurone layer	Layer 1-cell thick. Cells rectangular in T.S. Rounded-polygonal in surface view.	Cells are smaller and thicker walled.	2–4 rows of cells thick. In T.S., cells are square or radially extended but in surface section rounded-polygonal.	One cell thick. Thinner walled cells than in wheat, rye or barley.	Aleurone in a single layer.	Cells rounded—polygonal with extremely thin walls.
Starch	*Simple.* *Circular* grains appearing lenticular on edge view. Large grains 28–45μ. *Hilum:* central, appearing as a dot but usually indistinct. *Lamellæ:* generally indistinct; when present concentric. *Polarization:* cross indistinct; no play of colors with selenite plate.	*Simple.* Grains similar in shape to wheat starch but many are larger. Large grains 20–52μ in diameter. *Hilum:* Indistinct in, some grains, but a star-shaped central cleft in others. *Lamellæ:* concentric; often indistinct. *Polarization:* cross distinct.	*Simple.* Grains have a similar shape to those of wheat but frequently tending to bulge on one side and so appear subreniform Appear elliptical to lemon-shaped on edge view. Large grains usually 18 to 25μ and occasionally up to 30μ in length. *Hilum:* centric or circular or cleft, often indistinct. *Lamellæ:* concentric and often indistinct. *Polarization:* cross indistinct.	*Compound* or *Simple.* Grains polygonal in ellipsoidal or rounded aggregates (up to 60μ) of from 2 to many grains. Spindle-shaped forms may be present. Single grains up to 10μ in diameter.	*Simple.* Polygonal to rounded. 10–35μ in diameter, most over 15μ. *Hilum:* circular or a two- to five-rayed cleft. *Lamellæ:* indistinct. *Polarization:* cross distinct but no marked play of colors with selenite plate.	*Simple* or 2-to many compound. *Polygonal* 2–10μ in diameter. *Hilum:* usually indistinct but occasionally a central cleft. *Lamellæ:* indistinct. *Polarization:* cross distinct but no play of colors with selenite plate.

membranous epicarp, succulent mesocarp and soft succulent endocarp. The seeds are albuminous with the reserve food frequently in the form of hard cellulose, as in the date and ivory-nut-palm.

SABAL N.F. (SABAL)

Synonyms.—Saw Palmetto Berries, Dwarf Palmetto, Fan Palm.

Botanical Origin.—*Serenoa serrulata* (Michaux) Hooker filius.

Part Used.—The partially dried ripe fruit.

Purity Rubric.—It contains not more than 1 per cent. of foreign organic matter and should contain from 10 to 15 per cent. of its natural moisture when used for the manufacture of pharmaceutical preparations.

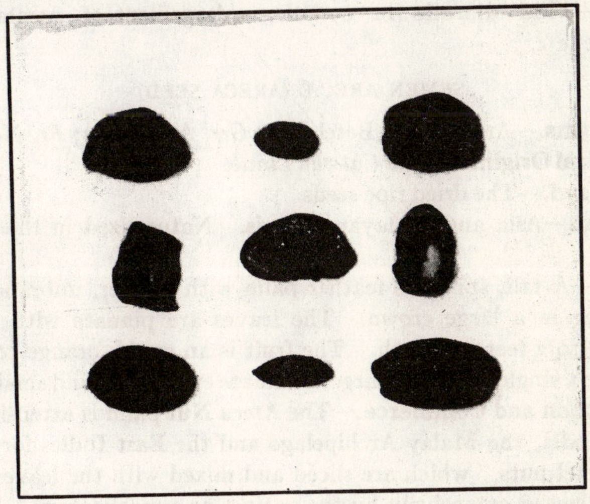

FIG. 25.—Sabal, × 1³⁄₂₀. *(Photograph by Stoneback.)*

Habitat.—In sandy soil from South Carolina to Florida, west to Arkansas and Texas.

Plant.—A fan palm, the main axis of which consists of a creeping rhizome, the anterior end of which arises a short distance from the soil and bears a dense cluster of leaves. Each leaf consists of an orbiculate blade with cleft segments and a long, stout, spiny-edged petiole. The inflorescence is a panicle. The fruit is a superior 1-seeded drupe.

Production and Commerce.—The palm thrives particularly well near the sea from South Carolina to Jupiter Inlet, Florida, where it forms in many places a dense growth stretching many miles inland. Collection of the fruit begins in August and lasts until January. The fruit is shaken into baskets and then partially dried artificially. It is then packed in barrels and preserved by adding a small quantity of alcohol to the contents thereof. The commercial supplies are obtained chiefly from the Cape Canaveral section of Florida.

Description.—A superior drupe of ellipsoidal or ovoid outline, 1.5 to 3 cm. in length and 1 to 1.5 cm. in diameter; externally brownish-black to bluish-black, smooth and somewhat oily, with a few large, more or less angular depressions, summit marked by the scar of the style, and the base either with a short stalk or stem-scar; epicarp and sarcocarp together forming a thin leathery shell, enclosing a hard, thin endocarp. The endocarp envelops an ellipsoidal or ovoid, somewhat flattened, reddish-brown seed. The odor is aromatic; the taste sweetish, aromatic, slightly acrid.

Constituents.—Volatile oil, fatty acids, resin, lipase, etc.

Uses.—Mild diuretic in cystitis, enlargement of prostate, senile impotence, etc.

SEMEN ARECÆ (ARECA SEED)

Synonyms.—Areca Nut, Betel Nut; *Ger.* Arekanuss; *Fr.* Noix d'arec.

Botanical Origin.—*Areca Catechu* Linné.

Part Used.—The dried ripe seeds.

Habitat.—Asia and Malayan Islands. Naturalized in the American tropics.

Plant.—A tall, spineless feather palm with slender, unbranched stem terminating in a large crown. The leaves are pinnate with numerous leaflets up to 2 feet in length. The fruit is an ovoid, orange colored nut containing a single seed with large, ruminate endosperm and small embryo.

Production and Commerce.—The Areca Nut palm is extensively cultivated in India, the Malay Archipelago and the East Indies for its seeds, called "Betel nuts," which are sliced and mixed with the leaves of *Piper betel* and chewed extensively by the natives as a masticatory. The seeds are separated from the fruits, usually boiled in water containing a small amount of lime and dried. They are packed in bags and shipped from Columbo, Ceylon, Padang and Penang to this country.

Description.—Seeds rounded conical, 20 to 25 mm. in length, externally grayish-brown and frequently showing portions of the silvery coat of the pericarp adherent; when cut showing a mottled surface of alternating dark brown and whitish tissues (ruminate albumen): odor slight; taste astringent and slightly bitter.

Constituents.—A colorless, oily, liquid alkaloid, arecoline, to which the vermifuge properties are attributed, the alkaloids arecaidine, guvacine, guvacoline and arecolidine; tannin and fat.

Uses.—Chiefly employed by veterinarians as a vermifuge and by orientals as a masticatory.

COCOANUT (COCONUT)

The Cocoanut palm (*Cocos nucifera* Linné), also known as the Coco palm and Cocoanut tree is the most valuable economic plant of the Palm family. While its habitat has been cited by authorities as the Cocos and Keeling Islands of the Indian Ocean, it is thought by O. F. Cook to be a native of tropical America. It is now found growing along the seacoasts of most tropical countries.

The Cocoanut is a feather palm with spineless stem, thickened at the base, that rises to 40 to 100 feet and bears a terminal crown of pinnate leaves with linear-lanceolate leaflets. The fruit is a large triangular-ovoid drupe with leathery epicarp, broad, fibrous mesocarp and stony endocarp containing a single large albuminous seed.

The most important pro 'ucts of the cocoanut fruit are the following:

Cocoanut.—The ripe fruit deprived of its husk (epicarp and mesocarp) and so consisting of the seed and stony endocarp to which a number of the mesocarp fibers usually ahere.

Copra.—The dried meat of the seed, consisting of the white, fleshy endosperm and small plug-like embryo embedded near its base. Under the microscope, sections of the endosperm show isodiametric to radially elongated cells with walls about 3 mm. thick and contents consisting of needle-shaped fat crystals and large aleurone grains. The aleurone grains possess a large phytoglobulin.

Shredded Cocoanut.—This product, also known as "dessicated cocoanut," represents the dried meat reduced to a coarse powder.

Cocoanut Oil.—(Oleum Cocois.) A fixed oil expressed from the seeds of the cocoanut. Much of the Copra of commerce is shipped to the United States and Europe where the oil is expressed. It is a white solid of the consistence of butter and is employed as a cosmetic, butter substitute and in the manufacture of soap.

Coir.—The fibers of the mesocarp of the cocoanut fruit. These are used in the manufacture of cocoanut mats, ropes and as stuffing material. Each fiber represents a fibrovascular bundle.

Cocoanut Shells.—These are obtained as a by-product in the preparation of copra and shredded cocoanut and have been used in powdered form or as charcoal to adulterate ground spices. Powdered cocoanut shells, while consisting in the main of stone cells of the endocarp, also contain tissues of the spermoderm and mesocarp. The diagnostic elements include elongated or more or less isodiametric, yellow, thick walled stone cells with branching pore canals and dark-brown contents, the latter becoming reddish-brown when treated with alkaline solutions, fragments of bast fibers with stegmata, thick walled, porous cells of the seed coat, and spiral, pitted and reticulate tracheæ.

The chief commercial source of Cocoanuts are the Philippines, Ceylon and the West Indies.

Allied Plants.—*Elæis guineensis* Jacquin, a West African palm cultivated in tropical America, yields palm oil. Palm oil which is obtained by heating the fruits with water and expressing the oil, is a fixed oil or solid fat of an orange-red color and possessing a violet odor and a bland taste when fresh. It is harder than butter, bleaches upon exposure to light or heat and rapidly becomes rancid with the development of an acrid taste. It is used in the preparation of some soaps, candles and ointments.

ARACEÆ (AROIDEÆ OR ARUM FAMILY)

Perennial herbs with colorless or milky, acrid or pungent sap and under-ground stems represented by rhizomes or corms; leaves either alternate or solitary, glabrous, with petiole sheathing at the base and usually swoolen, and the blade strongly palmately-, pedately- or peltately-nerved, cordate, or hastate, entire or variously cut. Inflorescence a spadix springing from the axil of the spathe; flowers usually imperfect, sessile and usually crowded on the spathe. Fruit a berry. Seeds with fleshy albumen or filled with a lrage fleshy embryo. Raphides of calcium oxalate are common in the group. Secretion sacs containing an aromatic oil occur in the genus *Acorus.*

CALAMUS (CALAMUS)

Synonyms.—Sweet Flag, Sweet Root, Sweet Cinnamon, Sweet Cane, Sweet or Grass Myrtle, Calamus Root, Radix Acori, Radix Calami Aromatici; *Ger.* Kalmus; *Fr.* Acore vrai.

Botanical Origin.—*Acorus Calamus* Linné.

Part Used.—The dried rhizome.

Habitat.—On the banks of swamps, streams or ponds of North America, Europe and Asia.

Plant.—A perennial herb with a horizontal, aromatic rhizome which gives rise to long sword-shaped, equitant leaves and scapes. From the upper part of each scape arises a yellowish-green spadix, from the point of insertion of which the scape is prolonged as a spathe.

Production and Commerce.—The rhizome system (usually a meter or more in length) is uprooted in the spring from the moist soil, washed, freed of roots, dried at a moderate heat and cut into segments of variable length. During drying it shrinks to about one-half its diameter and loses about 75 per cent. of its weight. In some collecting districts, notably Germany, it is peeled before being dried; but peeled rhizomes should not be employed for the manufacture of preparations, since they are deprived of a portion of the cortex containing a large number of oil cells. The commercial supplies of the drug come from Virginia, Michigan, North Carolina, Indiana, Germany, England, Russia and India. Both the peeled and unpeeled articles occur on the market.

Description.—Rhizome horizontal, in unpeeled or peeled, subcylindrical, entire or longitudinally split segments; when unpeeled, externally

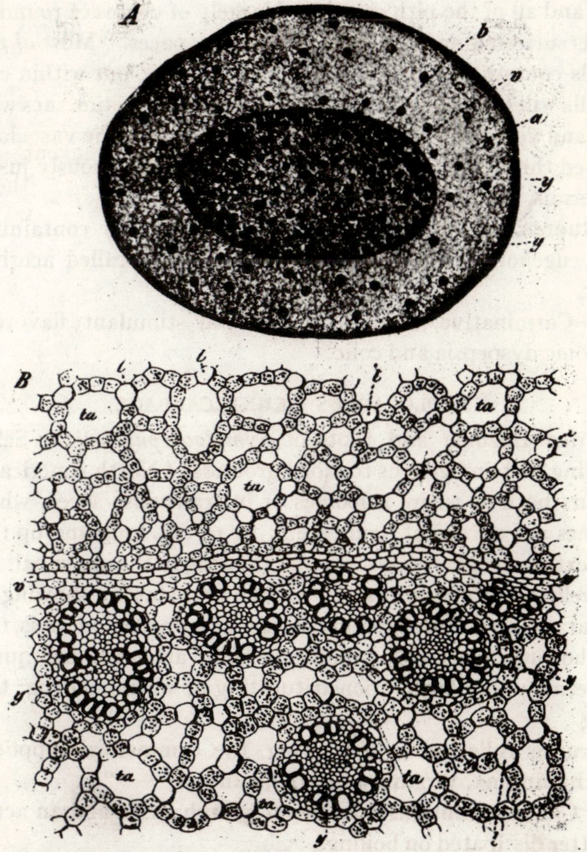

FIG. 26.—*Calamus Rhizome.* *A.* Transverse section. *B.* Portion of a transverse section in the region of the endodermis, ×65. *a*, cortex; *b*, central cylinder; *i*, starch parenchyma; *l*, secretion sacs containing volatile oil; *v*, endodermis; *ta*, intercellular-air-spaces; *y*, concentric fibrovascular bundle. (*After Berg.*)

reddish-brown (when peeled, pinkish-white), deeply wrinkled, somewhat annulate from remains of leaf sheaths, the upper surface marked with triangular leaf scars, lower surface with circular, pitted scars of rootlets arranged in irregular, zigzag lines; fracture short, sharp and corky; inner surface whitish or pinkish-white and spongy, showing an elliptical endodermis separating the outer cortex from the central cylinder, both of these regions exhibiting yellowish dots; odor aromatic; taste pungent and bitter.

Histology.—Transverse sections of the unpeeled Calamus exhibit an outer epidermis or cork beneath which is to be seen a broad cortex separated for a large central cylinder or stele by an endodermis. The outer region of the cortex consists of collenchyma cells, the inner region of the cortex and all of the pith comprised largely of chains of rounded parenchyma cells surrounding large intercellular-air-spaces. Most of the parenchyma cells contain small, spheroidal starch grains, but within each chain of these cells will be noted one or more spheroidal secretion sacs with suberized walls and yellowish volatile oil content. Concentric vascular bundles are scattered throughout the pith and occur more numerously just beneath the endodermis, where they appear crowded.

Constituents.—Volatile oil (1.5 to 3.5 per cent.) containing asaryl aldehyde, eugenol and asarone; a bitter glucoside called acorin, starch, tannin, etc.

Uses.—Carminative, aromatic bitter and stimulant; flavoring agent. Used in atonic dyspepsia and colic.

SYMPLOCARPUS (SKUNK CABBAGE)

The dried rhizome and roots of *Symplocarpus fœtidus* Salisbury, a fetid smelling herb indigenous to moist grounds of North America.

It occurs both as entire rhizomes or in transverse slices; when entire, the rhizomes are obconical, truncate, 5 to 10 cm. long and up to 4 cm. in diameter, externally grayish-brown and showing in the upper half numerous long, shrivelled rootlets; internally whitish and starchy showing a narrow cortex separated from a broad central cylinder by an endodermis, the central cylinder showing scattered bundles which are crowded just within the endodermis; odor fetid, upon triturating or warming drug; taste acrid and biting.

The drug is collected in the spring, the commercial supplies coming from North Carolina, Virginia and Michigan.

Skunk Cabbage contains volatile oil, starch, resin and an acrid principle, the latter dissipated on boiling.

It is employed in the form of a recent powder or infusion as an antispasmodic, emetic and diuretic; in asthma, chronic rheumatism, catarrh, dropsy and hysteria.

ARUM (INDIAN TURNIP)

The corm of *Arisæma triphyllum* (L.) Schott, commonly known as Jack-in-the-pulpit, an acaulescent herb indigenous to moist, shady woods of North America. It is gathered in the late spring.

It occurs as a depressed, globular corm from 2 to 5 cm. broad, externally covered with a wrinkled, brown cork and showing near the summit a whorl of numerous coarse rootlets; internally white, solid and mealy with scattered bundles.

It contains numerous long raphides of calcium oxalate, starch, mucilage, fat and an acrid volatile substance.

Indian Turnip has been used as a stimulant to the secretion in asthma, chronic catarrh and rheumatism.

LILIACEÆ (LILY FAMILY)

Herbs (*Lilium*), shrubs (*Yucca*), or trees (*Dracena Draco*), with regular and symmetrical almost always six-androus flowers. Stem either short, creeping, underground (*Polygonatum*), or swelling up and forming bulbs (Hyacinth), or corms (*Colchicum*) or stem may elongate above ground and become wiry and herbaceous or semi-shrubby as *Smilax*, or the stem may remain short giving rise to thick fleshy and sap-storing leaves as in *Aloe*. Leaves linear to lanceolate or ovate, rarely wider, divisible into sheathing base, narrow petiole and expanded blade. Venation, parallel, becoming in some ovate leaves parallel with oblique connections, reticulate or highly reticulate, as in *Smilax*, etc. The perianth is parted into six segments, the calyx and corolla being alike in color. Anthers introrse. Ovary three-locular with a single style. Fruit a three-locular, loculicidally dehiscent capsule (*Lilium*, etc.) or rarely a berry (*Asparagus*, etc.). Seeds usually numerous, albuminous. Many of the plants contain raphides of calcium oxalate.

SCILLA U.S.P. (SQUILL)

Synonyms.—Sea Onion, Squills, White Squills; *Fr.* Scille; *Ger.* Meerzwiebel.

Botanical Origin.—White variety of *Urginea maritima* (Linné) Baker.

Part Used.—The cut and dried fleshy inner scales of bulb.

Standard of Assay.—When squill in the form of the tincture is properly diluted and injected into the ventral lymph sac of a frog, it has a minimum systolic dose (minimum dose producing in one hour a stoppage of the ventricle of the heart in systole) of not more than 0.006 cc. of tincture, equivalent to 0.00,000,05 gm. of ouabain, for each gram of body weight of frog.

Habitat.—Mediterranean basin, in sandy and hilly localities.

Plant.—A perennial herb whose underground portion consists of a pear-shaped, tunicated bulb, bearing fibrous roots from its base and whose aerial parts consist of a succulent stem bearing a dense raceme of white flowers, in autumn, followed, in the spring, by a rosette of lance-ovate, deep green leaves. The fruit is an oblong, 3-lobed capsule, producing in each cell 6 purplish-brown, flattened seeds.

Production and Commerce.—Two varieties of Squill occur on the market, the white and red. The former has white scales, the latter, reddish-brown and rose colored; the white variety is preferred and is alone official in the U.S.P., since it imparts little color to preparations. The bulbs, which grow only half immersed in the sandy soil, near the sea, are collected in August, deprived of their dry, membranous outer scales, cut transversely into slices, sun-dried, and packed in casks for shipment. It has been found to absorb, in its dried condition, as much as 11 per cent. of moisture and, since it is apt to become moldy, should be kept in well-stoppered bottles. The commercial supplies are imported from Leghorn and Palermo, Italy. A small quantity of Red Squill is imported for use as rat poison.

Description.—It occurs on the market as irregular, more or less curved, flattened pieces of fleshy scales, from 0.5 to 5 cm. long, yellowish-white, somewhat translucent; brittle when dry, tough and somewhat flexible when damp; odor slight; taste mucilaginous, bitter, and acrid.

Microscopical Characteristics.—Epidermis of thin-walled cells and stomata; mesophyll of slightly elongated, thin-walled cells, many of which contain spheroidal aggregates of a sugar, when examined in alcohol or glycerin mounts. Scattered through the mesophyll are a few concentric fibrovascular bundles, with spiral and reticulate tracheæ and numerous elongated mucilage sacs containing raphides of calcium oxalate. These raphides may attain the length of 1 mm. and serve as the most important diagnostic character of the drug.

Powdered Drug.—Light-yellow to light yellowish-brown tending to cake in a moist atmosphere, and showing, under the microscope, fragments of thin-walled parenchyma, a few spiral and reticulate vessels, numerous acicular cystals and bundles of these in the form of long raphides.

Constituents.—The glucosides, scillin, scillain, scillipicrin and scillitoxin, mucilage (sinistrin), calcium oxalate, a trace of volatile oil, and sugar.

Uses.—Stimulating expectorant, cardiac stimulant and diuretic.

Substitutes.—Bulbs of several *Crinum* species growing in China, East Indies and Brazil.

ALLIUM N.F. (GARLIC)

Synonyms.—English Garlic: *Ger.* Gartenlauch, Knoblauch; *Fr.* Ail.

Botanical Origin.—*Allium sativum* Linné.

Part Used.—The fresh bulb.

Habitat.—Southern Europe. Naturalized and cultivated in the United States.

Plant.—A perennial, strong smelling, bulbous herb. Its underground portion consists of a compound bulb with numerous fibrous rootlets. The bulb gives rise above ground to a number of narrow, keeled, grass-like leaves and a stem which rises about a foot and terminates in a simple umbel of purple flowers. The flowers are later replaced by small bulbels.

Description.—Garlic occurs as a subglobular, compound bulb composed of from 8 to 15 or more bulblets envelcped by whitish, membranous scales which are attached to a short woody stem, the latter bearing on its under surface many yellowish-white rootlets; bulblets ovoid and 3 to 4 sided with an outer convex surface, each covered with a whitish scale leaf which encloses a thick, whitish fleshy scale within which are 1 to 2 translucent scales and, in the center, 2 or 3 yellowish to yellowish-green foliage leaves, the latter folded together lengthwise; odor, when bruised, strongly alliaceous; taste persistently pungent.

The dry membranous scales, rootlets and shrivelled leaf remnants should be removed before the drug is used in the manufacture of pharmaceutical preparations.

Constituents.—Up to 0.9 per cent. of volatile oil containing diallyl disulphide and allylpropyl disulphide; the glucoside, allin, which is hydrolyzed by the enzyme, allisin, to form volatile oil and fructose.

Uses.—Garlic is chiefly used in the form of the syrup as a diaphoretic, diuretic and expectorant. It is also employed as a poultice in bronchitis and as a seasoning agent.

VERATRUM VIRIDE U.S.P. (VERATRUM VIRIDE)

Synonyms.—American Hellebore, Green Hellebore, Swamp Hellebore, Indian Poke. *Ger.* Grüner Germer; *Fr.* Vératre vert.

Botanical Origin.—*Veratrum viride* Aiton.

Parts Used.—The dried rhizome and roots.

Limit of Impurities.—5 per cent. of its stems or other foreign matter and 4 per cent. of acid-insoluble ash.

Habitat.—In rich, wet woods, moist meadows, and swamps of Eastern and Central United States.

Plant.—A perennial herb with a stout stem 6–24 dm. high, bearing oblong-ovate, acuminate, sheathing, prominently veined leaves below, and terminating in a panicle of dense spike-like racemes of yellowish-green flowers. The fruit is a 3-celled, many-seeded capsule.

Commercial.—The rhizome and roots are dug in early summer, washed, usually cut into 2 to 4 longitudinal pieces and carefully dried. The chief source of supply of this drug is Michigan, Illinois, North Carolina and Virginia.

Description.—Rhizome erect, obconical, generally in the form of longitudinal slices from 2 to 7 cm. in length and from 1.4 to 3 cm. in diameter, externally varying from light brown to dark brown, often crowned with closely arranged leaf bases, somewhat annulate from scars of bud scales and bearing along the outer surface numerous light brown to yellowish-brown, deeply transversely wrinkled rootlets; fracture of rhizome hard and horny; internally grayish-white, showing numerous scattered fibrovascular bundles; fracture of roots, short, exhibiting a whitish interior; without odor but sternutatory; taste bitter and acrid.

Histology.—Transverse sections of the **rhizome** exhibit the following structures, passing from periphery toward the center:

1. *Epidermis* of brown-walled cells.

2. *Cortex*, a moderately broad zone composed of a matrix of parenchyma, the cells of which are rounded, more or less isodiametric and pitted. Most of the cells contain spherical or ellipsoidal, single or 2- to 3-compound starch grains, a few raphides of calcium oxalate, up to 150μ in length. Coursing outward through this region will be noted occasional fascicular bundles on their way to the rootlets.

3. *Endodermis*, a somewhat wavy layer of somewhat lignified cells, becoming 2 layered in parts, the inner and radial walls being more thickened than the outer wall, the U-shaped lumen being about one-half the width of the cell.

4. *Stele*, a broad parenchyma zone with cells resembling those of the cortex and showing fibro-vascular bundles arranged in irregular interrupted circles or scattered.

Transverse sections of the **root** present the following structure:

1. *Epidermis* of more or less quadrangular cells with lignified and thickened outer and radial walls.

2. *Hypodermis* of a layer of more or less compressed cells, beneath which are two to three layers of collenchyma.

3. *Aerenchyma*, consisting of air-spaces surrounded by parenchyma cells.

4. *Cortical parenchyma*, a broad zone of spherical cells which become gradually smaller toward the central cylinder. Most of the cells contain spherical or ellipsoidal, single or 2- to 3-compound starch grains, a number contain raphides of calcium oxalate.

5. *Endodermis*, consisting of a layer of endodermal cells with slightly lignified inner and radial walls and with U-shaped lumen about one-third to one-half the cell width.

6. *Pericambium* of a layer or two of meristematic cells.

7. *Radial Fibrovascular Bundle* of many alternating xylem and phloem patches.

8. Pith, a small central zone of starch and calcium oxalate containing parenchyma.

Powdered Drug.—The powder varies in color from grayish-brown to dark brown. It is strongly sternutatory. When examined under the microscope the following histological elements are exhibited: Raphides of calcium oxalate from 15μ to 150μ in length; numerous spheroidal or ellipsoidal starch grains from 3μ to 20μ in diameter, single or 2- to 3-compound; fragments of scalariform and reticulate tracheæ often adherent to

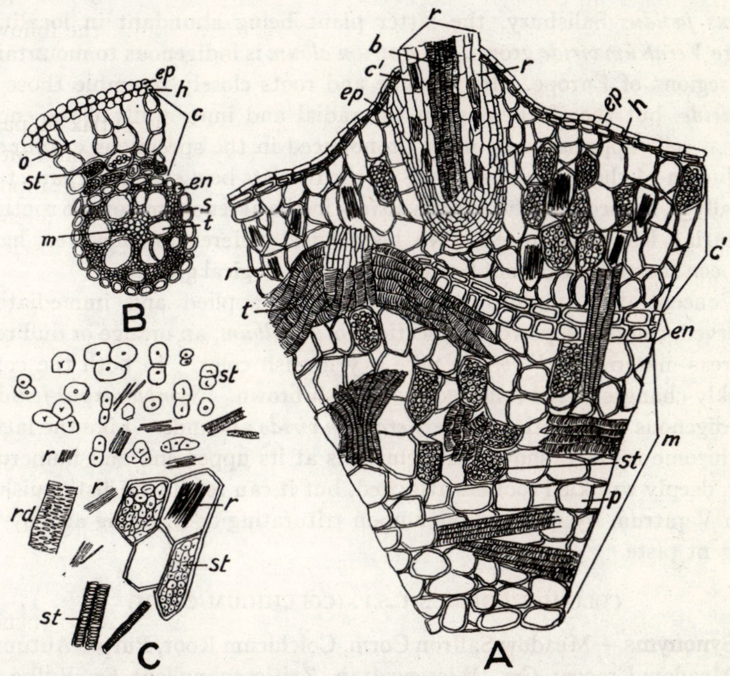

FIG. 27.—*Veratrum Viride*. *A*. Rhizome as observed in cross-section showing outgrowth of lateral rootlet (*r*); epidermis (*ep*); hypodermis (*h*); cortex (*c*); endodermis (*en*); pith (*m*); bundle of root (*b*); raphides in cells (*r*); starch (*st*); parenchyma (*p*); and tracheæ (*t*). *B*. Root as observed in cross-section showing epidermis (*ep*); hypodermis (*h*); oxygen chamber (*o*); starch parenchyma (*st*); endodermis (*en*); pith (*m*); sieve tissue (*s*) and tracheæ (*t*) of a radial fibrovascular bundle. *C*. Elements of powdered drug. Starch grains (*st*); raphides of calcium oxalate (*r*); reticulate duct (*rd*); and spiral ducts (*st* at lower left).

sclerenchyma fibers; fragments of reddish-brown to brownish-black suberous tissue, and many parenchyma cells or the walls thereof.

Constituents.—The alkaloids protoveratrine, jervine, pseudojervine, rubijervine and probably cevadine; jervic acid, resin, fat, gum, and starch.

Uses.—Cardiac, respiratory and vaso-motor depressant; the powdered drug is used as an insecticide.

Substitutes.—The rhizome and roots of *Helleborus niger* (Fam. *Ranunculaceæ*) have appeared on the market under the label "American Hellebore." This drug is a powerful cardiac stimulant, having a therapeutic action just opposite to that of Veratrum Viride. It can be readily detected by the grayish-black, knotty, external appearance of the rhizome, its dicotyledonous internal structure and its absence of raphides of calcium oxalate.

Adulterants.—Rhizomes and roots of European or White Hellebore, *Veratrum album* Linné; rhizomes and roots of Skunk Cabbage, *Symplocarpus fœtidus* Salisbury, the latter plant being abundant in localities where *Veratrum viride* grows. *Veratrum album* is indigenous to mountainous regions of Europe. Its rhizome and roots closely resemble those of *V. viride,* but the thickening on the radial and inner walls of the endodermal cells appears to be more pronounced in the specimens examined, the lumen of the endodermal cells of the rootlets being usually characteristically V-shaped and the oxygen spaces in the aerenchyma of the rootlets appearing less pronounced. No histological differences, however, have yet been shown that cannot be explained on ecological grounds.

Concentrated sulphuric acid, when first applied and immediately observed, colors the powder or sections of *V. album*, an orange or dull red, whereas material of *V. viride* take a yellowish color. In both the color quickly changes to red followed by reddish-brown. *Symplocarpus fœtidus* is indigenous to localities where *Veratrum viride* abounds. Like the latter its rhizome is erect, shows leaf remnants at its upper end and numerous long, deeply wrinkled rootlets attached, but it can readily be distinguished from Veratrum by its fetid odor upon triturating or warming and by its pungent taste.

COLCHICI CORMUS U.S.P. (COLCHICUM CORM)

Synonyms.—Meadow Saffron Corm, Colchicum Root, Purple-Autumn- or Meadow-Crocus; *Ger.* Wiesensafran, Zeitlosenknollen; *Fr.* Bulbe de Colchique.

Botanical Origin.—*Colchicum autumnale* L.

Part Used.—The dried corm.

Standard of Assay.—Not less than 0.35 per cent. of colchicine.

Habitat.—In meadows and pastures of Central and Southern Europe and Northern Africa.

Plant.—A perennial herb with a habit somewhat like the Tulip. The underground portion consists of an ovoid corm which is convex on one side and somewhat flattened with a groove on the other side. From this there first arises, in autumn of the first year, two to six, long tubed, lilac-purple flowers, the peduncles and lower portion of corolla tubes being surrounded by a spathe. In the spring of the second year there arise 3–5 dark green, long, lance-ovate shaped leaves and a 3-valved capsule containing many subglobular, small brownish seeds. A new corm is formed each year on the lateral inferior surface of the old one.

Production and Commerce.—The year-old corms have been found to contain the maximum amount of colchicine (active principle). These are dug up before the flowering of the plant, which varies in different latitudes from July to the end of October. The outer brown membranes and rootlets are removed and the corms usually sliced transversely and dried

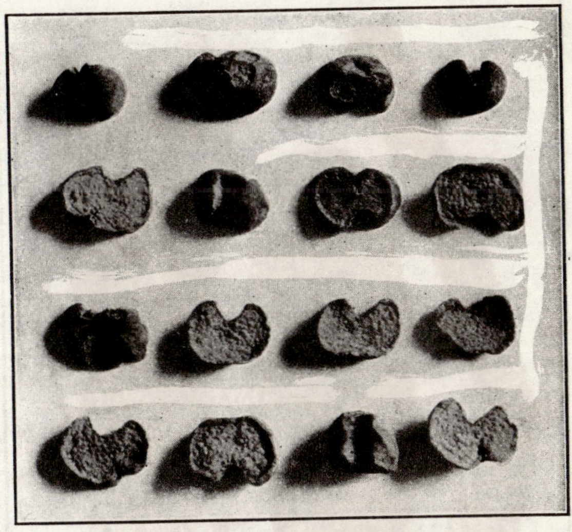

FIG. 28.—Colchicum Corm. Note the prevailing reniform slices of the corm. The groove, shown in both transverse and longitudinal view, is formed by the growing stem. × 2/3.

by the sun or in ovens. Most of the supply comes in bags from Leghorn, Italy, Trieste, Hamburg, Germany and Amsterdam, Holland.

Description.—In transverse and longitudinal slices, the transverse slices being reniform in shape, the longitudinal, ovate; from 2–5 mm. in thickness; flat surfaces whitish and of a crystalline appearance under a simple microscope; epidermis thin, light brown and wrinkled; fracture short and mealy; odor indistinct; taste starchy, bitter and acrid.

Powdered Drug.—Grayish brown to light-brown. Starch grains single or 2–6 compound; the individual grains spherical or polygonal and exhibiting a triangular or stellate central hilum; fragments of epidermis with thin, reddish-brown walls; tracheæ few with spiral or scalariform markings. Concentrated sulphuric acid colors the powder reddish-yellow.

Constituents.—The alkaloid colchicine ($C_{22}H_{25}NO_6$) 0.5 to 0.6 per cent.; starch. Colchicine is itself official in the U.S.P.

Uses.—Antirheumatic in acute gout and rheumatism.

COLCHICI SEMEN U.S.P. (COLCHICUM SEED)

Synonyms.—Meadow Saffron Seed; *Ger.* Zeitlosensamen; *Fr.* Semences de Colchique.

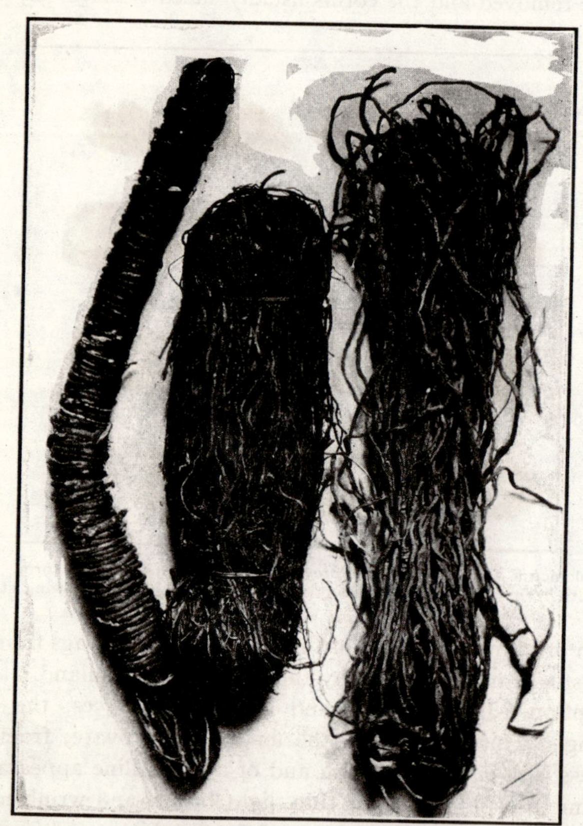

FIG. 29.—Mexican Sarsaparilla (to right); Jamaica Sarsaparilla (in center); Honduras Sarsaparilla (to left).

Botanical Origin.—*Colchicum autumnale* L.

Part Used.—The dried ripe seed.

Standard of Assay.—Not less than 0.45 per cent. of colchicine.

Commercial.—The seeds are collected from the capsules in late summer or early autumn and should be carefully dried. Recent supplies have been imported in a moist condition. They are shipped to this country from Holland, Germany, Italy and Trieste.

Description.—Seeds albuminous, ovoid or irregularly globular, somewhat beaked; from 2 to 3 mm. in diameter; externally dark brown, finely pitted; of almost bony hardness; internally grayish or light brown; odorless; taste bitter and acrid.

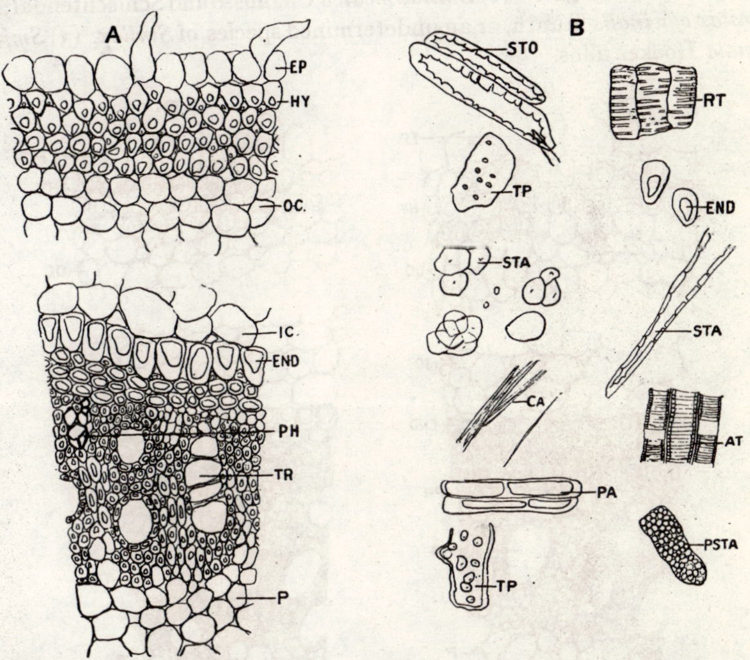

Fig. 30.—Mexican Sarsaparilla. A. Transverse section, showing epidermis and 2 root hairs (*ep*); hypodermis (*hy*); outer cortex (*oc*); inner cortex (*ic*); endodermis with radial and inner walls thicker than outer walls (*end*); phloem (*ph*); tracheæ (*tr*) and pith (*p*). B. Powdered Sarsaparilla. Reticulate tracheæ (*rt*); fragment of trachea with simple pores (*tp*); stone cells from stem (*sto*); sclerenchyma fiber (*sta* on right); starch (*sta* on left); raphide of calcium oxalate (*ca*); parenchyma cell with starch content (*psta*); annular tracheæ (*at*); endodermal cells (*end*); parenchyma (*pa*).

Microscopical Characteristics.—Transverse sections show a spermoderm of several layers of somewhat collapsed cells with thin, reddish-brown walls; the endosperm taking up most of the room within the seed coat and consisting of thick-walled, porous reserve parenchyma cells which contain oil globules and aleurone grains, the latter varying from 3 to 15μ; in diameter; a small embryo embedded in the endosperm. The beak or caruncle of the seed, when sectioned, shows parenchyma cells containing numerous ovoid, ellipsoidal or polygonal starch grains from 5μ to 20μ in diameter.

Constituents.—Colchicine (U.S.P.) 0.4 to 0.6 per cent., colchicoresin, tannin, fixed oil, starch, etc.

Uses.—Antirheumatic in rheumatic and gouty affections.

SARSAPARILLA U.S.P. (SARSAPARILLA)

Botanical Origin.—(1) *Smilax medica* Chamisso and Schlechtendal; (2) *Smilax officinalis* Kunth, or an undetermined species of *Smilax;* (3) *Smilax ornata* Hooker filius.

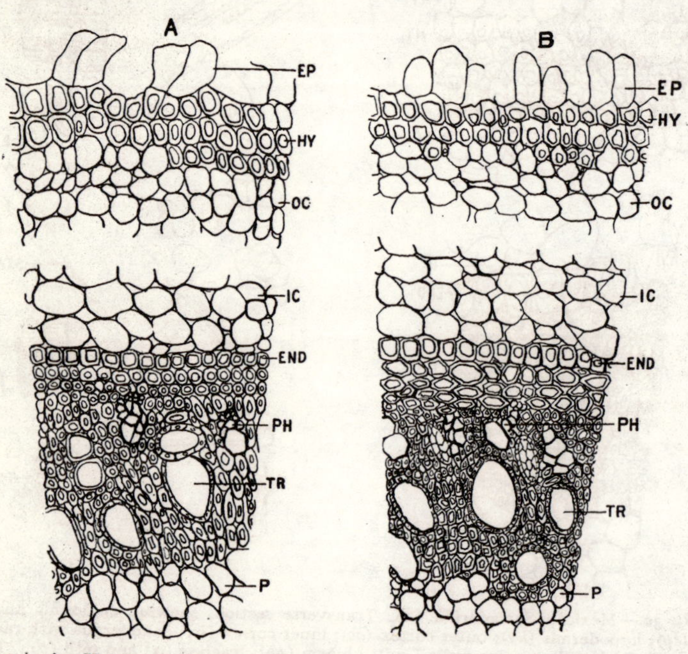

FIG. 31.—A, Honduras Sarsaparilla. Transverse section of root. Epidermis (*ep*); hypodermis (*hy*); outer cortex (*oc*); inner cortex (*ic*); endodermis (*end*); phloem (*ph*); trachea of xylem (*tr*) flanked by thick-walled wood fibers; pith (*p*). *B.* Native Jamaica Sarsaparilla. Transverse section of root. Epidermis (*ep*); hypodermis (*hy*); outer cortex (*oc*); inner cortex (*ic*); endodermis (*end*); phloem (*ph*); trachea of xylem (*tr*); pith (*p*).

Synonyms.—(1) Mexican, Vera Cruz, Tampico or Gray Sarsaparilla; (2) Honduras or Brown Sarsaparilla; (3) Central American, Jamaica, Costa Rica, Lima or Red Sarsaparilla; *Ger.* Sarsaparilla; *Fr.* Salsepareille.

Part Used.—The dried root.

Purity Rubric.—It contains not more than 2 per cent. of foreign organic matter, excepting the rhizome and crown, which must be removed before the root is ground and powdered. The Mexican variety yields not more than 4 per cent. of acid-insoluble ash, the other official varieties yield not more than 2 per cent. of their weight of acid-insoluble ash.

Plants.—Climbing evergreen shrubs with prickly stems. The leaves are alternate, coriaceous, ovate-oblong, 3-nerved and reticulate in venation, with a cordate base and stipules modified as tendrils. The flowers occur in axillary clusters. The fruit is a small, globular berry.

Commercial.—There are three commercial varieties of Sarsaparilla on the American market, namely: Mexican, Honduras, and Central American or Jamaica.

Distinctions Between the Official Sarsaparillas

Mexican	Honduras	Central American
Occurrence: Clusters of long roots attached to a crown with stem bases or stems.	Clusters of long folded roots compactly bound together with roots of same plant to within a short distance of end of cylindrical bundle.	Folded roots loosely bound together with roots of same plant into somewhat flattened bundles.
Color (externally): Grayish-brown to dark brown.	Reddish-brown to dark brown.	Yellowish- or reddish-brown.
External markings: Longitudinally furrowed, the furrows containing more or less of a blackish earth.	Longitudinally furrowed, the furrows usually free from earth.	Longitudinally wrinkled more or less furrowed and bearing numerous coarse fibrous rootlets.
Fracture: Brittle in cortex, tough, fibrous in central cylinder portion.	Short in cortex, sometimes tough and fibrous in central cylinder.	Short, or tough and fibrous in central cylinder.
Internal characteristics: The cortex is light brown, and whitish or brownish and horny. The central cylinder is porous and brownish-yellow. The pith is grayish and starchy.	The cortex is reddish-brown, dark brown or grayish-white and starchy. The central is light yellow and porous. The pith is grayish-white and starchy.	The cortex is light brown and non-mealy. The central cylinder is brownish-yellow and porous. The pith is grayish-white and starchy.
The outer and radial walls of the hypodermal cells are more thickened than the inner walls.	The cell walls of the hypodermis are almost uniformly thickened.	The walls of the hypodermal cells are almost uniformly thickened.
The inner and radial walls of the endodermal cells are more thickened than the outer walls.	The walls of the endodermal cells are nearly uniformly thickened.	The walls of the endodermal cells are nearly uniformly thickened.
Taste: Mucilaginous, somewhat sweetish and acrid.	*Taste:* Mucilaginous, starchy and slightly acrid.	*Taste:* Somewhat sweet, slightly mucilaginous, and slightly bitter.

Mexican Sarsaparilla is exported to this country either as rhizomes and roots or as roots, only, from Tampico, Mexico City and Vera Cruz. It is frequently imported in large bales bound with wire. Honduras Sarsaparilla is shipped from Puerto Cortez and Santa Barbara, British Honduras, packed in burlap, with the ends protected by green hides which are sewed on to the end of the package. Each package contains a number of cylindrical rolls bound firmy and closely around with roots of the same plant. Central American or Jamaica Sarsaparilla is imported from Costa Rica through Panama in bales. This variety should not be confused with the Native Jamaica Sarsaparilla which is cultivated on the island of Jamaica and whose endodermal and hypodermal cells show thickenings very similar to the Mexican variety.

Powdered Drug.—Light to dark grayish-brown. Starch grains from 3μ to 24μ in diameter, spheroidal, biconvex or spherical-tetrahedral, single, or 2–4 compound, frequently exhibiting a central cleft. Calcium oxalate in raphides up to 150μ in length. Hypodermal and endodermal cells with lemon-yellow or reddish-yellow porous walls and in the case of Mexican Sarsaparilla showing a distinctly irregular thickening; fragments of vessels with simple and bordered pores or scalariform or reticulate thickenings associated with sclerenchyma fibers possessing thin, slightly lignified and porous walls.

Constituents.—The glucoside sarsasaponin; parillin, smilacin, starch, resin, calcium oxalate, etc.

Uses.—As an alterative in syphilis, rheumatism and other blood diseases usually in combination with potassium iodide and other ingredients.

Adulterants and Substitutes.—(1) Rhizomes of tropical species of *Pteris;* (2) roots of a *Philodendron;* (3) rhizomes and aerial stems of same plant.

ALOE U.S.P. (ALOES)

Botanical Origin.—*Aloe Perryi* Baker, *Aloe vera* Linné and *Aloe ferox* Miller.

Synonyms.—(1) Socotrine Aloes; (2) Curaçao Aloes, Bitter Aloes, (3) Cape Aloes, Great Hedge Hog Aloes, *Ger.* Aloë; *Fr.* Aloes.

Part Used.—The inspissated juice of the leaves.

Purity Rubric.—Aloe yields not more than 4 per cent. of ash, not more than 10 per cent. of moisture, and not less than 50 per cent. of water-soluble extractive.

Habitat.—Africa.

Plants.—*Aloe Perryi* which yields Socotrine Aloe, is a perennial herb indigenous to Socotra. Its underground portion consists of an extensive fascicled root system. Its aerial portion comprises a trunk, rosette of thick succulent leaves and a raceme of flowers. As observed by Baker, the trunk attains a length of a foot and a diameter of 1½ to 2 inches. The succulent, lanceolate leaves are 12 to 20 in number and form a dense rosette at the summit of the trunk. They are pale green, becoming later frequently reddish, somewhat striate but not mottled. They attain a length of 15 in. and a breadth of 3 inches at the base, from which they taper gradually to an acuminate apex. They are channeled on their upper surface and exhibit small, deltoid, brown-tipped, marginal spines about a quarter of an inch apart. From the center of the leafy rosette there arises a raceme 1½ to 2 feet long. The peduncle portion of this is purplish, the pedicels red. The flowers which are borne upon the pedicels are tubular. They exhibit

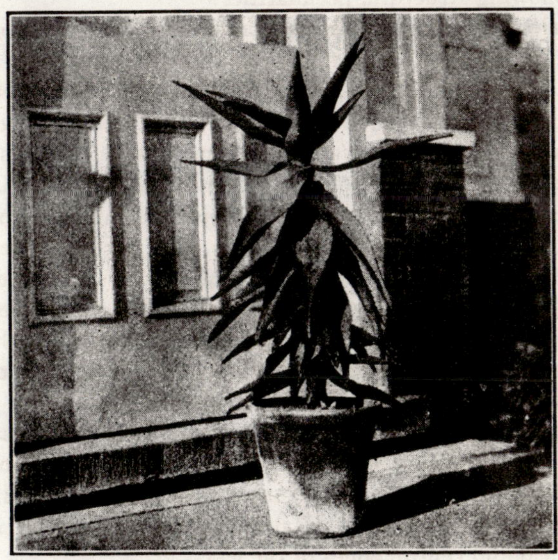

Fig. 32.—An Aloe plant.

a cylindrical perianth of a brilliant red color with a green tip in their early stage, turning yellow upon maturity. The stamens are unequal. Both stamens and style are slightly exserted. The fruit is a membranous capsule.

Aloe vera, the source of Curaçao Aloe, somewhat resembles in habit the preceding species. Its leaves are long and narrow, with repand and spiny margin, about 2 inches in thickness, 4 inches broad at the base and 12 to 20 inches long, when full grown. In color they are pea-green and when young are spotted with white. Its bright yellow tubular flowers are arranged along a slender loose spike. The stamens frequently project beyond the perianth tube.

Aloe ferox which yields Cape Aloe, is the loftiest of the whole genus. It sometimes attains a height of nearly 20 feet, the trunk below the rosette of leaves having been observed up to 3 feet long. The leaves are lanceolate, glaucous, becoming reddish and produce spines from every part, but stouter, longer, sharper and more curved ones are produced along the purplish margins and in a line along the middle of both the ventral and dorsal surfaces. The greenish-yellow to whitish flowers are tubular and borne upon a paniculate inflorescence.

Histology of the Leaves.—The leaves of all species of the genus *Aloe* are of the succulent, xerophytic, centric type. Either of the plants furnishing the official drug has leaves which, when examined microscopically, exhibit the following structural peculiarities:

A covering layer or epidermis containing scattered stomata, each surrounded in *Aloe ferox* by four neighboring cells. The outer walls of the epidermal cells are strongly cutinized. Beneath the epidermis is the mesophyll which is differentiated into an outer cortical and an inner central zone. The outer cortical zone comprises several layers of chlorenchyma cells containing chloroplasts; the inner (central) zone is composed of large, clear, thinner walled cells with abundant mucilage content.

On the border of the clear central and outer cortical zones are to be noted fibrovascular bundles arranged in the form of an ellipse. Each of these is accompanied by a number of long, tubular, thin-walled cells containing a bitter juice which, when inspissated, constitutes the drug. I have observed cells in the bundles of a large number of sections, the contents of which took on a red coloration, when a 5 per cent. solution of potassium hydroxide was applied. This would seem to indicate that the bitter juice containing anthraquinone derivatives is found not only in the cells accompanying the bundles, as previously recorded, but in certain cells of the bundles themselves.[1] Raphides of calcium oxalate are present in both cortical and central zones of the leaf.

Production and Commerce.—In the preparation of the drug, although the leaves of aloe-yielding plants are cut from nine, ten or twelve month old plants, they are not usually in the best of shape until the second or third year. When the soil is properly manured the plants have, in many instances, been found productive for ten or twelve years.

In March or early April workers go out into the aloe fields. Each begins by grasping a bunch of blades and cutting them off at their bases. In the Dutch West Indies they are then quickly placed, cut end downward, in a V-shaped trough several feet long and a foot or more thick. This is then arranged on an incline, so that the juice, in trickling from the leaves, runs down the sides of the trough and through an aperture at its lower end into a receptacle placed beneath. When the receptacle is filled with juice, the latter is poured into a cask and evaporated spontaneously or

[1] Youngken, H. W., "The Pharmacognosy of Aloes," *Pharm. Era*, p. 120, May, 1918.

reserved for later evaporation with the aid of heat. The latter process is accomplished by bringing the juice to a boil in copper vessels. As soon as the juice has thickened to a sufficient degree, it is poured into large gourd shells or boxes and allowed to harden.

An inferior method sometimes employed is that of expressing the juice from the leaves, afterwards boiling it with water, evaporating and pouring into gourds. The resulting product is usually known as the "common" or "ground" aloes.

In Cape Colony the worker prepares a hollow in the ground and spreads therein a goat skin. He then cuts off the aloe leaves and arranges them, cut surface inward, around the margin of the excavation until there are several radial series of leaves. The skin, upon being nearly filled with the juice from the leaves, is lifted from the ground, its contents emptied into a cast-iron pot and boiled until the proper consistency has been reached. It is then poured into the shells of squirting cucumbers or more usually into casks or barrels and allowed to harden.

In Zanzibar the juice, after being collected and boiled to the proper point, is poured into skins which are sewed up subsequent to its introduction.

At the present time the Socotrine Aloes is produced largely in Zanzibar, and is usually shipped in casks, kegs or skins to Europe, thence to the United States. Socotrine aloes is usually very wet, when imported, containing up to 20 per cent. or more of moisture. The Curaçao or West Indian Aloes, produced on the islands of Curacao, Bonaire and Aruba of the Dutch West Indies, is shipped direct to the United States. Most of the aloes which was received by the United States within recent years was this commercial variety. Cape Aloes, produced in Cape Colony, is shipped from Mossel Bay and Port Elizabeth to Cape Town and thence exported to Europe and the United States.

Description.—Socotrine aloes is found in the form of yellowish-brown to blackish-brown, opaque masses, sometimes soft. It is readily broken into pieces with a somewhat conchoidal fracture and sharp edges. Its odor when recent is disagreeable, but upon ageing it develops an odor resembling a mixture of saffron and myrrh. Its taste is nauseous and bitter.

Curaçao, or West Indian aloes, occurs in orange to blackish-brown opaque masses. Its fracture is irregular, exhibiting an uneven, waxy, sometimes resinous surface. Its odor is characteristic and its taste bitter and nauseous.

Cape aloes comes into the market in olive-black or reddish-brown masses frequently covered with a yellowish powder. Its fracture is sharp, exhibiting pieces with a smooth and vitreous broken surface. It has a distinct sour odor and bitter taste.

There occur on the market, in addition to the official commercial varieties described, certain sub-varieties of each of the official grades known as "hepatic or livery varieties." These are all opaque, darker in color, and obtained by allowing a partial fermentation of the juice to take place and then slowly evaporating it in the sun.

Zanzibar aloes is the hepatic (liver-colored) variety of Socotrine aloes. It is dark brown in color and has an opaque waxy fracture.

Barbadoes aloes is the hepatic variety of Curaçao aloes and occurs in deep chocolate brown, opaque, brittle masses.

Uganda or Crown aloes is the hepatic variety of Cape aloes. It comes into the market in the form of reddish-brown masses, which are more or less opaque.

Powdered Drug.—Powdered Socotrine Aloes is yellowish- to dark-brown. When mounted in a fixed oil and examined microscopically, it exhibits numerous reddish-brown to yellowish-brown, irregular fragments. When treated with nitric acid on a white surface, it forms a yellowish-brown to reddish-brown solution.

Powdered Zanzibar Aloes is reddish-yellow and when treated with nitric acid forms a yellowish-brown to reddish-brown solution.

Powdered Curaçao Aloes is reddish-brown and more or less opaque. When mounted in a fixed oil and examined microscopically, it shows numerous reddish-brown to blackish, opaque, angular fragments. It dissolves quickly in nitric acid forming a deep red solution.

Powdered Barbadoes Aloes is yellowish. Like that of Curaçao Aloes, it forms a deep red solution with nitric acid.

Powdered Cape Aloes is pale greenish-yellow becoming light brown on ageing. When mounted in a fixed oil and examined under the microscope, it shows numerous yellow angular fragments. Nitric acid dissolves it forming at first a reddish-brown solution which changes to purplish-brown and finally becomes green.

Powdered Uganda Aloes is yellowish-brown and forms a yellowish-brown solution with nitric acid.

Constituents.—Barbaloin ($C_{21}H_{20}O_9$), a pale yellow glucoside (absent in Natal aloes) aloe-emodin, bitter resin; isobarbaloin is present in addition to the foregoing in Curaçao and Barbadoes aloes; in Cape aloes there also is found an isomeric substance termed β-barbaloin. When barbaloin is boiled with alcohol acidified with hydrochloric acid, emodin ($C_{15}H_{10}O_5$) is yielded. The resin of Curaçao aloes consists of barbaloresinotannol combined with cinnamic acid; that of Cape, Uganda, Natal and Socotrine aloes of capaloresinotannol combined with paracumaric acid. Natal aloes contains as its chief active principle the glucoside, nataloin.

Use.—Purgative in constipation.

CONVALLARIÆ RADIX N.F. (CONVALLARIA ROOT)

Synonyms.—Lily-of-the-Valley Root; *Fr.* Muguet; *Ger.* Maiglöcklein.

Botanical Origin.—*Convallaria majalis* Linné.

Part Used.—The dried rhizome and roots.

Impurities.—Not more than 5 per cent. of leaves or other foreign matter and not more than 6 per cent. acid insoluble ash.

Habitat.—Mountainous regions of Europe, Asia and southeastern United States.

Plant.—A low, acaulescent, perennial herb widely cultivated for the beauty and fragrance of its flowers. Its subterranean portion consists of a branched, creeping, horizontal rhizome bearing 3 to 5 fibrous rootlets from the under and side portions of its nodes. Its aerial portion consists of 2 to 3 oblong, parallel veined leaves and later a slender scape bearing a one-sided raceme of small, white, bell-shaped, nodding flowers. The fruits are red berries.

Production and Commerce.—The rhizome and roots should be dug up during July and August, washed and dried. The commercial supplies of the drug used in this country come from Virginia, North Carolina and South Carolina.

Description.—Rhizome horizontal, elongated, usually branched, cylindrical, variable in length, from 1 to 3 mm. in diameter; externally light yellow to pale brown, with a few circular stem scars, and from the under and side portions at the nodes usually arise from three to five thin, tortuous, dark brown, branching roots; fracture short or fibrous; internally whitish. Odor indistinct; taste sweetish, becoming bitter and acrid.

Histology.—Transverse sections of the rhizome present the following structures for examination:

1. Epidermis of a layer of epidermal cells whose outer walls are highly cutinized.
2. Hypodermis of a layer of collenchyma cells.
3. Cortex of about 20 rows of parenchyma cells, some of which contain more or less spherical starch grains, others raphides of calcium oxalate.
4. Endodermis of usually 2 layers of endodermal cells, the radial and inner walls of which are strongly thickened and lignified.
5. Stele, a broad central region consisting of a matrix of starch and crystal-bearing parenchyma through which course closed collateral and concentric fibrovascular bundles.

The closed collateral bundles are arranged in an interrupted circle just within the endodermis. The woody portion of each is somewhat V-shaped. The concentric bundles are arranged in a somewhat irregular interrupted circle inside of these.

Powdered Drug.—Brown. It consists chiefly of cellular fragments and a few starch grains and raphides of calcium oxalate; cells of endodermis with slightly oblique ends and considerably thickened, lignified, porous walls; fragments of tracheæ with spiral and scalariform thickenings, or with porous walls; starch grains single or compound, mostly nearly spherical, and from 3μ to 12μ in diameter; raphides of calcium oxalate few, usually from 20μ to 60μ, rarely up to 150μ in length.

Constituents.—The glucosides convallarin and convallamarin; starch, calcium oxalate, etc.

Use.—Cardiac stimulant, usually in the form of fluidextract.

CONVALLARIÆ FLORES (CONVALLARIA FLOWERS)

Synonyms.—Lily-of-the-Valley Flowers; *Fr.* Muguet; *Ger.* Maiblumen.

Botanical Origin.—*Convallaria majalis* Linné.

Part Used.—The dried inflorescence.

Description.—The drug occurs as entire and broken inflorescences. Each entire inflorescence is up to 25 cm. in length and consists of an angled, dull green peduncle and rachis, the latter bearing about 8 or 10 drooping pedicels, each subtended by a small lanceolate bract and terminating in a brownish-colored, bell-shaped flower. Each flower consists of a campanulate perianth with 6 short recurved lobes, 6 stamens inserted on the base of the perianth and a syncarpous pistil having a 3-celled ovary, elongated style and a 3-lobed stigma. The odor is fragrant. The taste is sweet and slightly acrid.

Constituents.—The glucosides convallamarin and convallarin; volatile oil, resin, etc.

Use.—Cardiac stimulant.

TRILLIUM N.F. (TRILLIUM)

Synonyms.—Beth Root, Wake Robin, Birthroot; *Ger.* and *Fr.* Trillium.

Botanical Origin.—*Trillium erectum L.* and closely allied species of *Trillium*.

Part Used.—The dried rhizome.

Purity Rubric.—Not more than 2 per cent. of foreign organic matter.

Habitat.—Woodland of eastern and central North America.

Plants.—Perennial herbs with shortened tuber-like rhizomes from each of which arises an aerial stem bearing at its summit a whorl of 3 broadly rhombic or ovate leaves and a large terminal flower, which, in *Trillium erectum*, varies from brownish-purple to white to greenish or even pink.

Commercial.—The supplies of this drug come largely from North Carolina, Virginia, Indiana and Missouri.

Description.—Rhizome oblique, globular, oblong or obconical, truncate below, terminated by a small bud surrounded by a sheath of scarious leaf bases, annulated by leaf scars and fissured by stem scars; from 0.6 to 5 cm. in length and from 0.6 to 2.5 cm. in width, more or less compressed laterally, rootlet scars in several concentric rows on the under side in the upper portions; externally yellowish to reddish-brown; internally of a pale yellow; fracture somewhat uneven with either a hard and close texture or a more or less spongy appearance. Odor distinct; taste bitter and acrid with a sensation of warmth in the throat, and when chewed causing an increased flow of saliva.

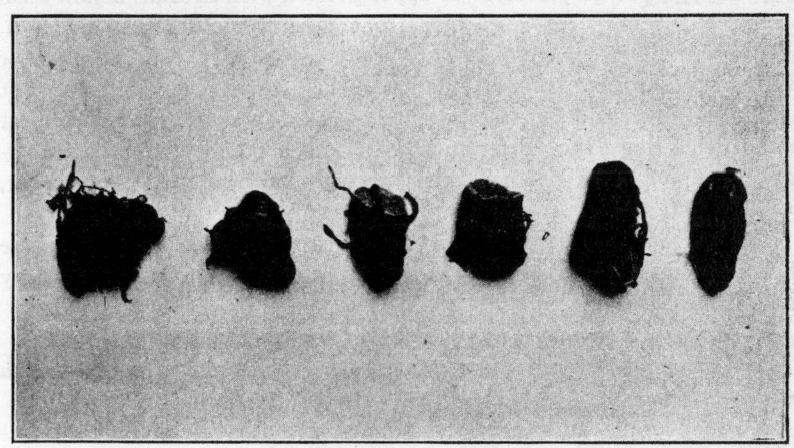

FIG. 33.—Beth Root, × 19/32.

Powdered Drug.—Yellowish-white; numerous parenchyma fragments, some of which contain raphides of calcium oxalate up to 225μ in length, others spheroidal altered or unaltered starch grains, the unaltered grains up to 20μ in diameter; fragments of reddish-brown epidermis; spiral and reticulate tracheæ and short, porous sclerenchyma cells.

Constituents.—A saponin principle called "trillin"; resin, tannin, starch, etc.

Uses.—Astringent, irritant, emmenagogue and expectorant.

ALETRIS N.F. (ALETRIS)

Synonyms.—Unicorn Root, Star Grass, Starwort, Ague Root, True Unicorn Root, Colic Root; *Ger.* Mehlige Aletris; *Fr.* Aletris farineux.

Botanical Origin.—*Aletris farinosa* L.

Part Used.—Dried rhizome and roots.

Purity Rubric.—Not more than 5 per cent. foreign organic matter and not more than 10 per cent. of acid-insoluble ash.

Habitat.—Eastern United States in sandy and grassy woods.

Plant.—A perennial herb with a spreading rosette of thin lanceolate leaves from the center of which arises a slender scape bearing a spike-like raceme of small, white, tubular flowers. The fruit is an ovoid capsule inclosed by the perianth. The seeds are minute and ribbed.

Commercial.—The commercial supplies of this drug are obtained from North Carolina, Virginia and Tennessee.

Description.—The drug occurs in the entire and broken condition. Rhizome horizontal or slightly oblique, nearly cylindrical or laterally compressed above, up to 4 cm. in length and 12 mm. in diameter; externally grayish-yellow to grayish-brown, upper portion with circular, hollow stem scars, leaf bases or stem bases, the latter frequently up to 8 mm. in length, the sides and lower portion showing many tough, wiry, pale yellowish or whitish, flexible roots, some of which have their cortex removed and exhibit a reddish-brown endodermis; fracture of rhizome short; internally light brown exhibiting a thin cortex and broad central cylinder, the latter showing numerous scattered yellowish fibrovascular bundles; odor slight, acetous; taste starchy, sweetish and somewhat bitter.

Microscopical Characteristics.—Transverse sections of the rhizome show the following microscopical peculiarities, passing from periphery toward the center:

1. Epidermis of a layer of yellowish-brown epidermal cells.

2. Cortex of several layers of starch parenchyma, through which course leaf trace bundles of the closed collateral type.

3. Endodermis, an interrupted zone of several layers of yellow thick-walled cells, readily separating from the cortex.

4. Central cylinder, a broad zone of starch parenchyma containing scattered bundles, each of which is surrounded by several layers of thick-walled lignified cells, possessing large oblique pores. The tracheæ are reticulate and porous.

Many of the parenchyma cells of the cortex and central cylinder contain raphides of calcium oxalate, but most possess spherical or elliptical starch grains up to 16μ in diameter.

Powdered Drug.—Light gray to yellowish-brown; fragments of epidermis, some with glandular hairs, numerous orange-yellow sclerenchyma fibers with pointed ends; fragments or porous and reticulate tracheæ, numerous fragments of parenchyma containing starch grains of a spherical or ellipsoidal shape, up to 16μ in diameter, numerous acicular crystals and raphides of calcium oxalate up to 50μ in length.

Constituents.—Bitter principle, starch, calcium oxalate, etc.

Use.—Uterine tonic, usually in the form of an elixir or fluidextract.

HELONIAS N.F. (HELONIAS)

Synonyms.—False Unicorn, Blazing Star.

Botanical Origin.—*Chamælirium luteum* (Linné) A. Gray.

Part Used.—The dried rhizome and roots.

Purity Rubric.—Not more than 5 per cent. of foreign organic matter.

Habitat.—In low grounds, Massachusetts to Florida, west to Nebraska and Arkansas.

Plant.—A perennial diœcious herb with a smooth stem 3–12 dm. high which arises from a tuberous rhizome and which is terminated by a spiked raceme of small white flowers. The leaves are lanceolate, the lower ones spatulate. The fruit is an ellipsoid, loculicidally 3-valved capsule up to 10 mm. long and containing numerous linear-oblong seeds.

Commercial.—Helonias is collected for the market chiefly in North Carolina, Virginia and Michigan.

Description.—Rhizome vertical or oblique, subcylindrical, from 0.5 to 3 cm. in length and about 1 cm. in diameter; externally grayish brown, annulate from scars of bud scales; upper portion with leaf bases enclosing a small bud; oblique rhizomes with a few stem scars up to 7 mm. in diameter; lower portion with numerous whitish or pale yellowish, nearly straight or slightly curved, wiry roots, from 5 to 8 cm. in length; fracture hard and horny; internally grayish-yellow exhibiting a narrow cortex and a broad central cylinder with 3 to 4 circles of small fibrovascular bundles; odor distinct; taste bitter and slightly astringent.

Microscopical Characteristics.—Transverse and longitudinal sections of the rhizome show a lignified cork zone, a broad cortex, through which extend, outwardly from the central cylinder, numerous lateral rootlet tissues; parenchyma cells with many spheroidal or ellipsoidal starch grains from 2–15μ in diameter, numerous raphides of calcium oxalate up to 40μ in length; the fibrovascular bundles are concentric and arranged in 3 or 4 irregular circles, the tracheæ showing either annular, porous or reticulate markings. A cross section of the root exhibits a cortex of starch-parenchyma, an endodermis of radially elongated cells with lignified walls and a central cylinder showing 5 to 7 mestome strands.

Adulterants.—The rhizome and roots of *Liatris* species which possess a somewhat terebinthinate odor and bitter taste.

Constituents.—Chamælirin (a glucoside), starch, calcium oxalate, etc.

Uses.—Uterine tonic, diuretic and anthelmintic.

DIOSCOREACEÆ (YAM FAMILY)

Herbs or shrubs with twining herbaceous stems arising from large tuberous roots or knotted rootstocks. Leaves broad, frequently cordate and palmate-reticulate and varying from simple to compound. Flowers small, diœcious, regular, having a 6-cleft, calyx-like perianth, six stamens and a 3-celled ovary. Fruit usually a membranous, three-angled or winged capsule containing winged seeds.

DIOSCOREA N.F. (DIOSCOREA)

Synonyms.—Wild Yam Root, Rheumatism Root, Colic Root, China Root.

Botanical Origin.—*Dioscorea villosa* Linné.

Part Used.—The dried rhizome.

Purity Rubric.—Not more than 2 per cent. of foreign organic matter.

Habitat.—North America west to Kansas in thickets.

Plant.—A perennial herb with matted, woody rhizome bearing slender aerial stems which twine over bushes. The leaves are mostly alternate, cordate, acuminate, villous beneath, 9 to 11 ribbed, otherwise reticulate. The flowers are greenish-yellow and of two kinds, viz.: sterile and fertile. The sterile flowers occur in drooping panicles, the fertile in drooping racemes. The fruit is a 3-winged capsule.

Commercial.—Wild Yam root is gathered in autumn and prepared for the market in Virginia, North Carolina, Indiana and Michigan.

Description.—Rhizome horizontal, knotty, often compressed, bent and branched, usually broken into pieces of varying length and up to 12 mm. in diameter, bearing scattered nodular lateral projections, tough filiform rootlets beneath and depressed stem scars and occasionally slender twisted portions of aerial stems above; externally pale brown, somewhat scaly; fracture very tough and short; fractured surface whitish or pale yellowish, with many small scattered yellowish bundles; odor indistinct; taste starchy and acrid.

Powdered Drug.—Whitish; numerous fragments of thick-walled, lignified, parenchyma cells most of which contain starch, a few calcium oxalate crystals in raphides; numerous spheroidal and oval starch grains, up to 35μ in diameter; few isolated acicular crystals or raphides; fragments of fibrovascular bundles, the tracheæ and tracheids of which possess bordered pores; fragments of yellowish or brownish epidermis and lignified sclerenchyma fibers; a few endodermal fragments with slightly lignified radial and inner walls; a few fragments of thin-walled parenchyma cells.

Constituents.—Resin, a saponin-like principle, starch, calcium oxalate, etc.

Uses.—Dioscorea is employed by the elecctics in the treatment of bilious colic and by others as an antirheumatic.

IRIDACEÆ (IRIS FAMILY)

Perennial herbs with equitant, 2-ranked leaves and regular or irregular flowers which are showy. Fruit a 3-celled, loculicidal, many-seeded capsule. Rootstocks, tubers, or corms mostly acrid. Fibrovascular bundles concentric. Calcium oxalate crystals occur in the form of long prisms (styloids) within mucilage cells.

CROCUS N.F. (CROCUS)

Synonyms.—Saffron, Spanish Saffron, True Saffron; *Fr. Gr.* Safran.

Botanical Origin.—*Crocus sativus* Linné.

Part Used.—The stigma.

Limit of Impurities.—10 per cent. of the yellow styles or other foreign matter, and 14 per cent. of volatile matter when dried at 100°C. (U.S. Dept. of Agriculture). Nor more than 2 per cent. of other foreign matter (N.F. v).

Ash.—Not more than 7.5 per cent. Ash is non-fusible. [Not more than 6 per cent. of total ash, nor more than 1 per cent. of ash insoluble in hydrochloric acid (U.S. Dept. of Agric.).]

Habitat.—Southern Europe and Asia.

Plant.—A perennial, low-growing, bulbous plant with an underground globular corm producing 6 to 9 sessile leaves surrounded in its lower part by 4 or 5 broad membranous scales. The flowers are borne on the terminal region of a scape. Each consists of a pale reddish-purple perianth showing a cylindrical tube about 4 in. long and 6 oblong oval segments, an androecium of 3 stamens and a gynœcium of 3 syncarpous carpels. The ovary is inferior, and 3-celled. The style is slender, elongated and pale yellow in the perianth tube and divided in its upper part into 3 drooping deep red stigmas.

Production and Commerce.—The bulbs are planted usually in late spring about 6 inches apart and from 5 to 6 inches deep in soil of medium fertility, care being taken to thoroughly cultivate. The purplish-blue flowers appear in October and the leaves the following spring. The flowering period lasts from 2 to 3 weeks during which time the flowers are collected every morning, as they open. The deep red stigmas are then collected either by pulling them out or cutting them off with the finger nail, after which the flowers are discarded. The stigmas are dried by spreading them in a thin layer on a sieve suspended over a low fire, after which they are placed in linen bags and stored in a dry place. The yield per acre of saffron varies from 10 to 30 pounds. It is estimated that 50,000 flowers are required to produce a pound of the dried drug.

Most of the supplies of the drug come from Spain where the crocus plant is cultivated on a large scale. The plant is also cultivated for the drug in Italy, Germany, France, Greece, Austria, and Persia. It was formerly grown in various localities of the United States as a garden crop, notably in Lebanon and Lancaster counties, Pennsylvania.

The two most important commercial varieties are Valencia and Alicante Saffrons, the former being preferred because it consists almost entirely of stigmas. The foreign drug is imported in tin containers averaging 1 pound each chiefly from Alicante and Valencia, Spain. Some commercial supplies have recently been received from Greece and Japan.

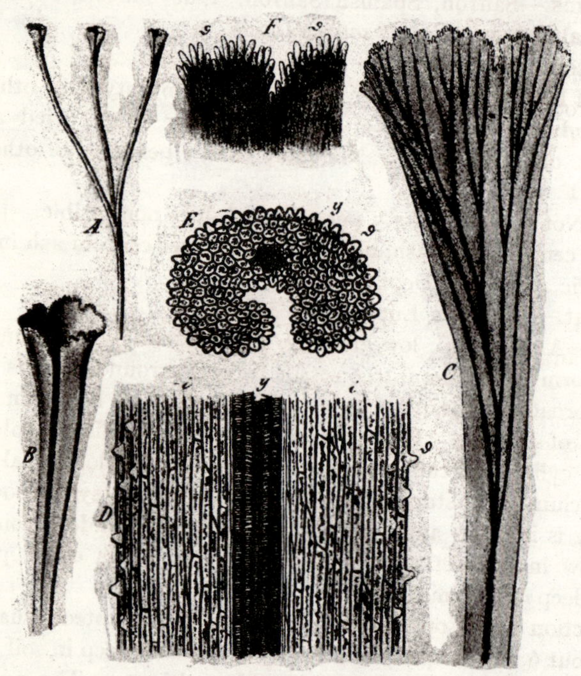

FIG. 34.—*Crocus sativa*. *A*. Upper end of style with its 3 stigmas (nat. size). *B*. A stigma, ×4. *C*. The same, macerated, spread out and enlarged. *D*. Longitudinal section of the lower portion of stigma, × 50. *E*. Transverse section through lower portion of stigma, × 50. *F*. A portion of the epidermis of the upper end of stigma showing papillæ, × 50. *i*, parenchyma; *ϑ*, papillæ; *y*, fibrovascular bundle. (*After Berg*.)

Description.—Stigmas 3, united or separate, attached to the top of the style; usually about 25 mm. in length, cornucopia-shaped, of a dark red color, the margin fimbriate or dentate; styles about 10 mm. in length, more or less cylindrical, solid, yellowish. Odor strong, characteristic; taste bitter, aromatic. Upon chewing the drug, the saliva is colored a bright orange-yellow. Saffron should not be exposed to light and should be preserved in amber-colored bottles or tin boxes.

When placed in sulphuric acid, saffron stigmas are immediately colored blue, gradually changing to violet, and finally to a deep wine color.

Microscopical Characteristics.—The distal end of the stigma shows numerous bladdery, cylindric papillæ about 150μ in length, among which occur a few smooth, spherical pollen grains from 40μ to 90μ in diameter and occasionally pollen grains showing outgrowths in the form of pollen tubes.

Powdered Drug.—Orange-red. Fragments of stigma showing elongated, thin-walled cells containing red coloring matter and some showing more or less cylindrical papillæ up to 150μ long. Pollen grains, spheroidal with reddish, granular contents.

Constituents.—Crocin (a red coloring principle), a colorless glucoside termed picrocrosin, volatile oil (trace only), dextrose, etc.

Uses.—Chiefly as a flavoring and coloring agent but also, by the laity, in the form of a tea as a stimulant, antispasmodic, diaphoretic (in measles) and emmenagogue.

Adulterants and Substitutes.—The crude drug has been adulterated with the ligulate flowers of *Calendula officinalis* that have first been colored with methyl orange or a red dye. *Calendula* may readily be distinguished by the ligula or strap-shaped portion of its corolla being 4 or 5-nerved and 3-toothed and by its epidermal cells containing yellowish droplets of an oil.

The tubular florets of *Carthamus tinctorius*, commonly known as American Saffron or Safflower, have long been substituted for Saffron. These are of a deep orange-red color, 25 to 40 mm. long, and exhibit a thin, cylindrical corolla tube, terminating in a 5-cleft limb, each lobe being up to 6 mm. long. From the throat of the corolla tube projects the yellow anther column and through the center of this the stigma. The pollen grains are spheroidal and spinose.

The tubular florets of *Onopordon Acanthium* L., the Cotton- or Scotch-Thistle, artificially dyed with a mixture of Ponceau 3R and tartrazined an weighted with a mixture of ammonium nitrate or potassium nitrate, borax and glycerin, represent a recent adulterant.

Basal portions of the styles and dyed floral parts, such as stamens and petals, of Crocus have also been employed as adulterants of the crude drug.

The powdered drug has been found adulterated not only with the aforementioned adulterants in ground form but also with glycerin, mineral or vegetable oil, colored emery, chalk and gypsum.

The presence of an added oil may be detected by pressing the suspected material between filter paper, when transparent spots will be noted.

The presence of an added aniline dye may be usually acertained by macerating 0.01 gm. of the suspected sample in 5 cc. of either ether, chloroform or petroleum benzine and noting more than a light lemon-yellow color in the solvents.

IRIS N.F. (ORRIS)

Synonyms.—Orris Root; *Ger.* Veilchenwurzel; *Fr.* Iris de Florence.

Botanical Origin.—*Iris florentina* L., *Iris germanica* L., or *Iris pallida* Lamarck.

Part Used.—The rhizome, freed from roots, peeled and dried.

Purity Rubric.—Not more than 1 per cent. of foreign organic matter.

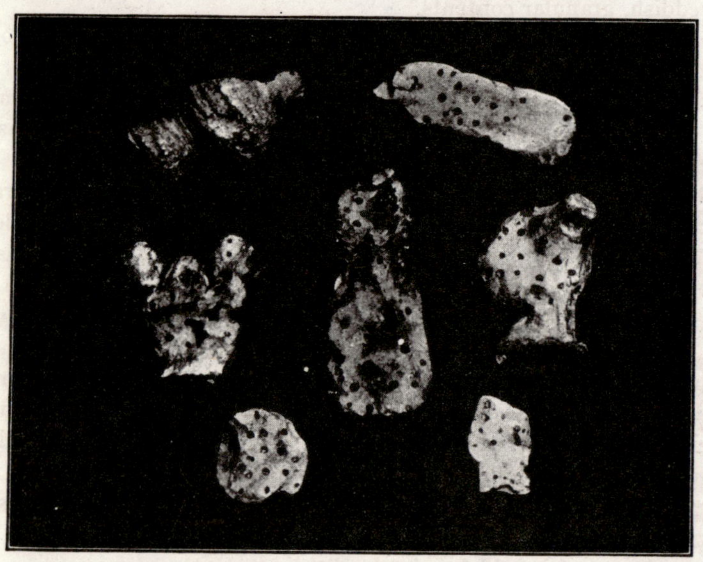

FIG. 35.—Orris, × ½. (*Photograph by Stoneback.*)

Habitat.—Mediterranean region.

Plant.—*Iris germanica*, commonly known as Fleur-de-Lis, is a perennial herb widely cultivated as an ornamental plant in the United States and growing wild in Virginia and West Virginia. Its subterranean portion consists of a horizontal branching, thick annulated rhizome system, bearing numerous equitant broad sword-shaped leaves, and later, long peduncled, 2 to 3-flowered spathes of flowers, the drooping sepals of which are dark violet purple with a brilliant yellow beard, the petals lilac colored and of about the same size as the sepals. There are 3 distinct stamens, the anthers of which are overarched by the 3 style arms, the latter bearing their stigmas as thin lips beneath the apices of the arms. The fruit is a 3-angled capsule.

Iris pallida differs from the preceding species by bearing pale blue flowers. *Iris florentina* bears large white flowers and has the most fragrant root.

Production and Commerce.—The chief commercial varieties of Orris are the Florentine, Verona and Mogadore. The three species are culti-

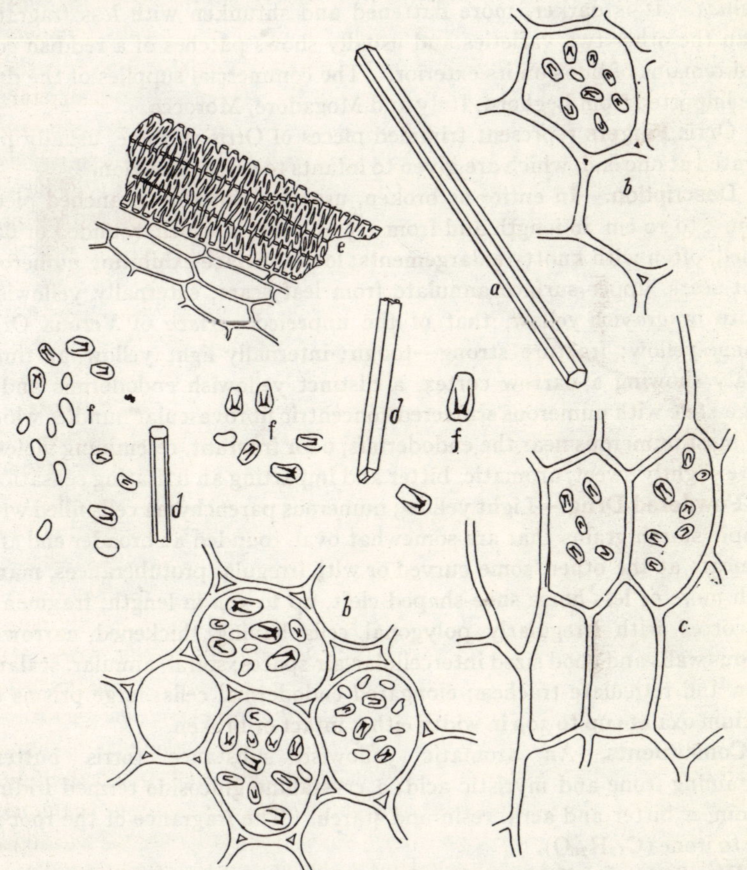

FIG. 36.—Powdered Iris florentina. (*a*) Large crystals of calcium oxalate; (*b*) parenchyma with starch; (*c*) parenchyma, longitudinal view; (*d*) broken prisms of calcium oxalate; (*e*) reticulate ducts; (*f*) starch grains showing characteristic horse-shoe shaped hilum. (*Schneider.*)

vated chiefly in Italy for the drug. The rhizomes of 2 or 3 year old plants are dug up in late summer or early fall, deprived of their roots and outer cortex and dried in the sun. The fresh rhizomes are devoid of odor and possess an acrid taste, but during the drying process, they lose their acridity and develop their peculiar fragrance. *Iris florentina* yields the commercial variety known as Florentine Orris. This is the lighter and most plump and fragrant of the three varieties and demands the highest price. Verona Orris is yielded by *Iris germanica* and *Iris pallida*. It is more yellow in color, less often branched and is generally not as carefully peeled as the Florentine variety. Mogadore Orris is yielded chiefly by *Iris germanica*. It is darker, more flattened and shrunken with less fragrance than the other two varieties and usually shows patches of a reddish cork and remains of buds on its exterior. The commercial supplies of the drug are imported from Leghorn, Italy and Mogadore, Morocco.

Orris Fingers represent trimmed pieces of Orris rhizome, usually perforated at one end, which are given to infants to assist dentition.

Description.—In entire or broken, usually jointed or branched pieces from 5 to 10 cm. in length and from 1.5 to 3 cm. in width, rounded or flattened, often with knotty enlargements; lower surface exhibiting numerous root scars, upper surface annulate from leaf scars; externally yellowish-white or grayish-yellow, that of the unpeeled surface of Verona Orris orange-yellow; fracture strong—tough; internally light yellow, at times mealy showing a narrow cortex, a distinct yellowish endodermis and a large stele with numerous scattered concentric fibrovascular bundles which are most numerous near the endodermis; odor fragrant, resembling violets; taste slightly sweet, aromatic, bitter and imparting an irritating sensation.

Powdered Drug.—Light yellow; numerous parenchyma cells filled with simple starch grains that are somewhat oval, rounded at broader end and truncate at the other, some curved or with irregular protuberances, many with more or less horse shoe-shaped cleft, up to 50μ in length; fragments of cortex with irregularly polygonal cells having thickened, narrowly porous walls and good sized intercellular-air-spaces; spiral, annular, scalariform and reticulate tracheæ; elongated endodermal cells; large prisms of calcium oxalate up to 30μ in width either intact or broken.

Constituents.—An aromatic yellowish substance (orris butter) containing irone and myristic acid; a crystalline glucoside termed iridin; tannin, a bitter and acrid resin and starch. The fragrance of the root is due to irone ($C_{13}H_{20}O$).

Uses.—In dentifrices and sachets.

IRIS VERSICOLOR N.F. (BLUE FLAG)

Synonyms.—Blue Flag, Larger Blue Flag; *Ger.* Amerikanische Schwertel; *Fr.* Rhizome d'Iris varié.

Botanical Origin.—*Iris versicolor* Linné and *Iris caroliniana* Watson.

Part Used.—The dried rhizome.

Purity Rubric.—Not more than 5 per cent. of its roots and leaf bases or other foreign matter.

Habitat.—In wet soil of eastern North America.

Plant.—*Iris versicolor* is a perennial herb whose underground portion consists of a horizontal rhizome system. Its aerial portion consists of sword-shaped, glaucous leaves and short pedicelled, showy, violet-blue flowers which are variegated with green, yellow and white toward the center. The fruit is a 3-celled, loculicidally dehiscent, subcylindrical capsule with obtuse angles.

Iris caroliniana which grows in swamps from Virginia to Georgia and Louisiana differs from the preceding species in possessing bright green leaves and lilac colored flowers variegated with yellow brown and purple.

Description.—Rhizome simple or branched, up to 15 cm. in length and 2 cm. in thickness, usually in longitudinally cut and broken pieces; outer surface gray-brown to purple brown, annulate, the upper surface exhibiting markings of leaf bases, the lower with numerous root scars and remnants of roots; fracture short and brittle; fractured surface pale purplish-brown and showing a thick porous cortex, a distinct endodermis and a broad central stele with scattered whitish fibrovascular bundles.

Histology.—Tranverse sections exhibit the following structures:

1. An *epidermis* with brownish walls and often partially detached.

2. A *hypodermis* of about 2 rows of hypodermal cells with uniformly thickened, strongly lignified walls, some of the cells containing a reddish-brown resinous substance.

3. A narrow *cortex* composed of a matrix of cortical parenchyma cells and large intercellular-air-spaces, coursing through which will be noted a few concentric fibrovascular bundles. Some of the parenchyma cells contain spherical or elliptical, simple or 2- to 4-compound starch grains, others a reddish-brown resinous substance, still others elongated prisms (styloids) of calcium oxalate.

4. An *endodermis* of a single layer of endodermal cells whose radial and inner walls are thickened and lignified.

5. A *central cylinder* composed of a matrix of somewhat spheroidal parenchyma cells between which are intercellular-air-spaces smaller than those of the cortex, The parenchyma cells contain similar contents to those of the cortex region. Scattered throughout the central cylinder are numerous concentric fibrovascular bundles of the monocotyl type.

Powdered Drug.—Reddish-brown; numerous resin cells containing a reddish-brown amorphous content; starch grains simple or 2- to 4-compound, the simple grains spheroidal or ellipsoidal and up to 22μ in diameter; calcium oxalate in styloids up to 350μ in length; tracheæ with annular, spiral, reticulate or bordered pore markings; few sclerenchyma fibers.

Constituents.—Volatile oil, acrid resins, tannin, sugar, starch, etc. "*Iridin*" is an oleoresin obtained by precipitating the tincture of this drug with water, "*Irisin*" is similarly prepared but the oleoresin is stiffened by the addition of some powdered root.

Uses.—Cathartic and diuretic.

ZINGIBERACEÆ (GINGER FAMILY)

Tropical plants, perennial herbs, with fleshy rhizomes and thickened roots which usually contain secretion sacs with volatile oil content, the latter frequently colored yellow by curcumin. The leaves vary from lanceolate to elliptic and are pinnately veined or parallel veined. They are either all radical or, in a few instances, alternate on a simple stem. The petiole generally forms a split sheath, sometimes ligulate. The leaf sheaths are folded tightly around each other, so as to often give the appearance of a stem. The flowers are hermaphrodite, irregular and trimerous and arranged in racemes, spikes or panicles. Sepals 3, short, often green; petals 3, elongate, often fused below; stamens 3 to 4 abortive, petaloid, one often absent, a sixth alone fertile and stamen-like. The petaloid stamens constitute the most attractive parts of the flower. Pistil inferior, tricarpellary. Fruit a capsule, generally loculicidally dehiscent and crowned with the remains of the perianth. Seeds numerous, angular or nearly rounded, frequently possessing an aril and containing perispermic and endospermic albumen. The fibrovascular bundles of the stems and leaves are either collateral or concentric. The starch grains are characteristically beaked at the hilum end of the grains.

ZINGIBER U.S.P. (GINGER)

Synonyms.—Ginger Rhizome; *Ger.* Ingwer; *Fr.* Gingembre.

Botanical Origin.—*Zingiber officinale* Roscoe.

Part Used.—The dried rhizome.

Standard of Assay.—Not less than 2 per cent. of a non-volatile ether-soluble extractive and not less than 12 per cent. of cold water-extractive.

Habitat.—S. Asia.

Plant.—A perennial herb with subterranean, digitately branched rhizome that sends up stems that are covered by leaf sheaths. Leaves alternate, smooth, pale green and lanceolate. Flower stems shorter than leaf stems and bearing a few flowers, each surrounded by a thin bract and situated in axils of large, greenish-yellow obtuse bracts, which are closely arranged at end of flower stem forming collectively an ovate oblong spike. Each flower shows a superior tubular calyx, split part way down one side; an orange-yellow corolla composed of a tube divided above into 3 linear-oblong, blunt lobes; 6 staminodes in 2 rows, the outer row of 3 being inserted at mouth of corolla, the posterior 2, small, horn-like, the anterior petaloid, purple and spotted and divided into 3 rounded lobes; and an inferior, 3-celled ovary with tufted stigma.

Production and Commerce.—Ginger is extensively cultivated in tropical and sub-tropical localities of both the Eastern and Western Hemispheres. Chief amongst those producing it are the West Indies, Africa, India and Japan. It is propagated from rhizome cuttings each containing a bud, which are planted from March to May, depending upon the latitude, about 1 ft. apart. The plants mature in about 9 or 10 months. The rhizomes are dug up upon the death of the aerial portions of the plants and washed. They are then prepared in different ways for the market. In some instances they are peeled and then washed in clean water, often containing lime juice, after which they are dried in the sun. In Jamaica this is the method employed in preparing "Unbleached Jamaica Ginger." In others, they are peeled on the flattened sides, treated with boiling water and subsequently dried, as is the case with the African and Indian varieties ("Coated or Unscraped Ginger"). Again, they may be peeled or scraped and then coated with carbonate or sulphate of lime to protect against attacks of insect larvæ. Limed gingers should be regarded with suspicion for "liming" has been resorted to by unscrupulous dealers to cover up defects in the "wormy" drug. Moreover, the rhizomes may be first peeled and then bleached by the use of sulphurous acid or chloride of lime ("Bleached Ginger").

The peel and off-fall in Jamaica Ginger preparation is occasionally imported for oil distillation.

The principal commercial varieties are the following: Natural Jamaica, Bleached Jamaica, African, Calcutta, Calicut, Cochin and Japanese. Most of the Ginger coming to this country at present consists of the Jamaica, Cochin and African varieties. These 3 varieties are alone recognized by the U.S.P. x.

Description of Commercial Varieties. Jamaica Ginger.—Rhizomes devoid of outer suberized layers, in horizontal, laterally compressed, irregularly branched pieces up to 16 cm. in length and up to 20 mm. in thickness; externally pale yellowish-buff or light brown, longitudinally striate, ends of branches with depressed stem scars; fracture brittle and uneven, mealy, fibrous and resinous; internally yellowish-brown, cortex thin, endodermis a thin yellow layer enclosing a large stele with numerous groups of fibrovascular bundles and yellowish oil cells; odor agreeably aromatic; taste aromatic and pungent.

African Ginger.—Rhizomes with cork partly removed on the flattened sides, the surfaces without cork smooth and of a light brown color, the surfaces with cork reticulately or longitudinally wrinkled and dark grayish-brown; fracture short or short fibrous; internally lemon-yellow or dark blue with yellow oil cells and reddish-brown resin cells; odor strongly aromatic; taste intensely pungent.

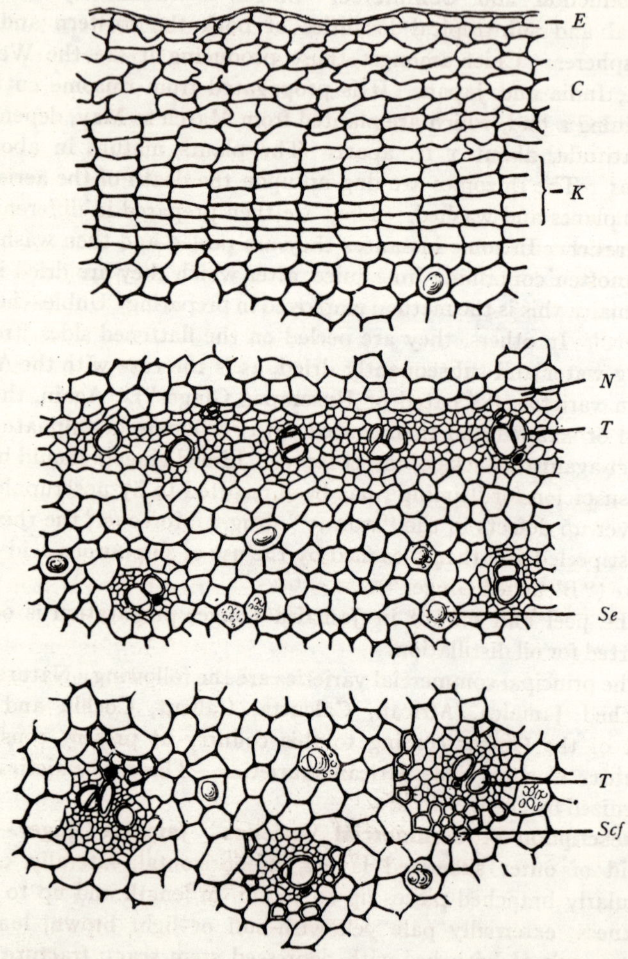

FIG. 37.—Transverse section through a representative portion of an unpeeled Ginger rhizome. Epidermis (*E*); cortex (*C*); cork (*K*); endodermis (*N*); tracheæ of fibrovascular bundle (*T*); secretion sac containing oil and resin (*Se*); sclerenchyma fibers (*Scf*). (*Tschirch and Oesterle.*)

Cochin Ginger.—Rhizomes with most or all of the corky layer removed on the flattened sides; externally light brown or grayish-yellow; fracture short and mealy; internally yellowish-white with numerous yellowish oil cells and brownish-red to black resin cells; odor aromatic; taste strongly aromatic and pungent.

Calcutta Ginger (Race Ginger).—Rhizomes somewhat resembling African Ginger, the branches being usually larger, and with a considerable portion of shrivelled pieces, externally grayish-brown or grayish-blue; fracture short and brittle, mealy, or horny; internally light yellow or light brownish-yellow with many yellowish oil cells and yellowish-brown resin cells; odor aromatic; taste starchy, strongly aromatic and pungent.

Calicut Ginger (Lemon Ginger).—Rhizomes resembling African Ginger, but more of the periderm is usually removed; externally dark yellow, orange or reddish-brown; fracture brittle and uneven, mealy; internally light yellow or brownish-yellow with large stele and numerous yellow oil and resin cells; odor aromatic; taste strongly aromatic and pungent.

Japanese Ginger (from *Zingiber Mioga* Roscoe).—Rhizomes usually with a thin coating of lime; externally nearly smooth and of a whitish color; fracture short, brittle and very mealy; internally yellowish-white to light brown with numerous brownish-red resin cells; odor aromatic; taste strongly aromatic and pungent.

Microscopical Characteristics.—Transverse sections of Jamaica Ginger, cleared by warming in chloral hydrate solution, show the following structure, passing from periphery toward the center: (see Fig. 37.)

1. *Cortex* of several layers of ordinary parenchyma cells with intercellular-air-spaces and containing gelatinized starch (due to warming in chloral). Scattered among the typical cells of this region will be noted secretion sacs which contain a yellowish oil (if rhizome is recent) or brownish resin insoluble in alcohol (if rhizome is old). Leaf-trace bundles cut obliquely or transversely will also be seen coursing through this region.

2. *Endodermis*, a pale brownish layer of cells whose walls are somewhat collapsed, the radial walls of which appear highly refractive upon warming the section in strong potash solution. Upon washing out the potash solution with water and adding a drop or two of concentrated sulphuric acid, these radial walls do not dissolve and so are suberised.

3. *Stele*, a broad central zone of ordinary parenchyma cells, air spaces and secretion sacs, similar in character to the cortex. In this region, just inside of the endodermis, will be observed a circle of crowded, closed collateral fibrovascular bundles, some possessing a single trachea, others groups of two or more tracheæ. Scattered irregularly throughout the remainder of the stele are larger closed collateral bundles of more or less rounded form with sclerenchyma fibers partially surrounding them.

Longitudinal-radial sections mounted in water exhibit elongated parenchyma cells filled with starch grains. Some of the starch grains can be observed outside the margin of the section and will be found to vary in shape and size. Ovoid, elongated-ovoid, and irregularly rounded forms can be made out, some of which are beaked at one end. The hilum is near the beak. They vary in size from 20μ to 40μ, usually, rarely attaining 50μ to 60μ in the long axis.

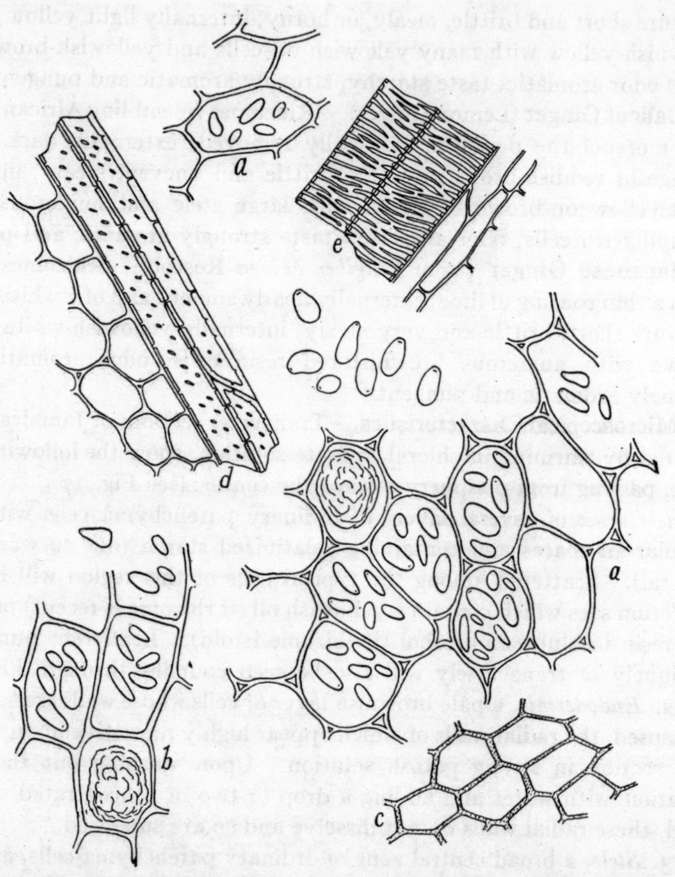

FIG. 38.—Powdered zingiber. (*a*) Parenchyma with starch, transverse view; (*b*) parenchyma, longitudinal view, showing one secretion sac containing a mass of resin; (*c*) cork, vertical view; (*d*) tracheids; (*e*) reticulate tracheæ. (*Schneider.*)

Two kinds of secretion sacs will be observed: one being rounded and containing a yellowish oil or oleoresin or reddish-brown resin, another adjacent to tracheæ and narrowly elongated with yellowish-brown contents.

The tracheæ vary in character, most being reticulate, others spiral, still others scalariform. The sclerenchyma fibers are elongated, more or less wavy-walled and possess oblique pits. The ends of the fibers are either tapered, rounded or square.

Longitudinal sections mounted in sulphuric acid dissolve with exception of the walls of the secretion sacs and radial walls of endodermal cells which, accordingly, must be suberised. Mounts made in phloroglucin and hydrochloric acid show no red coloration of the walls of many of the sclerenchyma fibers; some, however, take a pinkish tint, showing slight lignification.

Powdered Ginger.—Light yellow (Jamaica Ginger), light brown (Cochin Ginger) or brown (African Ginger). In water mounts starch grains of ovoid, spherical and elliptical to irregularly rounded or ovoid shape will be seen, many with one end beaked, 20μ to 50μ, rarely 60μ, in long diameter and showing excentric hilum near smaller end and striations. Adhering to many of the starch grains are granular particules of proteid matter or fill starch. Mounts of material, cleared by warming in 5 per cent. potassium hydrate solution or 1 per cent. hydrochloric acid and washing with water, show long, thin-walled, frequently non-lignified sclerenchyma fibers, distinctly undulate on one side and with oblique pores, reticulate, spiral and scalariform tracheæ, as well as oleoresin cells, the latter with suberised walls. Fragments of thin-walled parenchyma cells are also evident. Yellowish or brownish, thin-walled, cork cells are only occasional in Jamaica Ginger but numerous in African and Cochin Gingers. Japanese Ginger shows numerous compound starch grains in addition to simple starch grains.

Constituents.—Volatile oil, 1 to 3 per cent., consisting for the most part of a sesquiterpene, phellandrene and dextro-camphene; gingerol (a yellowish, oily, mixture of phenolic substances) up to 1.5 per cent., which gives to the drug its hot pungent taste; resins and starch.

Standard of Purity.—The United States Department of Agriculture has ruled that products labeled Ginger must conform to the following standard. Ginger is the washed and dried, or decorticated and dried, rhizome of *Zingiber officinale* Roscoe It contains not less than 42 per cent. of starch, not more than 8 per cent. of crude fiber, not more than 1 per cent. of lime (CaO), nor less than 12 per cent. of cold water extract, nor more than 7 per cent. of total ash, not more than 2 per cent. of ash insoluble in hydrochloric acid, nor less than 2 per cent. of ash soluble in cold water.

Jamaica ginger is ginger grown in Jamaica. It contains not less than 15 per cent. of cold water extract, and conforms in other respects to the standards for ginger.

Limed ginger (bleached ginger) is whole ginger coated with carbonate of calcium. It contains not more than 4 per cent. of carbonate of calcium, nor more than 10 per cent. of total ash, and conforms in other respects to the standards for ginger.

Uses.—Condiment, carminative and stimulant.

Adulterants.—Powdered Ginger has been frequently adulterated with exhausted ginger. This may be detected by the diminution in the ash soluble in cold water (which should not be lower than 2 per cent.) as well as by the decreased yield of cold water and alcoholic extract. Wheat Middlings and Wheat Flour have also found admixed with the ground or powdered drug. Ground turmeric has sometimes been added to the adulterated article to bring up its color to that of the genuine.

GALANGA N.F. (GALANGA)

Synonyms.—Galangal, Chinese Ginger, East India Root; Lesser Galangal, Rhizoma Galangæ; *Ger.* Galgant; *Fr.* Racine de Galanga.

Botanical Origin.—*Alpinia officinarum* Hance.

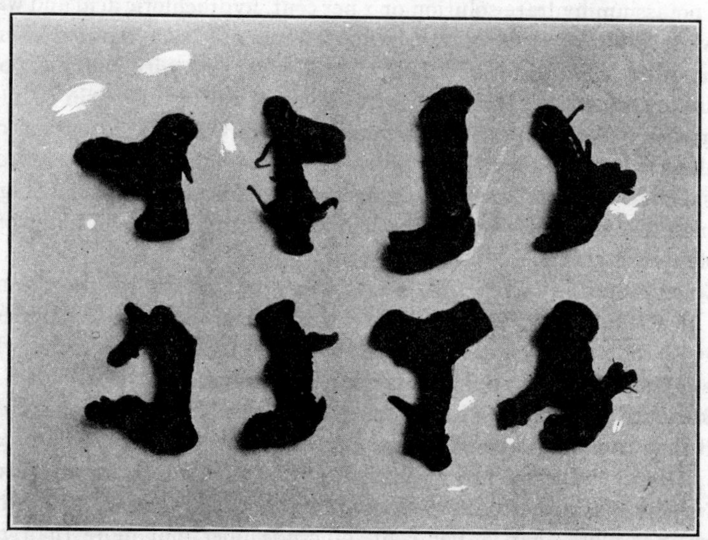

FIG. 39.—Galanga, × ½. (*Photograph by Stoneback.*)

Part Used.—The dried rhizome.

Purity Rubric.—Not more than 2 per cent. of foreign organic matter and not more than 3 per cent. of acid-insoluble ash.

Habitat.—China.

Plant.—A perennial reed-like herb bearing stems about 1 m. in height which are covered by the leaf sheaths of narrow lanceolate leaves. The inflorescence is a short raceme of white flowers that are shaded and veined with dull red.

Production and Commerce.—The plant is cultivated for the drug on the island of Hainan to the south of China. The rhizome is dug in late summer or early autumn, washed, trimmed, cut into segments and carefully dried. The commercial supplies of the drug are shipped from Shanghai and Hang-Chow, China in bales made of split cane and bound with cane. Much of the supply recently imported into the United States came through Hamburg, Marseilles and London and arrived in burlap bags.

Description.—The drug occurs in the form of branched or simple segments of the rhizome up to 11 cm. in length and 2 cm. in diameter, marked with wavy annulations of the leaf bases which possess a lighter color than the remainder of the surface; externally reddish or cinnamon-brown; internally orange-brown; fracture fibrous and uneven; odor agreeably aromatic; taste aromatic spicy and pungent.

Histology.—Cross sections of Galanga exhibit the following internal features:

1. *Epidermis* with thin-walled cells, some of which contain a reddish-brown amorphous substance.

2. *Cortex*, a broad region consisting chiefly of starchy parenchyma and numerous scattered secretion sacs with yellowish oil and reddish-brown resinous content.

3. *Endodermis*, a narrow zone of thin-walled cells.

4. *Central Cylinder*, a broad region composed of tissues similar to the cortex but showing numerous closed collateral bundles just beneath the endodermis and many scattered concentric bundles throughout the inner region.

Powdered Drug.—Reddish-brown. Numerous simple starch grains, the large grains up to 60μ in length, narrowly ellipsoidal, often broadened at one end, truncate, frequently curved, having a circular or cleft, excentric hilum, (often indistinct) and mostly indistinct lamellæ; numerous yellow oil cells and especially reddish resin cells; fragments of thick walled fibers; fragments of reticulate, scalariform and porous tracheæ.

Constituents.—Volatile oil containing cineol; resin containing galangol; the tasteless yellow crystalline bodies called kæmpferide and galangin; starch, etc.

Uses.—Aromatic stimulant, carminative and condiment.

CURCUMA (TURMERIC)

Synonyms.—Turmeric Rhizome, Yellow Root; *Ger.* Kurkuma; *Fr.* Safran des Indes.

Botanical Origin.—*Curcuma longa* Linné.

Part Used.—The prepared rhizome.

Habitat.—Southern Asia and East Indies.

Plant.—A perennial herb whose underground portion consists of an erect, ovate or pyriform, fleshy rhizome which gives rise to less fleshy elongated branches (secondary rhizomes), roots and leaves.

Production and Commerce.—Turmeric is grown extensively in China, India, Cochin China and Java from rhizome cuttings. The rhizomes are dug up at the close of the season's growth, washed and then prepared for the market either by scalding or boiling. During this process the starch becomes more or less altered, the contents of many of the cells becoming swollen to form pasty masses that are colored yellow by the curcumin also present in the cells. The rhizomes are then quickly dried in the sun. There are two important commercial forms on the market, viz.: *Round tumeric* representing the ovate or pear-shaped, fleshy main

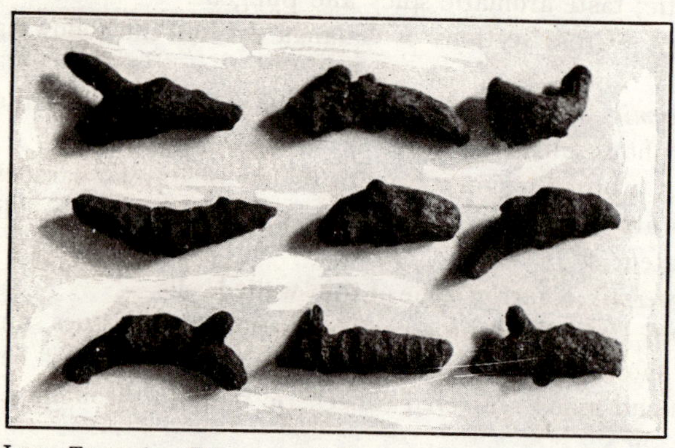

FIG. 40.—Long Turmeric. Rhizomes of *Curcuma longa* (Fam. *Zingiberaceæ*) showing branches and leaf scars, the latter represented by the annulations which appear on the surfaces of several of the rhizomes in the figure. × 3/8.

rhizomes and *Long turmeric*, the more slender, elongated, somewhat cylindrical and branched secondary rhizomes. The commercial supplies of this drug are imported from China and India.

Description.—Ovate, oblong or pyriform (round turmeric) or cylindrical and often short-branched (long turmeric); the round about half as broad as long, the long form from 2 to 5 cm. long and 1 to 1.8 cm. thick; externally yellowish to yellowish-brown, with root scars and annulations, the latter from the scars of leaf bases; fracture horny; internally orange-yellow to orange, waxy, showing a cortex separated from a central cylinder (about twice as broad as cortex) by a distinct endodermis; in both cortex and central cylinder scattered bundles are seen; odor aromatic; taste warmly aromatic and bitter.

Powdered Drug.—Deep yellow. See Fig. 41.

Constituents.—About 5 per cent. of volatile oil; curcumin, starch, resin, etc. Curcumin in a yellow crystalline substance which dissolves in alcohol forming a deep yellow solution; boric acid colors it reddish-brown, which upon the addition of alkalies becomes greenish-blue; an alcoholic solution of sulphuric acid imparts a deep crimson color to all tissues containing it.

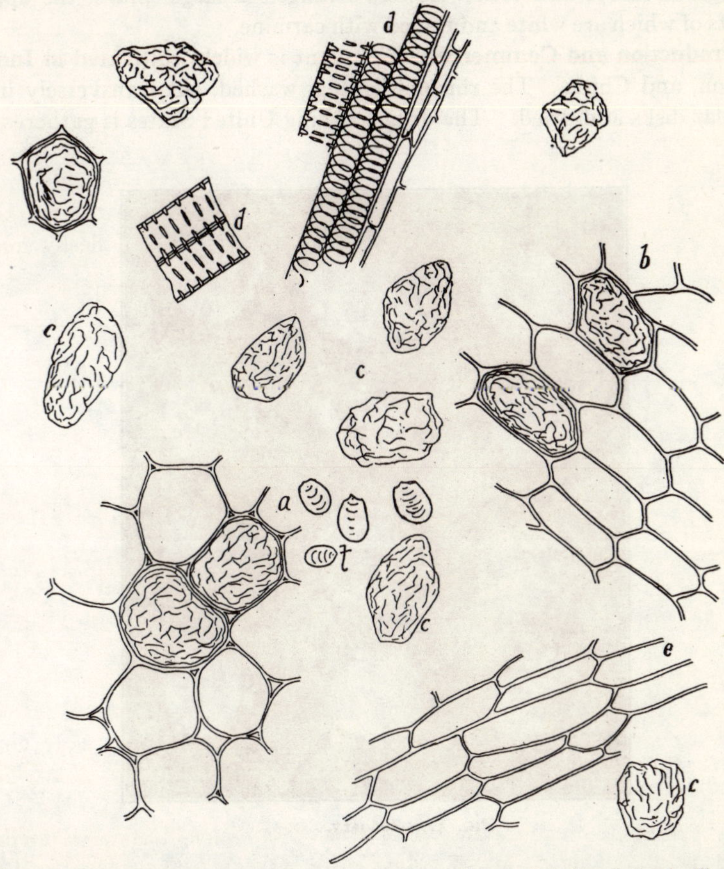

FIG. 41.—Powdered turmeric (curcuma). (*a*) Parenchyma with altered starch; (*b*) parenchyma, longitudinal view; (*c*) masses of altered starch; (*d*) ducts; (*e*) parenchyma; (*f*) normal starch granules. (*Schneider.*)

Uses.—Turmeric is a stimulant, coloring agent and condiment. It is an ingredient of many curry powders. Turmeric paper is prepared from the tincture and used as a test for boric acid and alkalies.

ZEDOARIA N.F. (ZEDOARY)

Synonyms.—Zedoary Root; *Ger.* Zittwerwurzel; *Fr.* Zedoarie.
Botanical Origin.—*Curcuma Zedoaria* (Bergius) Roscoe.
Part Used.—The dried rhizome.

Purity Rubric.—Not more than 2 per cent. of foreign organic matter.

Habitat.—India.

Plant.—A perennial herb with thick tuberous rhizome, handsome variegated leaves and yellow flowers arranged in large spikes, the upper bracts of which are white and tinged with carmine.

Production and Commerce.—The plant is widely cultivated in India, Ceylon, and China. The rhizome is dug, washed, cut transversely into circular disks and dried. The drug reaching United States is gathered in

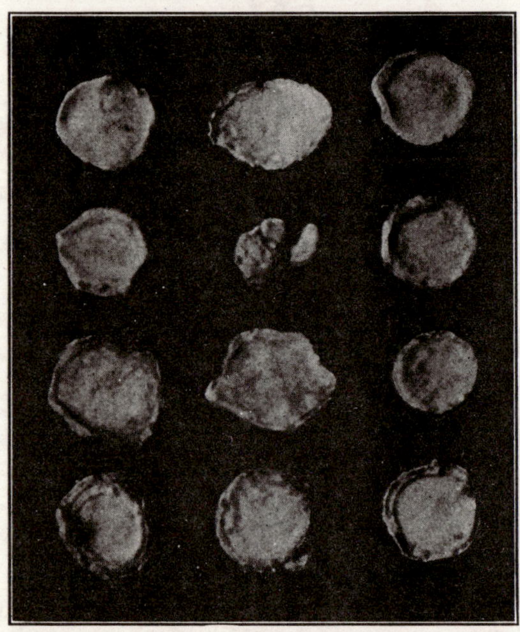

FIG. 42.—Zedoary. × ½.

Ceylon and India, shipped to Bombay and thence to Trieste, from which port it is exported to the United States.

Description.—In transverse (rarely longitudinal), rounded and frequently twisted slices of the rhizome up to 4 cm. in diameter and 15 mm. in thickness; externally grayish-brown, hairy, rough, with a few root scars; transverse surface pale red- to gray-brown; a clearly demarcated dark, circular endodermis, which is 2–5 mm. wide, separates the cortex which contains a few bundles from the broader stele which shows numerous orange-colored resin cells and scattered vascular bundles of a lighter color; odor aromatic, camphor-like; taste warmly aromatic and bitter.

Powdered Drug.—Numerous ovoid starch grains, up to 70μ in length with excentric hilum in smaller end of grain; numerous characteristic, 1- to 6-celled, thick-walled hairs, numerous fragments of starch-parenchyma, some with oil cells imbedded; very few sclerenchyma fibers; no stone cells or calcium oxalate crystals.

Constituents.—Volatile oil containing cineol; resin, fixed oil, mucilage and starch.

Uses.—Aromatic stimulant and carminative.

CARDAMOMI SEMEN U.S.P. (CARDAMON SEED)

Synonyms.—Cardamon; *Ger.* Kardamomen; *Fr.* Cardamomes.

Botanical Origin.—*Elettaria Cardamomum* White et Maton.

Part Used.—Dried seed, recently removed from the capsules.

Purity Rubric.—Not more than 5 per cent. of acid-insoluble ash.

Habitat.—Indo-China, in mountainous districts. Cultivated in Ceylon and near the Malabar coast, and recently in Guatemala.

Plant.—A perennial zingiberaceous herb attaining a height of 3 m. Its leaves are lanceolate and borne on long sheathing stems. The flowers are borne on horizontal racemes that arise from the stem near the ground. The fruit is an ovoid, loculicidally dehiscent capsule, the seeds of which are covered by an aril.

Production and Commerce.—The fruits (capsules) are gathered before maturity from October to late in December. Either the entire raceme may be cut or only nearly ripe fruits may be plucked from the rachis. They are cured on trays by sun or the shade of houses, graded by sieves, bleached by exposure to dew and sunlight or sulphurous acid and steam, and finally dried in the sun. The drug is exported both in the fruit (capsular) and seed form in chests. Seeds which have been removed from their capsules become inferior in time to those that have been retained. The greater bulk of the drug imported into this country is either shipped direct from Colombo, Ceylon, and from Bombay, and Delhi, India, or through London. Malabar and Mysore Cardamons come from Colombo; Mangalore from Bombay or Delhi. Smaller supplies have recently been coming forward from San Cristobal, Colban and Livingstone, Guatemala.

There are several varieties of Caradomon capsules which may be classified under two captions, based upon size and commercial source respectively. Thus, there are the "Shorts" (12 mm. long, 6 mm. broad) that are broad and plump, "Short-longs" (18–25 mm. long, 6 mm. broad) that are finer ribbed and lighter than the shorts, and "Longs" (25–30 mm. long, 4 mm. broad). According to the growing district or shipping port there are the following named varieties: 1. Malabar. 2. Mangalore. 3. Mysore. 4. Guatemala

Malabar Cardamon is recognized as the finest grade. It consists of "shorts" and "short-longs," of ellipsoidal or ovoid shape, light buff in color, with 15–18 aromatic and pungent seeds.

Mangalore Cardamon closely resembles the Malabar variety but the fruits are frequently larger, nearly spherodial and have a rough coat.

Mysore Cardamon, the second best grade, consists mostly of "shorts" that are ovoid-oblong, cream colored with nearly smooth surface and con-

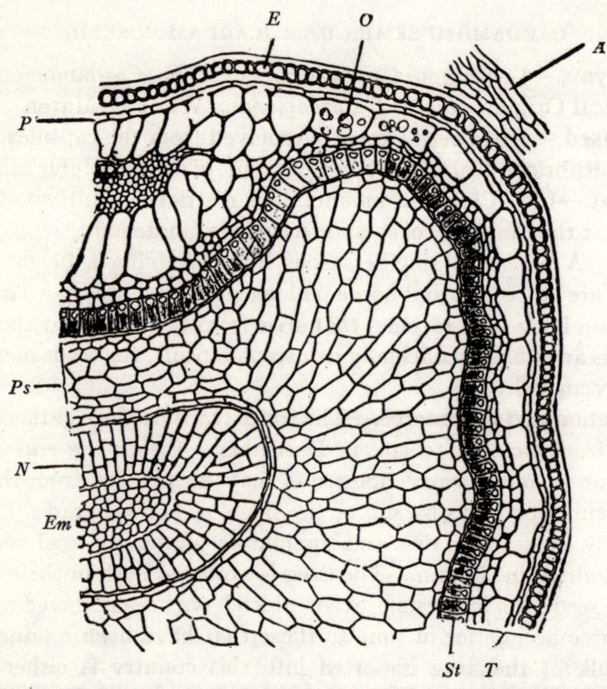

FIG. 43.—Transverse section of Cardamon Seed. Arillus (*A*); epidermis (*E*); parenchyma (*P*); oil cells containing oil globules (*O*); testa from outer integument (*T*); stone cells (*St*); with greatly thickened inner and radial walls, many containing a nodule of silica; perisperm (*Ps*); endosperm (*N*); embryo (*Em*). (*After Tschirch and Oesterle.*)

taining 9–12 seeds which are not as pungent as those of Malabar Cardamon.

The following varieties, obtained from various other species, have an inferior flavor:

Ceylon Cardamon, yielded by *Elettaria Cardamomun* var. *β major* Smith, consists of the fruits of wild plants. These are shrivelled, up to 40 mm. long, dark gray-brown, display a beak about 15 mm. in length and possess a slightly bitter taste. Used as a source of oil of cardamon.

Round Cardamon, from *Amomum Cardamomum*. L of Siam and Java, and *A. globosum* Loureiro, of China, is globular to globular-ovate; up to 15 mm. in diameter with seeds having a camphoraceous taste.

Bengal Cardamon, from *Amomum aromaticum* Roxburgh, has 9 wings near the summit of the capsule. Its seeds are about 3 mm. long and possess an aromatic, camphoraceous taste.

Winged Java Cardamon, from *A. maximum* Roxburgh, has 9–12 wings that extend from base to summit.

The U.S. Dept. of Agriculture requires that Cardamon fruits contain 64 per cent. of sound seeds and that Cardamon seed contain not more than 8 per cent. of total ash, nor more than 3 per cent. of ash insoluble in hydrochloric acid.

Physical Characteristics of Seeds.—These are mostly agglutinated in small groups by the adhering membranous aril, the individual seeds, oblong-ovoid, 3–4 sided, 4 mm. or less in length, 3 mm. or less in diameter, prominently longitudinally grooved on one side; gray, red, or brown in color, the surface being transversely furrowed and tuberculated; internally whitish, exhibiting a small reniform cavity containing an embryo; odor aromatic; taste aromatic and pungent.

Microscopical Characteristics.—Transverse sections of the seed show the following tissues passing from periphery toward the center: Fig. 43.

1. *Arillus*, a loosely attached membrane of tangentially elongated thin-walled cells.

2. *Spermoderm*, consisting of (*a*) an outer layer of epidermal cells with thickened angles, (*b*) a layer of pigment cells with brownish tannin contents, (*c*) a layer of large clear cells containing the volatile oil of cardamon, (*d*) a layer or two of thin-walled, tangentially elongated parenchyma cells and (*e*) a layer of brown, greatly thickened stone cells with minute triangular lumen near outer wall. Many of these contain a small nodule of silica.

3. *Perisperm*, a broad zone consisting of an outer layer of small aleurone cells loaded with aleurone grains and many layers of polygonal cells loaded with masses of minute spheroidal and polygonal starch, each grain of which is 1μ to 4μ in diameter. In about the center of many of these masses one or more crystals of calcium oxalate occur.

4. *Endosperm*, a small zone surrounding the central embryo. Both of these regions are composed of very small, thin-walled cells containing aleurone grains and fixed oil.

Powdered Drug.—Brown. Numerous fragments of seed coat with dark brown, polygonal cells, as observed in surface view; very numerous fragments of perisperm and endosperm, the cells filled with small starch grains from 1 to 4μ in diameter or containing one or more prisms of calcium oxalate from 10 to 25μ in diameter; few spiral tracheæ and accompanying sclerenchyma fibers.

Constituents.—Volatile oil (4 to 5 per cent.), fixed oil, starch, protein and calcium oxalate.

Uses.—Carminative and flavoring agent.

Adulterants.—Cardamon capsules are chiefly adulterated with immature fruits, mouldy or insect-infested fruits and Cardamon "Splits" (partially opened fruits). The principal adulterants of Cardamon Seed are small pebbles and seeds of *Amomum* species.

MARANTACEÆ (ARROWROOT FAMILY)

Perennial herbs chiefly of tropical climes with fleshy rhizomes or tubers rich in starch content The leaves are radical and cauline, usually long petioled, with a sheathing base and pulvinus at the summit of the petiole. The inflorescence is a panicle or raceme bearing irregular trimerous flowers with a one celled ovary. Calcium oxalate occurs in the form of rod-shaped crystals.

AMYLUM MARANTÆ (ARROWROOT STARCH)

Synonyms.—Arrowroot, West India-, Jamaica-, Bermuda- and St. Vincent Arrowroot, Maranta Starch.

Botanical Origin.—*Maranta arundinacea*, L.

Habitat.—West Indies and northern part of South America.

Plant.—A perennial herb with a long, thick, fleshy rhizome growing to the height of 2–6 feet. The leaves are green, pubescent beneath, ovate-oblong to ovate-lanceolate with acute apex and rounded base. The flowers are white.

Production and Commerce.—The rhizomes are gathered from plants cultivated chiefly in Bermuda and the West Indies, washed, beaten into a pulp and mixed with water and the starch separated by passing through copper sieves. The starch is then dried and placed in kegs which are exported from Bermuda and St. Vincent.

Description.—In whitish masses or granules up to 6 mm. in diameter (Bermuda) or 20 mm. (St. Vincent), velvety when rubbed between the fingers; starch grains ovoid, ellipsoidal, pear shaped or broadly spindle shaped from 10–65μ in diameter, hilum in center or toward broader end of grain and in the form of a transverse or two curved cleft resembling the wing of a bird in flight; lamellæ concentric and excentric but not as distinct as potato starch. Polarization crosses distinct; the grains show a marked play of colors with the selenite plate.

Uses.—Maranta starch is employed as a nutrient in dietary preparations for infants and convalescents, also as an ingredient in certain brands of ice cream.

Allied Products.—The term arrowroot has been applied to a number of other starches. East Indian Arrowroot represents the starch obtained from *Curcuma angustifolia* and *C. leucorhiza* (Fam. *Zingiberaceæ*). Brazilian Arrowroot is the starch obtained from the Sweet Potato, *Ipomoea Batatas* (Fam. *Convolvulaceæ*) or from *Manihot utilissima* (Fam. *Euphorbiaceæ*). Queensland Arrowroot is the starch obtained from *Canna edulis* and other species of *Canna*. Tahiti Arrowroot is the starch obtained from *Tacca pinnatifida* (Fam. *Taccaceæ*). Portland Arrowroot represents starch prepared from various species of *Arum* (Fam. *Araceæ*).

ORCHIDACEÆ (ORCHID FAMILY)

Perennial herbs of terrestrial or terrestrial saprophytic or epiphytic growth, having grotesque flowers. Roots fibrous to tuberous, often saprophytic in relation, or aerial with velamen. Stems and branches upright, in epiphytic types, often forming pseudobulbs. Leaves alternate, entire, parallel-veined, sheathing at base, rarely reduced to yellowish or pale scales in saprophytes. Flowers irregular, usually attractive, entomophilous, arranged in elongated spikes or racemes, trimerous. Sepals, 3 usually similar; petals 3 of which 2 often resemble sepals, third is variously, often greatly, modified and fused with 2 outer petaloid stamens as a labellum or lighting-board for insects. Third stamen of outer whorl fertile (*Orchideæ*) or a barren knob (*Cypripediæ*); pollen of fertile anther agglutinate as pollinia. Three stamens of inner circle barren and petaloid or one absent (*Cypripediæ*). Stamens all epigynous and often 3 are fused with the style as gynandrium. Carpels 3, syncarpous, with inferior, 3- rarely 4-, one (usually)-celled ovary. Fruit a capsule, 3 valved and one-celled. Seeds minute, abundant and wind disseminated.

VANILLA N.F. (VANILLA)

Synonyms.—Vanilla Bean; *Ger.* Fructus Vanillæ; *Fr.* Vanille.

Botanical Origin.—*Vanilla planifolia* Andrews.

Part Used.—The cured, full-grown, unripe fruit.

Standard of Assay.—Not less than 12 per cent. extractive yielded to dilute alcohol.

Habitat.—In damp woods and forests of eastern Mexico.

Plant.—*Vanilla planifolia* is a perennial, climbing epiphyte which arises from soil roots by means of a fleshy, dark-green, succulent stem that attaches itself to the trunks and branches of trees by means of aerial rootlets. The leaves arise from the nodes of the stem in alternate fashion. They are ovate to ovate-lanceolate in shape, dark green and fleshy. The inflorescence is an axillary raceme bearing pale yellowish-green flowers. The fruit is a unilocular capsule containing numerous minute blackish-brown seeds and a blackish-brown pulp.

Production and Commerce.—In the eastern provinces of Mexico the Vanilla plants are mostly cultivated from cuttings or seeds. In order to secure a good crop of fruits, artificial pollination is practiced, this work being done chiefly by women who use a bamboo ladder to reach the flowers and a feather with which to carry the pollen from the male to the female plant. The plants bear fruit the third year and continue until about 35 or 40 years old. The fruits are gathered in autumn as they commence to turn yellow. They are placed in heaps in sheds protected from rain and allowed to undergo a partial fermentation. They are then exposed to the

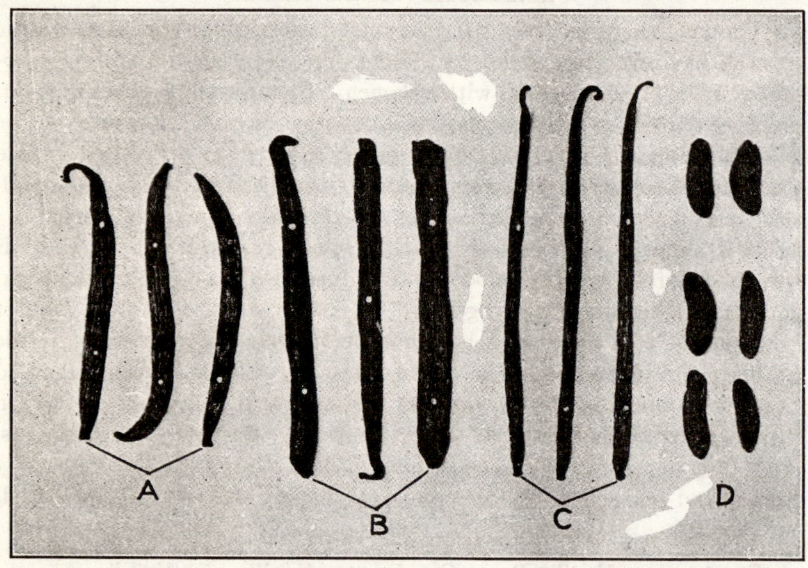

FIG. 44.—*A*, Tahiti Vanilla; *B*, Pompona Vanilla; *C*, Mexican Vanilla; *D*, Tonka seeds, × ⅓. (*Photographed by W. J. Stoneback.*)

sun or artificial heat and repeatedly sweated for a month or longer until a chestnut-brown color is noticed and the odorous principle, vanillin, has developed. They are then sun-dried for about 2 months, assorted according to length, coated with oil, tied in bundles of 80 to 120 beans with thread, wrapped, and shipped to the markets in tin cases, each holding about 40 pounds. The cultivation of the Vanilla plant also takes place in the Isle of Reunion, the Seychelles, Java, Madagascar, Hawaii, Tahiti and Guadeloupe. Mexican beans are considered the best (see description), attaining a length of 30 to 35 cm. This variety is principally consumed in Mexico and the United States. Bourbon or Reunion Vanilla, from the Isle of Reunion, is about two-thirds as long as the Mexican variety, blacker in

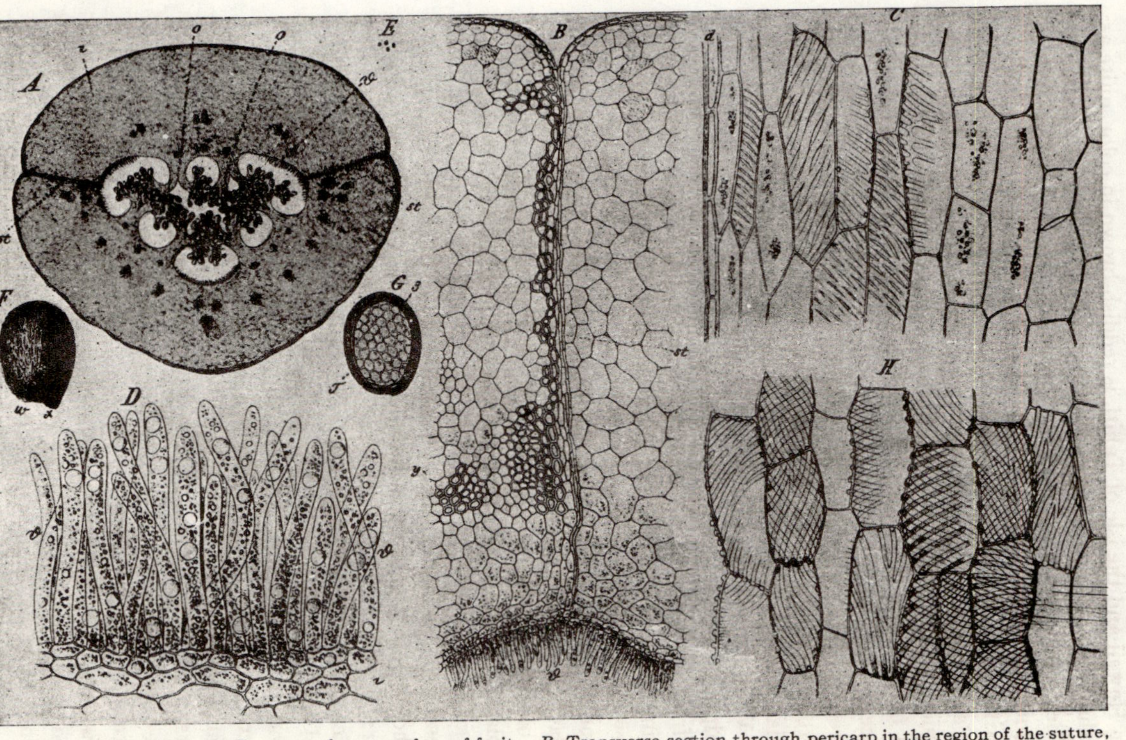

FIG. 45.—*Vanilla.* *A*, Transversely cut surface of fruit. *B*, Transverse section through pericarp in the region of the suture, × 40. *C*, Radial-longitudinal section of the outer portion of the pericarp showing parenchyma cells in mesocarp with reticulate markings and slits, × 190. *D*, Section through inner portion of pericarp showing balsam hairs, × 290. *E*, Seeds. *F*, Seed, × 65. *G*, the same, longitudinally cut. *H*, Tangential section through the outer portion of the pericarp showing spiral parenchyma, × 190. *E*, Epidermis, *d*; fibrovascular bundle, *y*; balsam hairs, *d*; pericarp, *i*; micropyle, *w*; hilum, *x*; placenta, *o*; seed coat, *j*; endosperm, 3; sutures, *st*. (*After Berg.*)

color, has a somewhat tonka-like odor, and its surface shows numerous needle-shaped crystals. The crop goes chiefly to France. Tahiti Vanilla, grown in Hawaii and the isle of Tahiti, is reddish-brown in color, quite as long as the Mexican, but broad in the middle and tapering toward either end. The capsules are twisted in the lower portion. The odor is unpleasant which makes the variety unsuitable for flavoring.

Mauritius Vanilla, from the Seychelles, consists of cylindrical pods about 15 cm. in length, lighter in color than the Mexican and having but a faint odor. The product goes chiefly to London. Vanilla Splits represent the fruits which are picked when more mature and show marked dehiscence.

The present commercial supplies of vanilla are shipped to this country mainly from Mexico City, Mexico, from Tahiti, and Madagascar.

Vanilla should be preserved in a cool place where it is not apt to become brittle. Vanilla which has become brittle should not be used.

Description.—Mexican Vanilla occurs in the form of linear, flattened capsules from 15 to 35 cm. in length and from 5–7 mm. in breadth; summits ending in flat circular scars; gradually tapering toward both ends, bases curved or hooked with a circular scar; externally blackish-brown, longitudinally wrinkled, moist-glossy; frequently with narrow, elliptical or irregular, somewhat wrinkled, dark-brown patches of cork; soft leathery and flexible; one-locular, containing a blackish-brown pulp with many minute blackish-brown seeds therein imbedded. The odor is aromatic and the taste agreeable.

Microscopical Characteristics.—Transverse sections of the capsules of Vanilla show the following characteristics, passing from periphery toward the center:

1. **Epicarp,** consisting of *epidermis* and *hypodermis.* The *epidermis* consists of a layer of thick-walled epidermal cells whose outer walls show the presence of a thin yellow cuticle. Stomata are present in this tissue. The epidermal cells contain protoplasm and brownish bodies. Some also contain small prisms of calcium oxalate and a few, vanillin crystals. The *hypodermis* is composed of one to several layers of collenchymatic cells with dark-colored contents. Its cells are somewhat larger than those of the epidermis and thicker walled.

2. **Mesocarp,** a broad region of somewhat loosely arranged large, thin-walled parenchyma cells, becoming smaller in the inner zone of this region. Most of these cells contain brownish contents and oily globules but some possess long raphides of calcium oxalate. Some of the cells of this region possess long oblique slit-like pores, others broad, spiral, band-like thickenings. An interrupted circle of fibrovascular bundles, each showing a central phloem more or less surrounded by a few spiral or

pitted tracheæ will be seen coursing through the mesocarp. Surrounding each bundle will be noted a circle of lignified sclerenchyma fibers. If the section be mounted in phloroglucin solution (5 per cent.) and a drop of strong sulphuric acid is added, a carmine-red color will be observed, showing the presence of vanillin in this region.

3. **Endocarp,** an irregular line of inner epidermal cells which is differentiated into two regions, the interplacental region and the placental region. The interplacental (inner) epidermis shows its cells elongated into numerous thin-walled glandular hairs which contain an abundance of balsam; the placental region covers the six bifid *placentæ* which extend into the cavity of the capsule. Its (inner) epidermis is composed of mucilaginous cells.

4. **Seeds.**—These are minute blackish to brownish-red bodies attached to the placental twigs of the placentæ. They are embedded in a dark-colored balsamic fluid secreted by the glandular hairs of the endocarp. Some of them may have been torn off in cutting the section. If some of these are mounted in chloral hydrate solution and examined they will be found to possess a strongly reticulate seed coat.

Powdered Drug.—The color is blackish-brown. The histological elements to be observed include fragments of the interplacental region characterized by unicellular glandular hairs containing globules of balsam, sclerenchymatous fibers with thick lignified walls and simple pores, tracheæ with pitted or spiral markings, polygonal stone cells of seed coat, fragments of parenchyma of the mesocarp with simple pores, or long oblique slit-like walls, or broad spiral bands, and calcium oxalate crystals in raphides up to 400μ in length and in monoclinic prisms up to 35μ long. Upon treating the powder with phloroglucin solution and sulphuric acid it takes on a carmine-red color, due to the presence of vanillin.

Constituents.—Vanillin (U.S.P.), (an odoriferous principle) 1.5 to 3 per cent., balsam, resin, sugar, fixed oil, etc. Vanillin occurs in the balsamic fluid formed in the hairs of the endocarp. This fluid is secreted into the cavity of the fruit and, upon curing, permeates the whole fruit, the vanillin crystallizing out in the form of needles. Vanillin also occurs in Benzoin, Balsam of Peru, Balsam of Tolu, Asafœtida and other drugs. It is produced commercially from Eugenol.

Use.—Flavoring agent.

Adulterant.—The powdered drug has frequently been adulterated with powdered Tonka, the powdered ripe seeds of *Coumarouna odorata* (Dutch Tonka) and *C. oppositifolia* (English Tonka). Tonka contains an aromatic principle known as coumarin, fixed oil, starch and aleurone. It may readily be detected microscopically in powdered Vanilla both by its spheroidal, eroded starch grains, which range from 4–8μ in diameter, and by examination of the crystals from a sublimate of a suspected sample on the thermo-stage. Coumarin melts at from 54–56°C. while vanillin melts at between 80–82°C.

Allied Drugs.—Vanillons, the fruits of wild plants of *V. planifolia*, are up to 12 cm. long and from 1.5 to 2.5 cm. in diameter, more or less triangular in outline, tapering toward both ends, reddish-brown to dark brown in color, often showing transverse markings and dehiscence. They possess a heliotrope-like odor, due to a phenol aldehyde, heliotrôpin. These fruits are employed in the flavoring of tobacco and manufacture of certain sachets.

Pompona Vanilla, from Guadeloupe, consists of the fruits of *Vanilla pompona*, which resemble Vanillons in appearance and Tahiti Vanilla in their disagreeable taste.

CYPRIPEDIUM N.F. (CYPRIPEDIUM)

Synonyms.—Lady Slipper Root, Moccasin-Plant or Flower, American Valerian, Yellow Ladies' Slipper; *Ger.* Gelbfrauenschuhwurzel; *Fr.* Racine de Cyprièpde jaune.

Botanical Origin.—*Cypripedium hirsutum* Miller, *Cypripediun pubescens* Willdenow, and *Cypripedium parviflorum* Salisbury.

Part Used.—The dried rhizome and roots.

Limit of Impurities.—3 per cent. of other parts of the same plant or other foreign organic matter.

Ash.—Not more than 6 per cent. acid-insoluble.

Habitat.—In woods and wet mossy places of United States and Canada.

Plants.—*Cypripedium hirsutum* or Showy Lady Slipper is a perennial orchid having ovate, acute leaves, round-ovate, white sepals, and a white saccate lip, pinkish-purple in front. A tuft of whitish hairs, is present in the throat.

Cypripedium pubescens or Common Yellow Lady Slipper possesses ovate, acute, green leaves, greenish-yellow, ovate-lanceolate sepals spotted and streaked with madder-purple and a golden-yellow saccate lip.

Cypripedium parviflorum or Small Yellow Lady Slipper somewhat resembles *C. pubescens* species but possesses a smaller flower of a bright yellow color.

Production and Commerce.—The rhizome and roots are dug up after the plant has flowered, washed, and dried. The commercial supplies are obtained from wild plants growing in North Carolina, Kentucky, Virginia, Indiana, Michigan and Missouri.

Description.—Rhizome horizontal, curved, 3–10 cm. in length and 4–10 mm. in width, orange-brown to dark brown, the upper side showing numerous circular, cup-shaped scars, densely covered below with wiry roots that vary from 3–15 cm. in length; fracture of rhizome short, white, that of roots somewhat fibrous; odor heavy and distinct; taste sweetish, bitter and pungent.

Powdered Drug.—Yellowish brown. Calcium oxalate in raphides up to 70μ long, frequently occurring as acicular (isolated) crystals; starch simple, spheroidal or more or less angular, up to 14μ in diameter, or compound; spiral, scalariform or pitted tracheæ; sclerenchyma fibers long, thin-walled and mostly lignified; tracheids few; fragments of thick-

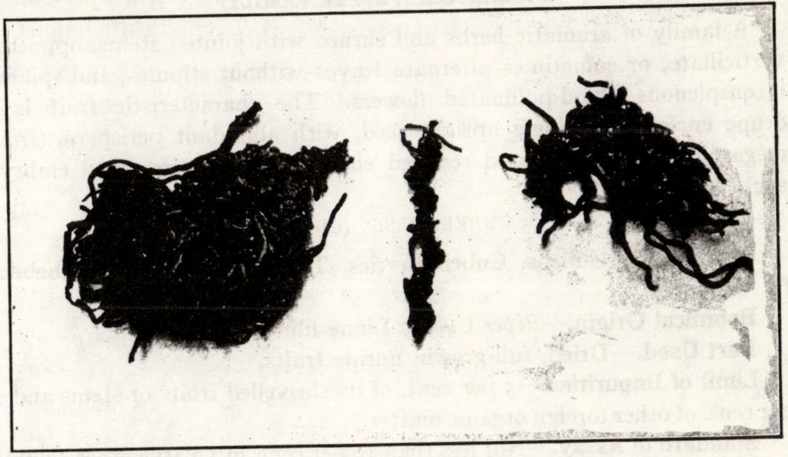

FIG. 46.—Cypripedium, × 1/12. (*Photograph by Stoneback.*)

walled parenchyma with simple pores, with starch, calcium oxalate or resin content.

Constituents.—Volatile oil, a bitter glucoside, tannin, gallic acid. resins, starch, calcium oxalate, etc.

Use.—Antispasmodic.

CLASS B—DICOTYLEDONEÆ

Plants having the following characteristics:

Two-seed leaves (cotyledons) in embryo.

Netted-veined leaves.

Stems, and roots of secondary growth with open collateral fibrovascular bundles, in stems, radially arranged about pith.

Exogenous stems.

Medullary rays present.

Cambium.

Roots developing secondary structure.

Flowers tetramerous or pentamerous (parts of each whorl, 4 or 5 or multiple thereof).

SUB-CLASS A—ARCHICHLAMYDEÆ

Those dictoyledonous plants in which the petals are distinct and separate from one another or are entirely wanting. That group of the Archichlamydeæ whose flowers show the absence of petals and frequently of sepals is called the *Apetalæ*. The group whose plants have flowers showing the parts of their corolla (petals) separate and distinct is called the Choripetalæ.

PIPERACEÆ (PEPPER FAMILY)

A family of aromatic herbs and shrubs with jointed stems, opposite, verticillate, or sometimes alternate leaves without stipules, and spiked, inconspicuous, wind-pollinated flowers. The characteristic fruit is a drupe enclosing a single upright seed, with abundant perisperm (from megasporangial tissue) and reduced endosperm (from matured embryo sac).

CUBEBA U.S.P. (CUBEB)

Synonyms.—Cubebs, Cubeb Berries, Tailed Pepper; *Ger.* Kubeben; *Fr.* Cubèbe.

Botanical Origin.—*Piper Cubeba* Linné filius.

Part Used.—Dried, full-grown, unripe fruits.

Limit of Impurities.—5 per cent. of its shrivelled fruits or stems and 2 per cent. of other foreign organic matter.

Standard of Assay.—Not less than 10 per cent. of volatile ether-soluble extractive.

Habitat.—Java, Sumatra and Borneo. Cultivated in Java, Sumatra, Ceylon and West Indies.

Plant.—A climbing perennial vine having a woody, jointed stem that roots at the joints and bears alternate, coriaceous, petiolate leaves and diœcious flowers in spikes; fruit a globular drupe, which when young is sessile but as maturation proceeds is gradually elevated on a slender stalk (*thecaphore*) formed by a basal development of the pericarp of the fruit.

Production and Commerce.—The plants are grown on special and coffee plantations, being planted against shade trees for support. The fruits, numbering up to 50 or more on each spike, are gathered while still green but full grown and dried in the sun. They are then taken to Batavia and Singapore from whence the commercial supplies are exported in bags. The article used in this country either comes direct from Singapore, Dutch East Indies, or through London and Amsterdam.

Description.—Drupe globular from 3–6 mm. in diameter, with a straight, slender stem-like portion up to 7 mm. in length; apex with remains of 4 stigmas, outer surface brownish, grayish or bluish-black and coarsely reticulate; one chambered, one seeded; the reddish-brown seed

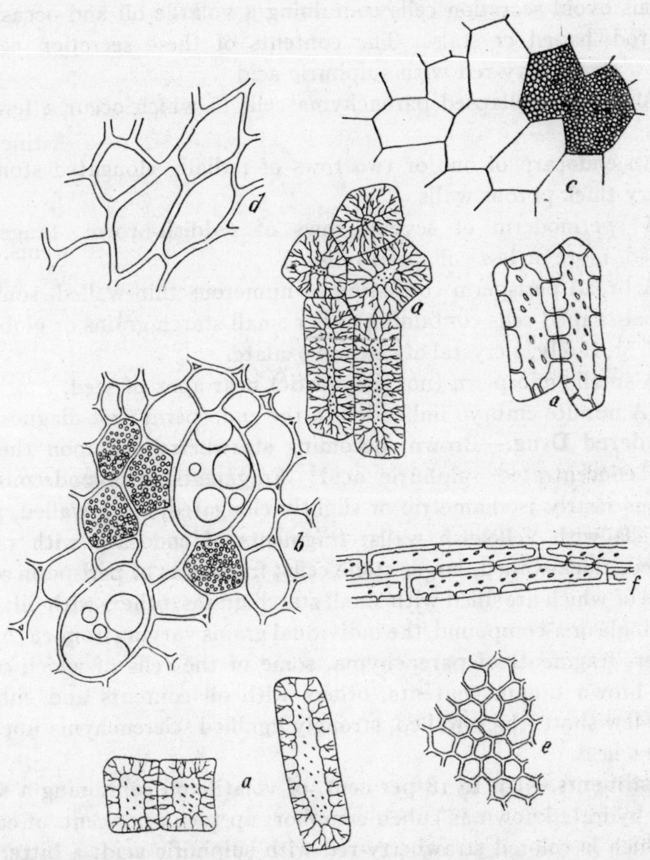

FIG. 47.—Powdered Cubeba. (*a*) Stone cells; (*b*) endosperm, with oil globules and proteid granules; (*c*) cells of perisperm; (*d*) parenchyma of stalk; (*e*) epidermal cells, vertical view; (*f*) tracheids. (*After Schneider.*)

attached to base of pericarp; odor aromatic; taste characteristically aromatic and pungent.

Microscopical Characteristics.—Passing from periphery toward the center, the following structures are noted in microscopic sections:

1. An epicarp of tabular epidermal cells having thick, wavy, outer walls and olive-green contents; beneath this

2. A hypodermis of two rows of thick-walled stone cells with yellowish, porous walls, the inner row being interrupted by intervening parenchyma cells.

3. A few layers of collapsed cells.

4. A broad zone of parenchyma cells, scattered among which are numerous ovoid secretion cells containing a volatile oil and occasionally short, rod-shaped crystals. The contents of these secretion cells are colored a strawberry-red with sulphuric acid.

5. A zone or collapsed parenchyma cells in which occur a few small bundles.

6. An endocarp of one or two rows of radially elongated stone cells with very thick porous walls.

7. A spermoderm of several rows of reddish-brown, tangentially elongated, more or less collapsed cells.

8. A broad perisperm consisting of numerous thin-walled, somewhat polygonal-shaped cells containing either small starch grains or globules of fixed oil, or, rarely, a crystal of calcium oxalate.

9. A small endosperm (not diagnostic) near apex of seed.

10. A minute embryo imbedded in the endosperm (not diagnostic).

Powdered Drug.—Brown, becoming strawberry-red upon the addition of concentrated sulphuric acid. Fragments of hypodermis with numerous nearly isodiametric or slightly elongated, thick-walled, porous stone cells with yellowish walls; fragments of endocarp with radially elongated, thick-walled, larger stone cells; fragments of perisperm some of the cells of which are filled with small starch grains, others with oil; starch grains single or 2-compound, the individual grains varying from 2μ to 12μ in diameter; fragments of parenchyma, some of the cells of which contain reddish-brown tannin contents, others with oil contents and suberised walls; a few short, thick-walled, strongly lignified sclerenchyma fibers and spiral tracheæ.

Constituents.—Up to 18 per cent. of volatile oil containing a sesquiterpene hydrate known as cubeb camphor; up to 3.5 per cent. of cubebic acid, which is colored strawberry-red with sulphuric acid; a bitter principle called cubebin which is colored cherry-red with sulphuric acid; resins, fixed oil, gum and starch.

Uses.—Diuretic, expectorant and genito-urinary antiseptic.

Adulterants and Substitutes.—(1) Fruits of *Piper ribesioides* which are light gray to dark brown, 5 to 8 mm. in diameter, have long, stem-like portions up to 14 mm. in length, isodiametric or nearly isodiametric stone cells in the endocarp, and give a brownish coloration with sulphuric acid. (2) Fruits of *Piper cubela* var. *rinæ badak* which are grayish, 3 to 6 mm. in diameter, with stem-like portion about 5 mm. in length; have stone cells scattered through parenchyma and give a dark brown coloration with sulphuric acid. (3) Fruits of other allied species of *Piper*, all of which thus far examined give a greenish to brown coloration upon crushing and adding sulphuric acid. (4) Superfluous rachis and stems. (5) Fruits of *Embelia ribes*, an Indian tree belonging to the *Myrsinaceæ*. These resemble somewhat black pepper drupes but contain embelic acid, which, in alcoholic solution is colored red with ammonia.

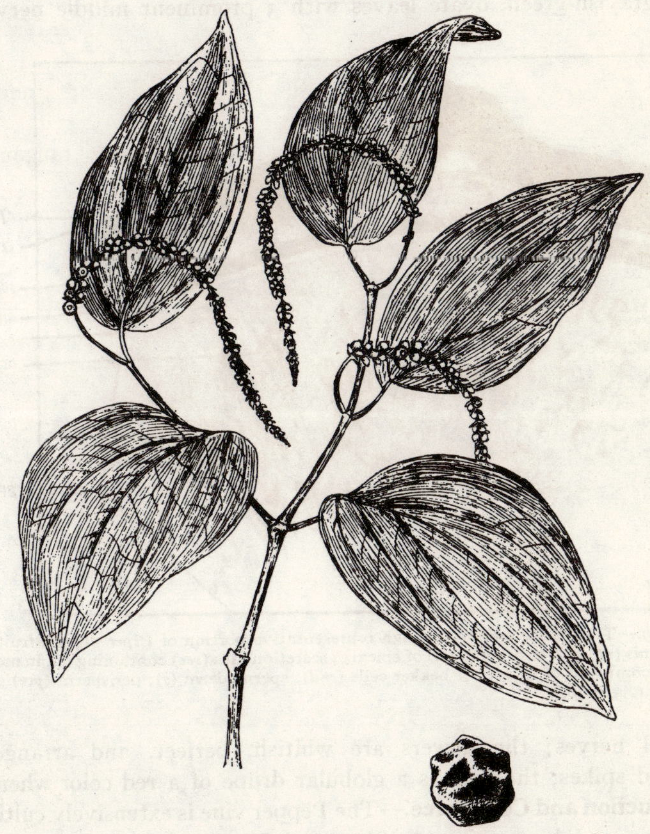

FIG. 48.—*Piper nigrum*—Branch and fruit. (*Sayre.*)

PIPER N.F. (PEPPER)

Synonyms.—Black Pepper, Pepper Corn; *Ger.* Schwarzer Pfeffer; *Fr.* Poivre noir.

Botanical Origin.—*Piper nigrum* L.

Part Used.—Dried unripe fruit.

Limit of Impurities.—2 per cent. of stems or other foreign matter.

U.S. Dept. of Agriculture Standard of Purity.—Circular 136 specifies not less than 6.75 per cent. of non-volatile ether extract, not more than 7 per cent. total ash and 1.5 per cent. acid-insoluble ash.

Habitat.—Malabar and Travencore. Cultivated in Singapore, Penang, Ceylon, Siam, India, Johore, Sumatra, Rioux-Lingga Archipelago, South America and the West Indies.

Plant.—A perennial climbing or trailing woody vine that has coriaceous, grayish-green, ovate leaves with 3 prominent middle nerves and

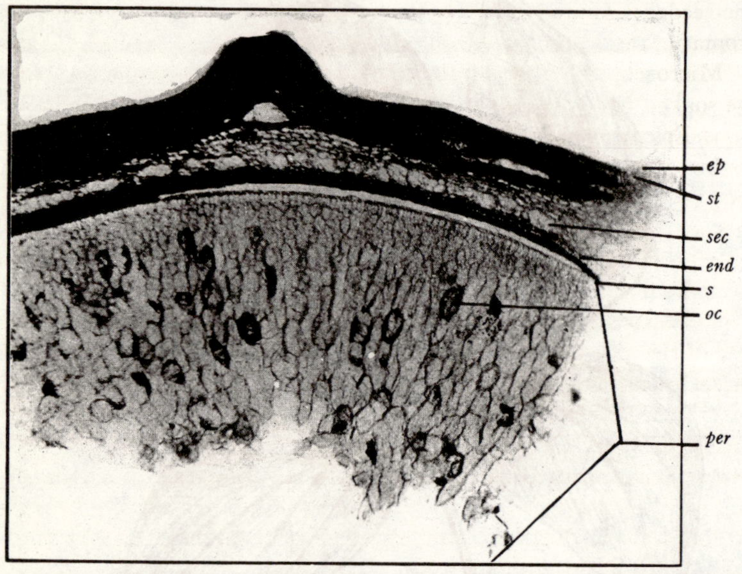

FIG. 49.—Transverse section through representative portion of *Piper nigrum* fruit, showing epidermis (*ep*) and stone cells (*st*) of epicarp; secretion sacs (*sec*) containing oil, in mesocarp; endocarp, composed of a layer of beaker cells (*end*); spermoderm (*s*); perisperm (*per*) containing oleoresin cells (*oc*).

2 lateral nerves; the flowers are whitish, perfect, and arranged on elongated spikes; the fruit is a globular drupe of a red color when ripe.

Production and Commerce.—The Pepper vine is extensively cultivated in Singapore, Johore, Sumatra, Siam and Penang, trees being planted to provide the requisite support and shade for its growth. The fruits are developed on spikes which are cut from the vines as soon as the lowest drupes on the axis begin to change in color from green to red. The entire spikes bearing unripe fruits are then dried in the sun or over fires, after which the fruits are separated from the rachis, garbled and placed in bags for shipment. A number of grades of black pepper are found on the markets. These are named after the ports of shipment or regions of growth, viz.: Singapore, Tellicherry, Siam, Penang, Acheen, Trang, etc. The best grades are fire-dried and possess a smoky odor and taste. Of these Singapore appears to be in most esteem. Most of the drug imported into the United States comes from Batavia, Singapore and Penang through London.

Acheen pepper represents the poorest grade. It consists of small, light-weighted fruits often admixed with pepper shells, dirt and small stones.

Physical Characteristics.—In entire nearly globular drupes, 6 mm. or less in diameter; grayish, brownish or black; surface coarsely reticulate; one-seeded; seed nearly white, hollow and adhering to the pericarp; odor aromatic; taste aromatic and strongly pungent.

Microscopical Characteristics.—Transverse sections made through the soaked fruit show the following structural peculiarities:

1. **Epicarp,** consisting of (*a*) an outer layer of polygonal cells having a distinct cuticle and containing dark-brown to blackish contents, and (*b*) a zone varying in thickness of from 2 to 3 layers and composed of thin-walled parenchyma cells intermingled with greatly thickened isodiametric to radially elongated stone cells. This region is termed by some authors the hypodermis.

2. **Mesocarp,** a comparatively broad zone constituting the greater area of the pericarp. The outer 7 or 8 layers of cells are for the most part parenchymatous and contain small starch grains and chlorophyll. Scattered here and there among these cells will be noted larger secretion sacs with suberised walls and oil or resin contents. The next several layers of cells appear more or less compressed and it is through this region that fibrovascular bundles ramify. Beneath the region of compressed cells will be noticed a layer of large oil cells having suberised walls and then a zone of two layers of small parenchyma cells.

3. **Endocarp,** consisting of a single layer of stone cells ("beaker cells") whose radial and inner walls are more strongly lignified than the outer ones.

4. **Spermoderm,** consisting of 2 or 3 layers of compressed, elongated cells beneath which is a pigment layer containing a dark-brown tannin substance that takes the blue color with ferric chloride solution.

5. **Perisperm,** of 3 regions, viz.:

(*a*) An outer layer of clear thin-walled cells called the "hyaline layer."

(*b*) An aleurone zone of 2 or 3 layers of cells containing protein granules.

(*c*) A broad zone of radially elongated, reserve parenchyma cells containing masses of minute starch grains imbedded in protein substance. The individual grains are more or less polyhedral in outline and have a diameter of 1–6μ. Scattered among the cells of this region are somewhat rounded oleoresin cells containing globules of oil, masses of resin and piperine. The last-mentioned substance can best be studied by mounting sections in alcohol, then allowing the alcohol to evaporate and remounting in water.

In the center of this zone a cavity 1 mm. or more in diameter will be noted.

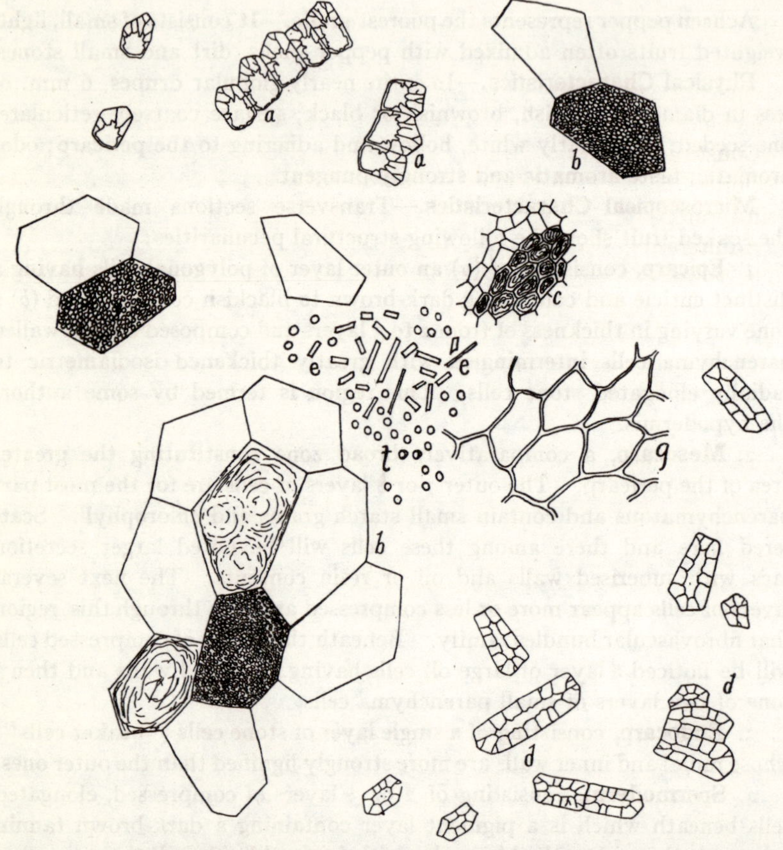

FIG. 50.—Powdered Black Pepper. (*a*) Stone cells with unequally thickened walls. (*b*) perisperm tissue with starch and resin; (*c*) epidermal cells; (*d*) typical stone cells; (*e*) crystals of piperin; (*f*) starch granules; (*g*) pericarp parenchyma. (*After Schneider.*)

6. **Endosperm,** a very small region of thin-walled cells and only seen when sections are cut through the upper part of the seed.

7. **Embryo,** very minute and imbedded in the endosperm.

Sections mounted in sulphuric acid display a deep red color due to piperine.

Powdered Drug.—Dark gray. The chief diagnostic elements in the ground or powdered drug are (1) compact masses of minute starch grains, composed of individual grains, rounded to angular in outline and 1–6μ in diameter, and oval aggregates; (2) stone cells of epicarp, varying from isodiametric to more or less columnar to irregular shaped with thick porous walls and reddish-brown contents, and (3) horseshoe-shaped stone cells of endocarp ("beaker cells") having usually thin outer walls and thickened radial and inner walls. Other histological elements include fragments containing the oil cells with brownish suberised walls, yellowish oil globules and needle-shaped piperine crystals. The latter frequently separate from oil globules.

Constituents.—A crystalline, feebly basic principle called piperine, a colorless liquid alkaloid—piperidine, a yellowish volatile oil, a pungent resin termed chavicin; starch and proteins.

Adulterants.—Whole black pepper has been adulterated with pepper hulls, consisting of the broken outer portions of the pericarp of the ripe fruit, a by-product in the preparation of white pepper. These are grayish-black in color and when sectioned show numerous characteristic stone cells of the epicarp.

Acheen Peppers (see Commercial).

Powdered black pepper has been adulterated with the following substances; Ground nutshells, buckwheat hulls, cocoa shells, leguminous seeds, pepper hulls, pepper stems, exhausted spices, cereals, mustard hulls, olive pits, flaxseed and sawdust. Charcoal has been added to light colored, fraudulent mixtures of pepper and adulterants, to bring up the color and capsicum to give necessary pungency.

Arancini, the small fruits of the sweet orange. These are about 100 mm. in diameter and have been recently found in ground form as an admixture in powdered black pepper. Their presence may be detected by treating the suspected powder on a slide with 4 per cent. sodium hydroxide solution, washing with water, adding a drop of Congo-red solution and removing excess of stain by washing with water. Red-colored cells and closely arranged spiral tracheæ, the latter appearing as a scalariform mass, indicate arancini.

Allied Products.—*White pepper* is the dried mature berry (more properly, drupe) of *Piper nigrum* L. from which the outer coating, or the outer and inner coatings have been removed. It contains not less than 7 per cent. of non-volatile ether extract, not less than 52 per cent. of starch, not more than 5 per cent. of crude fiber, not more than 3.5 per cent. of total ash, nor more than 0.3 per cent. of ash insoluble in hydrochloric acid. (U.S. Dept. Agric. Standard.)

Long Pepper is the dried entire spikes of immature fruit of *Piper longum* L., a shrub indigenous to Bengal and the Phillippine Islands and *P. officinarum* C.DC., a shrub indigenous to the Malay Peninsula. These compound fruits are elongated, up to 40 mm. long, about 5 to 7 mm. thick, of a grayish-black color and composed of numerous small immature drupes and bracts imbedded in the axis. Their taste and odor somewhat resembles black pepper but is distinctive and less strong. They contain about 1 per cent. of volatile oil, 6 per cent. of piperine, a pungent resin termed chavicin and starch.

Powdered long pepper has occasionally been found as an adulterant and substitute for powdered black pepper. Its diagnostic elements are large, elongated, porous, sclerenchyma cells of the endocarp, polygonal and rounded starch grains from 2 to 10μ in diameter, and averagely larger than those of black pepper, and masses of starch and chlorophylloid parenchyma from the mesocarp devoid of oil cells. The absence of oil cells and "beaker cells" together with the presence of larger starch grains and typical sclerenchyma cells distinguish this article from powdered black pepper.

MATICO N.F. (MATICO)

Synonyms.—Soldier's Shrub, Pepper Elder; *Ger.* Maticoblätter; *Fr.* Feuilles de Matico.

Part Used.—The dried leaves.

Botanical Origin.—*Piper angustifolium* Ruiz et Pavon.

Limit of Impurities.—5 per cent. of stems, flower spikes or other foreign matter.

Ash.—Not more than 6 per cent. acid-insoluble.

Habitat.—Tropical South America.

Plant.—A shrub attaining a height of 3 m. with stems characterized by large nodes and quadrangular branches. The leaves are short-petioled, alternate and lanceolate. The inflorescence is a long slender spike bearing small yellow flowers and bracts, that are hairy on the margins. The fruit is a small, hard, reddish-brown drupe containing a single albuminous, reddish-brown and reticulate seed.

Description.—The drug generally occurs in matted masses, the leaves being more or less broken. The entire leaves are short-petioled, lanceolate, from 10 to 20 cm. long and from 2 to 5 cm. broad; summit tapering and acute; base unequally cordate; margin crenulate; venation palmate-pinnate; upper surface dark green, scabrous and finely bullate; lower surface pale green, reticulate with prominent yellowish-brown, densely pubescent midrib and veins forming quadrangular meshes; odor aromatic; taste aromatic, pungent, somewhat pepper-like.

Microscopical Characteristics.—The upper epidermis consists of polygonal cells devoid of stomata. The lower epidermis possesses somewhat wavy-walled cells and numerous stomata surrounded by usually 5 neighboring cells. The mesophyll outside of the midrib exhibits a layer of clear, sub-epidermal cells adjacent to the upper epidermis, 2 or 3 layers of palisade cells, showing here and there a spherical internal gland possessing a yellowish oil content, and a spongy parenchyma zone that is marked by the presence of fibrovascular bundles. In many of the cells of this region reddish-brown tannin masses occur, in others raphides or monoclinic prisms of calcium oxalate. The midrib region is somewhat oval in cross section and shows a zone of collenchyma beneath upper and lower epidermis, and fibrovascular bundles arranged in a semicircle. The upper epidermis shows relatively few hairs as compared with the lower. The non-glandular hairs are uniseriate, 6–10 cells, with joints, the terminal cell being pointed. The glandular hairs consist of a unicellular stalk and a unicellular head.

Powdered Drug.—Greenish-yellow. Hairs of non-glandular type 6–10 cells long, jointed and striate, with distinctly pointed end cells; numerous yellowish or reddish masses of oleoresin and resin; fragments of mesophyll containing resin glands and cells with chloroplasts or crystals of calcium oxalate; fragments of epidermis, the lower showing numerous stomata and characteristic neighboring cells; fragments of seeds, occasionally, with reddish-brown reticulated spermoderm.

Adulterants.—The leaves of various other species of *Piper*.

Substitute.—The leaves of *Eupatorium glutinosum* Lam. (*Compositæ*). These differ from Matico in being opposite, longer petioled, with pinnate-reticulate venation, serrate margin and cordate base. The upper surface of the leaves is scabrous and coarsely bullate while the lower surface is woolly, exhibiting many long, twisted, non-glandular hairs and short glandular hairs. If flowers be present they are arranged in flower heads on a panicle of cymes. The fruits are 5-angled, truncate akenes, each with a bristly pappus.

Constituents.—An acrid resin, volatile oil (2 to 3.5 per cent.) containing matico-camphor; bitter principle, artanthic acid, tannin, etc.

Uses.—Aromatic astringent in diarrhœa and genito-urinary diseases, styptic, and stimulant.

KAVA N.F. (KAVA)

Synonyms.—Kava Kava, Methysticum, Ava; *Ger.* Kawakawawurzel.

Botanical Origin.—*Piper methysticum* Forster.

Parts Used.—The dried rhizome and roots.

Purity Rubric.—Not more than 1 per cent. of foreign organic matter.

Habitat.—Sandwich Islands.

Description.—The drug occurs in irregular, transverse, oblique and longitudinal slices of the rhizome up to 20 cm. in length and 10 cm. in width. Pieces showing the knotty crown are soft, light, starchy and spongy, partly scraped and light brown to gray. Portions of stem bases often adhering to this are hollow and woody. Cylindrical segments of tough roots are sometimes present. Externally dark brown or blackish; fracture of thin slices short and mealy and of thick slices, tough and uneven; odor faint, characteristic; taste aromatic slightly bitter and pungent, followed by a sensation of numbness.

Powdered Drug.—Light yellowish-brown. Numerous simple or 2- to 3-compound starch grains, the individual grains being spheroidal or plano-convex and up to 45μ in diameter, many showing radial or triangular central clefts; yellow resin and oil cells; sclerenchyma fibers narrow, with thin lignified walls; tracheæ with scalariform or reticulate markings, up to 150μ broad. Upon treating sections of the drug or powder with alcohol and examining under the microscope, pale yellow crystals of methysticin separate out which take on a violet-red color when concentrated sulphuric acid is added.

Constituents.—Resins, methysticin, pseudomethysticin, yangonin, kavaine (an alkaloid), glucosides, starch, etc.

Uses.—Diuretic and genito-urinary antiseptic.

SALICACEÆ (WILLOW FAMILY)

A family of anemophilous shrubs or trees of temperate or cold regions, including the Willows and Poplars, whose bark often contains bitter principles (salicin, etc.). Leaves alternate, simple, entire, stipulate; stipules rarely green, persistent, usually functioning as winter bub-scales and falling in spring. Inflorescences diœcious spikes, so on separate plants. Staminate spikes forming deciduous catkins of yellowish flowers, pistillate as persistent spikes of green flowers. Flowers of catkins numerous, each of 2 to 5 (Willow) or 6 to 15 (Poplar) stamens in axil of a small bract leaf, sometimes with small nectar knob or girdle at base. Pistillate flowers green, each of a bicarpellate pistil in axil of bract, ovary one-celled with parietal placentation, style simple, stigma bilobed. Fruit a capsule dehiscing longitudinally. Seeds small, exalbuminous, surrounded by a tuft of hairs for dissemination.

Microscopically, the plant axis is characterized by the occurrence of isolated groups of sclerenchyma fibers in the pericycle, the presence of layers of hard and soft bast in the phloem, the superficial development of cork, narrow medullary-rays in the wood and tracheæ with simple pores. In several species of *Populus* stone cells occur in the primary cortex, forming a ring in *P. alba*. In this species stone cells also occur in the hard bast. Calcium oxalate occurs in the form of solitary crystals, crystal-fibers and rosette aggregates. The leaves frequently show stomata on both surfaces with parallel neighboring cells. The epidermis often shows mucilaginous modification of the inner, occasionally the outer wall of its cells. Glandular hairs are absent. Non-glandular hairs are abundant and are unicellular in character. The glucoside salicin U.S.P., occurring in the bark of many species of *Salix* and *Populus*, imparts a red color to sulphuric acid.

POPULI GEMMÆ N.F. (BALSAM POPLAR BUDS)

Synonyms.—Balm of Gilead Buds, Tacamahac, Black Poplar Buds, Willow Poplar Buds.

Botanical Origin.—*Populus balsamifera* Linné (Balsam Poplar), *Populus candicans* Aiton (Balm of Gilead), and *Populus nigra* Linné (Black Poplar).

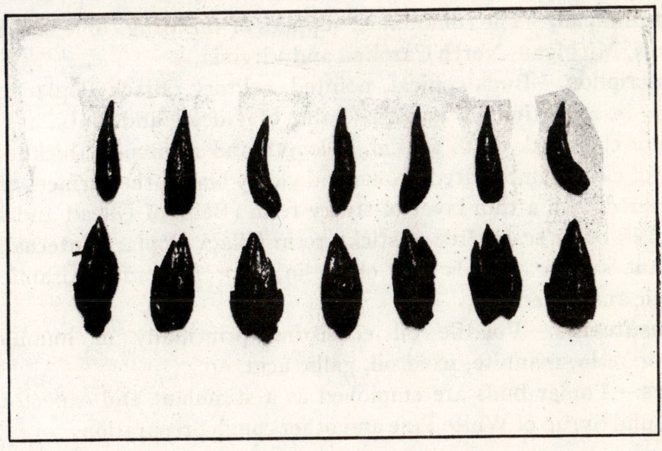

FIG. 51.—Poplar buds, $\times \frac{3}{5}$. (*Photograph by Stoneback.*)

Part Used.—The air-dried, closed winter leaf buds, collected early in the spring.

Purity Rubric.—Not more than 10 per cent. of flower buds and not more than 1 per cent. of acid-insoluble ash.

Habitat.—Balsam Poplar, northern United States and Canada. Black Poplar—Europe. Naturalized in U. S. A.

Plants.—*Populus balsamifera*, commonly known as Balsam Poplar, or Tacamahac, is a tree, pyramidal in shape, which rises to the height of 45 to 90 feet. Its leaves are alternate, deciduous, ovate-lanceolate or cordate-ovate, smooth, serrulate, bright green on upper surface, whitened beneath. Its leaf buds are good-sized, reddish-brown and abundantly covered with fragrant resin. Its branches are ridged below the leaves. Its flowers appear in the early spring before the leaves have opened, and are arranged in long drooping catkins. Its fruits are small pods enclosing seeds covered with a cottony down.

Populus balsamifera var. *candicans* (*P. candicans* Ait.), the true Balm of Gilead, differs from the preceeding species with which it has often been confused by not possessing the pyramidal habit of growth of the Balsam Poplar, its top being broad and spreading and by its leaves being broader and more cordate.

The Black Poplar (*Populus nigra*) is a large spreading tree attaining a height of 80 feet in some localities. Its leaves are deltoid, acute with serrate, glandular margins. Its leaf stalks are compressed. Its buds are very sticky, yellowish-brown and usually more slender than those of the former species.

Commercial.—The commercial supplies of this drug come largely from Missouri, Michigan, North Carolina and Virginia.

Description.—Buds conical, pointed, solitary (Black Poplar) or, solitary or in agglutinated masses (Balm of Gilead and Balsam Poplar), simple or clustered, up to 2.5 cm. in length and 13 mm. in thickness, consisting of closely imbricated brown and glossy scales, the surfaces of which are covered with a thin layer of sticky resin (Balm of Gilead and Balsam Poplar) or outer scales free of sticky resin (Black Poplar); internally with abundant salicin crystals and oleoresin, odor fragrant, balsamic; taste aromatic and bitter.

Constituents.—Volatile oil consisting principally of humulene; a balsamic resin, mannite, fixed oil, gallic acid, etc.

Uses.—Poplar buds are employed as a stimulant and expectorant in Compound Syrup of White Pine and other cough preparations.

CARBO LIGNI U.S.P. (WOOD CHARCOAL)

Synonyms.—Charcoal, Carbo Ligni Pulveratus, Soft Wood Charcoal; *Ger.* Holzkohle; *Fr.* Charbon de bois.

Botanical Origin.—Various soft-wooded genera, mainly *Salix* and *Populus*, *Acer*, and *Tilia*, *e.g.*, the Willow, Poplar, Maple and Linden groups.

Part Used.—The charred wood.

Ash.—Not more than 7 per cent.

Production.—Two methods are largely employed for the production of charcoal, viz. the "stack" and "retort" methods. Both of these are dependent on the principle that organic matter burnt without the access of air is carbonized.

The first of these methods, which dates from a remote period, consists of piling billets of wood on ends into a conical pile or stack and covering this with earth or sod, leaving several openings at the bottom and one at the top so that a draught may insure a proper beginning of combustion.

A fire is started at the bottom of the stack and, when under way, the hole at the top is closed. As soon as the wood is all ignited the openings at the bottom are closed. The effect of this process is to drive off the volatile substances of the wood such as water, wood spirit, oxygen, etc., carbon alone remaining. In districts where wood is plentiful this method is frequently practised.

The modern method consists of burning wood without access of air in cast-iron retorts connected with condensers. This process insures the collection of valuable by-products such as tar, acetic acid, methyl alcohol, acetone, cresol, guaiacol, creasote, naphthalene, paraffine, etc.

Description.—A dull black, odorless and tasteless powder which should be free from grittiness. If 1 Gm. of charcoal is boiled with 3 cc. of potassium hydroxide test solution and 10 cc. of distilled water for a half minute and filtered, the filtrate should not show more than a slight brown color. A colorless filtrate would indicate complete carbonization.

Uses.—Wood Charcoal is employed as an absorbent and deodorant.

MYRICACEÆ (WAX MYRTLE AND BAYBERRY FAMILY)

Diœcious or sometimes monœcious, aromatic shrubs or trees with watery juice and possessing underground branches which arch downward, then upward producing many suckers. Roots fibrous and bearing many short rootlets upon which are frequently found coralloid clusters of tubercles containing the *Actinomyces Myricarum* Youngken. Leaves alternate, revolute in vernation, serrate, irregularly dentate, lobed or entire, rarely pinnatifid, pinnately and reticulately veined, pellucid punctate, evergreen (*Myrica cerifera*) or deciduous (*Myrica carolinensis*, *Comptonia*) generally exstipulate, rarely stipulate. Flowers naked, unisexual, monœcious or diœcious, in the axils of unisexual or androgynous aments from scaly buds formed in the summer in the axils of the leaves of the year, remaining covered during the winter and opening in March or April, before or with the unfolding of the leaves of the year.

Staminate flowers in elongated catkins, each consisting of 2 to 8 stamens inserted on the torus-like base of the oval to oval-lanceolate bracts of the catkin, usually subtended by 2 or 4, rarely by numerous bracteoles; filaments short or elongated, filiform, free or connate at the base into a short stipe; anthers ovoid, erect, 2 celled, extrorse, showing longitudinal dehiscence. Pistillate flowers in ovoid or ovoid-globular catkins. Gynœcium of 2 united carpels on a bract. Ovary sessile, unicellular, subtended by 2 lateral bracteoles which persist under the fruit, or by 8 linear-subulate bracteoles, accrescent, and forming a laciniate involucre inclosing the fruit; styles short and dividing into 2 elongated style arms which bear stigmatic surfaces on their inner face;

ovule orthotropous, solitary, with a basilar placenta and superior micropyle. Fruit an akene (*Comptonia*) or ceriferous nut (*Myrica*). Pericarp covered with glandular emergences which secrete wax or fleshy emergences, smooth and lustrous or smooth, glandular. Seed erect, exalbuminous, covered with a thin testa. Embryo straight, cotyledons thick, plano-convex; radicle short, superior.

There are two distinct genera of this family, *e.g.*, *Myrica* and *Comptonia*.

Among the outstanding histological characteristics might be mentioned the following: Superficial development of cork, feebly developed wood-parenchyma, narrow medullary-rays in wood, broadening out in wedge-shaped fashion in the phloem, a discontinuous to continuous band of sclerenchyma fibers in the pericycle, leaf epidermis showing stomata with 5–10 neighboring cells, unicellular non-glandular hairs and stalked glandular hairs with balloon-, bowl-, or saucer-shaped oil or resin containing heads. Rosette aggregates and monoclinic prisms of calcium oxalate, tannin, and gummy lignin occur in the axis of many of the species.

MYRICA N.F. (BAYBERRY)

Synonyms.—Wax Myrtle, Bayberry Bark, Candleberry, Candlewood, Wax Berry, Tallow-shrub, Tallow-Bayberry, Sweet-oak; *Ger.* Wachs-myrtel; *Fr.* Arbe à suif.

Botanical Origin.—*Myrica cerifera* Linné and *Myrica carolinensis* Miller.

Part Used.—The dried bark.

Limit of Impurities.—5 per cent. of adhering wood or other foreign organic matter.

Habitat.—*M. cerifera* or Wax Myrtle is indigenous to brackish marshes, sandy soil on the border of brackish ponds, estuaries and near the sea, from as far north as the Tuckahoe River, N. J., through southern Jersey, Maryland, Virginia, as far south as Southern Florida, west through the Gulf States to the shores of Arkansas Bay in Texas and northward in the region of the Mississippi to the valley of the Washita River in Arkansas. *M. carolinensis* or Bayberry is found chiefly near the coast but also in inland swamps and pine forests from Nova Scotia to Florida and Louisiana, on the borders of the Great Lakes and in Indiana.

Plants.—*Myrica cerifera* is an evergreen diœcious shrub or tree from 1 to 12 m. high, erect to ascending in habit with a tall crooked trunk and upright or spreading crooked branches which form a round-topped head. The recent shoots are greenish or reddish-brown, densely covered with yellowish or reddish glands, twigy elongate at the ends of branches and bearing numerous leaf buds above and flower buds below during the season.

The leaves are coriaceous, simple, alternate, exstipulate, lanceolate or oblong-lanceolate, pinnate-reticulate in venation, acute, mucronate, obtuse or notched at apex, long cuneiform at base and decurrent on the short stout petiole, glandular-punctate with orange-red sunken and golden yellow raised glandular hairs on both surfaces and shining dark green on

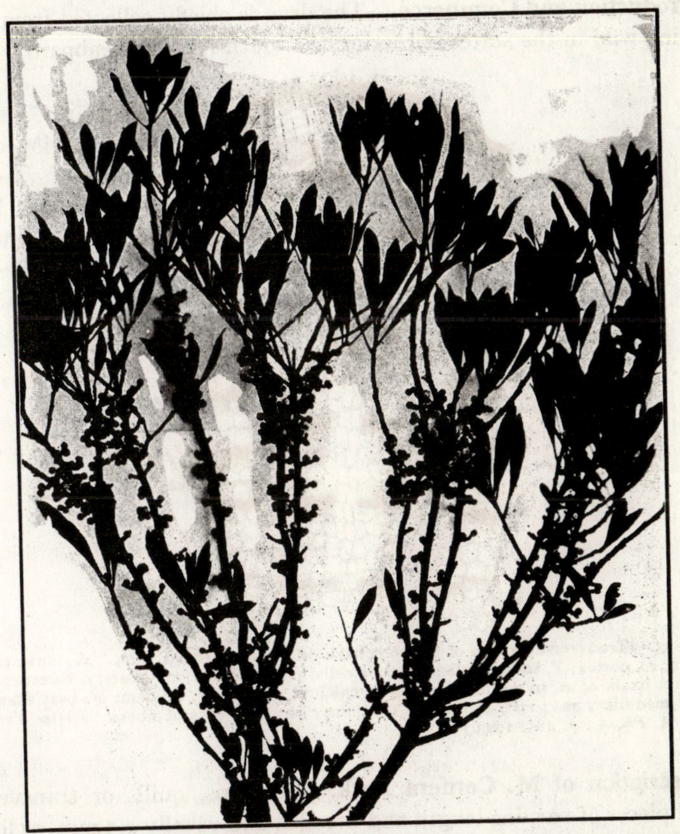

FIG. 52.—*Myrica cerifera* (Wax Myrtle). Fructiferous branches, showing evergreen leaves which persist over the winter. The ceriferous nuts of this and allied species are employed in the manufacture of the fragrant "Bayberry" candles.

upper surface. The inflorescences are male and female catkins on separate plants, partly formed the year before flowering below the leaves on the previous season's wood. The fruits are small, spherical, bluish-white, ceriferous nuts, the pericarp of which is covered with glandular emergences which secrete wax. They are employed in the manufacture of the fragrant Bayberry candles. The seed is erect and exalbuminous.

Myrica carolinensis is a deciduous shrub attaining a height of 2 to 3 m. with elliptic-obovate, membranous leaves which, while bearing golden yellow, balloon-shaped, glandular hairs, are devoid of the orange-red depressed, bowl- and saucer-shaped glandular hairs which are found along with the former type on *M. cerifera* and hybrids between *M. cerifera* and *M. carolinensis* (*M. Macfarlanei* Youngken).

Production and Commerce.—The drug is chiefly collected from plants growing wild in the states bordering the south Atlantic seaboard.

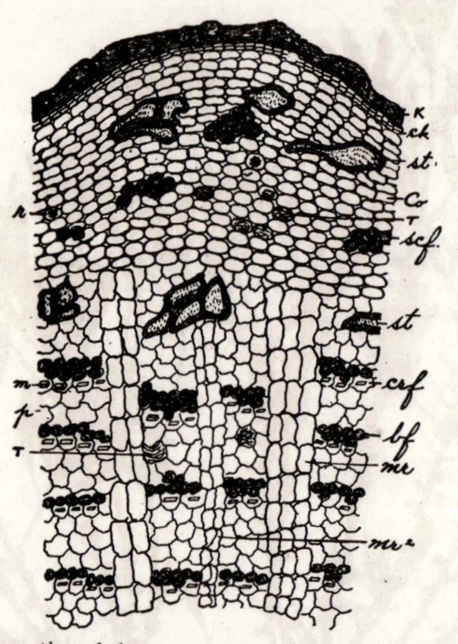

FIG. 53.—Transverse section of the root bark of *Myrica cerifera*, ×75. *K*, cork; *ck*, cork cambium; *co*, cortex; *T*, tannin cells; *st*, stone cells; *scf*, sclerenchyma fibers; *r*, rosette crystals of calcium oxalate; *m*, monoclinic prisms of calcium oxalate; *p*, phloem; *bf*, bast fibers; *mr*, primary medullary ray; *mr*², secondary medullary ray; *crf*, crystal fibers. (*After Youngken in Jour. A. Ph. A., p.* 485, 1923.)

Description of M. Cerifera Bark.—In strips, quills or transversely curved pieces of varying length and breadth and usually 2.5 mm. or less in the thickness, rarely up to 5 mm. in thickness (aerial stem bark); outer surface either silvery-gray, reddish brown or grayish brown, scaly in rhizome and root barks, bearing occasional warts or slight transverse ridges, that of the aerial stem bark exhibiting a number of raised oval lenticels, inner surface deep rusty brown to brown, finely longitudinally striated, somewhat roughened (rhizome and root barks); fracture short, weak and uneven; fractured surface brown with short projecting fibers near or along inner border of root bark; odor characteristic; taste astringent, mildly bitter and slightly acrid.

Histology of Root Bark (*M. cerifera*).—1. Cork of several layers of irregular brick-shaped cells which vary in their staining capacity. Many of the cells have highly suberized walls which stain green with extract of chlorophyll. Some, however, have all of their walls lignified, while others show lignification only on their inner walls.

2. Phellogen of meristematic cells, usually collapsed.

3. Secondary cortex whose cells are tangentially elongate and smallest in the outermost portion, becoming larger as one passes toward the phloem. Usually 3 or 4 of the outer layers of the exocortex region are devoid of intercellular-air-spaces. The remaining layers show numerous air-spaces which are for the greater part small and angular. Most of the cortical parenchyma cells contain starch grains with a central, cleft hilum being either simple and spheroidal or 2–4-compound. The individual grains are up to 12μ in diameter. Some, however, contain rosette aggregates and monoclinic prisms of calcium oxalate, while others have their walls thickened and are filled with a yellowish-brown substance which presents the following reactions: It is insoluble in cold or boiling water, cold concentrated potash solution, ammonia; alcohol or xylol. It is soluble in boiling nitric acid, boiling concentrated potash solution and hot solution of sodium hypochlorite. This substance has been termed "lignine-gommeuse" by Tison and Chevalier.

The rosette aggregates are from 11 to 45μ in diameter.

Sclerenchyma fibers which are quite narrow are few and usually isolated singly or in small groups of 2, 3 or rarely 4 amongst the cells of the cortex. Stone cells occur singly or in groups within this region.

4. Endodermis whose cells do not differ materially from those of the adjacent cortex.

5. Phloem, a comparatively broad zone of irregular phloem patches and medullary-rays, the latter often broadening out toward the cortex in fan-shaped fashion. The primary medullary rays are mostly 1 to 4 cells, rarely 1–5 cells broad. The secondary medullary rays are 1 to 2 cells broad. The bast fibers are arranged singly or in groups forming interrupted circles. They are more numerous in the metaphloem than in the protophloem region. Crystal fibers containing monoclinic prisms of calcium oxalate accompany the bast fibers. Stone cells occur in both this region and the cortex and are arranged both singly or in groups. They are of variable shape, have lamellated, porous, lignified walls and vary in length from 24μ to 129μ and in breadth from 15 to 59μ. Starch grains and tannin are found both in the phloem cells and the phloem medullary-rays. Many of the phloem cells and air spaces contain monoclinic prisms of calcium oxalate 7 to 22μ in length. Frequently several crystals are present in one cell or space.

Histology of Aerial Stem Bark (*M. cerifera*).—The cork consists of several layers of brick-shaped cells, whose walls are for the greater part suberized. The contents of these cells stain variously with safranin and methyl green.

Separating the cork from the cortex one notes a phellogen layer of tangentially elongated cells. The cortex is usually narrow and shows comparatively small, angular intercellular-air-spaces. Its cells are tangentially elongate. Some of them contain gummy lignin and tannin, while many are filled with starch grains, or crystals of calcium oxalate which may be in the form of monoclinic prisms or rosette aggregates.

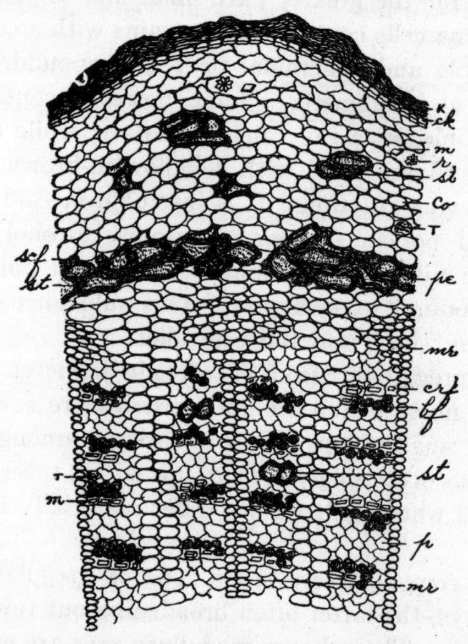

FIG. 54.—Transverse section of the aerial stem bark of *Myrica cerifera*, ×75. *K*, cork; *ck*, cork cambium; *co*, cortex; *pe*, pericycle, containing a nearly continuous band of stone cells and sclerenchyma fibers (*scf*), the stone cells predominating; *p*, phloem; *bf*, bast fibers; *crf*, crystal fibers; *T*, tannin cells; *mr*, medullary rays; *r*, rosette crystals and *m*, monoclinic prisms of calcium oxalate. (*After Youngken in Jour. A. Ph. A., p.* 485, 1923.)

Occasionally these crystals may also be seen in the air spaces. Stone cells of irregular form and size, arranged singly or in small groups, are scattered throughout this region. The outer 3 or 4 layers of exocortex are composed of collenchymatic cells and show no air-spaces. A continuous zone of sclerenchyma fibers and cells is present in the pericycle of older barks, a discontinuous one in younger one. The sclerenchyma cells are of different sizes and shapes and show varying degrees of lignification. Frequently cells containing crystals of calcium oxalate are found adhering to them. Some of the stone cells contain gummy lignin. The phloem region is traversed by numerous primary and secondary medullary-rays which generally broaden out toward the cortex, arching in many phloem masses. The primary medullary-rays are usually 1–3 rows of cells in width in this region. The secondary medullary-rays of the phloem vary from 1–2 rows of cells in breadth. The sieve tubes show oblique sieve plates. Their walls show numerous transverse pits. Tannin and crystals are quite abundant in the phloem parenchyma. Both stone cells and narrow bast fibers are sparsely scattered either singly or in small groups among the other phloem elements. The bast fibers are accompanied by crystal fibers. Each cell of the crystal fibers contains a monoclinic prism of calcium oxalate. The cambium line is somewhat wavy.

Histology of Rhizome Bark (*M. cerifera*).—The bark of the rhizome of *Myrica cerifera* differs histologically from the aerial stem and root barks in the following particulars: In transverse section the cortex cells appear

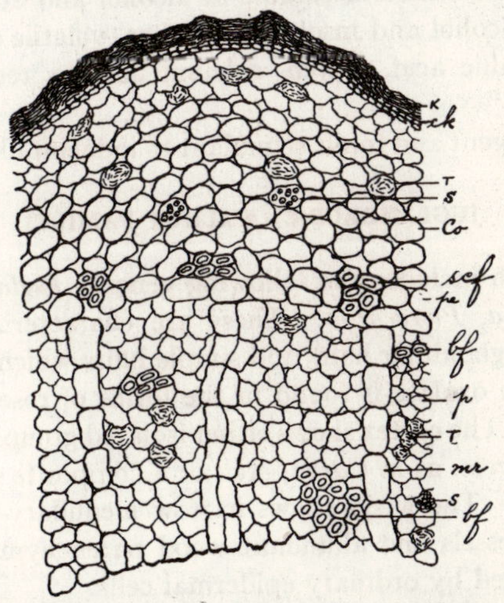

FIG. 55.—Transverse section of rhizome bark of *Myrica cerifera*, ×75. *K*, cork; *ck*, cork cambium; *co*, cortex; *pe*, pericycle, containing islets of sclerenchyma fibers (*scf*); *p*, phloem, separated into phloem patches by medullary-rays (*mr*); *bf*, bast fibers in phloem patches; *s*, starch; *T*, tannin. (*After Youngken in Jour. A. Ph. A., p.* 486, 1923.)

more rounded, less tangentially elongate. The intercellular-air-spaces are somewhat larger. No crystals of calcium oxalate have been found in the cortex. There are generally more cells containing gummy lignin. Sclerenchyma elements are entirely wanting in the cortex. A discontinuous zone of sclerenchyma is present in the pericycle composed of numerous widely separated small islets of comparatively thin-walled pericyclic fibers. The phloem region averagely shows fewer bast fibers. The medullary-ray cells are broader and have thinner walls.

Powdered Drug.—Reddish-brown; numerous crystals of calcium oxalate in monoclinic prisms up to 25μ in length, or in rosette aggregates up to 35μ, rarely 45μ in diameter; numerous simple, or 2- to 3- or rarely 4-compound starch grains, the individual grains being spheroidal or plano-convex, often with a central cleft and up to 12μ in diameter; strongly lignified, porous sclerenchyma fibers with walls up to about 13μ in thickness, often accompanied by crystal fibers containing monoclinic prisms; rounded or irregular stone cells up to 125μ in length, usually in groups, with thick, lignified, lamellated, porous walls; cork cells polygonal in surface view, some with brownish walls and filled with reddish contents; fragments of parenchyma, some of the cells rich in starch; cells containing gummy lignin; tracheæ with bordered pores from adhering wood very few or absent.

Constituents.—Tannin (giving a bluish-black precipitate with ferric chloride T.S.), an acrid resin soluble in alcohol and ether, an astringent resin soluble in alcohol and insoluble in ether, volatile oil, myricinic acid, gummy-lignin, gallic acid, starch, calcium oxalate, red coloring matter, etc.

Uses.—Astringent and tonic, stimulant to indolent ulcers.

JUGLANDACEÆ (WALNUT FAMILY)

A family which includes the following genera: *Juglans*, *Carya*, *Platycarya*, *Engelhardtia*, *Pterocarya*. These are characterized histologically by having peltate glandular hairs and simple hairs which frequently occur in tufts. Calcium oxalate is found in the forms of rosette aggregates or solitary crystals. The cortex shows either isolated groups of sclerenchyma fibers in the pericycle, as in *Carya*, etc., or a composite sclerenchymatous ring (in *Juglans*). The wood shows narrow medullary-rays, simple perforations in the vessels and abundant wood parenchyma. The leaf stomata are surrounded by ordinary epidermal cells.

JUGLANS N.F. (JUGLANS)

Synonyms.—Butternut Bark, White Walnut; *Ger.* Graue Wallnussrinde; *Fr.* Ecorce de Noyer.

Botanical Origin.—*Juglans cinerea* L.

Part Used.—Dried bark of the root with the outer bark more or less removed.

Limit of Impurities.—Not more than 2 per cent. of adhering wood or other foreign organic matter.

Habitat.—Eastern United States in rich woods from New Brunswick and Quebec to Georgia, west to Minnesota and Kansas.

Plant.—A forest tree with short trunk and broad, deep, round-topped, open crown. The bark varies from nearly smooth, light gray on the branches and young trunk to roughened by black fissures separating broad light gray ridges on older trunks. The wood is light brown, soft and coarse grained. The leaves are alternate, imparipinnate leaves with 11–17 ovate-lanceolate, serrate leaflets that are glabrous above and pubescent beneath. The fruit consists of an elongated-ovate drupe containing a 4-ribbed nut pointed at one end. The kernel is sweet, oily and edible.

Production and Commerce.—The inner bark is separated from the roots, after they have been collected in autumn, and dried. When first uncovered this bark is white but gradually changes on exposure to a lemon color, then to dark brown. The commercial supply comes chiefly from North Carolina, Virginia and Michigan.

Description.—It occurs in quills, curved pieces or in chips of variable length and up to 10 mm. thick. The color is deep brown throughout. The outer surface is smooth or warty; the inner surface, smooth and striate, with stringy fibers adhering. The fracture is short and fibrous. The odor is faintly aromatic. The taste is bitter, astringent and acrid.

Powdered Drug.—Dark brown. Under the microscope it exhibits numerous long, narrow, thick-walled sclerenchyma fibers, some of which are accompanied by crystal fibers, containing monoclinic prisms of calcium oxalate from 10μ to 50μ in length; fragments of epidermis composed of polygonal cells with yellowish-brown walls and brownish contents; numerous fragments of parenchyma containing brown tannin masses and oil; numerous rosette aggregates of calcium oxalate up to 55μ in diameter, monoclinic prisms of calcium oxalate; starch grains that are either simple and globular or 2–4-compound, the simple grains being up to 15μ in diameter; stone cells with simple or branching pores, up to 125μ in length and 70μ in width.

Constituents.—A yellow crystalline acrid substance, juglandic acid, oily extractive, gum, resin, etc.

Use.—Mild cathartic in habitual constipation.

FAGACEÆ (BEECH FAMILY) (CUPULIFERÆ)

Beeches, Chestnuts, Oaks.—The trees of this family are found in the temperate forests of the eastern and western hemispheres and comprise about 368 species. North America has over 50 species of oaks; 2 species of chestnuts; 1 species of beech and 1 species of golden-leaved chestnut. The most important American oaks used for building, for furniture, for cooperage, for wagons, for tanning leather, etc., are white oak, *Quercus alba;* chestnut oak, *Q. prinus;* black oak, *Q. velutina;* live oak, *Q. virginiana;* swamp white oak, *Q. platanoides;* cow oak, *Q. Michauxii,* and the two

Pacific coast oaks, *Q. chyrsolepis* and post oak, *Q. garryana.* The uses of the fast disappearing chestnut, *Castanea dentata*, are well known. The wood of the beech, *Fagus grandifolia*, is used for chairs, toolhandles, plane stocks, shoe lasts and for fuel. The nuts (mast) fatten hogs and feed wild animals and birds. The cork of commerce is obtained from the bark of *Quercus Suber* and *Quercus occidentalis*, plants indigenous to Spain and France.

The above trees are all monœcious, that is, the staminate (male) and pistillate (female) flowers are distinct from each other, but borne on the same tree. Most of the species are trees, a few oaks are shrubs. The leaves are simple, netted-veined and alternate. A pair of deciduous stipules are found at the base of the leaf-stalk (petiole). The margins of the chestnut and beech leaves are sharply cut with large teeth. The leaves of the oaks divide the genus into two groups, viz.—the white oaks with rounded lobed leaves and annual acorn production, and the black oaks with sharp bristle-tipped lobes and biennial acorn production. The male flowers are in dangling heads (beech), or in catkins (chestnut and oaks). The male flowers have a united perianth, which is 4–6 parted and encloses an indefinite number of undivided stamens. The female flowers have a superior 6-parted perianth, the pistil consisting of 3 carpels with a corresponding number of stigmas. The ovary is 3–6-celled and each cell has 2 pendulous ovules. The fruit is a one-seeded nut. The cup, or cupule, in the beech is 4-sided, is covered externally with weak spines and encloses two 3-sided seeds. The cupule in the chestnut forms the spiny bur, which splits into 4 valves at maturity, enclosing 3 nuts. The cupule in the oak is saucer-, or cup-shaped, and encloses a single rounded nut, or acorn. The seeds are exalbuminous and the cotyledons are thick and fleshy, edible in the beech, chestnut and a few of the oaks.

The principal histological peculiarities of this family are as follows: Subepidermal cork development; wood fibers with bordered pits; a sclerenchyma ring in the pericycle; non-glandular hairs unicellular or uniseriate or tufted; glandular hairs of varying shape; stomata devoid of neighboring cells; calcium oxalate in rosette aggregates, often in crystal fibers, or as solitary crystals; numerous tannin cells; tracheæ with scalariform markings numerous.

GALLA U.S.P. (NUTGALL)

Synonyms.—Galls, Aleppo Galls, Smyrna Galls; *Ger.* Gallapfel; *Fr.* Galla de chêne.

Botanical Origin.—*Quercus infectoria* Olivier (*Quercus lusitanica* Lam.) and other allied species of *Quercus*.

Part Used.—The gall from the young twigs.

Habitat.—Mediterranean Basin from Greece to Persia.

Production and Commerce.—The female of *Cynips tinctoria*, gall-fly, (Class *Insecta*, order *Hymenoptera*, family *Cynipidæ*) punctures the young leaf buds of the dyer's oak with her ovipositor and deposits one or more eggs in the wound. The egg hatches and a young insect or larva emerges in the plant tissue. The larva secretes a fluid (probably from its salivary glands) which contains an enzyme capable of converting starch into sugar. The cells immediately surrounding the larva contain considerable starch

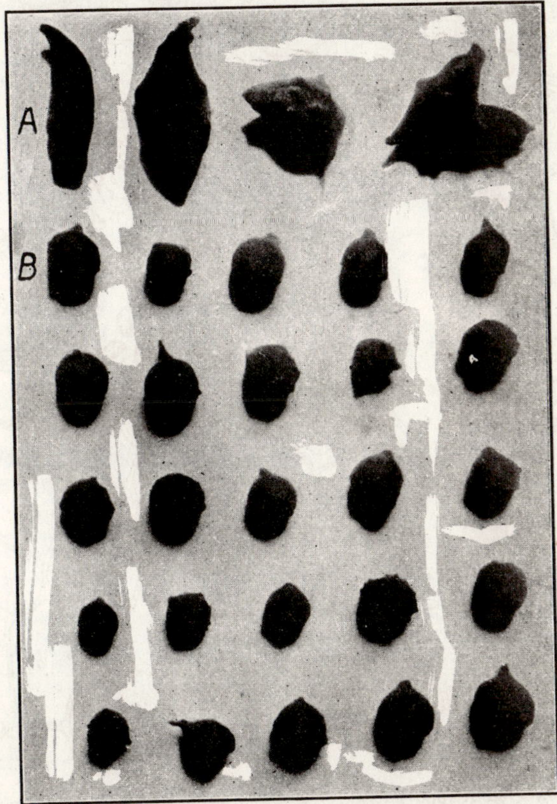

FIG. 56.—Chinese galls (*A*); Aleppo galls (*B*).

and are termed the nutritive zone. This starch is gradually changed to sugar by the enzyme which makes more food available than usual to the growing plant cells. The protoplasm of these is, accordingly, stimulated toward greater cell-reproduction as the rate of change from starch to sugar is accelerated, and a hypertrophied growth, tumor or gall is the result. In the gall the insect undergoes a metamorphosis, passing from the larva or "worm" stage to the chrysalis or pupa stage and thence to the imago or adult stage. In this last stage it channels its way out leaving a tubular canal communicating with a central hollow cavity. While the insect is in the early larval stage most of the cells of the gall contain numerous tiny starch grains. By the time the larva is transformed to a chrysalis, gallic

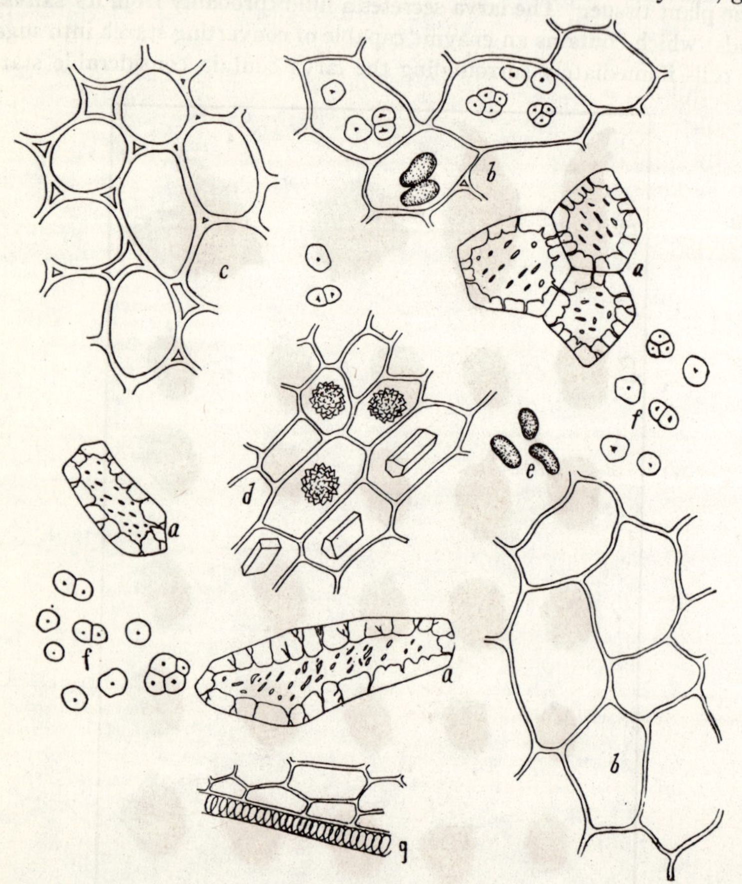

FIG. 57.—Powdered Aleppo nutgall. (*a*) Stone cells; (*b*) parenchyma with starch and tannin bodies; (*c*) parenchyma; (*d*) parenchyma with crystals; (*e*) tannin bodies; (*f*) starch granules; (*g*) spiral duct. (*After Schneider.*)

acid has taken the place of considerable of the starch in the cells near the middle of the gall, while tannic acid in masses is abundantly present in the cells at the center and near the outer margin. When the imago or adult winged insect is developed, most of the cells of the gall contain masses of tannin together with a small amount of gallic acid. After the imago has emerged from the gall, the tannin constituent of the cells undergoes oxidation which results in replacement by an insoluble product. The gall becomes lighter in weight and color and more spongy in texture. The so-called "White Galls" of commerce represent this last stage. The galls should be collected before the insect has emerged. Most of the official galls are gathered by the peasants of Asia Minor and Persia who dry them in the sun. During this time they lose about 50 per cent. in weight. The product is then sold to dealers in small villages or bartered for articles of European manufacture. On account of different stages of maturity, the galls vary in color from black, through green and blue, to white. The black galls contain the most tannin, the white the least. The galls are graded by the exporter. Nutgalls are exported from Persia, Aleppo in Asiatic Turkey and from Greece. They come to this country mainly from Aleppo.

Description.—Nearly globular from 0.8 to 2.5 cm. in diameter; externally blackish-olive-green or blackish-gray, more or less tuberculated on upper portion, the basal portion nearly smooth and contracted into a short stalk; heavy, sinking in water, excepting smaller galls; breakable and short horny; internally grayish or dark brown, consisting of a central slightly radiating and resinous portion, occasionally hollow and traversed by a narrow radial canal extending to the exterior as shown by the hole in the whole gall; odor slight; taste strongly astringent.

Powdered Drug.—Brownish-yellow; numerous fragments of thick-walled starch parenchyma; numerous simple, spheroidal, ellipsoidal or polygonal starch grains up to 30μ in diameter or length, and compound grains; few stone cells with thick lignified walls and branching pore canals; a few spiral and reticulate tracheæ; oval or bean-shaped tannin masses; monoclinic prisms and rosettes of calcium oxalate, the latter up to 40μ in diameter.

Constituents.—Tannic acid U.S.P. (50 to 70 per cent.), gallic acid, resin and starch.

Use.—Astringent, chiefly in the form of an ointment.

Adulterants.—The whole drug frequently is admixed with White Galls. The powdered drug has been admixed with ground nut shells and olive pits.

Allied Drug.—**Chinese Galls** are produced on the leaves of *Rhus semialata* Murray by the sting and deposited ova of an *Aphis* (plant louse). They are quite irregular in shape, irregularly lobed with a number of protuberances and have a thin wall and large hollow interior. They contain 70 to 80 per cent. of tannin. The powdered drug is brownish ash gray and shows under the microscope numerous unicellular trichomes with pointed ends that are frequently recurved, greenish-yellow resin masses, fragments of thin-walled parenchyma and spheroidal starch grains.

12

QUERCUS N.F. (QUERCUS)

Synonyms.—White Oak Bark; *Fr.* Ecorce de chêne; *Ger.* Eichenrinde.

Botanical Origin.—*Quercus alba* Linné.

Part Used.—The dried inner bark of the trunk and branches.

Purity Rubric.—Not more than 2 per cent. of its outer bark or wood or other foreign organic matter.

Habitat.—United States from Maine to Minnesota, south to Florida and Texas.

Plant.—A large tree with an average height of 70 to 80 feet which, when grown in the open, has a crown of gnarled and twisted, lateral, leafy branches. Its leaves are alternate, obovate with 3- to 9- but usually 7-ascending, round-ended lobes, which are separated by deep round-based sinuses. The yellow staminate flowers open in May when the leaves are partly developed and are found on hairy aments. The pistillate flowers occur on short axillary stalks with hairy, involucral scales and possess red spreading styles. The fruit is an acorn with ovoid, shining glans, and bowl-shaped cupule.

Commercial.—The commercial supplies of oak bark come chiefly from Michigan and Germany. The imported article usually comes in the form of the cut and sifted drug and is shipped in bags.

Description.—In nearly flat pieces up to 10 mm. in thickness; externally light brown, darkening with age, rough splintery; fracture uneven and coarsely fibrous; odor faint; taste strongly astringent, not tingeing the saliva yellow when chewed.

Powdered Drug.—Light brown. Numerous thick-walled, lignified sclerenchyma fibers; numerous crystal fibers containing prismatic crystals or rosette aggregates of calcium oxalate; stone cells with thick, lamellated walls, up to 100μ in length; starch grains up to 10μ in diameter; fragments of parenchyma with yellowish-brown amorphous contents; few fragments of cork with brownish amorphous content.

Constituents.—Quercitannic acid (about 10 per cent.), oak red, quercit, pectin, resin, calcium oxalate, etc.

Use.—Astringent. Chiefly used in the tanning industry.

Adulterant.—The bark of the Black Oak, *Quercus velutina* Lam., which is reddish-brown and tinges the saliva yellow on chewing.

CASTANEA N.F. (CASTANEA)

Synonyms.—Chestnut Leaves; *Fr.* Feuilles de chataignier; *Ger.* Kastanien-blätter.

Botanical Origin.—*Castanea dentata* (Marshall) Borkhausen.

Part Used.—The dried leaves.

Limit of Impurities.—5 per cent. of its stems or other foreign matter.

Habitat.—North America, from Maine to Michigan, south along the mountain ranges to Alabama, Mississippi and Arkansas.

Plant.—A large spreading tree growing to a height of 60 to 100 feet and having a trunk diameter of 3 to 10 feet. The bark on old trunks is deeply fissured, the fissures separating oblique ridges that possess dark brown scales. The leaves are smooth, simple, alternate, oblong-lanceolate, sharp pointed at apex, and serrate along margin. The staminate flowers are crowded on lower aments. The pistillate flowers appear at the base of the

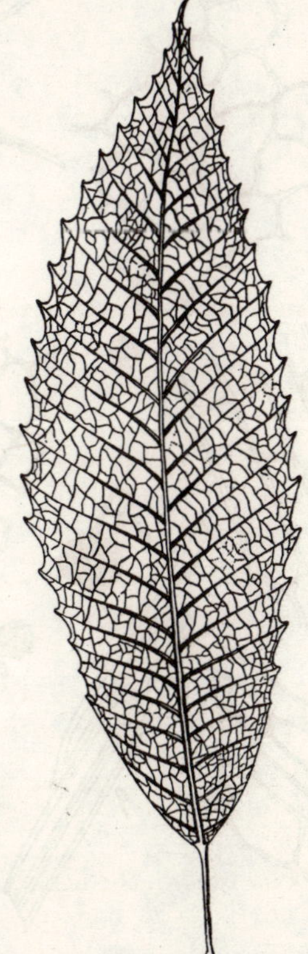

FIG. 58.—Chestnut leaf. (*After Sayre.*)

upper aments as globular structures. The fruit is a spiny bur containing from 1 to 5, usually 2 or 3, nuts.

Collection.—The leaves are gathered in autumn and carefully dried.

Description.—Leaves usually folded and matted together or broken; when spread out and entire, petiole about 12 mm. in length; lamina oblong-lanceolate, sharp pointed at apex, acute at base, coarsely serrate along margin, the teeth being attenuated; nearly smooth; coriaceous; upper surface dark green or yellow green; lower surface light green; pinnately veined, the veins of the first order ending in the teeth; odor slight; taste astringent.

Powdered Drug.—Olive green to greenish-brown. Few long, yellow, simple non-glandular hairs; few stellate hairs, each of from 3 to 8 units

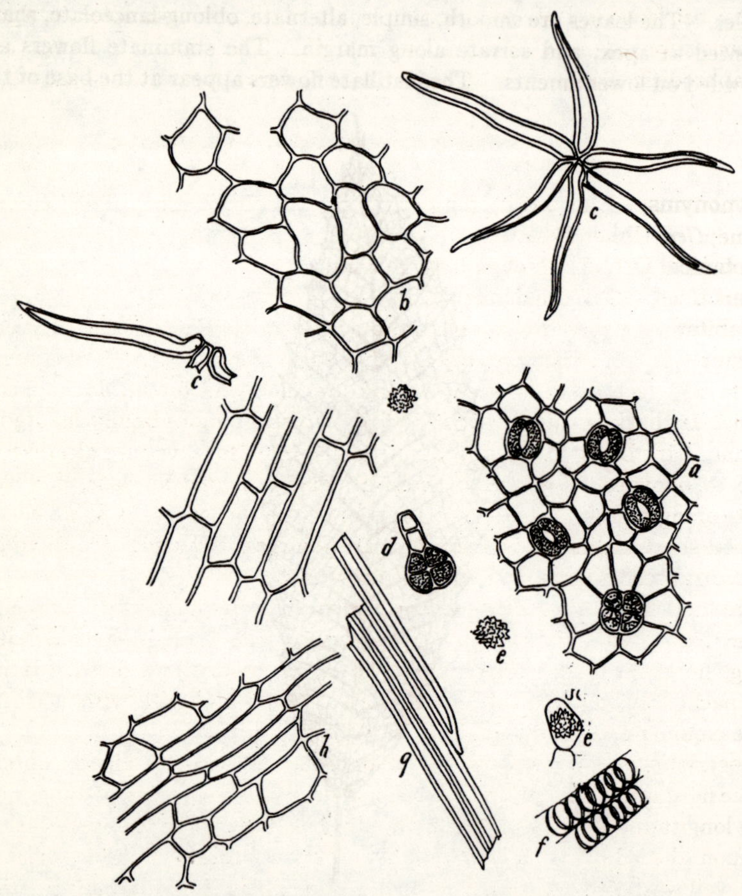

FIG. 59.—Castanea. Leaf elements. (*a*) Lower epidermis; (*b*) upper epidermis; (*c*) stellate trichomes; (*d*) glandular trichome; (*e*) rosette crystals; (*f*) spiral ducts; (*g*) sclerenchyma fibers; (*h*) parenchyma. (*Schneider.*)

and spreading at the base; numerous rosette aggregates and monoclinic prisms of calcium oxalate up to 50μ in diameter; crystal fibers containing monoclinic prisms, numerous fragments of parenchyma, many with chloroplasts, others with yellowish-brown tannin masses, colored blue with ammonio-ferric alum T.S.

Constituents.—Tannin, mucilage, resin, etc.
Use.—Astringent.

ULMACEÆ (ELM FAMILY)

Forest trees indigenous to the temperate and tropical zones, characterized by being woody plants, with alternate pinnately veined leaves and caducous stipules and without milky juice. Their flowers are unisexual or hermaphroditic with 6 or 4 parts to the perianth. Fruit a samara.

ULMUS U.S.P. (ELM)

Synonyms.—Elm Bark, Slippery Elm, American Elm; *Fr.* Ecorce d'Orme; *Ger.* Ulmenrinde.

Botanical Origin.—*Ulmus fulva* Michaux.

Part Used.—The dried inner bark.

Habitat.—Quebec to North Dakota, south to Florida and Texas.

Plant.—A tree attaining a height of 50 to 60 feet and a trunk diameter of 1 to 2½ feet, with stout ascending branches and broad, flat-topped crown. Its bark is thick, tough, dark brown and longitudinally fissured, the inner bark being fragrant and mucilaginous. Its leaves are alternate, ovate to obovate, dark green, acute at apex, unequal at base, doubly serrate along margin. The flowers appear before the leaves, in April, clustered on short stalks. The fruit is a short-stalked, flat samara consisting of a central seed surrounded by a yellowish wing.

Production and Commerce.—The Elm trees are found in large numbers in the New England States and Michigan. The bark is collected in spring, deprived of its cork, sawed into oblong pieces and dried. It is then packed in bundles which are bound at either end with wire. Most of the commercial supply comes from Michigan.

Description.—In sawed or cut oblong, flat or slab-like pieces; outer surface light brown or buff with occasional dark brown patches of adhering cork, longitudinally striate and with adhering bast fibers, colored blackish upon the addition of very dilute iodine test solution; inner surface light yellowish-brown, nearly smooth and finely longitudinally striate; fracture fibrous; fractured surface porous; odor distinct; taste mucilaginous.

Histology.—Transverse sections show for the most part a broad phloem composed of alternating interrupted bands of bast fiber groups and soft bast. Running at right angles to these are medullary-rays from 1 to 6 cells in width. The bast fiber groups are surrounded by crystal fibers containing monoclinic prisms or twin crystals of calcium oxalate 10 to 35μ in length. In each soft bast zone (between 2 medullary-rays) occurs 1 or more mucilage sacs. Many of the medullary-ray cells and phloem parenchyma cells and the majority of cortical parenchyma cells, adhering to phloem, contain small spheroidal to polygonal starch grains from 3μ to 25μ in diameter.

Powdered Drug.—Pale brown. Numerous long, thick walled, bast fibers, usually broken, up to 25μ in diameter with non-lignified or only slightly lignified walls, starch grains spheroidal or polygonal, usually from 3μ to 15μ in diameter, occasionally up to 25μ; monoclinic prisms of calcium oxalate up to 35μ in length; numerous fragments of parenchyma with embedded mucilage cells; odor resembling powdered foenugreek.

Constituents.—Mucilage, starch and calcium oxalate.

Uses.—Demulcent and emollient; the powdered drug as a poultice.

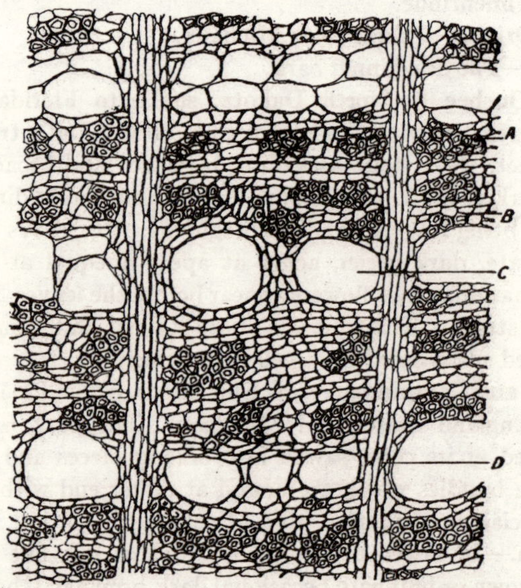

FIG. 60.—Ulmus—Cross-section of bark. *A*, Bast fibers; *B*, phloem parenchyma; *C*, mucilage sacs; *D*, medullary rays. (*Sayre.*)

MORACEÆ (MULBERRY FAMILY)

Herbs, shrubs or trees characterized for the greater part by containing a milky juice. This exists in laticiferous tubes that pervade the entire plant or are limited to the fibrovascular regions only, as in several species of *Ficus*. The leaves are ovate with serrate margins and caducous stipules. The flowers are small, unisexual, solitary or clustered and variously colored. The fruit is an akene enclosed by the perianth.

CANNABIS U.S. (CANNABIS)

Synonyms.—Cannabis Indica, Guaza, Ganjah, Hashish, Indian Hemp; *Ger*. Hanf; *Fr*. Chanvre.

Botanical Origin.—*Cannabis sativa* Linné.

Parts Used.—The dried flowering tops of pistillate plants.

Limit of Impurities.—10 per cent. of its fruits, large foliage leaves, stems over 3 mm. in diameter, and not more than 2 per cent. of other foreign matter.

Ash.—Not more than 5 per cent. acid-insoluble.

Standard of Assay.—Cannabis, in the form of the fluidextract, administered by mouth to dogs in doses not exceeding 0.1 cc. for each kilogram of body weight of dog, produces a degree of incoördination equal to that caused by the same dose of the standard fluidextract (see U.S.P. x, p. 95–96).

Habitat.—Asia. Cultivated in United States, Africa, India, Europe and Brazil.

Plant.—A tall, roughish, annual, diœcious herb thriving in waste and cultivated ground. The stem is angular, may attain a height of 4.5 m., and bears numerous palmately-compound leaves. The leaflets are linear-lanceolate, serrate and 5–7 in number. The flowers are greenish and borne on axillary panicles (staminate) or catkins (pistillate). The ovarian portion of the pistillate flower is one-celled and contains a pendulous ovule that forms with the ovarian wall a small glandular akene, upon maturation.

Production and Commerce.—*Cannabis sativa* is grown in temperate countries for its bast fibers which constitute "hemp" and for its fruits known as "hemp seed." It is cultivated extensively in both tropical and temperate countries for its tops. Its foliage leaves and young twigs, when dried, constitute the drug known as "*bhang;*" its resin is separately collected and marketed in India under the name of "*churrus*" or "*charas*." The dried flowering tops constitute "*guaza*" or "*ganjah*." Several varieties of Cannabis have been found on the market, taking their names from the countries in which the plants were grown. Of these the most important have been the Indian, American and African.

Indian Cannabis is obtained from plants grown in various districts of India, chiefly north of Calcutta. There the plants are cultivated in rows, collection of the drug taking place as soon as the flowering tops have assumed a brownish color. These are then cut off, the fruits shaken out, allowed to wilt and then subjected to the process of rolling and treading, in order to work resinous matter from the stems into the inflorescences. There are two grades of Indian Cannabis—(1) Round and (2) Flat. The round, sometimes called "Bengal ganjah" or "gauza," is prepared near Calcutta by kneading the tops into cylindrical or rounded resinous masses.

This grade is mostly consumed in India and the West Indies. The flat grade is kneaded into a compressed flattened form. The color is grayish-brown. The commercial supplies of the Indian grown drug are imported into this country in cases from Bombay, India.

American Cannabis, representing the chief variety used in the United States today, is yielded by *Cannabis sativa* plants cultivated in various sections of the United States. It occurs on the market in the form of broken segments of the inflorescences and more or less crumpled and broken leaves varying in color from brownish-green to light brown. The commercial supplies of this variety come from North and South

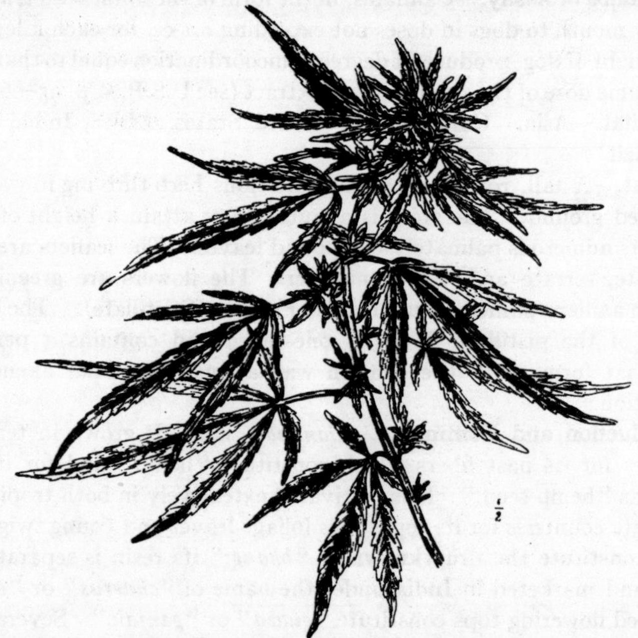

FIG. 61.—*Cannabis*—Branch. (*Sayre.*)

Carolina, Illinois, Indiana, New York, Wisconsin, Kentucky, Texas and Missouri. It is shipped in bags.

African Cannabis, from *Cannabis sativa* plants growing near the eastern and western coasts and central regions watered by the Congo and Zambesi rivers, comes into the market in the form of broken leaves and flowering tops of a greenish-brown color which are shipped in bags chiefly from Zanzibar.

Description.—In addition to the characteristics previously mentioned for the several commercial varieties, the drug presents the following for examination:

The stems are longitudinally furrowed, not more than 3 mm. in diameter, pubescent and of a light green or light brown color. The short stems (twigs) bear leafy bracts and pistillate flowers, a number of these being replaced by fruits. The foliage leaves are palmately 5–7 compound, the leaflet portions, when soaked in water and spread out, being linear-lanceo-

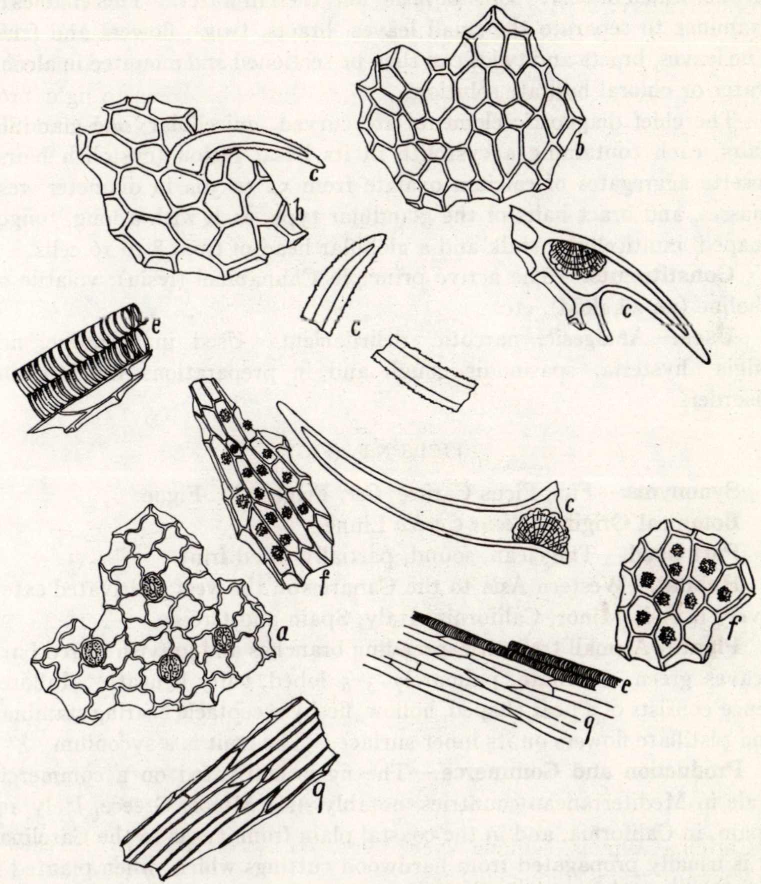

FIG. 62.—Powdered Cannabis. (*a*) Lower epidermis of leaf; (*b*) upper epidermis of leaf; (*c*) trichomes with cystoliths; (*e*) spiral ducts; (*f*) parenchyma with minute rosette aggregate crystals; (*g*) phloem tissue. (*After Schneider.*)

late in outline, with acuminate apex and coarsely serrate margin. The bract leaves are ovate-lanceolate, pubescent, each enclosing one or two pistillate flowers, or more or less developed fruits. The calyx is dark green, pubescent and somewhat folded around the ovary or fruit. The ovary is one-chambered and contains a single campylotropous ovule.

Attached to it are 2 slender, pubescent styles. The fruit is light green to light brown, broadly ellipsoidal, about 3.5 mm. long and finely wrinkled. The odor is agreeably aromatic. The taste is pungent and resinous.

Histology.—The compressed, agglutinated flowering tops can best be prepared for microscopical examination by soaking these first in strong alcohol which dissolves some of resin, and then in water. This enables the examiner to separate the small leaves, bracts, twigs, flowers and fruits. The leaves, bracts and twigs can then be sectioned and mounted in alcohol, water or chloral hydrate solution.

The chief diagnostic elements are curved, unicellular, non-glandular hairs, each containing a cystolith in its basal region (cystolith hairs); rosette aggregates of calcium oxalate from 5μ to 30μ in diameter, resin masses, and bract hairs of the glandular type, each with a long, tongue-shaped, multicellular stalk and a globular head of from 8 to 16 cells.

Constituents.—The active principle Cannabinol (resin); volatile oil, choline (an alkaloid), etc.

Uses.—Analgesic, narcotic, delirifacient. Used in migraine, neuralgia, hysteria, spasmodic cough and in preparations for intestinal disorders.

FICUS N.F. (FIG)

Synonyms.—Fici, Ficus Caricæ; *Ger.* Feigen; *Fr.* Figue.

Botanical Origin.—*Ficus Carica* Linné.

Part Used.—The clean, sound, partially dried fruit.

Habitat.—Western Asia to the Canaries on the west; cultivated extensively in Asia Minor, California, Italy, Spain and Greece.

Plant.—A small tree with spreading branches and grayish or red bark. Leaves green, alternate, palmately 3–5 lobed, hairy beneath. Inflorescence consists of a pear-shaped, hollow, fleshy receptacle bearing staminate and pistillate flowers on its inner surface. The fruit is a syconium.

Production and Commerce.—The fig is cultivated on a commercial scale in Mediterranean countries, notably Asia Minor, Greece, Italy and Spain, in California, and in the coastal plain from Texas to the Carolinas. It is usually propagated from hardwood cuttings which, when planted in heavy soil, form trees bearing fruit in 2 to 4 years. The average fig tree will not produce good fruit unless caprified. Caprification consists of attaching branches of the caprifig (wild fig) to the cultivated fig tree. The fruit of the caprifig, which is seedless and gall-like, contains large numbers of the eggs of a small wasp, *Blastophaga grossorum.* These, upon hatching, develop either into adult male or female wasps. The wingless males eat their way out of the galls in which they were developed and into the galls occupied by developing females. Here copulation is followed by the death of the male wasps while the females escape. Spreading themselves over the staminate flowers of the caprifig, they become dusted with pollen. Some of them, chancing to visit the half-grown fruits of the cultivated fig, cut their way through the scaly orifice at the summit and enter the hol-

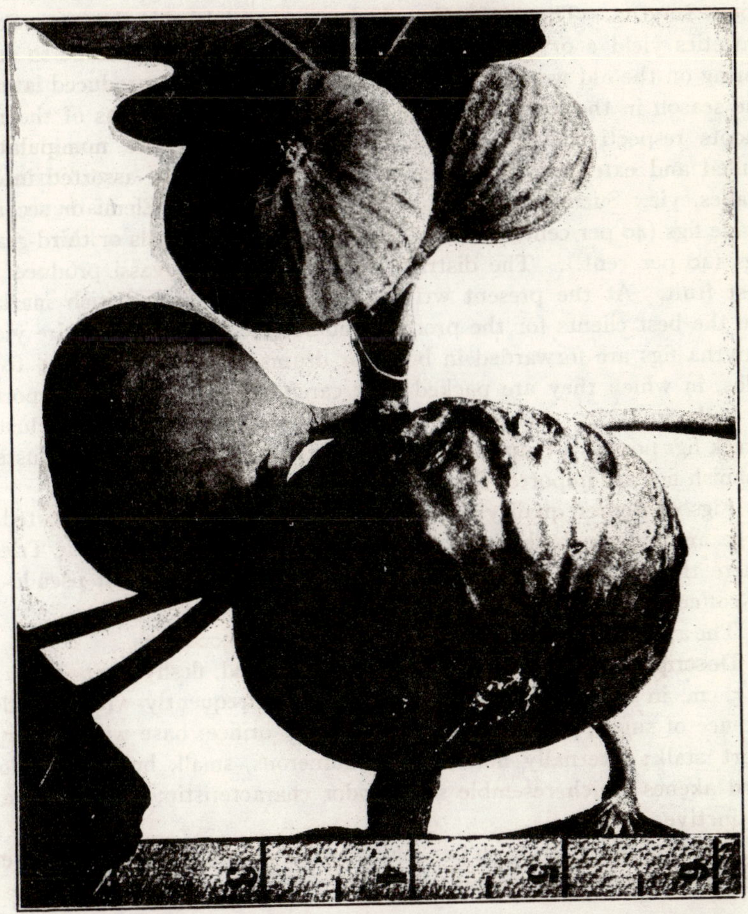

FIG. 63.—Smyrna figs on fruiting-branch. The large fig is fully mature, the others partly so. (*After Rixford, Bull. 732, Bureau of Plant Industry, U. S. Dept. of Agriculture.*)

lowed interior, there to pollinate the female flowers lining its margin. Pollination is followed by fertilization which enables the fruits of the cultivated fig to fully mature. The female wasp dies within the cultivated fig fruit, leaving no progeny. Only those have progeny which visit caprifigs.

Natural figs are those which are either allowed to dry on the tree or gathered and dried by artificial heat or by the sun. *Pulled figs* are those which are rendered pliant by pulling and kneading.

Most of the figs used in the United States come from Smyrna and California. Smyrna figs are obtained from trees cultivated in the district about Smyrna. They are gathered when ripe and dried in the sun. Some varieties yield 2 or 3 crops annually. The first crop is borne in early spring on the old wood; the second and third crops are produced later in the season in the leaf axils on the lower and upper portions of the new shoots respectively. Smyrna figs of better quality are manipulated, pulled and extended by armies of workers. They are assorted into 3 grades, viz.: Suzini or first-grade figs (20 per cent.), Elemi or second-grade figs (40 per cent.), a mixture of Elemis and naturals or third-grade figs (40 per cent.). The districts of Erbeyli and Inovassi produce the best fruit. At the present writing the American and British markets are the best clients for the product and receive almost the entire yield. Smyrna figs are forwarded in boxes or drums containing from ½ to 20 kilos, in which they are packed very carefully; some are also exported in bulk, in sacks, such being generally threaded into a string cluster. Greek figs possess a tough skin and usually are imported in string clusters. Spanish figs are imported from Malaga and Valencia.

Figs of poorer quality are called "hordas." These are exported in large amounts in bulk, in sacks, mainly to Central Europe via Trieste where they are used in distilleries or in the manufacture of pseudo- or fig-coffee.

The average annual harvest of Smyrna figs is 20,000 tons.

Description.—Compressed, irregularly rounded, fleshy fruits from 2.5 to 5 cm. in diameter, light brown to yellow; frequently with an efflorescence of sugar; summit with a small scaly orifice; base with a scar or short stalk; internally hollow, with numerous, small, brownish-yellow, hard akenes which resemble seeds; odor characteristic; taste sweet and distinctive.

Constituents.—Up to 62 per cent. of dextrose; fat, proteins, starch, etc.

Uses.—Laxative and food.

HUMULUS N.F. (HOP)

Synonyms.—Hops, Hop Vine, Lupulus; *Ger.* Hopfen; *Fr.* Houblon.

Botanical Origin.—*Humulus Lupulus* L.

Part Used.—The carefully dried strobile, bearing its glandular trichomes.

Limit of Impurities.—Two per cent. of stems, leaves, or other foreign matter.

Ash.—Nor more than 5 per cent. acid insoluble.

Habitat.—North America, Europe and Asia.

Plant.—A perennial, diœcious, twining herb whose aerial portion consists of several long, angular, entwining stems bearing cordate, palmately 3–5-lobed, scabrous, dark green, stipulate leaves. Its yellowish-white staminate flowers are borne in racemes. Its pistillate flowers are pale

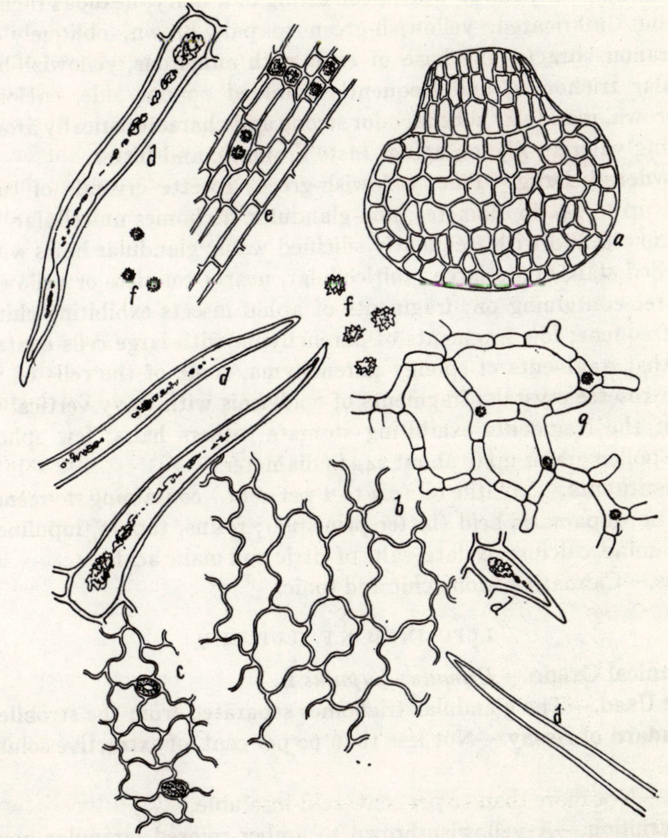

FIG. 64.—Ground Humulus. (*a*) Gland (lupulin); (*b*) upper epidermal cells; (*c*) epidermal tissue with stomata; (*d*) trichomes; (*e*) parenchyma with crystals; (*f*) rosette aggregate crystals of calcium oxalate; (*g*) spongy tissue cells with crystals. (*Schneider.*)

green and borne on a leafy conical spike. Its fruit is an ovate to ovate-cylindrical strobile which consists of a flexuous rachis bearing yellowish-green to pale brown, ovate, membranous, scaly bracts, each enclosing a brown glandular akene.

Production and Commerce.—Hops are cultivated in various sections of the United States, Europe, Australia and South America. The strobiles are gathered from the vines when mature in September, carefully dried in kilns by fire and packed in hemp bags or bales for the market. They are unfit for use in pharmacy when they develop a valeric acid odor. The commercial supplies used in the United States are chiefly obtained from Michigan, Indiana and Illinois.

Description.—Strobile ovate or ovoid-cylindrical, from 3 to 5 cm. in length and up to 3 cm. in width, consisting of a hairy, flexuous rachis and numerous imbricated, yellowish-green to pale brown, obliquely ovate, membranous bracts, the base of each with numerous, yellowish-brown, glandular trichomes, and frequently infolded on one side, enclosing a light brown, glandular achene; odor strong and characteristically aromatic, becoming valerian-like on aging; taste aromatic and bitter.

Powdered Drug.—Pale yellowish-green; rosette crystals of calcium oxalate up to 24μ in diameter; non-glandular trichomes unicellular, somewhat curved and with frequently silicified walls; glandular hairs with a 3 to 4-celled stalk and a large multicellular, nearly colorless or yellow head the latter containing oil; fragments of aphid insects exhibiting chitinous walls, frequent; few fragments of parenchyma with large cells containing cystoliths; fragments of spongy parenchyma, some of the cells of which contain rosette crystals; fragments of epidermis with wavy vertical walls, some of the fragments exhibiting stomata, others hairs; few spherical, spinose pollen grains up to about 24μ in diameter.

Constituents.—Volatile oil (0.3 to 1 per cent.) containing myrcene and humulene; lupamaric acid (bitter principle); resins, tannin, lupuline, trimethylamine, calcium oxalate, salts of citric and malic acids, etc.

Uses.—Calmative, stomachic and tonic.

LUPULINUM N.F. (LUPULIN)

Botanical Origin.—*Humulus Lupulus* L.

Part Used.—The glandular trichomes separated from the strobiles.

Standard of Assay.—Not less than 60 per cent. of extractive soluble in ether.

Ash.—Not more than 10 per cent. acid-insoluble.

Description.—A yellowish-brown to amber-colored, granular powder, having the characteristic odor and taste of hops, becoming dark red in color and valerian-like in odor on aging, when it is unfit for use. It floats when placed in water. The best lupulin is amber colored.

Microscopical Characteristics.—The glandular trichomes, when viewed from the side, resemble in outline the sporophore of a toadstool just before the veil has been rent. In this view each consists of a cup- or bowl-shaped, multicellular head consisting of a single layered wall of angular secreting cells and an upraised thin cuticle, beneath which is a globular mass of yellowish or yellowish-brown oleoresin. When viewed from the top, each has a circular outline. In this view a marginal layer of cells of the bowl of the head is in sharp focus while the other parts are not clear.

Constituents.—Volatile oil, resin, tannin, asparagin, choline, etc.

Use.—Calmative, chiefly in the form of fluidextract.

Adulterant.—Floor sweepings of hop bins, which are low in ether-soluble resin and high in ash.

SANTALACEÆ (SANDALWOOD FAMILY)

Herbs, shrubs or trees having entire exstipulate leaves, cymes of flowers and oil seeds. Many are parasitic on the roots of other plants.

SANTALUM ALBUM N. F. (SANDAL WOOD)

Synonyms.—White Sandalwood, Yellow Sandalwood, Lignum Santali, White Saunders; *Fr.* Santal Citrin; *Ger.* Sandelholz.

Botanical Origin.—*Santalum album* Linné.

Part Used.—The heartwood.

Purity Rubric.—Not less than 3.5 per cent. of volatile oil and not more than 1 per cent. of foreign matter.

Habitat.—India.

Plant.—A small tree growing to the height of about 30 feet, with grayish-brown bark, smooth ovate leaves and small, yellow, pink or violet flowers borne in cymes.

Production and Commerce.—The trees are cultivated on a large scale in Mysore under government supervision. The heartwood is obtained by uprooting trees with thick trunks, removing the bark and sapwood from the trunk and larger branches and roots and sawing or cutting the heartwood into billets or logs. Most of the drug entering this country is imported from Cochin and Bombay, India through London.

Description.—In billets, pieces or chips of varying shapes and sizes, heavy, hard but splitting easily, color light yellow; transverse sections yellow to light reddish-brown, with alternating light and dark concentric zones nearly equal in diameter, with numerous pores and traversed by many very narrow medullary-rays; odor characteristic, aromatic, persistent; taste peculiar, strongly aromatic.

Histology.—When examined under the microscope, sections show the medullary-rays from 2 to 4 rows wide, the cells thick-walled and radially marked; the wood wedges consisting largely of wood fibers with pointed ends, large parenchyma and thick-walled secretion vessels and cells containing single crystals of calcium oxalate up to 30 μ in length; the oil in globules adhering to the walls of the ducts and parenchyma cells. The powder is rich in the medullary-ray cells.

Constituents.—Volatile oil (3 to 5 per cent.) official in the U.S.P. as *Oleum Santali.*

Use.—Sandalwood is used in the arts and as a source of oil of santal, the latter being a genito-urinary stimulant and disinfectant.

ARISTOLOCHIACEÆ (BIRTHWORT FAMILY)

Herbs or twining semi-woody or woody plants, having more or less swollen nodes from which spring cordate or reniform or ovate leaves. Flowers regular (*Asarum,* etc.) or irregular (*Aristolochia*) often offensively smelling. Fruit a capsule. Seeds with copious albumen and minute embryo.

SERPENTARIA U.S.P. (SERPENTARIA)

Synonyms.—(1) Virginia Snakeroot; (2) Texas Snakeroot; *Ger.* Virginische Schlangenwurzel; *Fr.* Couleuvrée de Virginie.

Botanical Origin.—(1) *Aristolochia Serpentaria* Linné and (2) *Aristolochia reticulata* Nuttall.

Part Used.—The dried rhizome and roots.

Limit of Impurities.—10 per cent. of overground stems and 2 per cent. of other foreign matter, not more than 10 per cent. acid-insoluble ash.

Habitat.—(1) Connecticut to Florida, west to Michigan and Missouri, in rich woods. (2) Louisiana to Arkansas, south to Texas, in rich woods.

Plants.—Low perennial herbs with slender stems branched at the base, alternate, ovate or cordate or hastate leaves, and purplish flowers borne on short stalks near the ground with no corolla and with a calyx shaped like the letter S. The fruit is a 6-valved, septicidally dehiscent capsule containing flat seeds. *Aristolochia reticulata* differs from *A. Serpentaria* in having a larger rhizome with fewer and thicker rootlets, and thicker leaves with more prominent reticulations and shorter petioles.

Production and Commerce.—There are two commercial varieties of the drug, viz.: Virginia Snakeroot and Texas Snakeroot. The chief bulk of the drug is collected in Virginia, North and South Carolina, Tennessee and Georgia, and represents Virginia Snakeroot. Texas Snakeroot comes largely from Texas.

Description.—Rhizome oblique, subcylindrical, curved, from 10 to 30 mm. in length and from 1 to 2.5 (Virginia Snakeroot) or 2 to 4 mm. (Texas Snakeroot) in diameter; externally dark brown with short stem bases on upper surface and bearing numerous long, thin, yellowish-brown roots on its lower and lateral surfaces; fracture short; internally yellowish-white, wood with broad excentric wedges; odor camphoraceous, terebinthinate; taste aromatic and bitter.

Histology.—Transverse sections of the rhizome are characterized by a suberized epidermis, a cortex of 10 to 15 rows of parenchyma, a narrow inner bark, exhibiting a more or less continuous arc of sclerenchyma, a cambium, a broad, porous xylem with wood wedges separated by medullary-rays, up to about 8 cells wide, the walls of the latter being lignified and porous, and an eccentric pith with its cells showing lignified and porous walls.

The aerial stem exhibits a more or less continuous arc of sclerenchyma fibers in the pericycle, a few non-glandular hairs whose terminal cells are often recurved and an interrupted circle of 6 to 10 bundles. Simple and 2–4-compound starch grains, the individual grains of which are spherical or plano-convex and up to 18μ in diameter occur in the cells of the cortex, pith and medullary rays.

Constituents.—Volatile oil containing borneol; bitter principle, resin. tannin, starch, etc.

Use.—Aromatic bitter.

ASARUM N.F. (ASARUM)

Synonyms.—Canada Snakeroot, Wild Ginger; *Ger.* Canadische Haselwurzel; *Fr.* Asaret du Canada.

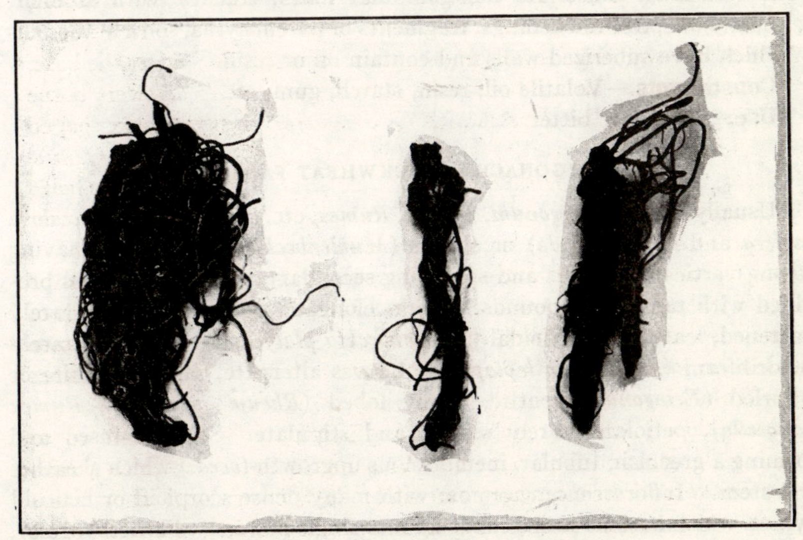

Fig. 65.—Asarum, × 9/18. (*Photograph by Stoneback.*)

Botanical Origin.—*Asarum canadense* Linné.

Part Used.—The dried rhizome and roots.

Limit of Impurities.—5 per cent. of foreign organic matter.

Habitat.—North and central United States, in rich woods.

Plant.—A soft, pubescent, perennial herb whose aromatic bitter rhizome bears several kidney-shaped membranous leaves with long petioles and bell-shaped flowers having a brownish-purple calyx. The fruit is a capsule.

Collection.—The rhizomes are dug in the spring, cleaned, most of the roots removed and dried. The commercial supplies come from Indiana, North Carolina, Michigan and Virginia.

Description.—Of horizontal growth, occasionally branched, two-edged when young, quadrangular when older, finely striate, usually more or less twisted, from 5 to 17 cm. in length and from 2 to 4 mm. in thickness; nodes enlarged with irregular scars from petioles and remains of pedicels; internodes with annular scars from scales; dark purplish-brown externally; fracture short, internally whitish, starchy or resinous; attached roots few, from 5 to 7 cm. in length and not over 1 mm. in thickness, having from four to six radial fibrovascular bundles. Odor aromatic, non-irritating upon heating; taste pungent and slightly bitter.

Powdered Drug.—Yellowish brown; numerous simple and 2- to 4-compound starch grains, many with a distinct central hilum, the individual grains from 4μ to 20μ in diameter; fragments of brownish epidermal cells with occasional uniseriate non-glandular hairs; tracheæ with annular, reticulate or spiral thickenings; fragments of parenchyma, some of the cells of which have suberized walls and contain oil or resin.

Constituents.—Volatile oil, resin, starch, gum, etc.

Use.—Aromatic bitter.

POLYGONACEÆ (BUCKWHEAT FAMILY)

Usually herbs (*Polygonum*, *Rheum*, *Rumex*, etc.), rarely trees (*Coccoloba uvifera* and *C. platyclada*) or shrubs (*Muhlenbeckia*, *Brunnichia*) having strong vertical tap roots and spreading secondary roots more or less provided with tannin compounds. Stems elongate, green, to woody, rarely flattened, leathery, phylloidal (*Muhlenbeckia platyclada*), still more rarely tendriliform (*Antigonum leptopus*). Leaves alternate, rarely opposite or whorled (*Eriogonum*), entire, rarely lobed (*Rheum palmatum*, *Rumex acetosella*), petiolate, rarely sessile, and stipulate. Stipules fused and forming a greenish, tubular, membranous upgrowth (*ocrea*) which sheathes the stem. Inflorescence racemose with many dense scorpioid or helicoid cymes, which in some forms condense into single flowers. Flowers regular, pentamerous, with simple calyx, becoming trimerous with two whorls of 3 sepals each. Stamens varying from 15 or 12 to 9 or 6, more rarely to 5, 4, 3 to 1 (*Kœnigia*), hypogynous, more rarely by enlargement of receptacle and slight fusion of sepals, perigynous. Pistil tri- to bicarpellate, often 3- to 2-sided; ovary 1-celled with 1 ovule. Styles 3, rarely 2, radiating-penicillate in wind-pollinated inconspicuous flowers, becoming condensed, knob-like in conspicuous insect-pollinated flowers. Fruit a triangular or biconvex akene often crowned by persistent styles and surrounded by persistent closely applied sepals. Seeds solitary, albuminous, with straight embryo, or in *Rumex*, curved embryo.

The following histological features characterize this family: tracheæ with simple pores; wood fibers with simple pits; cork either superficial or internal; calcium oxalate in rosette aggregates or solitary crystals; mucilaginous epidermal cells in leaves. Vascular bundles occur in the pith of species of *Rheum* and *Rumex* with xylem and phloem inversely oriented.

RHEUM U.S.P. (RHUBARB)

Synonyms.—Rhubarb Root, Turkey- or Chinese-Rhubarb, Rhizoma Rhei; *Ger.* Rhabarberwurzel; *Fr.* Rhabarbarum.

Botanical Origin.—*Rheum officinale* Baillon, *Rheum palmatum* L. and other species of *Rheum* grown in China and Thibet.

Part Used.—The dried rhizomes and roots, deprived of periderm tissues.

Purity Rubric.—Not less than 30 per cent. of diluted alcohol-soluble extractive.

Habitat.—China, Thibet, and Chinese Tartary.

Plants.—Perennial herbs resembling our garden rhubarb but attaining a larger size. Their underground portion consists of a strong vertical rhizome with fleshy, spreading roots. The above-ground portion consists of a number of long petioled leaves that arise from the rhizome in the spring, and flower shoots bearing elongated leafy panicles that are crowded with greenish-white flowers. The lamina is cordate to somewhat orbicular, entire or coarsely dentate (*Rheum officinale*) or palmately lobed (*R. palmatum*) or deeply incised (*R. tanguticum*). The fruit is an achene with 3 broad thin wings and surrounded at its base by the remains of the perianth.

Production and Commerce.—The production of Rhubarb extends over a large area of China. The chief localities are the northern provinces, Shensi, Shansi, Chihli and Honan, the northwest province of Kansu, the Mongolian province of Tsing-hai, and the mountainous districts of the western province of Szechuen. *Rheum officinale* is collected chiefly in the mountainous country separating Thibet from the province of Szechuen and extending eastward to Hupeh. *Rheum palmatum* is abundant in the province of Kansu where it collected in commercial quantities. A large amount of rhubarb probably derived from this species is collected near Lake Kokonor in Thibet. The rhizome and roots are dug up late in September from plants 8–10 years old, washed, and, after the removal of most of the bark, are either cut into segments and kiln or sun dried, or the segments may be bored with holes and suspended on strings to dry. Most of the drug is shipped through Hankow to Shanghai from whence it is exported to Europe. Smaller quantities are exported from Tientsin, Canton, Amoy, Fuhchow and Ning-po. Shensi Rhubarb is esteemed as the best variety. "Black Hearted" Rhubarb consists of pieces of the drug that possess dark or hollow central areas, due to the decay of these regions in the process of drying by artificial heat. The exterior of the pieces becomes hardened before the interior has lost all of its moisture, and so the pieces decay in the center.

The commercial varieties of Chinese Rhubarb imported into this country are Shensi, Canton and High Dried. Each of these occurs in "flats" or "common rounds."

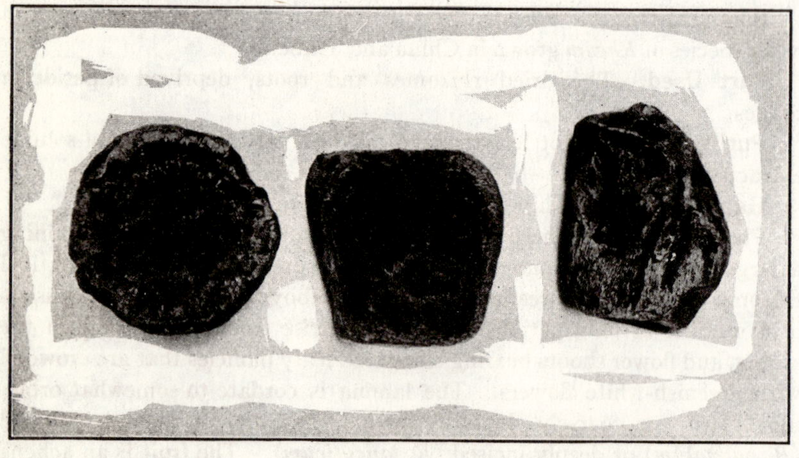

A *B* *C*

FIG. 66.—Shensi Rhubarb, ×⅜. *A* and *C*, two views of Round variety; *B*, Flat variety (*Photograph by Stoneback.*)

High Dried Rhubarb is dried on strings and shows a hole running through the rhizome or root.

Common Round Rhubarb consists of sections of the entire root and rhizome. Flats are large roots split in two lengthwise.

Shensi Rhubarb is esteemed as the finest variety. It is characterized by being firmer, heavier, deeper colored and more compact than the Canton variety, with a marbled often pink-colored interior, when fractured, and an agreeable odor and taste.

Canton Rhubarb is lighter in weight and color, less compact, and more fibrous in character. Its fractured surface is devoid of the strikingly

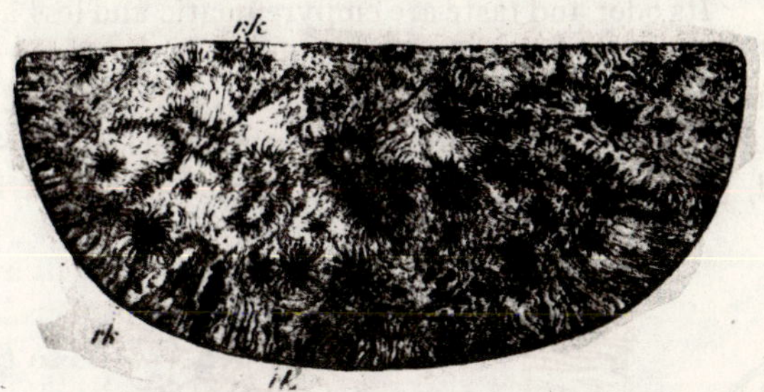

FIG. 67.—Rhubarb rhizome. Transversely cut surface showing stellate spots (*rk*) which represent compound fibrovascular bundles. Natural size. (*After Berg.*)

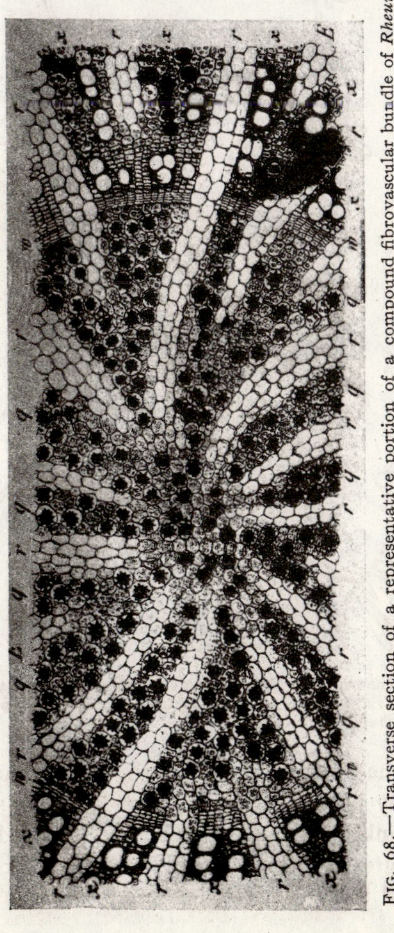

FIG. 68.—Transverse section of a representative portion of a compound fibrovascular bundle of *Rheum* showing cambium ring, *w*; medullary rays, *r*; xylem portions of bundles, *x*; and phloem portions of bundles *q*. Note rosette crystals of CaŌ in parenchyma cells. ×60. (*After Berg.*)

marbled character of the Shensi variety, appearing more uniformly granular in aspect. Its odor and taste are empyreumatic and less agreeable.

High Dried Rhubarb may be distinguished from the two preceding varieties by its rougher and duller coat and more empyreumatic odor.

Description.—The drug occurs on the market in sub-cylindrical, barrel-shaped, plano-convex or irregularly formed pieces, or in cubes or

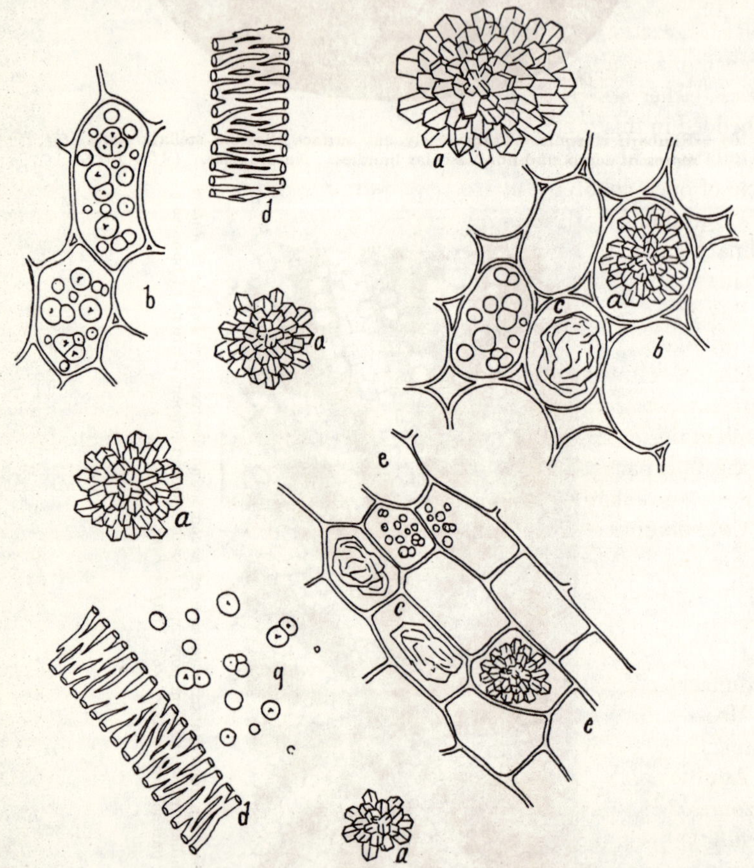

FIG. 69.—Powdered Rheum. (*a*) Rosette aggregates of calcium oxalate; (*b*) parenchyma with starch, resin and crystals; (*c*) resin; (*d*) reticulate ducts; (*e*) parenchyma, longitudinal view; (*g*) starch. (*Schneider.*)

rectangular pieces, the last commonly known as "rhubarb fingers." It is hard and moderately heavy. The outer surfaces are smooth, longitudinally wrinkled or sunken, yellowish-brown and mottled with alternating striæ of grayish-white parenchyma and brownish or reddish medullary-rays, while here and there may be seen reddish-brown cork patches and branched scars of fibrovascular bundles. The fracture is uneven and granular. The cut surface is mottled with irregular, radial, reddish-brown to brown medullary-rays and lighter colored parenchyma. The odor is aromatic. The taste is characteristically bitter and astringent. When chewed a gritty sensation is experienced and the saliva is colored yellow.

Histology.—Sections of Rhubarb are characterized by regular dicotyl structure, excepting the xylem region. This consists of a matrix of wood parenchyma similar to the phloem and cortex regions in that the cells possess either starch, tannin or large rosette crystals of calcium oxalate. Imbedded in this matrix near the cambium line are a number of compound ("stellate") fibrovascular bundles. Each of these consists of a small circle of open collateral bundles separated from each other by medullary-rays containing anthraquinone derivatives. The bundles differ from the ordinary open collateral bundle in showing phloem inside and xylem outside the cambium.

Powdered Drug.—Reddish-brown or yellowish-brown. It is colored red with alkalies. Under the microscope it shows numerous starch grains, spherical, single or 2–4 compound, from 2μ to 25μ in diameter, fragments of spiral and reticulate tracheæ, parenchyma cells containing starch grains or tannin masses, large rosette aggregates of calcium oxalate for the most part 50μ to 100μ in diameter, occasionally attaining a diameter of 150μ, and medullary-ray cells with anthraquinone derivatives.

Constituents.—Chrysophanic acid (di-hydro-oxy-methyl-anthraquinone), emodin, (tri-hydro-oxy-methyl-anthraquinone), rhein (tetra-hydro-oxy-methyl-anthraquinone), aloe-emodin, emodin monomethyl ether, rheo-tannic acid, glucogallum (a glucoside), tannin, gallic acid, calcium oxalate, starch, etc. The active principles are found in the cells of the medullary-rays.

Uses.—Purgative with secondary astringent action in indigestion; stomachic bitter, laxative.

Adulterants.—The crude drug has been found adulterated with the rhizomes and roots of *Rheum rhaponticum* and *R. undulatum* or *R. Compactum* hybrids, known as European, English or Garden Rhubarb. These are more astringent and mucilaginous and contain less calcium oxalate and so are not as gritty as the official article. They are likewise lighter in color and weight and contain the crystalline glucoside rhapontin, chrysophanic acid, etc., but no emodin, aloe-emodin or rhein. European Rhubarb has also been substituted for the official article.

It is distinguished microscopically from the official drug by showing a diffuse circle of isolated compound fibrovascular bundles ("stellate spots"). The medullary-rays are straighter, and the drug possesses none of the reddish color so characteristic of official Rhubarb.

RUMEX N.F. (RUMEX)

Synonyms.—Yellow Dock, Curled Dock (*R. crispus*), Bitter Dock or Broad-leaved Dock (*R. obtusifolius*).

Botanical Origin.—*Rumex crispus* L. and *Rumex obtusifolius* L.

Part Used.—Roots.

Limit of Impurities.—5 per cent. of its stem bases or other foreign organic matter.

Habitat.—Europe. Naturalized in the United States and Canada and found growing abundantly in waste and cultivated soil.

Plants.—Perennial herbs. *Rumex crispus* has a smooth stem either simple or branched above, from 0.9 to 1.5 m. high. Its leaves are acute, lanceolate with wavy-curled margins, the lower ones being truncate or cordate at the base. The greenish flowers are arranged in loose whorls on a panicled raceme. The calyx is composed of six sepals, the 3 outer being herbaceous, the 3 inner somewhat colored. The stamens are 6 in number. There are 3 styles bearing tufted stigmas. The fruit is a 3-angled akene with entire valves. *Rumex obtusifolius* somewhat resembles *R. crispus* but differs from it in possessing a rough stem, broader leaves with obtuse apex, and akenes, the valves of which show sharp, awl-shaped teeth at the base.

Commerce.—The commercial supplies of American grown Rumex are obtained largely from Virginia, North Carolina, Michigan and Indiana. Rumex is also imported from Europe, the chief shipping ports being Marseilles, Hamburg, Trieste and Leghorn. European Rumex comes in burlap bags and is usually cut. Occasionally it contains an excessive amount of dirt or stem bases.

Description.—The roots being fleshy are usually split longitudinally or cut into transverse segments during preparation. Entire roots simple or branched and twisted, up to 35 cm. in length and 7 cm. in diameter; externally dark reddish-brown (*R. crispus*) or pale yellowish-brown (*R. obtusifolius*), wrinkled longitudinally, marked with small root scars which are frequently transversely elongated and with remains of the stem or stem scars, the former being purplish, hollow and finely striated; fracture short and dusty; odor indistinct; taste astringent, and somewhat bitter.

Microscopical Characteristics.—Cross sections of *R. crispus* exhibit the following structures passing from periphery toward the center:

1. An outer zone of light brown cork cells beneath which is a collapsed phellogen.

2. Several rows of collenchyma cells.

3. A broader zone of cortical parenchyma cells with thin walls, some containing starch, others rosette crystals of calcium oxalate. Leaf-trace bundles are occasionally met with in this region.

4. A circle of small fibrovascular bundles characterized by few tracheæ and fibers.

5. Pith composed of parenchyma, some of the cells of which contain starch, others rosette aggregates of calcium oxalate.

Powdered Drug.—Dark brown; numerous ellipsoidal or elongated or truncate starch grains up to 25μ long; fragments of light brown cork cells; rosette crystals of calcium oxalate 25μ to 60μ in diameter; stone cells up to 200μ in diameter, lamellated and with few simple pores; sclerenchyma fibers few and with simple pores; tracheæ up to 100μ in width with reticulate and scalariform markings.

Constituents.—Chrysophanic acid (rumicin), a tannin colored green with iron, nepodin, lapodin, etc.

Uses.—Purgative and laxative in dyspepsia and diarrhœa; stomachic and tonic.

CHENOPODIACEÆ (GOOSEFOOT FAMILY)

Annual or perennial herbs or undershrubs of more or less succulent character and wide distribution, the greater number inhabiting the shores of oceans and salt lakes. Leaves mostly alternate, simple, usually flat, entire, sinuate-toothed or cut, sometimes fleshy, semi-cylindric to cylindric and exstipulate. Flowers small, inconspicuous and greenish, each with a free calyx of from 5 to 2 sepals, no corolla, as many hypogynous stamens as calyx lobes and a pistil with a one-celled ovary and 4 to 2 stigmas. Fruit a utricle. Seeds albuminous (*Chenopodium*) with curved or annular embryo surrounding the mealy albumen or embryo folded, dividing the albumen into two parts or seed exalbuminous with embryo forming a conical spiral (Saltwort). To this family belong the Spinach and Beet and a number of common sea-shore plants such as the Samphire, Sea Blite, Salt Bush, and Saltwort.

CHENOPODIUM (CHENOPODIUM)

Synonyms.—American W[illegible] Wild Wormseed, Jerusalem Tea, Goosefoot, Jerusalem Oak, S[illegible] Weed; *Ger.* Amerikanischer Wurmsamen; *Fr.* Ansérine Vermifuge.

Botanical Origin.—*Chenopod[illegible] ambrosioides* var. *anthelminticum* (Linné) A. Gray.

Part Used.—The dried fruits.

Habitat.—West Indies, Central and South America. Naturalized in the United States.

Plant.—An aromatic annual or perennial weed growing in waste localities in many sections of the United States and cultivated extensively in Maryland and to a lesser extent in South Dakota for its oil which is official in the U.S.P. as **Oleum Chenopodii.** Its leaves are lanceolate or oblong, strongly serrate, the lower being nearly laciniate-pinnatifid. Its flowers are minute, green and clustered in glomerules on almost naked, elongated spikes. Its fruit is a utricle with blackish akene enveloped by a bladdery calyx.

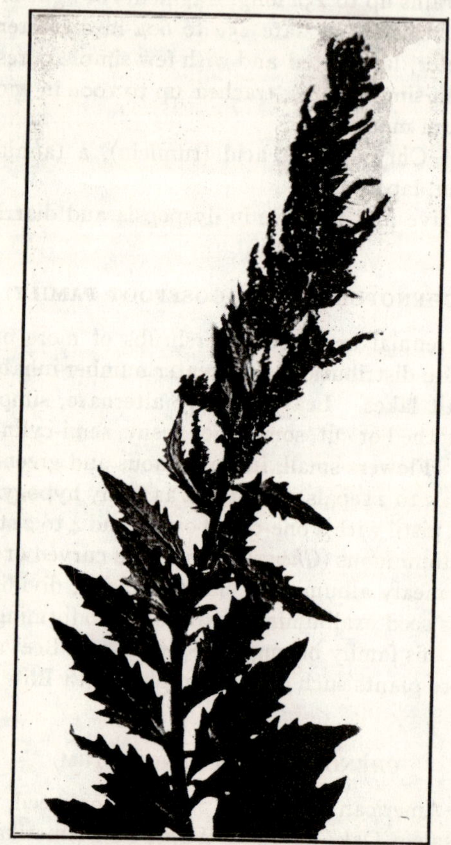

FIG. 70.—*Chenopodium ambrosioides* var. *anthelminticum* (Fam. *Chenopodiaceæ*) the fruits of which (utricles) constitute "American Wormseed."

Production and Commerce.—American wormseed is cultivated chiefly in Maryland, Virginia, North Carolina, Florida, Indiana and South Dakota. It thrives best when planted in pulverized loamy soil. The seeds are sown in the spring in rows 3 to 4 feet apart and lightly covered. When well up the plants are thinned to stand about 18 in. apart in the row. A pound of seed is sufficient for an acre. Shallow cultivation between the rows is essential for a good crop. When grown for the seeds, the crop should be harvested before the tops take on a brown color. The plants are mowed down and dried by the fire, after which the seed is thrashed out and cleaned by passing through wire sieves. When grown for the oil, the plants are cut when the tops are still green and the fresh overground parts of the flowering and fruiting plants subjected to steam distillation. The oil should yield not less than 65 per cent. of ascaridol. The yield of seed averages about 1000 pounds per acre. Most of the commercial supply of the seed comes from Florida, Virginia, North Carolina and Indiana, while the oil is largely produced in Maryland and South Dakota.

Description.—Fruit depressed globular, greenish-yellow or greenish-brown, about 1.5 mm. in diameter, consisting of an outer thin, bladdery and glandular calyx surrounding a lenticular, brownish-black to reddish-black, glossy, seed-like akene; odor distinct, aromatic; taste pungent and bitter.

Constituents.—Volatile oil containing ascaridol (anthelmintic principle) p-cymol, d-camphor and a terpene.

Uses.—Anthelmintic, for the round and hook worms.

PHYTOLACCACEÆ (POKE FAMILY)

A family of apetalous trees, shrubs, or woody herbs chiefly of tropical and subtropical climes with alternate entire leaves, and flowers resembling those of the goosefoot family (*Chenopodiaceæ*), but differing in having the several-celled ovary composed of many carpels united in a ring, and forming a berry in fruit. The genus Phytolacca is the sole representative in the United States.

PHYTOLACCA N.F. (PHYTOLACCA)

Synonyms.—Poke Root, Pigeon Berry, American Nightshade, Scoke, Pocan, Red Ink Plant; *Ger.* Kermesbeerenwurzel; *Fr.* Agouman, Racine de Phytolaque.

Botanical Origin.—*Phytolacca decandra* Linné.

Part Used.—The dried root.

Purity Rubric.—Not more than 5 per cent. of its stem bases or more than 2 per cent. of other foreign organic matter.

Habitat.—E. North America, in waste places. Naturalized in southern Europe and West Indies.

Plant.—A smooth perennial herb. The underground portion consists of a much-branched, fleshy root system. From the crown of the tap root arise one or more smooth, purplish-green, aerial stems that may attain a height of 2 to 2.5 m. The leaves are alternate, petiolate, entire, smooth, ovate, and acute at both summit and base. The inflorescences consist of racemes of greenish-white flowers. Each flower has 5 rounded, white sepals, 10 stamens and 10 short, green carpels arranged in a ring. The fruit is a compound berry composed of 10 ripened carpels and of a dark purple color when fully mature. Each matured carpel possesses a single lens-shaped black seed. The young tender shoots of Poke are edible. The leaves and roots have frequently been employed to adulterate Belladonna Leaves and Belladonna Root. The berries are poisonous.

Production and Commerce.—The root system is dug up in autumn. After the rootlets have been cut off, it is washed and the fleshy roots are then cut into transverse, longitudinal and oblique slices and dried. The thinner roots are generally cut into segments before drying. The commercial supplies are obtained largely from Michigan, Indiana, North Carolina and Virginia.

Description.—In nearly cylindrical segments or short fusiform roots (rarely), for the most part in transverse, longitudinal or oblique, often irregularly broken, slices; externally bark yellowish to dark brown, incompletely annulate and longitudinally or spirally wrinkled; texture fibrous; fracture tough; inner surface grayish to light brown, showing alternating circular zones of fibrovascular tissue and parenchyma, the latter being much retracted; odor slight; taste at first slightly sweet, then very acrid.

Microscopical Characteristics.—Transverse sections of the root are characterized by the presence of a narrow cortex, concentric series of open collateral fibrovascular bundles, numerous cells containing short raphides of calcium oxalate and some, crystal sand. Longitudinal radial sections exhibit tracheæ with characteristic diamond-shaped bordered pores.

Reticulate and scalariform tracheæ as well as wood fibers with oblique slits may also be observed See Figs. 241 and 242.

Powdered Drug.—Dark yellow to pale brown; sternutatory; calcium oxalate in raphides from 15 to 50μ long, or in micro-crystals (crystal sand), often filling up the cavities of certain cells; starch grains simple or 2-compound, the individual grains from 6μ to 35μ in diameter; sclerenchyma fibers with oblique slits; tracheids and tracheæ either with diamond-shaped bordered pores or reticulate or scalariform thickenings; fragments of parenchyma and cork.

Constituents.—A bitter saponin-like glucoside, free formic acid, 10 per cent. of a non-reducing sugar, traces of an alkaloid called phytolaccine, phytolaccic acid, starch, calcium oxalate, etc.

Uses.—Poke root has been used in the form of its fluidextract or as a resinoid (phytolaccin) as an alterative in rheumatism and as an emetic.

MAGNOLIACEÆ (MAGNOLIA FAMILY)

Trees and shrubs having alternate leaves and single large flowers with calyx and corolla colored alike. Sepals and petals dediduous, anthers adnate. Carpels and stamens numerous. Bark aromatic and bitter. Fruit a collection of follicles deshiscing dorsally.

ILLICIUM (ILLICIUM)

Synonyms.—Star Anise, Chinese Star Anise, Fructus Anisi Stellati; *Ger.* Sternanis; *Fr.* Anise étoilé, Badiane.

Botanical Origin.—*Illicium verum* Hooker filius.

Part Used.—The dried ripe fruit.

Habitat.—In mountainous districts of southeastern Asia.

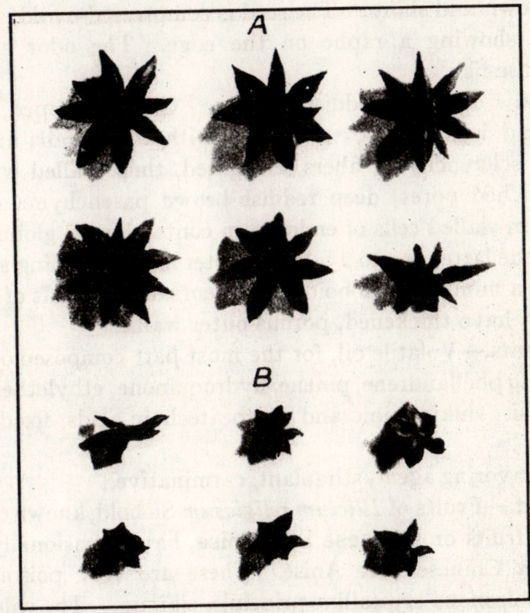

FIG. 71.—Chinese star anise (*A*); Japanese star anise (*B*). × ⅝.

Plant.—An evergreen tree growing to the height of 4 to 6 m. The leaves are entire, lanceolate, pellucid-punctate with acute apices. The flowers are greenish-yellow. The fruit consists of 6–8 dark brown, woody follicles arranged around a central axis, each containing a compressed-ovoid, shiny, brown seed.

Production and Commerce.—The fruits are gathered from trees growing wild as well as cultivated. Cultivation of the plant is practised extensively in mountainous regions of French Indo-China, Southwestern China, Japan, the Philippines and Jamaica. The fruits are picked just before maturity. Most of the drug is used for the production of volatile oil. In fact the most of the commercial oil of anise on the market consists of oil of star anise. This is distilled from the fruits while still recent. The greater bulk of the crude drug and the oil used in the United States comes from southern China.

Description.—The fruit is formed of 6 to 8 (rarely up to 11) one-seeded, boat-shaped, woody follicles arranged in a radiate whorl around a short central column which proceeds from a short pedicel. The latter is curved near the fruit. The follicles are usually of unequal length, broadly ovate, laterally compressed, the distal portion prolonged to a blunt, nearly straight beak. Their outer surface is reddish-brown. Their inner surface is pale yellowish-brown and shiny. The seed is compressed-ovoid, shiny, smooth and brown, showing a raphe on the edge. The odor and taste are aromatic, anise-like.

Powdered Drug.—Reddish-brown. Column-shaped, irregularly branching and isodiametric stone cells with thick walls and branching pore canals; sclerenchyma fibers, elongated, thick-walled with simple to slightly branched pores; deep reddish-brown parenchyma of mesocarp; polygonal thin-walled cells of endosperm containing oil globules and aleurone grains, the latter 10μ to 25μ in diameter and containing a large phytoglobulin and a number of globoids; fragments of epidermis of pericarp, the cells of which have thickened, porous outer walls.

Constituents.—Volatile oil, for the most part composed of anethol but also containing phellandrene, pinene, hydroquinone, ethylether and methyl chavicol; anisic, shikimminic and protocatechuic acids, fixed oil, protein, etc.

Uses.—Flavoring agent, stimulant, carminative.

Adulterant.—Fruits of *Illicium religiosum* Siebold, known commercially as **Shikimmi** fruits or **Japanese Star Anise,** have occasionally been found admixed with Chinese Star Anise. These are very poisonous. They contain the poisonous crystalline principle, sikimin. The chief diagnostic differences between Chinese and Japanese Star Anise will be noted in the following table:

Chinese Star Anise	Japanese Star Anise
1. Follicles with acute summit tapering to blunt, nearly straight beak.	1. Follicles for most part smaller than Chinese Anise, with acuminate summit tapering to short, upward curved beak.
2. Irregularly branching stone cells in central axis.	2. Stone cells of central axis somewhat rounded.
3. Aleurone grains of seed endosperm contain one large phytoglobulin and usually a number of globoids.	3. Aleurone grains contain 2 or 3 prismatic phytoglobulins and 2 or 3 globoids.
4. Powder becomes blood red when boiled in dilute potassium hydroxide.	4. Powder becomes yellowish-brown when similarly treated.
5. Odor resembling Anisum.	5. Odor resembling Sassafras or Cajuput.
6. Taste aromatic, like Anisum.	6. Taste aromatic, bitter and camphor-like.

RANUNCULACEÆ (CROWFOOT FAMILY)

Herbs, rarely shrubs (*Clematis*), with acrid, poisonous, watery juices and with alternate, rarely opposite, simple, rarely compound, exstipulate leaves. Flowers pentamerous, regular to irregular, incomplete to complete, aposepalous and apopetalous. Sepals 5—rarely more or less—green to petaloid, regular, passing to irregular (Larkspur, Monkshood). Petals none or 5, regular to rarely irregular, often nectariferous and with nectariferous petals often variously transformed. Stamens indefinite, hypogynous. Pistil of many to few apocarpous carpels, each carpel with one to several ovules. Fruit a collection of achenes (*Ranunculus*, *Anemonella*), or a collection of follicles (Columbine, Larkspur, Peony) or rarely a berry as in Baneberry (*Actœa*). Seeds albuminous.

ACONITUM U.S.P. (ACONITE)

Synonyms.—Monkshood, Aconite Root, Aconite Tuber, Wolfsbane, Cuckoo's Cap, Blue Rocket, Friar's Cap, Jacob's Chariot; *Fr.* Coqueluchon; *Ger.* Aconitknollen, Sturmhut, Eisenhut.

Botanical Origin.—*Aconitum Napellus* Linné.

Part Used.—The dried tuberous root.

Limit of Impurities.—5 per cent. of Aconite stems or 2 per cent. of other foreign matter.

Standards of Assay.—This drug is standardized biologically. By biological assay, when made into the tincture and administered subcutaneously to guinea pigs, it has a minimum lethal dose not exceeding 0.0004 cc. of tincture for each gram of body weight of guinea pig.

Habitat.—Mountainous districts of Europe and Asia.

Plant.—A perennial herb attaining the height of from 0.7 to 1.5 m. The underground portion consists of a fusiform, parent, tuberous root from which arise one or more lateral shoots, each forming a conical daughter tuberous root. The leaves are alternate, long stalked, with blades palmately cut into 5 or 3 segments which are in turn divided into narrow segments. The inflorescence is a terminal raceme of violet-blue flowers. The bracts are lanceolate, there being two beneath each pedicelled flower. The sepals are 5, bluish-purple, the upper one helmet shaped, laterally compressed, the 2 lateral ones blunt and ovate, the two lower oblong-lanceolate. The petals vary from 2–8 and are hammer-like, the 2 posterior ones being covered by the hood of the posterior sepal. The stamens are numerous and hypogynous. There are 3 or 4 carpels, with bilobed stigmas. The fruit consists of 3 to 4 beaked follicles containing numerous angular, wrinkled and acrid seeds.

Production and Commerce.—Aconite is largely collected from plants growing wild in cool regions of Germany, Spain, France and Switzerland,

It may be propagated from seeds or by divisions of roots. The latter method is preferable in localities where more than one species abounds, since hybridization is avoided. If seeds are employed they should be planted as soon as possible after they are gathered from the plants for, if allowed to completely dry, they lose in their power of germination and are

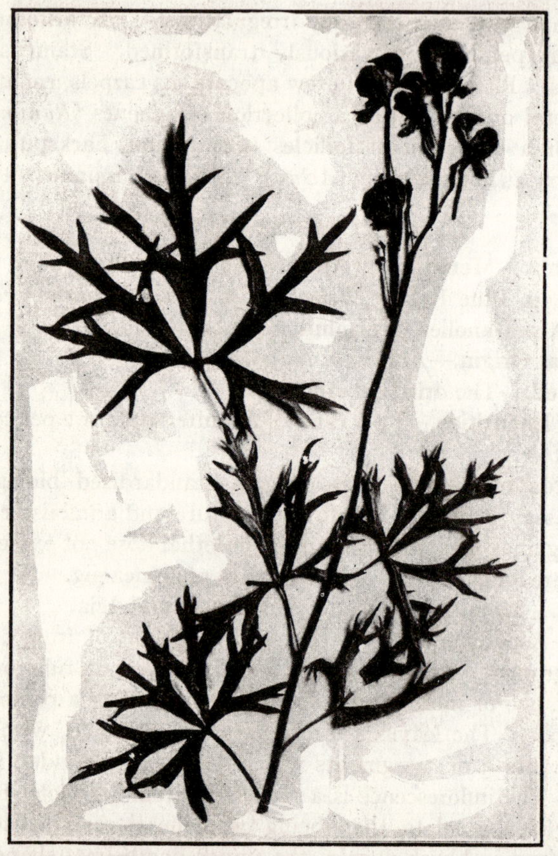

FIG. 72.—*Aconitum Napellus.* Note the palmately 3- to 5-cut leaf blades and the terminal raceme of flowers. In each flower, the posterior sepal is helmet- or hood-shaped and, in the incompletely expanded condition, arches over the rest of the flower. Hence, the common names, "Monkshood" and "Friar's Cap," assigned to the plant because of fancied resemblance.

mostly non-viable after a year's storage. Elevated situations, some shade, cool climate and well-drained gravelly loam are ideal conditions for a good crop. The tuberous roots are dug up in autumn, washed, freed from the rootlets and carefully dried. The present commercial supplies come to this country from Germany, Italy, Spain, France and Trieste.

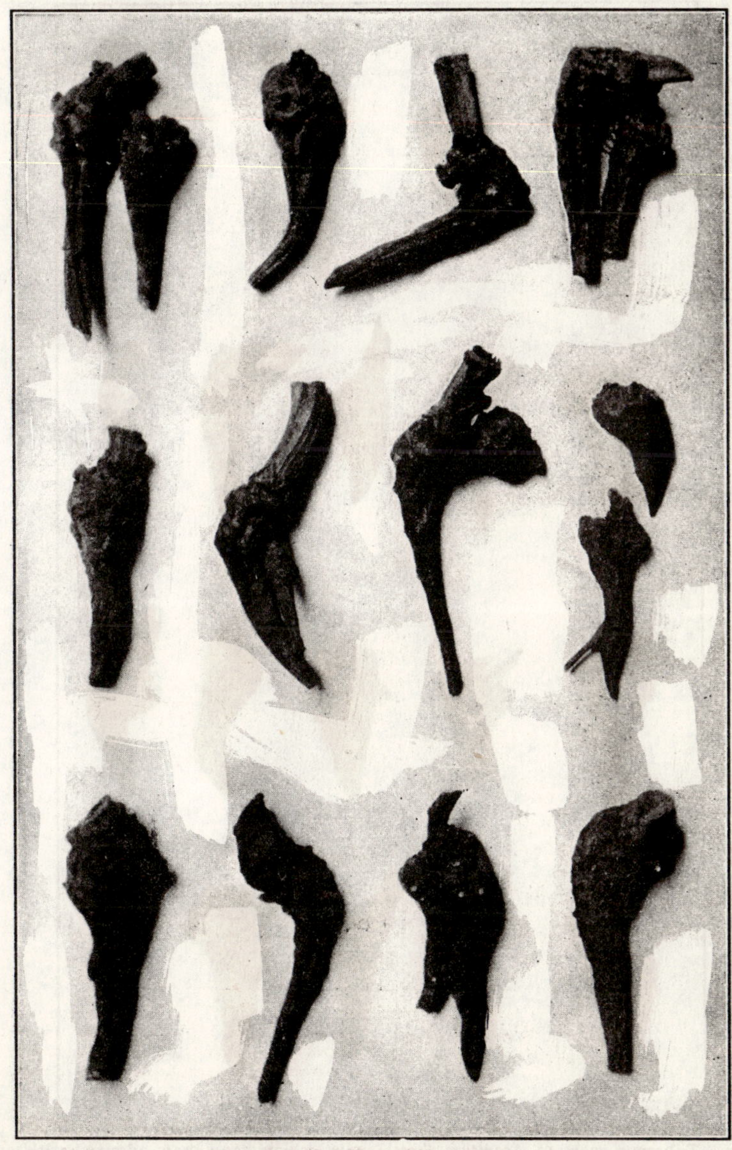

Fig. 73.—Tuberous roots of *Aconitum Napellus*. Note that several of these show parent and daughter tubers still joined together. × ½.

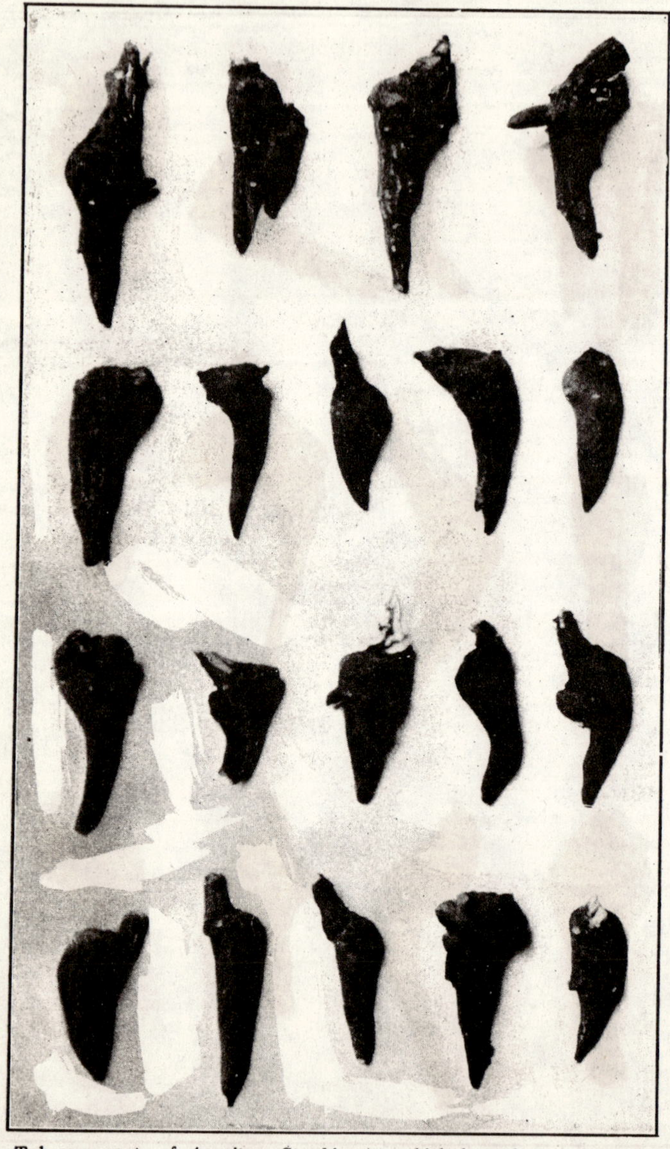

FIG. 74—Tuberous roots of *Aconitum Stoerkianum*, which have been admixed with and substituted for the official Aconitum. × ½.

Description.—The tuberous roots occur either singly or in clusters of 2 (or rarely 3), when the younger smoother root is connected with

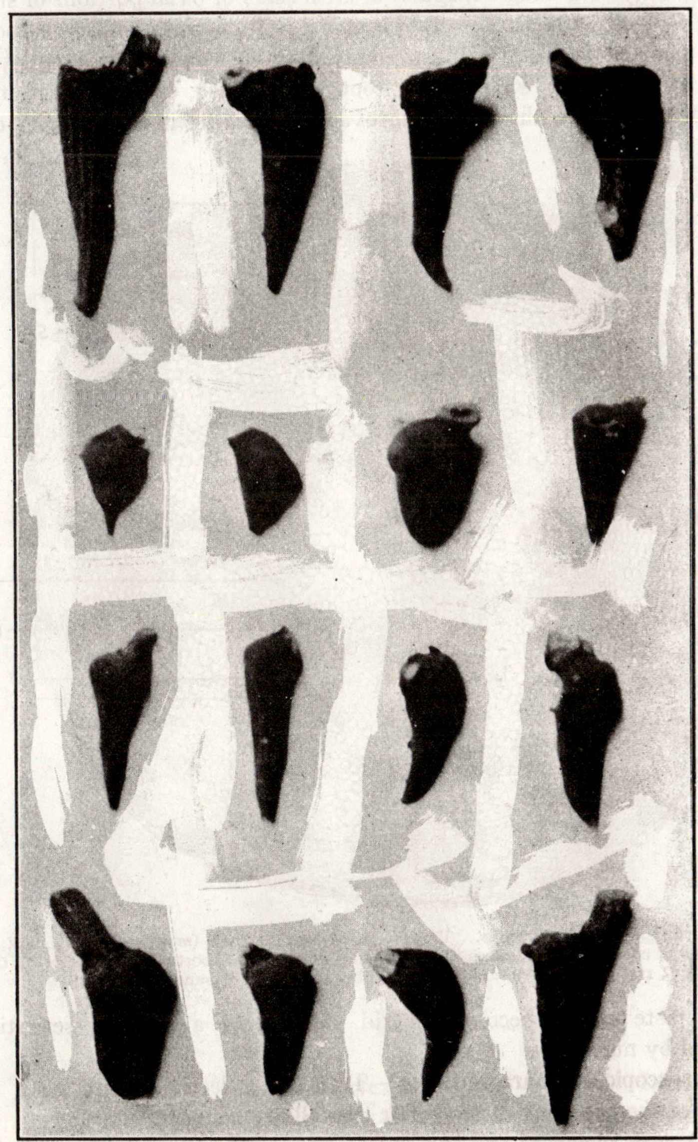

FIG. 75.—Japanese aconite. × ⅝.

the older deeply wrinkled root by means of a side branch. Each root is somewhat conical or fusiform, from 4 to 10 cm. in length and from 1 to 3.5

cm. in width at the crown; externally dark brown or grayish-brown, smooth or longitudinally wrinkled, the upper end with a bud or remains of bud scales (young daughter roots) or stem scars or basal portions of stems (older shriveled roots), the other external portions with numerous rootlet scars or short rootlets; fracture short, horny or mealy; internally, old roots are brownish while young roots are whitish, exhibiting a 5- to 8-angled cambium with a small fibrovascular bundle in each angle; odor

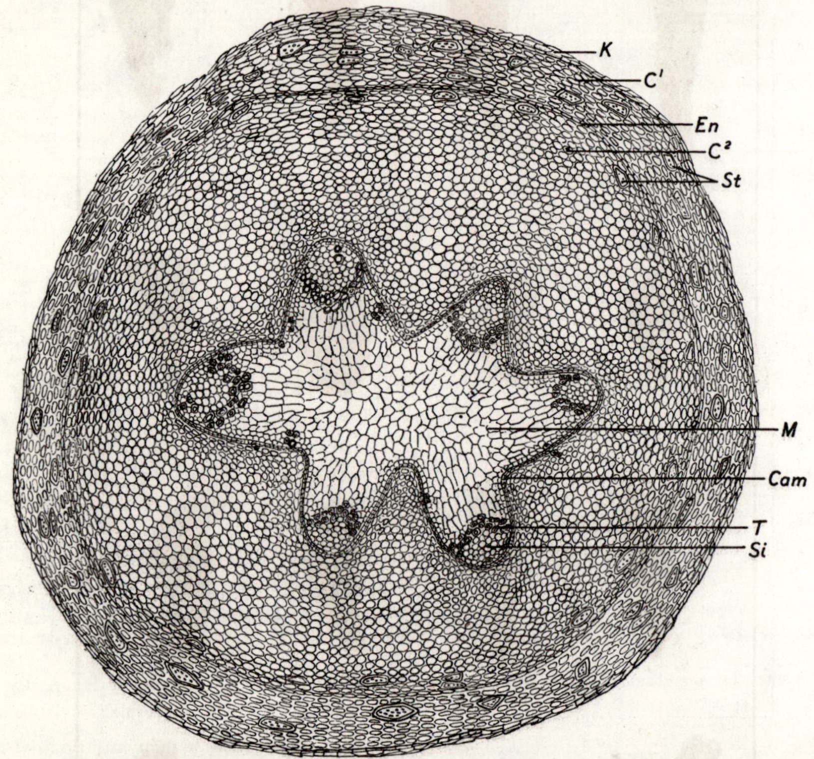

FIG. 76.—*Aconitum Napellus.* Transverse section of root (*magnified*). *K*, cork; C^1, outer zone of cortex; *En*, endodermis; C^2, broader inner zone of cortex; *St*, stone cells; *Cam*, cambium; *T*, tracheæ of xylem and *Si*, sieve tubes of phloem of bundle; *M*, pith.

slight; taste sweet, becoming acrid, developing a tingling sensation, followed by numbness.

Microscopical Characteristics.—Transverse sections, cut near the middle of the tuberous root, exhibit the following structure:

1. A cork region of one or more layers of blackish or brownish cells.

2. A broad cortex of two regions, viz.: an outer narrower and an inner broader zone. The narrower zone consists of from 8 to 15 layers of

parenchyma cells, interspersed among which are numerous stone cells of various shapes. Separating this zone from the broader, inner one is an endodermis of a single layer of tangentially elongated endodermal cells. The broader zone consists of about 20 layers of starch-containing parenchyma cells, interspersed among which are a few small fibrovascular bundles. Stone cells may also occur in this zone just beneath the endodermis.

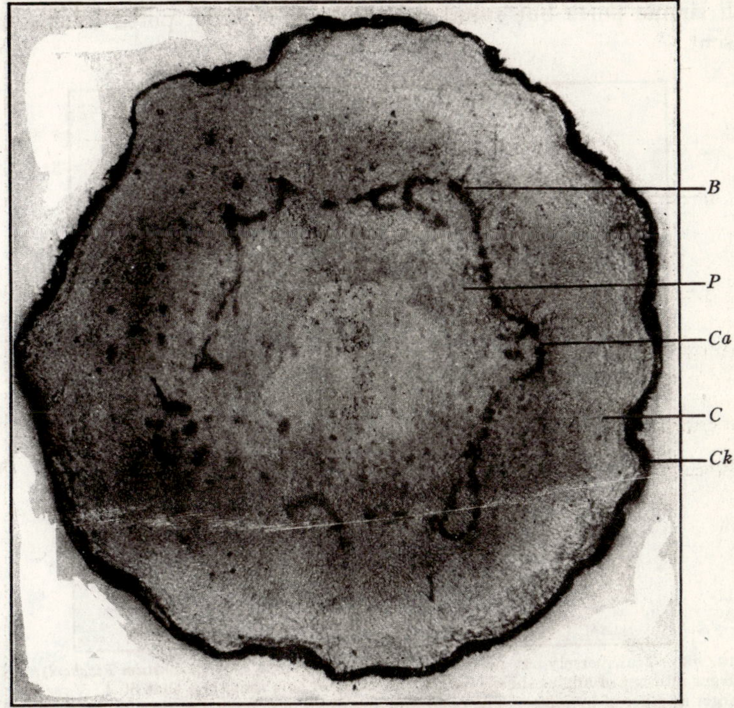

FIG. 77.—Transverse section of tuberous root of *Aconitum Stoerkianum*, showing cork (*Ck*); cortex (*C*); cambium (*Ca*); fibrovascular bundles (*B*); and pith (*P*). × 18.

3. A 5 to 8-angled cambium, more or less star-shaped, within the angles of which, and frequently scattered along the entire cambial line occur collateral fibrovascular bundles.

4. A broad 5 to 8-rayed pith composed of parenchyma cells. The parenchyma cells of both cortex and pith contain numerous single or 2–5-compound starch grains as well as active principles. Most of the active principles are localized in the cortex just outside of the angles of the cambium.

Powdered Drug.—Grayish-brown; starch grains abundant, spherical or plano-convex, single or 2- to 5-compound, the individual grains from 3μ to 20μ in diameter and frequently showing a central cleft hilum; stone cells of varying shape, strongly lignified or elongated to fibers up to 400μ long with porous walls up to 25μ thick; fragments of yellowish-brown cork; fragments of parenchyma filled with starch; sclerenchyma fibers from stems few, very long with lignified walls about 5μ or 6μ in thickness and showing oblique or transverse slit-like pores; tracheæ for the most part with simple pores but spiral, reticulate and border pored tracheæ also present.

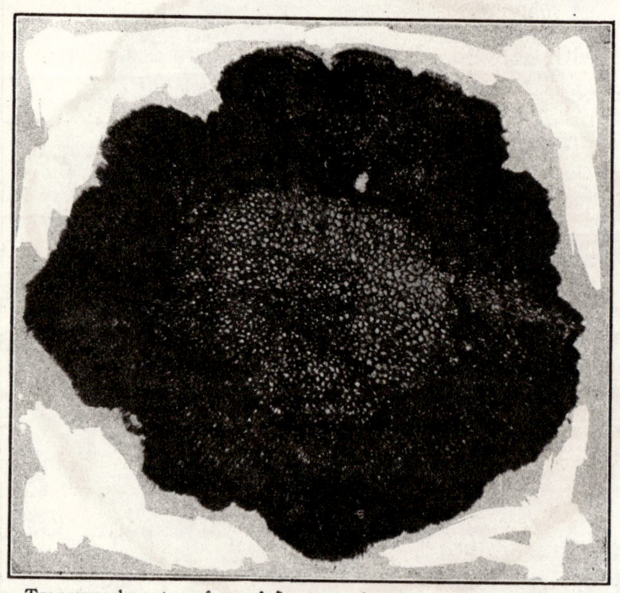

FIG. 78.—Transversely cut surface of Japanese Aconite root (*Aconitum Fischeri*). Note the larger number of angles shown by the cambium of this root than that of *A. Napellus*, also the larger number of bundles. The cambium angles are much smaller than those of the official aconite. × 20.

Constituents.—Aconitine ($C_{34}H_{47}O_{11}N$) aconine, benzaconine and napelline (alkaloids); aconitic acid, starch, mannitol and resin. Aconitine (U.S.P.) is the most important alkaloid and occurs up to 0.75 per cent. If 1 mg. of this alkaloid is mixed with 2 drops of H_2SO_4 containing 5 mg. of ammonium vanadate in a cc., an orange color is produced.

Uses.—Cardiac depressant in high arterial tension of cardiac origin; locally in form of diluted tincture as an analgesic in facial neuralgia, rheumatism, etc.

Substitutes and Adulterants.—1. *Japanese Aconite Root.* Two roots bearing this commercial designation occur on the market. The first of these, yielded by *Aconitum Fischeri* Reich., is of conical shape, smaller, less wrinkled, of lighter weight and more mealy than the official article. It is claimed to contain an alkaloid called *jesaconitine*. The second is yielded by *A. uncinatum* L. var. *japonicum* Regel. This root is also conical, smaller, starchy, and less wrinkled than U.S.P. aconite; the daughter tuberous root is dark-gray and nearly smooth while the parent root is brownish and marked with slightly raised longitudinal ridges. It contains *japaconitine*. Both of these Japanese Aconites have an uneven, wavy, ellipsoidal or circular cambium with numerous collateral fibrovascular bundles arranged along its course.

2. Root of *Aconitum chasmanthum* Stapf. This is averagely smaller and less wrinkled than the official root, about 2 cm. long and 0.75 cm. in diameter, with rootlet stubs mostly clustered at the basal end. It *contains indaconitine*.

3. *Indian or Nepaul Aconite* is the root of *A. laciniatum* Stapf. It is larger than the official root, being up to 15 cm. long and 4 cm. thick near the crown, brown and deeply wrinkled externally, generally horny internally and exhibiting gelatinized starch grains when scrapings are examined under the microscope. It contains *pseudaconitine*.

4. Root of *Aconitum ferox* Wallich. This is obtained from another Indian Aconite, native to the Himalayas. It is conical, up to 10 cm. long and 3 cm. in diameter, externally grayish-brown and deeply furrowed. The fracture is horny or mealy, the fractured surface being yellowish-brown or whitish and showing a 7 to 9 angled cambium. It contains *pseudaconitine*.

Allied Species.—*A. Lycoctonum* L., indigenous to Europe and N. Asia possesses a several headed rhizome which contains *lycaconitine* and *myoctonine*. *A. heterophyllum* Wallich of India possesses small fusiform or ovoid grayish roots which are bitter but not acrid or benumbing and contains the alkaloid, *atisine*. *A. paniculatum* Lam. contains *paniculatine* while *A. spicatum* Lam. contains *bikhaconitine*.

HYDRASTIS U.S.P. (HYDRASTIS)

Synonyms.—Golden Seal, Yellow Puccoon, Yellow Root, Orange Root Ground Raspberry, Indian Paint; *Fr.* Sceau d'Or; *Ger.* Canadische Gelbwurzel.

Botanical Origin.—*Hydrastis canadensis* Linné.

Part Used.—The dried rhizome and roots.

Limit of Impurities.—2 per cent. of its stems or leaves or 2 per cent. of other foreign organic matter.

Standard of Assay.—Not less than 2.5 per cent. of ether-soluble alkaloids of Hydrastis.

Ash.—Not more than 3 per cent. acid-insoluble.

Habitat.—In rich well-drained woodlands of North America, east of the Mississippi.

Plant.—A perennial herb, known to the Cherokee Indians who used its underground portion both for dyeing and as an internal remedy. Its valuable properties were presented by them to the early American settlers. The underground portion of the plant consists of a horizontal, branching

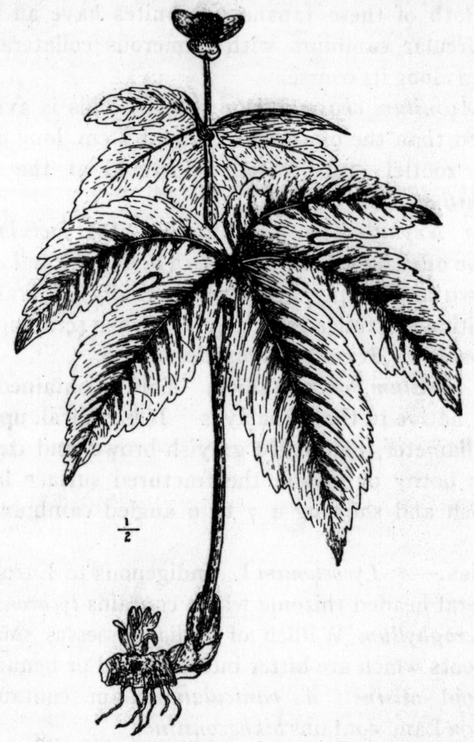

FIG. 79.—*Hydrastis canadensis.* (*From Sayre.*)

rhizome bearing numerous long slender roots. The aerial portion consists of a single radical leaf and a short stem 1 to 1.8 dm. in length which bears near its summit 2 petiolate, palmately 5–7-lobed, serrate leaves and ends with a solitary greenish-white flower that opens in April or May. The fruit consists of a compound crimson berry which has an appearance somewhat like that of the raspberry.

Production and Commerce.—Although plentiful in our virgin forests, Golden Seal, as a wild plant, has become very scarce during the past quarter of a century. Most of the drug is obtained from plants growing wild in Indiana, Ohio and West Virginia. Cincinnati is the leading

Hydrastis market. Some of the drug is obtained from plants cultivated in the Pacific northwest while scattering collections are made in Georgia, Missouri, Minnesota and West Ontario.

The plants are usually propagated by seedlings or by cuttings of the rhizome. Seedlings may be procured by sowing the seeds in mid-autumn in seed beds containing abundant leaf mold. After planting, the seeds should be covered with an inch of fine leaf mold and protected during the cold winter season by covering the beds with burlap. After the seedlings have developed to the height of about 2 inches, they can be set out in cold frames or transplanted to pots to harden their root-system. They are later planted out in the open in well-fertilized soil containing abundant leaf mold, being set 6 or 8 inches apart, and protected in summer against excessive light and heat by lath-shade or vines. The ideal location in which to grow Hydrastis either from seedlings or cuttings is on the sloping side of a woodland hill where shade is abundant and drainage excellent. The rhizomes and roots should be collected in autumn after the aerial portion of the plant has withered. Plants grown from rhizome cuttings are generally ready for collection the third or fourth year, while those grown from seed should not be collected until the fifth year. The rhizomes and roots are washed clean and then dried on a clean dry floor or in partial shade, protected from rain, outside. They are kept in loose masses until marketed, in order to prevent mold attack.

Description.—Rhizome horizontal or oblique, sub-cylindrical, from 1–6 cm. in length and from 2–9 mm. in diameter, occasionally with stem bases; externally yellowish-or grayish-brown, marked by numerous stem scars and more or less annulate from scars of bud-scales, otherwise deeply longitudinally wrinkled; on the under and lateral portions arise many long slender roots which are easily detached; fracture short, waxy; internally of a deep yellow color in center, greenish-yellow near margin and exhibiting an interrupted circle of small, radially elongated fibrovascular bundles; odor distinct; taste bitter.

Microscopical Characteristics.—Transverse sections of the rhizome exhibit the following internal peculiarities:

1. Epidermis or cork, depending on age, with thin, yellowish-brown, suberized cells.

2. Cortex of about 25 layers of cortical parenchyma cells frequently showing traces of root outgrowths.

3. A circle of elongated, open collateral, fibrovascular bundles separated by broad medullary-rays. In fully developed bundles, there is to be observed a more or less collapsed phloem and cambium and a radially elongated xylem with a prominent group of wood fibers near the pith.

The remainder of the xylem is composed of tracheæ, tracheids and wood parenchyma, some of the last containing yellowish contents.

4. Pith composed of parenchyma cells.

Transverse sections of Hydrastis roots show the following:

1. Epidermis of a single layer of yellowish-brown, elongated epidermal cells with suberized outer walls, some giving rise to root-hairs.
2. Cortex of thick-walled, starch-containing parenchyma.

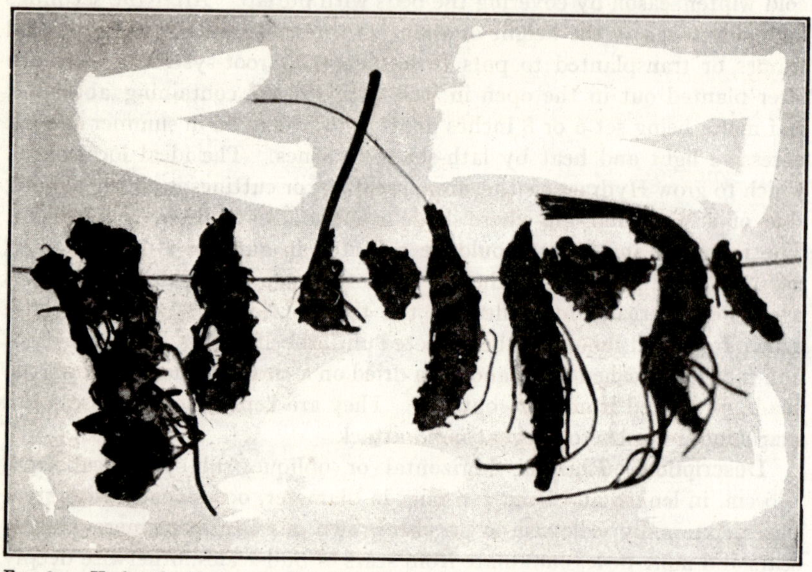

FIG. 80.—Hydrastis rhizomes, more or less deprived of many of their rootlets, ×1½. (*Photograph by Stoneback.*)

3. Endodermis of slightly lignified endodermal cells.
4. Pericambium of more or less collapsed thin-walled cells.
5. Radial fibrovascular bundle of 2 to 6 xylem patches alternating with as many phloem arms.

Sections prepared from the rhizome which has been macerated in water, when mounted in concentrated sulphuric acid and examined under the microscope, exhibit the formation of numerous needle- or rod-shaped crystals, some attaining a length of 200μ. These crystals represent sulphates of hydrastine and berberine.

Powdered Drug.—Brownish-yellow; numerous spherical simple starch grains, averagely 2μ to 15μ in diameter, the larger exhibiting a central hilum; a few 2- to 6-compound starch grains; fragments of starch parenchyma; fragments of fibrovascular tissue, the tracheæ with simple and bordered pores, some with spiral thickenings, the wood fibers short, thin-walled and with simple pores; a few fragments of cork tissue, the cells of which have reddish-brown walls.

Constituents.—The alkaloids hydrastine (colorless), berberine (yellow) and canadine; starch, etc.

Uses.—Hydrastis is an alterative to mucous membranes and a bitter tonic. It is employed in gastro-intestinal and nasal catarrh, in inflammation of the mucous membrane of the vagina, uterus and urethra, in menorrhagia, hemorrhoids, etc.

Adulterants.—Rhizomes and roots of *Jeffersonia diphylla*, *Cypripedium* species, and *Aristolochia Serpentaria*.

CIMICIFUGA U.S.P. (CIMICIFUGA)

Synonyms.—Black Snakeroot, Black Cohosh, Macrotys, Bugbane; *Ger*. Schwarze Schlangenwurzel; *Fr*. Racine d'Actèe à Grappes.

Botanical Origin.—*Cimicifuga racemosa* (Linné) Nuttall.

Part Used.—The dried rhizome and roots.

Limit of Impurities.—2 per cent. of its stems or other foreign matter.

Ash.—Not more than 4 per cent. acid insoluble.

Habitat.—In rich woods of eastern North America.

Plant.—A perennial herb whose subterranean portion consists of a thick, knotted rhizome system. Its aerial stem grows to the height of 1 to 2.5 m. Its leaves are decompound, the leaflets cut serrate along the margin and subcordate to subcuneate at the base. The inflorescence is a long wand-like raceme of white flowers.

Production and Commerce.—The drug is chiefly collected from plants growing wild in the Blue Ridge. Scattering collections are made in Indiana and Northern Pennsylvania. It is shipped either in bales or bags.

Description.—The drug occurs as a mixture of entire and broken rhizomes and roots. Rhizome horizontal, somewhat branched, from 2 to 15 cm. in length and from 1 to 3 cm. in thickness; externally dark brown, slightly annulate from circular scars of bud scales; the upper surface with several buds and numerous large stem bases terminated, frequently, by deep cup-shaped scars, each of which shows a radiate structure; or less frequently by fibrous strands, lower and lateral surfaces with numerous root scars and a few short roots; fracture horny; internally whitish and mealy or dark brown and waxy, bark thin, wood radiate and of about the same thickness as the pith; odor slight; taste bitter and acrid.

Roots cylindrical or obtusely 4-angled, up to 3 mm. thick; externally dark brown, longitudinally wrinkled; fracture short; internally bark brownish-black, wood yellowish and showing 3 to 6 rays.

Histology.—Transverse sections of the **rhizome** exhibit a yellowish-brown suberized epidermis, several layers of starch- and resin-containing cortical parenchyma, a circle of open collateral fibrovascular bundles whose xylem contains tracheæ with bordered pores and numerous strongly lignified wood fibers, medullary-rays separating the bundles and containing starch, and a central pith whose cells resemble those of the cortex.

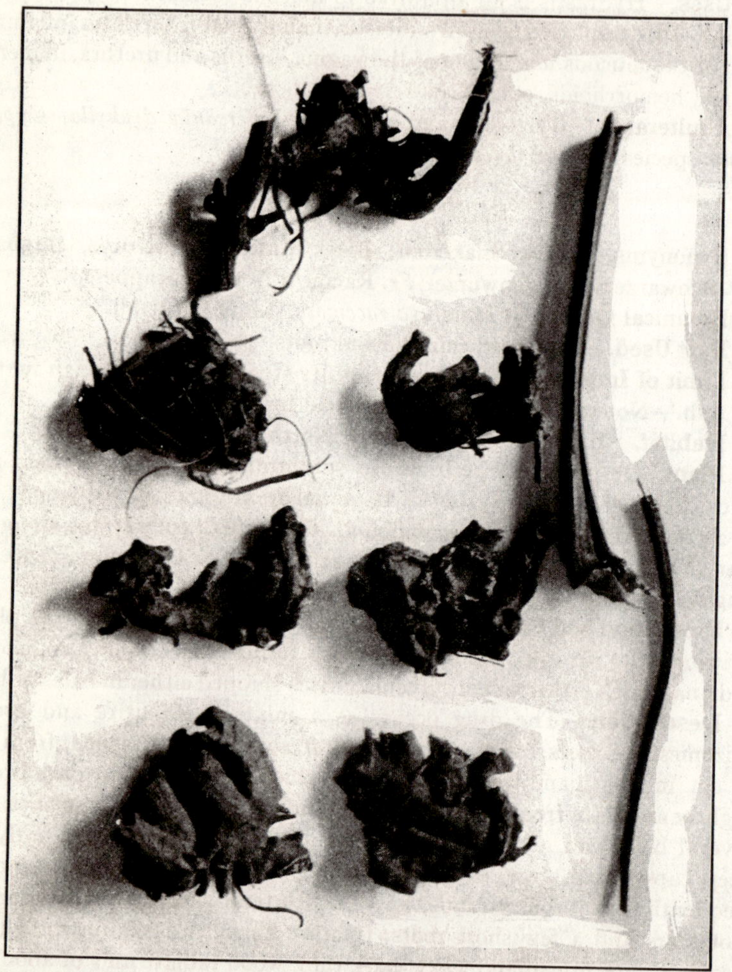

FIG. 81.—Cimicifuga. At right is portion of aerial stem (above) and root (below). × 5/8.

Transverse sections of the **root** exhibit a thin epidermis, a cortex, separated into two zones by a distinct endodermis, and 4 to 6, occasionally 3, fibrovascular bundles separated by broad wedge-shaped medullary-rays.

Constituents.—Resin, racemosin and 2 other crystalline principles, isoferulic acid, tannin, starch, etc. *Macrotin* or *cimicifugin* is a mixture of

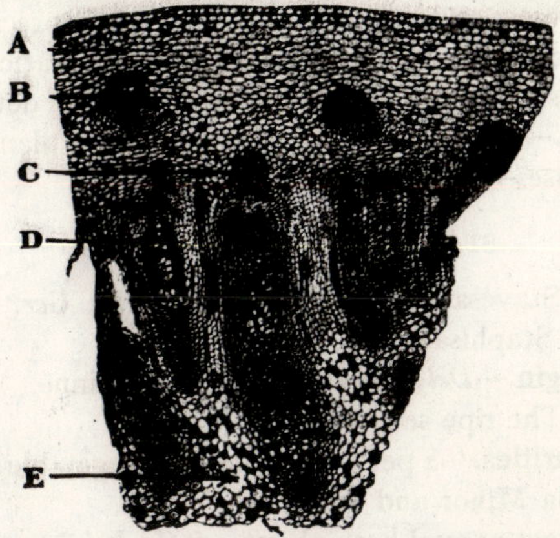

FIG. 82.—Transverse section of Cimicifuga rhizome (representative portion), ×18 diameters. *A*, cortex. *B*, fibrovascular bundle. *C*, phloem. *D*, xylem. *E*, pith. (*Photomicrograph, after Sayre.*)

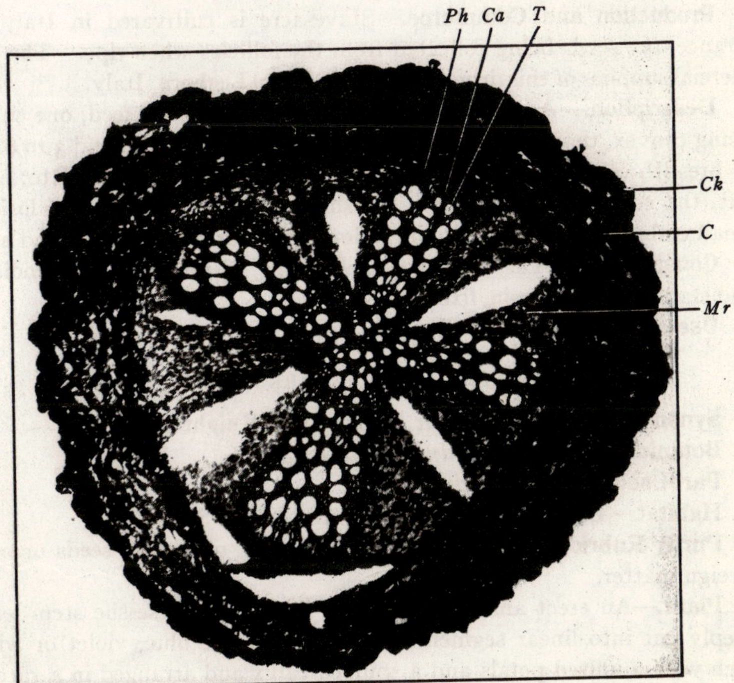

FIG. 83.—Transverse section of Cimicifuga root (highly magnified.) Cork (*Ck*); cortex (*C*); medullary-ray (*Mr*); phloem (*Ph*), cambium (*Ca*) and trachea in xylem (*T*) of an open collateral fibrovascular bundle.

resinous substances prepared by pouring a concentrated alcoholic tincture of the drug into water and separating and drying the precipitate.

Uses.—Cimicifuga is employed as an anti-rheumatic and as a remedy for dyspepsia, dysmenorrhœa, neuralgia, etc., but is of doubtful value.

Adulterants.—Excessive aerial stems of same plant and dirty roots are the chief causes of inferiority of this drug.

STAPHISAGRIA (STAPHISAGRIA)

Synonyms.—Stavesacre, Semen Pedicularis; *Ger.* Stephanskörner, Läusekörner; *Fr.* Staphisaigre.

Botanical Origin.—*Delphinium Staphisagria* Linné.

Part Used.—The ripe seed.

Limit of Impurities.—2 per cent. of foreign vegetable matter.

Habitat.—Asia Minor and Southern Europe.

Plant.—An erect annual herb about 4 ft. in height with palmate, 5–9-lobed, pubescent leaves. Its flowers are purplish with spurred calyx and borne in racemes. Its fruit consists of 3 downy follicles, each containing about 12 angled seeds.

Production and Commerce.—Stavesacre is cultivated in Italy and France, the seeds being collected from the follicles when ripe. The commercial supplies of this drug are imported from Leghorn, Italy.

Description.—A somewhat tetrahedral, albuminous seed, one surface being convex, the others plane, from 4 to 10 mm. in length and 3 to 8 mm. in breadth; externally dark brown, or grayish, coarsely reticulate; easily cut, the cut surface showing a bluish-gray oily endosperm, enclosing a small embryo at the pointed end; odor slight; taste very bitter and acrid.

Constituents.—The alkaloids delphinine, delphisine, delphinoidine, and staphisagroine; resin, fixed oil, etc.

Use.—Parasiticide in pediculosis.

DELPHINIUM N.F. (LARKSPUR SEED)

Synonyms.—Field Larkspur, Lark's Claw, Knight's Spur.

Botanical Origin.—*Delphinium Ajacis* Linné.

Part Used.—The dried ripe seed.

Habitat.—Europe. Naturalized in the United States.

Purity Rubric.—Not more than 2 per cent. of foreign seeds or other foreign matter.

Plant.—An erect annual, about 1½ ft. high with sessile stem leaves deeply cut into linear segments. The flowers are blue, violet or white, each with 2 united petals and a spurred calyx and arranged in a raceme. The fruit consists of a single pubescent follicle containing many small, ridged seeds.

Production and Commerce.—The commercial supplies of this drug are imported from Europe.

Description.—Seed albuminous, irregularly tetrahedral, about 2 mm. in diameter, seed coat crustaceous, its outer surface black, blackish-brown or grayish with from 8 to 12 rows of centrifugally elongated epidermal cells transversely encircling the seed and forming wavy ridges, occasionally intersecting and with narrow channels between; endosperm fleshy, whitish and oily; embryo-small, in endosperm; odor indistinct; taste bitter, later biting and acrid.

Constituents.—The alkaloid, delphinine; resin, fixed oil, etc.

Use.—Larkspur is employed externally in the form of its tincture as a parasiticide in pediculosis.

COPTIS N.F. (COPTIS)

Synonym.—Goldthread, *Ger.* Gelbe Niesswurz; *Fr.* Coptide.

Botanical Origin.—*Coptis trifolia* (Linné) Salisbury.

Part Used.—The dried plant.

Purity Rubric.—Not more than 3 per cent. of foreign organic matter.

Habitat.—Northern North America, south to Maryland, mountains of North Carolina and Tennessee and northeast Iowa.

Plant.—A low perennial herb found in woods and swamps. Its underground portion consists of a slender (filiform) rhizome of orange or deep golden-yellow color bearing several hair-like rootlets from the lower surface of each of its nodes. Its aerial portion consists of several radical leaves that are evergreen, long petioled and trifoliate, and a slender scape 7 to 12.5 cm. high which bears a small white flower from May to July. The fruit consists of 7 follicles containing small black seeds.

Production and Commerce.—Goldthread is collected when in flower, dried and marketed both in the form of entire plants and as rhizomes. Most of the commercial supplies are gathered in the "Blue Ridge" district.

Description.—It occurs in loose matted masses consisting of long, filiform, orange-colored, cylindrical, branched rhizomes, slender hair-like roots and leaves. The leaves are coriaceous, trifoliate, evergreen, with long slender petioles. The segments of the lamina are broadly obovate-cuneate, crenately lobed and toothed with sharp-pointed teeth, prominently veined, dark green and shining, often becoming brown upon drying. The flowers, when present, are small, solitary, terminating slender scapes, whitish or light brown, each with 5–7 small, petaloid, deciduous sepals, 5–7 small, club-shaped, pale yellow petals, numerous stamens and 7 carpels. The fracture of the rhizome is weak and brittle. The odor is indistinct. The taste is bitter.

Powdered Drug.—Yellowish-green; numerous mostly single, spheroidal starch grains up to 10μ in diameter; fragments of leaf epidermis, composed of cells with wavy vertical walls and broadly elliptical stomata; fragments of the nerved scales from the nodes, composed of cells with yellow walls; leaf parenchyma cells containing chloroplasts; non-glandular thick-walled hairs from the midrib of leaf up to 75μ in length; elongated epidermal cells

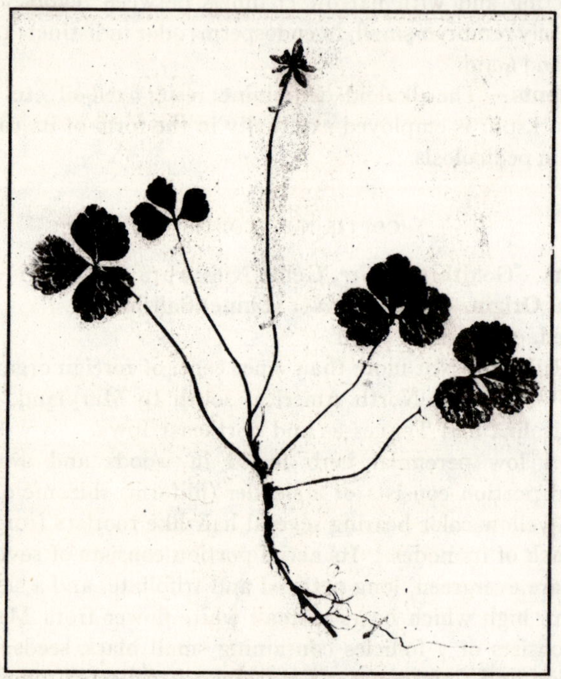

FIG. 84.—*Coptis trifolia.* Plant.

from the roots possessing yellow walls and reddish contents; fragments of epidermal and cortical parenchyma cells of rhizome often filled with yellowish contents, fragments of elongated ordinary parenchyma cells containing starch grains; spiral and pitted tracheæ; narrow thin-walled sclerenchyma fibers.

Constituents.—A yellow alkaloid (berberine) and another alkaloid (coptine), which gives a purple coloration when heated with sulphuric acid, starch, etc.

Uses.—Coptis is employed as a bitter tonic and for ulcerated mouth.

ADONIS N.F. (ADONIS)

Synonyms.—Pheasant's Eye, False Hellebore, Spring Adonis; *Ger.* Sommerteufelsauge.

Botanical Origin.—*Adonis vernalis* Linné.
Part Used.—The dried overground portion.
Limit of Impurities.—5 per cent. of foreign organic matter.
Habitat.—Northern Europe and Asia.
Plant.—A perennial herb.

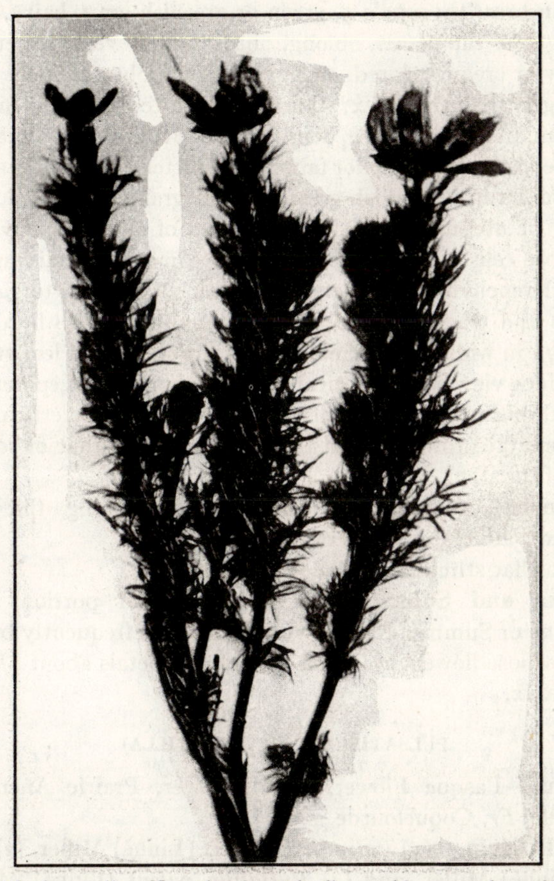

FIG. 85.—*Adonis vernalis.* Note the pinnately-dissected leaves and terminal flowers

Production and Commerce.—The drug is obtained during the late spring from plants which grow wild or are cultivated in central and southern Europe. It is dried and then tied in bundles for the market. The commercial supplies are imported from Hamburg, Germany.

Description.—Adonis occurs in bundles of the entire aerial portions of plants or pieces of the same. Stems up to 40 cm. in length, simple or branched, soft and weak, shining, the branches mostly from near the base and resembling the main stem; naked below, except for some scale-like leaf vestiges, densely foliaceous above; leaves up to 4 cm. long and about two-thirds as broad, pinnately-divided into several segments, the larger of which are again divided, the ultimate segments being linear and acute; flowers terminal, yellow usually, becoming cream colored on drying, from 3 to 6 cm. in breadth; sepals 5, green or greenish-gray, hairy, more than half the length of the petals, oblong, obtuse, finely veined; petals from 5 to 20, yellow or cream colored, concave, oblong, obtuse, finely veined and slightly longer than the calyx; stamens indefinite; pistils indefinite, forming in the fruit an ovoid, obtuse, dense head of ovoid akenes that are tipped with small persistent styles; odor faint; taste bitter and slightly acrid.

Powdered Drug.—Grayish-green; starch grains and calcium oxalate crystals few or absent; numerous fragments of the parenchyma of the medulla whose cells exhibit porous walls; fragments containing narrowly elongated sclerenchymatous fibers with lignified walls up to 7μ thick and oblique slits and tracheæ, the latter either spiral or with bordered pores and up to 17μ in width; epidermal cells of the stems and leaf stalks, elongated in surface view with elliptical stomata; portions of epidermis of the leaf blade exhibiting striated epidermal cells with wavy vertical walls and elliptical stomata; brown-colored tissue representing that of scales found at the base of the stem.

Constituents.—Adonidin (a compound containing the glucoside, picroadonidin), adonidinic acid, resin, etc.

Use.—Cardiac stimulant of the Digitalis group.

Adulterant and Substitute.—The overground portion of *Adonis æstivalis* Linné or Summer Adonis whose stems are frequently branched at the top and whose flowers are crimson with flat petals about 1½ times as long as the calyx.

PULSATILLA N.F. (PULSATILLA)

Synonyms.—Pasque Flower, Wind Flower, Prairie Anenome; *Ger.* Kuchenschelle; *Fr.* Coquelourde.

Botanical Origin.—(1) *Pulsatilla vulgaris* (Linnè) Miller, (2) *Pulsatilla pratensis* (Linné) Miller, and (3) *Pulsatilla patens* (Linné) Miller. (*A. patens* var. *Nuttaliana Gray.*)

Part Used.—The dried herb.

Limit of Impurities.—5 per cent. of foreign organic matter.

Habitat.—1. Europe and Asia. 2. Europe and Asia. 3. Canada and United States, west of the Mississippi.

Plants.—Perennial herbs with twice or thrice pinnately-divided or cleft basal leaves and erect stems whose sessile, cauline leaves form an involucre near the flower. The single flower which terminates the stem varies from blue to bluish-purple or reddish-purple. The fruit is an achene with a long feathery style.

Production and Commerce.—Pulsatilla is produced chiefly in Czecho-Slovakia and reaches this country in bags or bales shipped from Hamburg, Germany. American Pulsatilla was grown in fair sized lots in the Western United States during the World War.

Description.—Leaves and flowering scapes matted, silky-villous; basal leaves with petioles up to 30 cm. in length, the latter hollow,

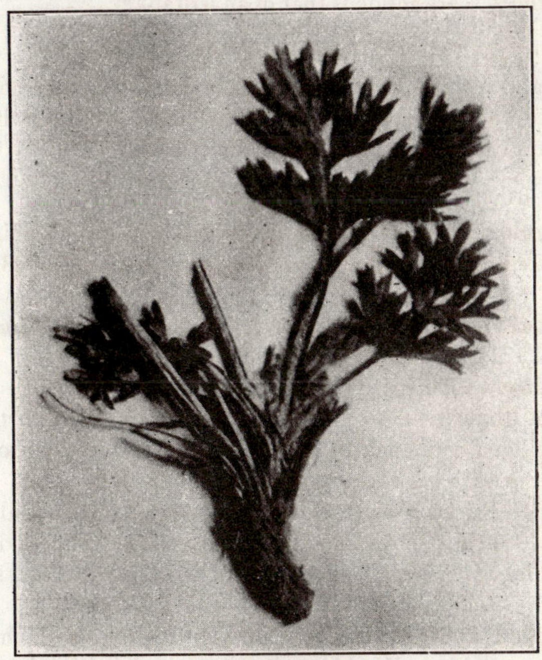

FIG. 86.—Pulsatilla.

often purplish in color, the blades twice or thrice deeply 3- or 4-parted or pinnately cleft, the lobes linear and acute, the base of the petiole more hairy than above and frequently attached to the short root-stock; flowering scapes up to 30 cm. in length, solid in the lower portion and hollow in the upper part, with sessile, involucral, dissected leaves near the flower, occasionally with remains of the dull purple hairy sepals and the dense-woolly, plumose-tailed akenes. Nearly odorless; taste very acrid, diminishing on keeping.

Powdered Drug.—Grayish-green; numerous simple, thick-walled hairs up to 2.5 mm. in length and up to 20μ in thickness; tracheæ up to 35μ in breadth with spiral markings or with simple or bordered pores; fragments of epidermal tissue with stomata, the latter being broadly elliptical and up to 50μ in length; some epidermal cells with wavy vertical walls; calcium oxalate crystals and starch grains few or absent.

Constituents.—Volatile oil containing anemonol (pulsatilla camphor); a crystalline vesicant principle which readily decomposed into anemonin and isoanemonic acid in the presence of water; bitter principle, tannin, etc.

Uses.—Pulsatilla is used in the treatment of amenorrhœa and dysmenorrhœa. Its action is that of an irritant.

BERBERIDACEÆ (BARBERRY FAMILY)

Herbs and woody plants with watery juices and alternate, or radical, simple or compound leaves often bearing spines or barbs, which give them a barbed appearance. Fruit a berry or capsule.

BERBERIS N.F. (BERBERIS)

Synonyms.—Oregon Grape Root, Barberry, Trailing Mahonial Rocky Mountain Grape; *Ger.* Gemeiner Sauerdorn, Berberitze; *Fr*, Vinettier.

Botanical Origin.—Various species of the Section *Mahonia* (Nuttal). De Candolle of the genus *Berberis* Linné.

Parts Used.—The dried rhizome and roots.

Limit of Impurities.—5 per cent. of the overground parts of the plant or other foreign organic matter. Pieces of the rhizome or root over 45 mm. in diameter or with bark removed should be rejected.

Habitat.—Rocky Mountain range of North America and westward.

Plants.—Shrubs with smooth stems, yellow wood and flowers, and compound leaves bearing leaflets with dentate margins and spines. Fruit a berry.

Production and Commerce.—Berberis is obtained chiefly from *B. Aquifolium* growing in Washington, Oregon and California. It is shipped in bags.

Description.—In simple or branched cylindrical segments of the rhizome and roots of variable length and up to 45 mm. in diameter; externally light yellowish-brown, longitudinally wrinkled and showing small irregular fissures in the cork; fracture strong and tough; internally showing a very thin, brownish-green, soft bark about 1 mm. in thickness, a broad yellowish wood, exhibiting numerous radiating narrow, medullary-rays and a narrow yellow pith (rhizome) or no pith (root); odor slight; taste bitter; on chewing it colors the saliva yellow.

Histology.—Transverse sections made through the rhizome exhibit the following internal structures:

1. Cork, a narrow irregular zone of brownish somewhat collapsed cells.

2. Cork cambium, of somewhat collapsed meristematic cells.

3. Cortex of only a few layers of tangentially-elongated parenchyma cells with yellowish amorphous contents.

4. Numerous radially elongated, open collateral fibrovascular bundles arranged in a circle and separated by starch-containing medullary-rays that are for the most part narrow. Each bundle consists of an outer phloem composed of alternating horizontal groups of bast fibers and soft bast, a cambium of more or less collapsed cells, and a very broad, porous xylem composed of numerous wood fibers intermingled with pitted and reticulate tracheæ.

5. Pith, a narrow central zone of parenchyma tissue. the cells of which contains simple or 2- to 3-compound starch grains and active principles.

Similar sections made through the root show curved medullary-rays and no pith. Otherwise they resemble the rhizome.

Powdered Drug.—Yellowish-brown, showing for the most part fragments of wood fibers and medullary rays associated with tracheæ having bordered pores or reticulate markings; starch grains single or 2- to 3-compound, the individual grains somewhat spheroidal and from 3–20μ in diameter; fragments of parenchyma, some containing starch, others a yellowish amorphous substance.

Constituents.—The alkaloids berberine, oxyacanthine, berbamine; resin and starch.

Uses.—Bitter tonic and antiperiodic.

Adulterant.—Aerial stem of lighter yellow color and having cork that detaches in long strips.

CAULOPHYLLUM N.F. (CAULOPHYLLUM)

Synonyms.—Blue Cohosh, Pappoose Root, Squaw Root.

Botanical Origin.—*Caulophyllum thalictroides* (L.) Michaux.

Parts Used.—Dried rhizome and roots.

Purity Rubric.—Not more than 3 per cent. of foreign organic matter and not more than 4 per cent. of acid-insoluble ash.

Habitat.—Eastern North America in deep rich woodlands.

Plant.—A perennial herb having a thick, crooked, horizontal rhizome that sends up in the spring a smooth stem 3 to 7 dm. high, which is terminated by a panicle of yellowish-green flowers. A short distance below the flower cluster the stem bears a large sessile, triternately compound leaf having 2 to 3-lobed leaflets.

Description.—Rhizome branched, crooked, horizontal, from 7 to 25 cm. long and from 5 to 15 mm. thick, showing on its upper surface broad cup-shaped stem scars and short bases of stems, and on its lateral and lower surfaces tough and wiry, grayish to yellowish-gray, matted together rootlets. Externally grayish-brown to brown; fracture tough and woody; internally whitish to grayish-brown with numerous narrow bundles inclosing a broad pith. Roots long, curved, tortuous, thin and tough with a 4-rayed xylem. Odorless but sternutatory. Taste very bitter and acrid.

Powdered Drug.—Light brown. It shows fragments of yellowish-brown cork, pitted tracheæ, fragments of sclerenchyma fibers and tracheids with bordered pores, fragments of starchy parenchyma, and numerous more or less spheroidal starch grains up to 16μ in diameter.

Constituents.—Caulophylline, caulosaponin, caulophyllosaponin, citrullol, volatile oil, resin, starch, etc.

Uses.—Blue cohosh is used as an antispasmodic, emmenagogue and oxytocic.

PODOPHYLLUM U.S.P. (PODOPHYLLUM)

Synonyms.—Mandrake, May Apple Rhizome, Wild Lemon, Umbrella Plant, Vegetable Mercury; *Fr.* Rhizome de podophyllum; *Ger.* Fussblattwurzel.

Botanical Origin.—*Podophyllum peltatum* Linné.

Part Used.—The dried rhizomes and roots.

Standard of Assay.—Not less than 3 per cent. of resin of podophyllum.

Habitat.—Eastern and central North America.

Plant.—A perennial herb whose underground portion consists of a long, brown, jointed and branched rhizome bearing thick fibrous roots from the lower surface of its various nodes. Its aerial portion consists of two kinds of stems which arise from separate nodes of the rhizome. One of these, the flowering stem, bifurcates at its summit to form 2-stalked 5 to 7-lobed leaves from the fork of which arises a stalked, nodding, white flower. The other, the flowerless stem, terminates in a peltate, 7- to 9-lobed leaf. The flower consists of 6 caducous sepals, 6 to 9 obovate white petals, 12 to 18 hypogynous stamens, a fleshy pistil with ovate ovary and sessile stigma. The fruit is an ovate berry about the size of a small lemon.

Production and Commerce.—The drug is collected in the spring or autumn. That which is collected in the spring yields the higher resin content. The rhizomes are dug up, washed, cut into cylindrical segments and carefully dried. The commercial supplies are chiefly obtained from plants growing wild in Virginia, North Carolina, Kentucky, Indiana and Tennessee.

Description.—In subcylindrical jointed pieces, usually showing a node and long internode region from 4 to 20 cm. in length, the node being up to

15 mm., the internode up to 9 mm. in diameter, compressed above and below; externally reddish-brown to dark brown, smooth or slightly longitudinally wrinkled; upper surface of nodes marked with deeply depressed, circular stem scars and sometimes with buds or stem bases; lower surface of nodes, and at times portions of internodes adjacent to them, showing numerous white root scars or roots that may attain a length of 7 cm. and a thickness of 2.5 mm.; fracture of both rhizome and root weak, brittle and even; internally, bark of rhizome grayish-white, of root white, wood of

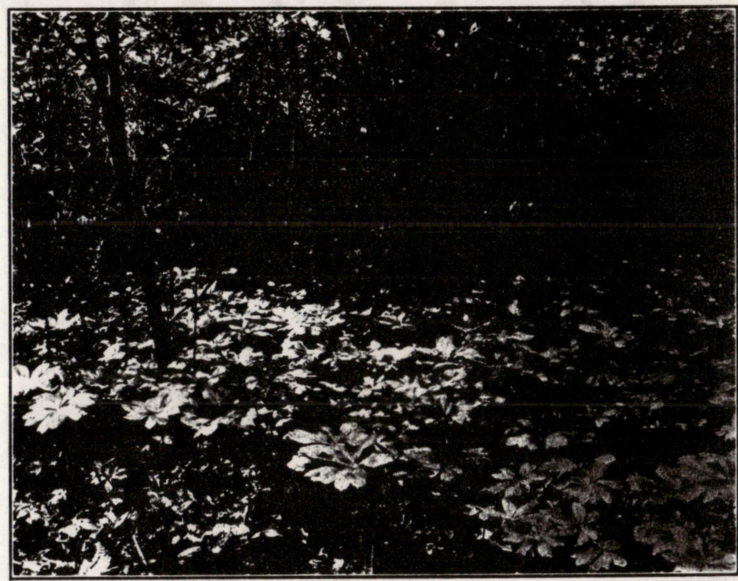

FIG. 87.—Colony of May Apple (*Podophyllum peltatum*) growing in an open area of woodland near Germantown, Pa.

rhizome, showing a circle or ellipse of isolated yellow xylem masses, within which region is a large grayish-white pith, central region of root showing a yellow bundle; odor indistinct; taste sweetish, bitter and acrid.

Microscopical Characteristics.—Transverse sections made through the internode of the rhizome show the following structures:

1. Epidermis of reddish-brown cells with suberized outer and radial walls.

2. Cortex of about 20 layers of rounded cortical parenchyma cells containing numerous spheroidal, polygonal or 2- to 6-compound starch grains.

3. Fibrovascular bundles of the open collateral type 16 to 34 in number and arranged in an interrupted circle or an ellipse. Medullary-rays separate the bundles and unite the cortex with the pith.

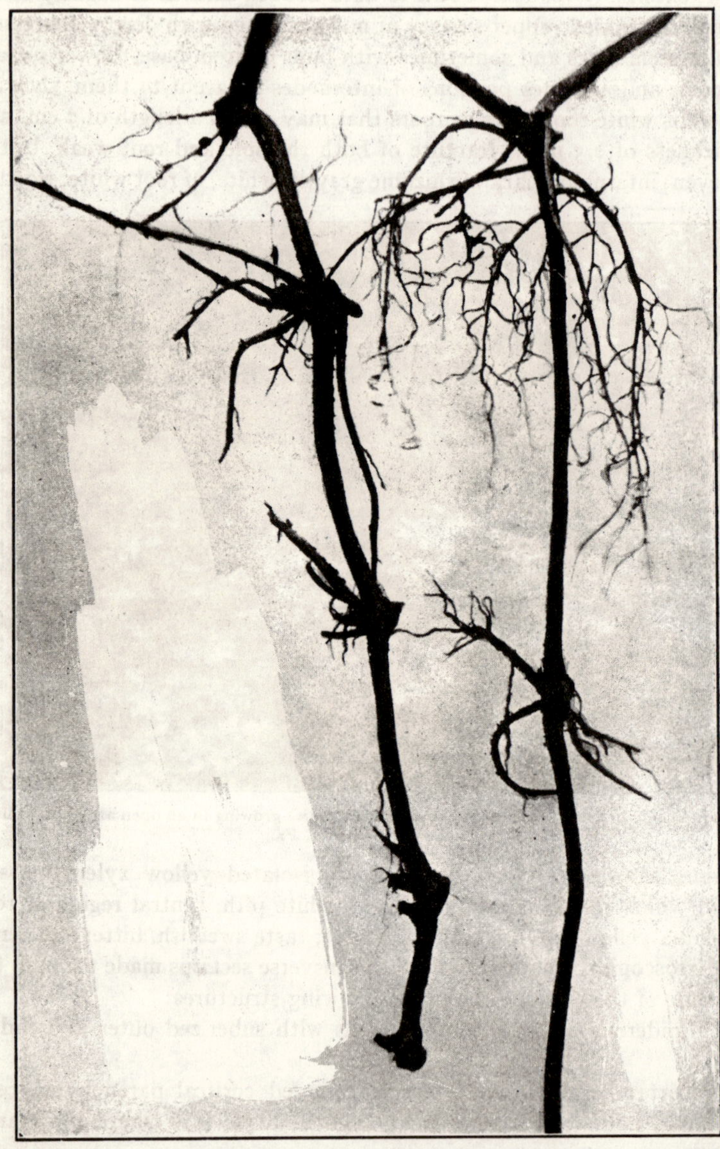

FIG. 88.—Two rhizome systems of *Podophyllum peltatum* Linné. Note prominent, enlarged nodes with undeveloped buds and rootlets and long internodes. At the anterior end of right hand system will be noted two young branches issuing from the distal node in furcate fashion. × ½.

4. Pith, a broad zone of parenchyma similar in nature to that found in the cortex.

Sections made through the nodes show the presence of rosette aggregates of calcium oxalate in certain of the parenchyma cells.

Powdered Drug.—Light brown with a distinct odor; starch grains numerous, spheroidal, polygonal or 2- to 6-compound, the individual grains from 3–20μ in diameter; calcium oxalate in rosette aggregates up to

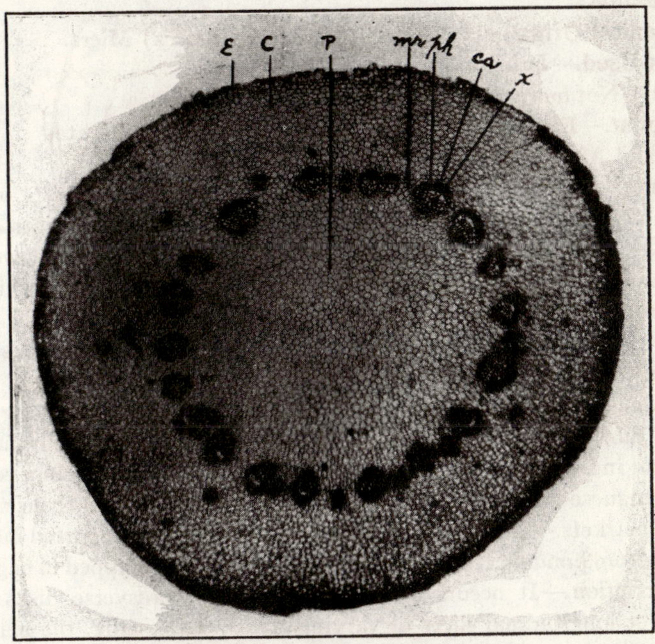

FIG. 89.—Transverse section cut through internode of Podophyllum rhizome showing epidermis (*e*); cortex (*c*); circle of fibrovascular bundles separated from each other by medullary rays, one of which is indicated by *mr*; phloem (*ph*), cambium (*ca*) and xylem (*x*) of a fibrovascular bundle; pith (*p*) filling up center of rhizome. Photomicrograph × 20.

80μ in diameter; which tracheæ with simple pores or spiral, scalariform or reticulate thickenings; fragments of parenchyma containing starch and reddish-brown epidermal cells.

Constituents.—3.5 to 5 per cent. of resin composed of podophyllotoxin ($C_{15}H_{14}O_6$), podophylloresin, picropodophyllin and quercetin (a yellow coloring principle); podophyllic acid, starch, calcium oxalate, and gallic acid.

Use.—Chologogue cathartic, chiefly in the form of Resin of Podophyllum (Podophyllin) U.S.P.

MENISPERMACEÆ (MOONSEED FAMILY)

Choripetalous, woody, climbing, tropical plants with alternate, extipulate, simple, often peltate, leaves. Flowers green to white. Fruit a one-seeded succulent drupe. Seeds albuminous. They usually contain tonic, narcotic or poisonous bitter principles.

CALUMBA U.S.P. (CALUMBA)

Synonyms.—Columba, Columbo, Colombo; *Ger.* Colombowurzel; *Fr.* Columbe.

Botanical Origin.—*Jateorrhiza palmata* (Lamarck) Miers.

Part Used.—Dried root.

Ash.—Not more than 2.5 per cent. acid-insoluble.

Habitat.—Eastern Africa and Madagascar. Cultivated in East Indies and Africa.

Plant.—A perennial climber clinging to trees in the forests of East Africa, Madagascar and other countries into which it has been introduced. Its leaves are simple, large and palmately 3- to 7-lobed. Its flowers are diœcious, small and inconspicuous and arranged in racemes, which are compound in the staminate plant and simple in the pistillate. The underground part consists of a short fibrous rhizome bearing numerous thick, fusiform roots.

Production and Commerce.—The underground portion is dug up in March, during dry weather; the thick roots are separated from the rootstock, cut into transverse slices and dried in the shade. It is shipped from the Portuguese possessions in Southeast Africa to India and thence to the world's markets. In 1924, about 100,000 pounds were imported into this country from London, Hamburg and Marseilles. It is shipped in bags.

Description.—It occurs in circular or ovate transverse disks or in oblique or longitudinal slices of varying sizes. Externally, the marginal cork is brown and irregularly wrinkled, the cut surfaces yellowish to yellowish-green brown, radiate and showing a distinct dark cambium in the outer portion and a depressed center. The fracture is short and mealy. The odor is slightly aromatic and the taste very bitter and aromatic.

Histology.—Thin transverse sections when examined microscopically are characterized by the following peculiarities:

1. Cork, arranged in alternating layers of small and large cells and showing fissures extending into the next layer.

2. Cork cambium of 2 or 3 layers of tangentially-elongated meristematic cells.

3. A broad cortex composed of tangentially elongated cortical parenchyma cells filled with ovoid, ellipsoidal or irregular starch grains. Among

the outer cells of this region will be noticed yellow stone cells with irregularly thickened, lignified, porous walls and containing calcium oxalate ether in the form of prisms or crystal sand (sphenoidal microcrystals).

4. Open collateral fibrovascular bundles, narrow and elongated, arranged in a circle and separated from each other by medullary-rays.

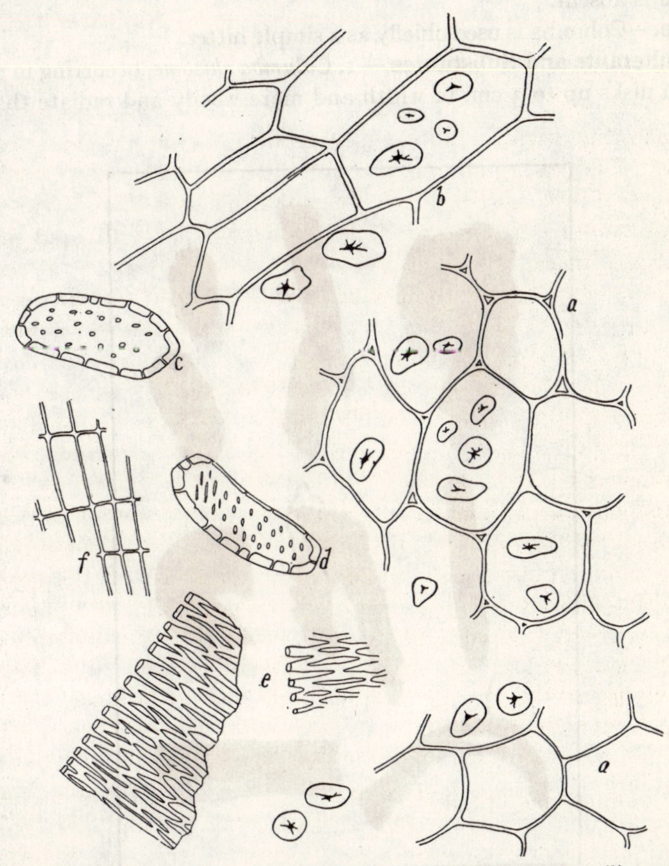

FIG. 90.—Powdered Calumba. (*a*) Parenchyma with starch grains; (*b*) parenchyma, longitudinal view; (*c*), (*d*) stone cells; (*e*) fragments of reticulate ducts; (*f*) cork cells, lateral view. (*Schneider.*)

Powdered Drug.—Greenish-brown to grayish-yellow; numerous starch grains mostly single, occasionallv 2- to 3-compound, the individual grains up to 85μ long, avoid, ellipsoidal or irregular with an excentric, linear, X-shaped or branching hilum; stone cells few with irregularly thickened, porous walls and often containing one or more prisms of calcium oxalate or numerous micro-crystals; fragments of tracheæ with bordered pores and reticulate markings associated with wood fibers and lignified wood parenchyma, the last having large pores.

Constituents.—The yellow alkaloids, columbamine, jateorhizine and palmatine; the bitter principles columbin and chasmantherin; starch, etc. Tannin is absent.

Use.—Columba is used chiefly as a simple bitter.

Adulterants and Substitutes.—1. *Columba rhizome*, occurring in deeper colored disks up to 3 cm. in width and more woody and radiate than the root.

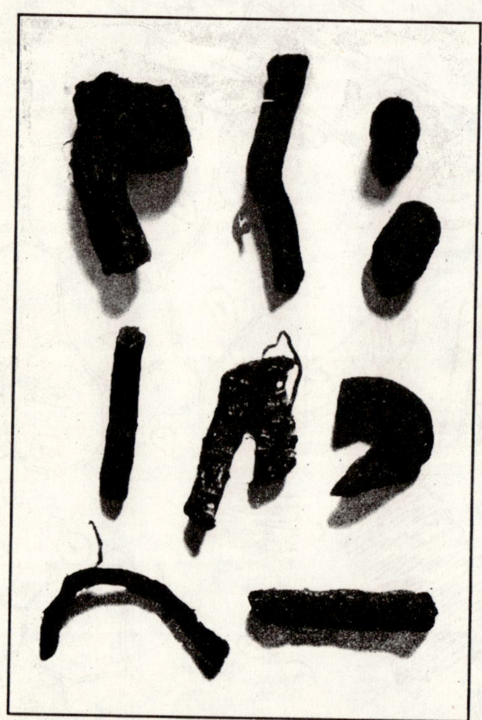

Fig. 91.—Pareira. × ⅓.

2. *Ceylon Columba*, the root of *Coscinum fenestratum* (Fam. *Menispermaceæ*), the slices of which are dark yellow, more woody and not depressed in the center.

PAREIRA N.F. (PAREIRA)

Synonyms.—Pareira Brava, Velvet Leaf; *Fr.* Butua. *Ger.* Grieswurzel.
Botanical Origin.—*Chondodendron tomentosum* Ruiz et Pavon.
Part Used.—The dried root.

Limit of Impurities.—5 per cent. of its stems or other foreign organic matter.

Habitat.—Brazil and Peru.

Plant.—A perennial diœcious climber with stem attaining a thickness of up to 10 cm. and with rough bark covered with warty protuberances. The leaves are long petioled, ovate, cordate, smooth on upper surface but tomentose with an ashy hue on lower surface. The inflorescence is a panicle of small flowers. The fruit is a purplish-black, one-seeded, oval drupe, occurring in bunches of 6.

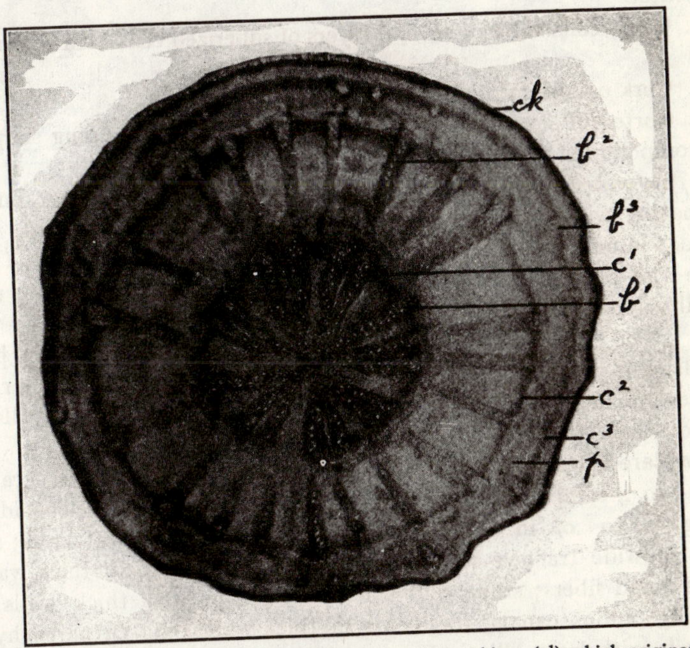

FIG. 92.—Transverse section of Pareira. Cork (*ck*); cambium (c^1) which originated first series of bundles (b^1); cambium (c^2) which originated second series of bundles (b^2); cambium (c^3) giving rise to third series of bundles (b^3), the last only slightly developed; parenchyma of cortex (*p*).

Production and Commerce.—The plants grow wild in various parts of Brazil and Peru where they are known as Abutua or Butua. They are particularly abundant on the hills separating the Copacabana from the basin of the Rio de Janeiro. The roots are dug at various seasons of the year, cut into transverse segments and dried. They are shipped to the various markets of the world from Rio Janeiro and Bahia, Brazil.

Description.—The drug occurs on the market in heavy segments of variable length and from 0.5 to 6 cm. in diameter. The segments are cylindrical, more or less tortuous; externally brownish-black or blackish-brown with transverse ridges or knot-like projections, occasionally fissured and furrowed or longitudinally wrinkled; hard and tough; having a waxy luster when recently cut; the transverse surfaces exhibiting several successive eccentric and distinctly radiate concentric zones of projecting fibrovascular bundles, separated from each other by concentric zones of parenchyma and stone cells; odor indistinct; taste bitter. An infusion of the drug turns bluish-black with tincture of iodine.

Histology.—Transverse sections of the root, examined under the microscope, show the following peculiarities, passing from periphery toward the center.

1. Cork, consisting of several layers of suberized cells with brown contents.

2. Cork cambium of meristematic cells.

5. Cortex of several layers of parenchyma cells containing simple or 2–4-compound starch grains.

4. Several concentric zones of open collateral fibrovascular bundles alternating with zones of parenchyma containing starch. Each fibrovascular bundle exhibits an outer semicircular phloem composed of sieve tissue and phloem parenchyma, a somewhat collapsed cambium and a radially elongated xylem composed of wide tracheæ surrounded by wood fibers. The fibrovascular bundles are separated from each other by broad medullary-rays whose cells contain abundant starch. Each circular zone of parenchyma shows on its inner face a nearly closed ring of stone cells, the walls of which are thick and porous.

Powdered Drug.—Dark brown. Starch grains mostly simple, occasionally 2- to 4-compound, the individual grains spheroidal, ellipsoidal or oblong, 5μ to 30μ in diameter, a number showing central clefts; fragments of wide tracheæ with slit-like pores and lignified, thick-walled, porous wood fibers; stone cells usually in groups with thick walls and radiating porous canals; fragments of thick-walled starch parenchyma, the walls with large elliptical pores; a few fragments of brownish-black cork cells.

Constituents.—A yellow alkaloid, pelosine (berberine) which is soluble in benzene, a crystalline and an amorphous alkaloid insoluble in benzene, starch, tannin, wax, etc.

Use.—Pareira has been used in chronic inflammations of the urinary tract.

Substitutes and Adulterants.—The roots and stems of *Cissampelos Pareira* L. (Fam. *Menispermaceæ*), frequently called "False Pareira" and found growing in the West Indies and South America, has been the most common substitute for the genuine article. The roots of this plant are dark brown in color externally, light brown internally, show but one circle of fibrovascular bundles and are devoid of a waxy luster when cut. The stems are in long cylindrical segments, some of which, in having trailed along the ground, show rootlets at the nodes. They are usually less than an inch in diameter, have light-brown bark showing longitudinal or spiral shallow furrows and wrinkles, a coarse fibrous fracture and no concentrically arranged bundles. Both roots and stems are bitter but devoid of astringency. An infusion of False "Pareira" is not colored bluish-black with iodine.

Stems of *Chondodendron tomentosum* Ruiz et Pavon are often admixed with the official roots or occasionally entirely substituted for the genuine article. These are of varying length, 1 to 4 inches in diameter, grayish in color, and show concentrically arranged series of bundles like the root, but differ from it in exhibiting a distinct pith, a tendency of the bundles to separate, in being frequently partially covered externally with foliaceous lichens bearing black apothecia and in the absence of a waxy luster of their cut surfaces. Some segments have stumps of roots springing from them.

Roots and stems of *Abuta rufescens* Aublet (Fam. *Menispermaceæ*) from Guiana, commonly known as "White Pareira," occur in segments ½ to 3 inches thick, exhibit concentric zones of whitish or pale yellow color, when cut, are very starchy and devoid of odor or bitter taste.

Roots and stems of *Abuta amara* Aublet (Yellow Pareira), a plant growing in Guiana, are characterized internally by their deep bright yellow color, their numerous concentric zones of bundles and very bitter taste. The woody stem segments are covered with a whitish bark.

COCCULUS N.F. (COCCULUS)

Synonyms.—Fish Berry, Indian Berry, Cocculus Indicus, Levant Berry; *Ger.* Kokkelskörner, Fischkörner; *Fr.* Coque du Levant.

Botanical Origin.—*Anamirta Cocculus* (Linné) Wight et Arnott.

Part Used.—The dried ripe fruit.

Purity Rubric.—Not more than 2 per cent of foreign organic matter.

Habitat.—Eastern India and the Malay Archipelago.

Plant.—A perennial, diœcious, woody climber bearing alternate, cordate, pinnately-veined leaves and axillary, pendulous panicles of small flowers. The fruit is a red drupe of reniform outline containing an urn-shaped seed.

Production and Commerce.—The fruits are collected, when ripe, from wild plants by the natives and dried in the sun. In India, Ceylon and the East Indies they have been used to stupefy fish after which the fish are readily caught by hand. Most of the product is sent to Calcutta, Madras and Bombay from which it is shipped to London and the United States.

Description.—Drupe grayish to blackish-brown, wrinkled, reniform, 8 to 13 mm. in length and 7 or 10 mm. in breadth and thickness, the base marked by a circular stem scar; seed yellowish-gray, urn-shaped, its longitudinal and cross sections crescent-shaped; odor indistinct; taste bitter and oily.

Microscopical Characteristics.—

I. *Pericarp:*

1. Epicarp of a layer of more or less cubical-shaped cells.
2. Mesocarp consisting of an outer region of thin-walled cells with brown granular contents which become reddish-brown with solution of potassium hydroxide, a zone of elongated brownish-red cells through which course fibrovascular bundles; several rows of yellowish cells.
3. Endocarp of strongly lignified, porous sclerenchyma fibers.

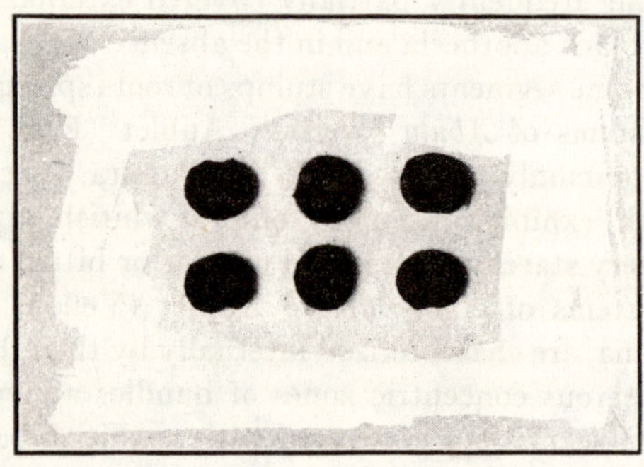

FIG. 93.—Fish Berries, × ⅞. (*Photograph by Stoneback.*)

II. *Seed:*

1. Endosperm composed of polygonal cells with thin walls containing aleurone and fixed oil, the latter frequently in the form of acicular crystals or prisms or aggregates.
2. Embryo.

Powdered Drug.—Brown. The diagnostic histological elements are: numerous-thick walled, porous, yellow sclerenchyma fibers, and thin-walled cells of the endosperm containing aleurone grains up to 50μ in length and acicular, prismatic or aggregate crystals of fixed oil, the latter soluble in ether and alkaline solutions. The taste is very bitter.

Constituents.—A bitter, crystalline neutral principle termed picrotoxin, which is poisonous and found in the seeds; the alkaloids menispermine and paramenispermine, found in the fruit wall; fat, resin, gum, etc.

Use.—Parasiticide in pediculosis.

MYRISTICACEÆ (NUTMEG FAMILY)

A family of tropical, apetalous and diœcious trees and shrubs having entire, alternate, petiolate evergreen leaves, small regular flowers, and capsular fruits. The seeds are albuminous and covered by a fleshy laciniate arillus. Secretory sacs with suberized walls and containing a yellowish, brownish or red oil are scattered throughout the plants. The hairs are stellate. Calcium oxalate has been found in a number of the plants investigated in the form of acicular crystals or aggregates of these.

MYRISTICA U.S.P. (MYRISTICA)

Synonyms.—Nutmeg; Round Nutmeg, *Ger.* Myristicasamen; *Fr.* Muscade.

Botanical Origin.—*Myristica fragrans* Houttuyn.

Part Used.—The dried ripe seed deprived of its seed coat and with or without a thin coating of lime.

Purity Rubric.—Not less than 25 per cent. of non-volatile, ether soluble extractive and not more than 0.5 per cent. of acid-insoluble ash.

Habitat.—Molucca Islands. Cultivated in tropical lands.

Plant.—An evergreen tree growing to the height of 25 to 50 feet. Its leaves are coriaceous, dark green, entire, oblong-ovate to ovate-lanceolate in outline with acute apex and base. Its pistillate flowers are small, yellow, and axillary. Its fruit is a yellow, nearly globular, tough, fleshy, 2-valved, longitudinally grooved capsule which contains a single ovoid seed. The seed is closely surrounded and almost completely covered by a fleshy, irregularly slit arillus.

Production and Commerce.—Nutmeg trees grow wild in the Dutch Banda and adjacent islands of the East Indies where the soil is light and the climate moist. They are cultivated in the Banda Islands, Java, Sumatra, Penang, Ceylon, Malacca and the West Indies. The trees bear fruit when 8 or 9 years old and yield annually for about 60 years. The fruit is collected, after it has split open, by means of a hook fastened to a long pole or by hand. The pericarp (fruit wall) is removed and the scarlet arillus ("mace") carefully stripped off, flattened and dried. The seeds are then taken to the drying house and placed on frames where they are exposed to a gentle heat for two months, being turned every 2 or 3 days. As soon as the kernels rattle within their shells, the shells (seed coats) are broken with a mallet, the kernels removed and assorted, and the best often coated with milk of lime or powdered slaked lime to prevent insect attacks. In Penang and Singapore the kernels are unlimed. Inferior kernels are employed for expressing the oil.

Nutmegs are imported into the United States both from the East Indies and West Indies. The importations during the last five years have ranged from 3,250,000 to 5,000,000 pounds. East Indian nutmegs are usually limed, the West Indian not limed. Shrivelled nutmegs and nutmegs in the shell are imported for distillation of the oil. East Indian nutmegs are shipped to this country from the ports of Padang, Batavia, Penang, Singapore and Surabaya, from Amsterdam, Rotterdam, Hamburg, and London. West Indian nutmegs are shipped from the port of Grenada. Approximately 50 per cent. of our supply comes from Grenada and 40 per cent. from Java. Moldy and insect-infested material is the chief cause of inferiority.

Physical Characteristics.—Globular, ovoid or ellipsoidal, 20 to 30 mm. in length, 15 to 24 mm. in diameter; externally light to dark brown, usually whitish on account of the lime coating, reticulately furrowed and deeply grooved on one side, the groove indicating the position of the raphe; at one end showing a white projection in the center of which is the micropyle; when cut, the exposed surfaces have a mottled appearance because of the ruminate albumen (dark brown outer perisperm penetrating by numerous branches into the light brown endosperm); odor strongly aromatic; taste warmly aromatic.

Powdered Drug.—Reddish-brown. Under the microscope it shows fragments of perisperm composed of small, thin-walled parenchyma cells with brown pigment and few spiral ducts imbedded in which are large reservoirs with volatile oil contents; fragments of the endosperm, composed of polygonal-shaped parenchyma cells, filled with starch and aleurone grains and occasionally brown pigment; starch grains simple or 2- to 20-compound, the individual grains being spheroidal, polygonal or plano-convex, from 3μ to 20μ in diameter with distinct hilum; aleurone grains with large phytoglobulin. The powder obtained from limed nutmegs, when examined in 25 per cent. sulphuric acid, shows small acicular or short rod-shaped crystals of calcium sulphate which have separated.

Constituents.—Up to 40 per cent. of a solid fat; up to 15 per cent. of volatile oil, containing myristicin (*Oleum Myristicæ*, U.S.P.); starch and proteins.

Uses.—Nutmegs are used as a spice and medicinally as a stimulant and carminative.

Substitutes.—1. *Papua or Macassar nutmegs* obtained from *Myristica argentea* Warburg of New Guinea. These are longer, narrower and less aromatic than the genuine with a feeble odor and disagreeable, acrid taste. Imported here in large amounts.

2. *Bombay nutmegs* from *Myristica malabarica* Lamarck, which are ellipsoidally-elongate and entirely devoid of odor.

Adulterants.—The powdered drug has been adulterated with exhausted nutmeg, corn meal, curcuma, powdered beans, ground olive pits and ground cocoanut shells.

MACIS (MACE)

Synonyms.—True Mace; *Fr.* Fleur de muscade; *Ger.* Muskatblüthe.

Botanical Origin.—*Myristica fragrans* Houttuyn.

Part Used.—The dried arillode of the seed.

Standard of Purity.—Not more than 3 per cent. total ash, 0.5 per cent. acid-insoluble ash and 20 to 30 per cent. of non-volatile ether extract (Circular 136, U.S. Dept. Agric.).

Commercial.—Upwards of 1,000,000 pounds of Mace are imported annually into this country from the East and West Indies. It is shipped in cases, barrels and bags. East Indian mace comes either direct from Amboyna, Banda, Padang, Papua, Batavia, Singapore and Surabaya or indirectly through Amsterdam, Rotterdam and London. West Indian mace is shipped from Grenada.

Description.—It occurs in buff to brownish-orange colored, oily, narrow bands, 25 mm. or more in length, somewhat branched and lobed above, united into broader bands below; odor fragrant; taste warmly aromatic.

Histology.—Transverse sections cut through the middle or upper part of Mace show the following microscopic structures.

1. Outer epidermis of tangentially elongated cells with thick walls and very thick outer cuticle.

2. Fundamental parenchyma of thin-walled cells containing numerous small amylodextrin granules of various shapes. These can be best seen in sections first cleared with ether or petroleum benzin. Through this zone fibrovascular bundles course. Large oil cells are found scattered among the parenchyma cells.

3. Inner epidermis, similar to the outer epidermis.

Powdered Drug.—Orange buff to orange brown and showing in microscopic mounts made in water the following: Elongated epidermal cells, fragments of parenchyma cells with small amylodextrin granules which take a red color with iodine, and large secretion sacs containing yellow oil.

Constituents.—Volatile oil, fixed oil, resin, mucilage, etc.

Uses.—Flavoring agent, stimulant.

Adulterant Of Powdered Mace: The ground arillode of *Myristica Malabarica* Lam; commonly called Bombay Mace. The distinctions between genuine powdered Mace and Bombay Mace are as follows:

Powdered True Mace	Powdered Bombay Mace
Orange buff to orange-brown.	Yellowish brown to deep brown.
Taste aromatic.	Taste non-aromatic.
Secretion sacs contain a yellowish oil, not greatly changed in color by addition of an alkali.	Secretion sacs contain an orange-red resinous substance which is dissolved by alkalies forming a blood red liquid.
HCl gives no greenish color.	HCl produces greenish color.

Powdered True Mace	Powdfred Bombay Mace
If potassium chromate T.S. is added to an alcoholic solution of Mace (1 in 10), the precipitate formed is yellow and does not change to red on standing, nor does the solution develop a red coloration.	Similar treatment of an alcoholic solution (1 in 10) of Bombay Mace or true Mace adulterated with the latter results in a yellow precipitate changing soon to red and the solution becomes red.
Oil · cells pale yellow after treatment with caustic alkali.	Oil cells showing blood-red liquid after treatment with caustic alkali.
Amylodextrin granules up to 12μ in length.	Amylodextrin granules attaining a greater length.

MONIMIACEÆ

Tropical aromatic shrubs and trees with opposite coriaceous leaves and cymose inflorescences. The plant axis and leaves contain cells or internal glands with hydrocarbon contents. Glandular hairs are absent, the non-glandular type common.

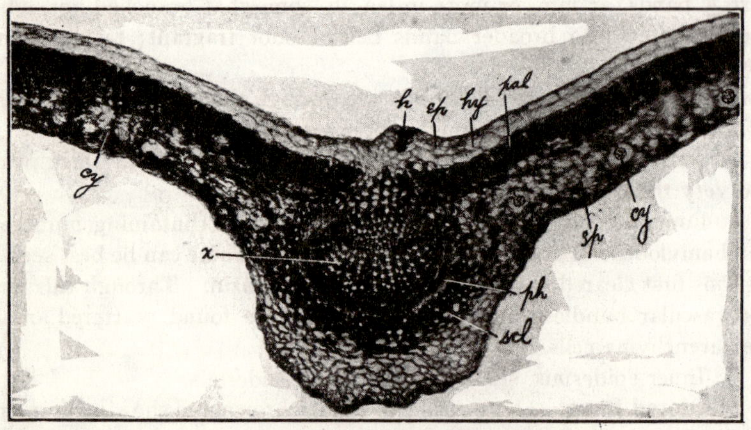

Fig. 94.—Boldo leaf as observed in a transverse section. Base of hair (*h*); epidermis (*ep*); hypodermis (*hy*); palisade parenchyma (*pal*); spongy parenchyma (*sp*); cystoliths (*cy*); xylem (*x*); phloem (*ph*); and arc of sclerenchyma fibers in pericycle (*scl*).

BOLDUS N.F. (BOLDO)

Synonym.—Boldo Leaves.

Botanical Origin.—*Boldu Boldus* (Molina) Lyons.

Part Used.—The dried leaf.

Purity Rubric.—Not more than 2 per cent. of its stems or other foreign organic matter and not more than 6 per cent. of acid-insoluble ash.

Habitat.—Mountainous districts of Chile.

Plant.—A diœcious evergreen shrub bearing opposite, ovate to ellipsoidal coriaceous leaves and cymose flowers.

Description.—Lamina broadly ovate or ellipsoidal, from 3 to 7 cm. in length and from 1 to 4 cm. in breadth, the base varying from rounded to very slightly indented; the apex varying from acute to rounded to slightly emarginate, the margin entire and sharply revolute; thick, coriaceous, rigid and brittle; from pale green to brownish-green, papillose, roughened on both surfaces, the principal veins coarsely reticulate, impressed above, prominent underneath, the petiole stout and rigid from 1 to 6 mm. in length, reticulate; odor peculiar; when crushed very strong and somewhat resembling oil of chenopodium; taste bitter, warm and pungent, camphoraceous and slightly terebinthinate.

Histology.—Transverse sections of the lamina show the following microscopic characteristics:

1. *Upper epidermis* of clear tangentially elongated cells with thick, more or less wavy, outer cuticle and thick walls and pits from the base of which groups of unicellular, thick-walled hairs emerge.
2. *Hypodermis* of usually 2 layers of clear elongated cells.
3. *Palisade parenchyma* of 2 layers of columnar, chloroplast-containing cells. In this region there occur spheroidal internal glands with hydrocarbon contents.
4. *Spongy parenchyma* of small irregularly rounded and elongated cells and large intercellular-air-spaces in which cystoliths are frequently observed.
5. *Lower epidermis* of a layer of clear tangentially elongated cells and stomata. In this epidermis pits are found which lodge groups of unicellular, thick-walled trichomes (stellate hairs).

Constituents.—An aikaloid termed boldine; a glucoside called boldoglucin; volatile oil, tannin and resin.

Uses.—Stimulant and diuretic in diseases of the genito-urinary tract.

LAURACEÆ (LAUREL FAMILY)

Aromatic trees or shrubs with alternate, coriaceous, pellucid punctate leaves containing considerable volatile oil. The flowers are polygamous with a petaloid calyx of 4 to 6 sepals and perigynous stamens, having anthers that dehisce by 2 to 4 recurved valves. The fruit is a drupe or berry. Represented by the Sassafras, Spice Bush, Red Bay, Pond Spice, Cinnamon and Camphor trees. Among the histological peculiarities of this family might be noted the following: Non-glandular unicellular hairs, acicular or spindle-shaped crystals of calcium oxalate, numerous secretion sacs containing either oil or mucilage and distributed through all parts of the plants.

SASSAFRAS N.F. (SASSAFRAS)

Synonyms.—Ague Tree, Saxifrax, Sassafras Bark, Cinnamon Wood; *Ger.* Sassafrasrinde; *Fr.* Ecorce de Sassafras.

Botanical Origin.—*Sassafras variifolium* (Salisbury) O. Kuntze.

Part Used.—The dried bark of the root.

Limit of Impurities.—4 per cent. of adhering wood, outer corky tissues or other foreign organic matter.

Ash.—Not more than 5 per cent. acid-insoluble.

Habitat.—United States in rich woods from Kansas eastward.

Plant.—A tree, 4 to 30 m. high, with spicy aromatic bark and greenish-yellow twigs. The leaves are entire, ovate, or 2 to 3 lobed. The flowers are diœcious, greenish-yellow and appearing in April in the Philadelphia neighborhood. The fruit is a blue ovoid drupe borne on the end of a thick reddish pedicel.

Production and Commerce.—The bark is gathered in the early spring or autumn, deprived of the outer corky layers and dried. The commercial supplies come largely from Virginia, Tennessee and Kentucky. The official oil of sassafras (U.S.P.) is distilled from the entire root.

Description.—In irregularly transversely curved or quilled pieces deprived of the grayish-brown cork, of variable length and from 1 to 4 mm. thick; outer surface orange-brown, nearly smooth; inner surface reddish-brown, finely striated; fracture short brittle, the fractured surface light yellow to reddish-brown; odor aromatic; taste slightly mucilaginous, astringent, aromatic and pungent.

Histology.—Under the microscope transverse sections of the drug mounted in water exhibit the following structures:

1. Cortex (secondary) composed of numerous layers of irregularly rounded parenchyma cells, some of which contain single or 2- to 4-compound starch grains and others yellowish-red tannin masses that become bluish-black with ferric chloride test solution. Scattered among the parenchyma cells will be noted numerous secretion sacs containing globules of oil or, at times, mucilage. Occasionally patches of cork cells may be found adhering to the outer margin of the cortex, due to imperfect peeling of bark. These cells appear tabular and are arranged in regular rows.

2. A broader phloem, separated into numerous phloem patches by wavy medullary-rays. Each phloem patch is composed of broader polygonal sieve tubes and narrower phloem parenchyma, interspersed among which are numerous isolated, angular, strongly lignified bast fibers and secretion sacs containing oil or mucilage. The phloem parenchyma cells and the medullary-ray cells contain either starch or tannin masses.

Powdered Drug.—Light reddish-brown and showing the following histological elements: 1. Spindle-shaped bast fibers with sharply pointed ends, up to 400μ long and with strongly lignified walls. 2. Simple or 2–4-compound starch grains, the separate grains being spheriodal or polygonal and often with a cleft, up to 20μ in diameter, some of the grains altered. 3. Fragments of parenchyma, some of the cells containing irregular yellowish-red tannin masses, others starch grains and still others oil globules. 4. Fragments of thin-walled, porous tracheæ associated with thin-walled wood fibers, these due to wood that frequently adheres to the bark.

Constituents.—Volatile oil (6 to 9 per cent.) containing safrol; tannin, sassafrid, starch, etc.

Uses.—Aromatic, stimulant, diaphoretic, flavoring agent.

Adulterant.—The bark of the stem of the same plant has often been found admixed with the root bark. It is distinctly fissured on the outer surface, less aromatic and more mucilaginous than the latter. When examined under the microscope, unlike the root bark, it shows bast fibers in groups, stone cells, and a large number of cells in the cortex that contain chloroplastids.

SASSAFRAS MEDULLA N.F. (SASSAFRAS PITH)

Synonyms.—Ague Tree Pith, Saxifrax Pith.

Botanical Origin.—*Sassafras variifolium* (Salisbury) O. Kuntze.

Part Used.—The dried pith.

Purity Rubric.—Not more than 1 per cent. of foreign organic matter and not more than 0.5 per cent. of acid-insoluble ash.

Habitat.—In rich woods from Kansas eastward.

Plant.—See under Sassafras.

Collection.—In late autumn.

Description.—In cut or broken straight or irregular pieces up to 10 cm. long and 6 mm. thick, externally whitish; fracture weak and brittle, the fractured surface being whitish and porous; odor slight; taste mucilaginous.

Microscopical Characteristics.—Under the microscope, cross sections show numerous large ordinary parenchyma cells separated by large angular intercellular-air-spaces. The walls of these cells are somewhat lignified and distinctly porous. Water mounts show the separation of a glary mucilage from their inner surface which is not precipitated by alcohol.

Constituents.—Mucilage and a mere trace of volatile oil.

Uses.—Sassafras pith is chiefly used for the preparation of Mucilage of Sassafras Pith N.F., the latter being employed chiefly as an emollient in eye lotions.

CINNAMOMUM U.S.P. (CINNAMON)

Synonyms.—Saigon Cinnamon, Saigon Cassia, Annam or China Cinnamon; *Ger.* Saigonzimmt; *Fr.* Cannelle de Saigon.

Botanical Origin.—*Cinnamomum Loureirii* Nees.

Part Used.—The dried bark.

Standard of Assay.—Not less than 2 per cent. of volatile extractive, soluble in ether.

Habitat.—Cochin China.

Commercial Source.—Saigon.

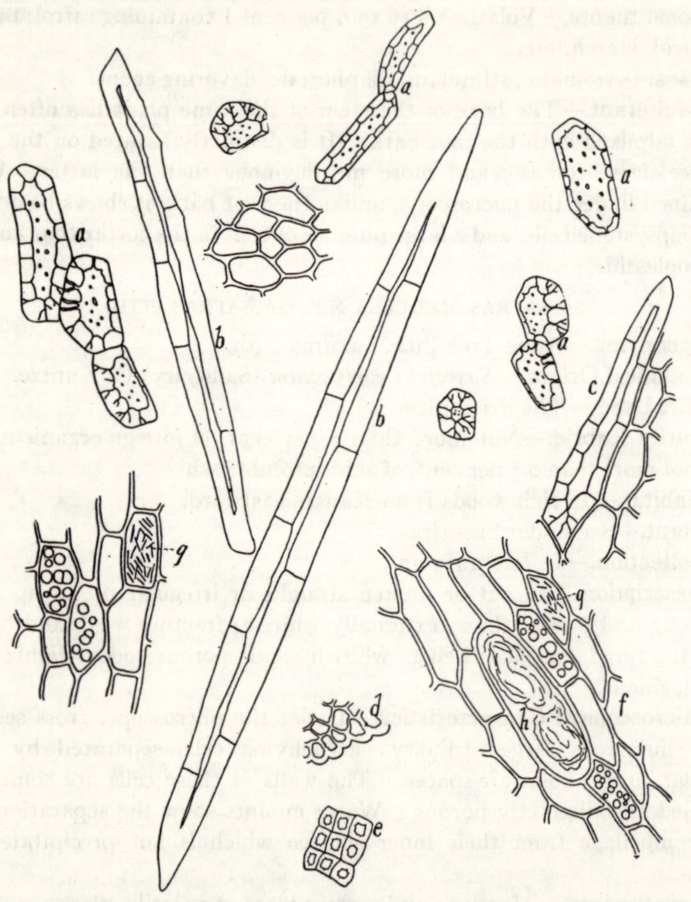

FIG. 95.—Powdered Cinnamon. Saigon. (*a*) Stone cells; (*b*), (*c*), sclerenchyma fibers; (*d*) epidermis, lateral view; (*e*) epidermis, vertical view; (*f*) parenchyma, longitudinal view with crystal bearing cell (*g*), resin cell (*h*) and starch. (*After Schneider.*)

Plant.—A glabrous evergreen tree of medium height with opposite or alternate, elliptic or oblong, short petioled, 3-nerved leaves with acuminate apex.

Description.—In single quills having a length of about 30 cm. and in chips and pieces of quills; the bark from .5 to 3 mm. in thickness; outer surface light brown to dark purplish-brown, often with grayish patches of lichens and numerous bud scars; finely longitudinally wrinkled on bark of younger twigs, rough from corky patches surrounding lenticels on bark of old stems; inner surface cinnamon brown to dark brown; fracture short; inner bark porous; odor aromatic, characteristic; taste sweetish, strongly aromatic and pungent.

Histology.—Sections of the older stem bark show the following microscopic peculiarities:

1. Cork, composed of several layers of more or less lignified cork cells.
2. Cork cambium of somewhat collapsed cells.
3. Cortex composed of several layers of more or less flattened parenchyma cells with brown walls, many of which contain round starch grains. Scattered about in this region are colorless stone cells and some oil and mucilage cells.
4. Pericycle, a nearly continuous zone, several layers in width, of stone cells among which are small groups of sclerenchyma fibers with slightly lignified walls. These contain reddish-brown contents.
5. Phloem, a broad zone traversed by medullary-rays averagely 1 to 3 cells wide, which divide this region into a number of more or less oblong, radial phloem patches. Each of these shows somewhat collapsed sieve tubes, isolated bast fibers (which like the stone cells contain a reddish-brown substance), and parenchyma, the latter either filled with single and compound starch grains or short raphides of calcium oxalate.

Powdered Drug.—Reddish-brown; numerous single and compound starch grains, the individual grains spheroidal, plano-convex or polygonal and up to 20μ in diameter; fragments with stone cells, the lumina frequently containing a reddish-brown amorphous substance; sclerenchyma fibers usually in groups with very thick and slightly lignified walls; fragments of lignified cork cells; fragments of reddish-brown parenchyma, some containing oil cells.

Constituents.—Volatile oil (3 to 6 per cent.) containing cinnamic aldehyde; starch, resin, tannin, mucilage, calcium oxalate, etc.

Uses.—Aromatic and flavoring agent.

CINNAMOMUM ZEYLANICUM (CEYLON CINNAMON)

Synonyms.—True Cinnamon, Cortex Cinnamomi, *Ger.* Zeylonzimmt; *Fr.* Cannelle de Ceylon.

Botanical Origin.—*Cinnamomum zeylanicum* Breyne.

Part Used.—The dried inner bark.

Limit of Impurities.—3 per cent. of the outer bark or other foreign matter.

Standard of Assay.—Not less than 0.5 per cent. of volatile extractive, soluble in ether.

Ash.—Not more than 5 per cent. The amount of ash insoluble in dilute hydrochloric acid does not exceed 2 per cent. of the weight of Ceylon Cinnamon taken.

Habitat.—Ceylon.

Plant.—A tree with 3- to 5-nerved evergreen, coriaceous, aromatic leaves which are glaucous beneath.

Production and Commerce.—The bark is obtained from plants which are cultivated in Ceylon in such a way that they develop slender shoots with little or no astringent cork. This is accomplished by cutting the crown of the tree down to form stools. The latter send forth adventitious shoots which lengthen at the rate of about a meter a year. When the shoots are about 1½ to 2 meters long, they are cut down during the rainy season and deprived of leaves and small twigs. Every 2 or 3 years a new crop of shoots are formed. The bark is then obtained by making 2 incisions lengthwise down the shoot with cross incisions every 2 feet or more apart and removing with the aid of a knife. It is then allowed to ferment for several days, at the end of which period it is sufficiently soft to remove the outer layers. This is accomplished by scraping the outer bark as far as the pericyclic fibers. Double quills are then formed by placing congeries of from 7 to 12 or more strips together and allowing to dry successively in the shade and sun. The quills are then usually made into bundles that are tied with split bamboo and exported from Colombo or Calcutta to the markets of the world.

Description.—In closely rolled double, flexible quills, composed of from 7 to 12 thin layers or inner bark, up to 50 cm. in length, the bark up to 1 mm. in thickness; outer surface yellowish-brown, smooth, longitudinally striate and showing circular or irregular brownish patches, occasionally with perforations that indicate the positions of the nodes; inner surface light brown with faint striæ; fracture short with projecting fibers; odor delicately aromatic; taste sweetish and warmly aromatic.

Histology.—Sections of this bark exhibit the following inner structure:

1. Pericycle, containing an almost continuous band of stone cells among which are small groups of bast fibers with thick, though slightly lignified walls.

2. Phloem, a broad zone traversed by medullary-rays averagely 1 to 2 cells wide and containing both starch and raphides of calcium oxalate. The parenchyma cells of each phloem patch contain ether starch, raphides, or reddish-brown contents. Scattered among these are bast fibers that are either isolated or in small groups, oil cells and mucilage cells.

Powdered Drug.—Light brown or yellowish-brown; simple or compound starch grains. The separate grains spheroidal, plano-convex or polygonal, mostly under 10μ in diameter; bast fibers mostly single, with thick walls and of spindle shape; stone cells with colorless walls and reddish brown contents, averagely longer and more uniformly thickened than in Saigon cinnamon; fragments with yellowish to reddish-brown walls and contents; no or very few cork cells; calcium oxalate in raphides up to 8μ in length.

Constituents.—Volatile oil (up to 1 per cent.) containing cinnamic aldehyde; resin, mucilage, starch, tannin, calcium oxalate, etc.

Uses.—Aromatic and flavoring agent.

CINNAMOMUM CASSIA (CASSIA CINNAMON)

Synonyms.—Cassia Bark, Chinese Cassia, Cassia Lignea, Canton Cassia; *Ger.* Chinesischer Zimmt; *Fr.* Casse.

Botanical Origin.—*Cinnamomum Cassia* (Nees) Blume.

Part Used.—The dried bark.

Ash.—Not more than 5 per cent. of total ash, nor more than 2 per cent. of ash insoluble in hydrochloric acid.

Habitat.—Southeastern China.

Plant.—An evergreen tree.

Production and Commerce.—The trees are cultivated for the bark and oil of cassia in the southeastern part of China. The bark is collected, usually scraped, and dried in the shade and sun. It is then made into bundles up to 40 cm. long and weighing from ½ K. to 1 K. These are tied with split bamboo, packed into bamboo cases which are covered with bamboo mats. Very frequently the bundles contain chips and dirt in the center and long quills of bark on the outside. The commercial supplies come in boxes from Calcutta and China. The leaves and twigs of this tree are gathered and distilled for *Oil of Cinnamon* U.S.P.

Description.—Cassia Cinnamon is similar in general microscopic appearance to Saigon Cinnamon but is usually partially scraped on the outer surface which is brownish-gray. Its odor and taste are less aromatic and pungent. It possesses relatively more starch and relatively fewer bast fibers than the other cinnamon barks on the market.

Constituents.—Less than 2 per cent. of volatile oil; mucilage, resin, tannin, calcium oxalate, etc.

Uses.—Aromatic and flavoring agent.

Adulterant.—The chief adulterant for both Saigon and Cassia Cinnamons is Fagot or Batavia Cassia, the bark of *Cinnamomum Burmanni.* This occurs mostly in double quills which are scraped, up to 3 mm. thick, reddish to light brown externally and possess a mucilaginous and less aromatic taste than the other cinnamons.

The powder forms a slimy mass with water and contains tabular and prismatic crystals.

The following is a summary of the chief differences between the important commercial varieties of cinnamon barks:

	Saigon	Ceylon	Cassia	Fagot
Quills	Single	Double with 7 to 12 pieces of bark	Single	Double (usually)
Outer surface	Unscraped	Cork and most of cortex removed	Partially scraped	Scraped
Taste	Pungently aromatic	Delicately and warmly aromatic	Mildly aromatic	Mucilaginous and mildly aromatic
Starch grains	Abundant and mostly over 10μ	Not abundant and usually under 10μ	Abundant, mostly over 10μ	Not abundant and usually under 10μ
Calcium oxalate in medullary-rays	Raphides	Raphides	Raphides	Tabular and prismatic crystals

CAMPHORA U.S.P. (CAMPHOR)

Synonyms.—Gum Camphor, Camphor Laurel; *Ger.* Kampher; *Fr.* Camphre.

Botanical Origin.—*Cinnamomum Camphora* (Linné) Nees et Ebermaier.

Part Used.—The dextrorotatory ketone.

Habitat.—China, Japan and Formosa.

Plant.—A large, much-branched evergreen tree, attaining a height of 60 to 100 feet and a trunk diameter of 20–45 inches; indigenous to Asia but naturalized in Mediterranean regions, Egypt, South Africa, Ceylon, Brazil, Jamaica and southern and southwestern United States. Its branches bear alternate, broadly lanceolate, entire, coriaceous leaves acuminate at both base and apex, shiny on upper surface and glaucous beneath. Its flowers are small and greenish-white to white. Its fruit is a purple, one-seeded drupe. The pedicels bearing the fruits end in a saucer-shaped disk.

Production and Commerce.—The camphor tree is cultivated on a large scale in Formosa and Japan for camphor, camphor oil and for its wood, which is used in cabinet work. It has been introduced into Southern and Southwestern United States, South America and Southern Europe for ornamental planting and into Mauritius, the Malay States, Florida California, Texas and Manilla for the production of camphor.

Camphor is found in crystalline form in the clefts of the roots and stems but most of it occurs dissolved in the volatile oil.

The bulk of the world's supply of this drug comes from Formosa and Japan. In these countries large natural forests of the camphor tree exist and production is under control of the Japanese government. A law of Japan requires a camphor tree planted for each one felled.

The methods employed in obtaining camphor vary in different districts. Those practised in the province of Tosa in Japan are reported by Dewey (Circular 12, U. S. Dept. of Agric., Div. of Botany) as follows: "The camphor trees are felled, and the trunk, larger limbs, and sometimes the roots are cut into chips by hand labor with a sharp concave adz. The fresh chips are placed in a wooden tub about 40 inches high and 20 inches in diameter at the base, tapering toward the top like an old-fashioned churn. The perforated bottom of the tub fits tightly over an iron pan of water on a furnace of masonry. The tub has a tight-fitting cover, which may be removed to put in the chips. It is surrounded by a layer of earth about 6 inches thick to aid in retaining a uniform temperature. A bamboo tube extends from near the top of the tub into the condenser. This consists of two wooden tubs of different sizes, the larger one right side up, kept about two-thirds full of water from a continuous stream which runs out of a hole in one side. The smaller one is inverted with its edges below the water, forming an air-tight chamber. This air chamber is kept cool by the water falling on the top and running down over the sides. The upper part of the air chamber is sometimes filled with clean rice straw, on which the camphor crystallizes, while the oil drips down and collects on the surface of the water. In some cases the camphor gum and oil are allowed to collect together on the surface of the water, and are afterward separated by filtration through rice straw or by pressure.

About 12 hours are required for distilling a tubful by this method. Then the chips are removed and dried for use in the furnace, and a new charge is put in. At the same time the camphor and oil are removed from the condenser. By this method 20 to 40 pounds of chips are required for 1 pound of crude camphor.

The principles generally held to be essential in distilling camphor of good quality are: (1) The heat must be uniform and not too great, producing a steady supply of steam; (2) the steam, after liberating the camphor, must not come in contact with metal, that is, the tub and condensing apparatus must be of wood."

The *crude camphor* thus produced is of a dirty, pinkish white-color and in a mass of crystalline granules. In this condition it is frequently shipped to the United States and Europe where it is purified by resublimation.

In California, *Ramona stachyoides*, *Artemisia trifolium* and *Artemisia frigida* are grown for Camphor. The volatile oil of the first of these contains about 40 per cent. of camphor. Camphor is imported into this country in tin-lined or zinc-lined cases. Crude camphor comes to the United States from Hongkong and Foochow, China, and from Formosa;

refined camphor from Shanghai, China, and from Formosa; synthetic camphor from Germany.

Description.—Camphor occurs in white, translucent cakes or granules of a tough consistence; surface is fissured and crystalline; fracture uneven, the fractured surface being irregular and transparent; odor penetrating and characteristic; taste pungent and aromatic. Its specific gravity is 0.990 at 25°C. It is freely soluble in alcohol, chloroform, ether, carbon disulphide, benzin, or in fixed and volatile oils, but only slightly soluble in water. When triturated with equal parts of either menthol, thymol, chloral hydrate, salol, phenol, naphthol or resorcin, it forms a liquid. It melts between 174° and 177°C. and volatilizes at ordinary temperatures.

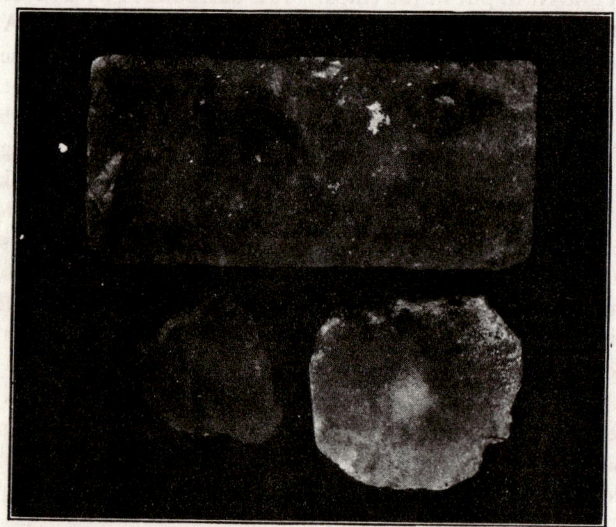

Fig. 96.—Camphor, × 1/3.

Powdered Drug.—White. When a drop of 1:100 solution of vanillin and a drop of concentrated sulphuric acid are added to powdered camphor on a glass slide over a white surface, a succession of colors, passing through yellow, red, violet and blue, is evident.

Constituents.—Chiefly a dextrogyrate modification of a saturated ketone, having a chemical formula of $C_{10}H_{16}O$.

Uses.—Camphor is employed externally in the form of spirit or liniment as a rubefacient; internally as an antiseptic and carminative and hypodermically as a cardiac stimulant. Large quantities are used in the manufacture of celluloid.

Substitutes.—**Borneo Camphor** is a camphor naturally deposited in the clefts and hollows of the wood of *Dryobalanops aromatica* Gaertner, a tree belonging to the *Dipterocarpaceæ* family and growing in Borneo and Sumatra. This product is almost entirely consumed in China and the East Indies. It consists mostly of dextro-borneol, a substance which can be transformed to true camphor by treatment with nitric acid.

Blumea or Ngai Camphor is a product resembling true camphor obtained by distillation from *Blumea balsamifera*, a shrub of the Malay Peninsula and Burmah.

Synthetic Camphor is produced from pinene by a process wherein pinene is converted into pinene hydrochloride from which isoborneol is prepared. The isoborneol is then reduced to form camphor. The synthetic article can be distinguished from natural camphor by its optical inactivity and by not giving the color reaction with vanillin-sulphuric acid.

Adulterant.—Stearic acid has occasionally been added to camphor. Ammonium chloride has been reported in a sample of camphor imported from Formosa.

PAPAVERACEÆ (POPPY FAMILY)

Herbs with milky or colored juices present in either laticiferous vessels (*Papaver*) or in laticiferous cells which are sac- or tube-like (*Chelidonium*). The flowers are regular with their parts in twos or fours. The fruit is a capsule containing numerous oily albuminous seeds. Calcium oxalate is wanting, except in *Bocconia frutescens*, where it is found in clustered crystals. Glandular trichomes are absent and uniseriate non-glandular trichomes are only present in some of the genera. Stomata occur either on both surfaces of the leaves or on the lower surface only. The guard cells of these are surrounded by ordinary epidermal cells. In several species of *Papaver* including *Papaver somniferum*, groups of water stomata are present in depressions on the lower surface of the leaf teeth.

OPIUM U.S.P. (OPIUM)

Synonyms.—Opium Poppy, Poppy, Succus Thebaicus, Gum Opium, Thebaicum, Meconium; *Ger.* Mohnsaft; *Fr.* Pavot officinal, Opium.

Botanical Origin.—*Papaver somniferum* L. and its variety *album* DeCandolle.

Part Used.—The air-dried milky exudation (latex) obtained by incising the unripe capsules.

Standard of Assay.—It yields in its normal, moist condition not less than 9.5 per cent. of anhydrous morphine.

Habitat.—Asia. Cultivated.

Plants.—Annual herbs with thick, branching, yellow root systems, the tap root of which gives rise to a smooth, glaucous, branched stem bearing alternate, dull green, ovate, clasping leaves that are irregularly cleft or toothed. The flowers are large and showy, solitary, varying in color from light pink to purplish-pink and purple (*P. somniferum*) to silvery white (*P. somniferum* var. *album*), and nodding in the bud stage. Each flower consists of a receptacle borne on the end of a long peduncle and bearing 2 green sepals, 4 colored petals, numerous stamens and an incompletely many-celled ovary bearing on its summit a radiate stigma. The fruit is a capsule, dehiscing by terminal pores beneath the stigma and containing numerous small, reniform, bluish, cream colored or white seeds, each with an oily endosperm. The bluish seeds obtained from ripe capsules are known in commerce as "*maw seeds.*"

Production and Commerce.—Opium is obtained from plants that have been cultivated in rich, well-manured soil in warm and temperate climes. The poppy seed, often mixed with sand, is sown broadcast over the tilled field in early autumn. About 13 ounces of seed is used in Asia Minor to the acre. The fields are weeded in the spring when the poppy has attained a height of about 6 inches and the plants thinned to stand about 2 feet apart. The plants flower in April and May and the capsules mature from June to July. While nearly all parts of the poppy contain a white milk juice or latex, the unripe capsules contain it in especial abundance. The capsular wall is traversed by a network of branching and anastomosing laticiferous vessels which contain the latex. In the green, unripe condition this latex is richest in morphine content, but as the capsules turn yellow and ripen, the morphine content diminishes while that of codeine and narcotine increases.

The drug is collected chiefly in Turkey, Macedonia, Bulgaria, Asia Minor, Persia, Jugo-Slavia, India and China. The method of collecting it is, in general, as follows: Shortly after the petals and stamens fall, generally in the late afternoon or early morning while the temperature is low, transverse, oblique or vertical incisions are made into the unripe capsules by means of a single-bladed knife with one saw edge (dgeezguee) or a several bladed knife (nushtur), care being observed not to cut through the inner wall of the capsule lest valuable juice be lost and the seeds injured. The white latex exudes and soon hardens on the outer surface of the capsule into brownish masses which are scraped off the following day on a wooden tray. The scrapings are later transferred to earthen vessels or larger trays or dumped on the ground, where the opium is kneaded by the hands to a uniform consistency. It is then shaped into balls, cakes or rarely sticks.

In Turkey, Asia Minor, Bulgaria and Macedonia the opium is generally made into compressed spheroidal or flattened cakes of varying size and usually weighing from 100 grams to several kilograms. These are covered with poppy leaves and dried for several days in the shade or sun. When sufficiently dry they are packed in wicker baskets or bags with the reddish-brown winged fruits of a *Rumex* species to prevent them from cohering. In Persia, after collection, the drug is kneaded, frequently with gum, into a uniform mass and then usually cut into brick-shaped masses which are dried and wrapped in red or white paper and tied with red or yellow string. In India the masses are partially dried in the sun and made into round

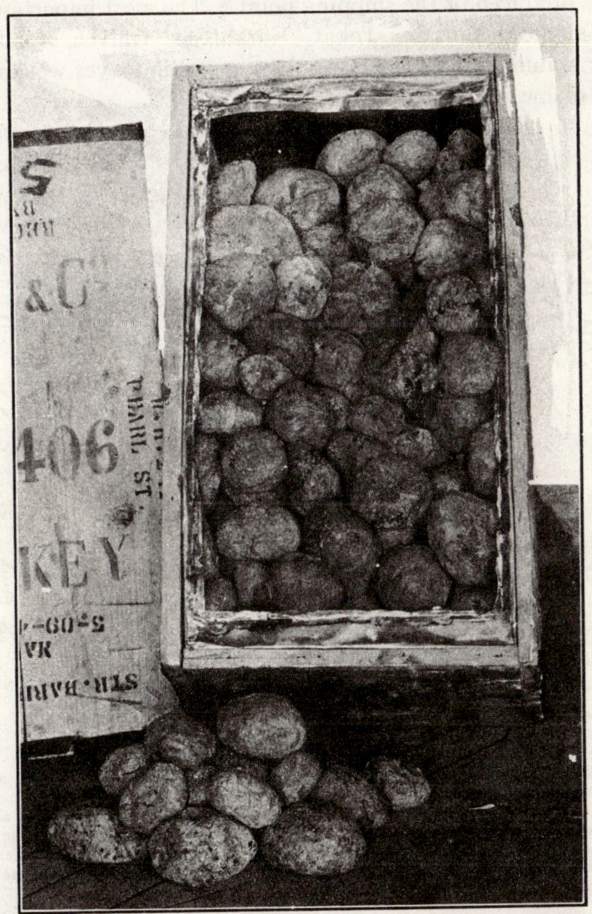

FIG. 97.—Original chest of opium, as imported from Turkey. (*Courtesy of Parke, Davis and Company.*)

balls (*Malwa opium*) or flat cakes (*Bengal abkari opium*) and wrapped in oiled paper.

The commercial varieties of opium are as follows: 1. Turkey, Smyrna, or Constantinople; 2. Persian; 3. Chinese; 4. Indian. The drug chiefly comes from Persia and Turkey in tin- or zinc-lined wooden cases.

Turkey Opium is generally recognized as the best grade and is the kind seen most commonly on the American and English markets. It is produced in various parts of Turkey, Asia Minor, Bulgaria and Macedonia. Constantinople, Smyrna and Salonica are the chief opium centers. There are several sub-varieties of this named either after the districts in which the drug is produced or the shipping point. The most important of these are the Salonica, Malatia, Tokat, Karahissar, Ghiveh, Balukissar and Boghaditz opiums. The Malatia opium comes in loaves weighing 4 to 5 ozs. and is of low morphine content.

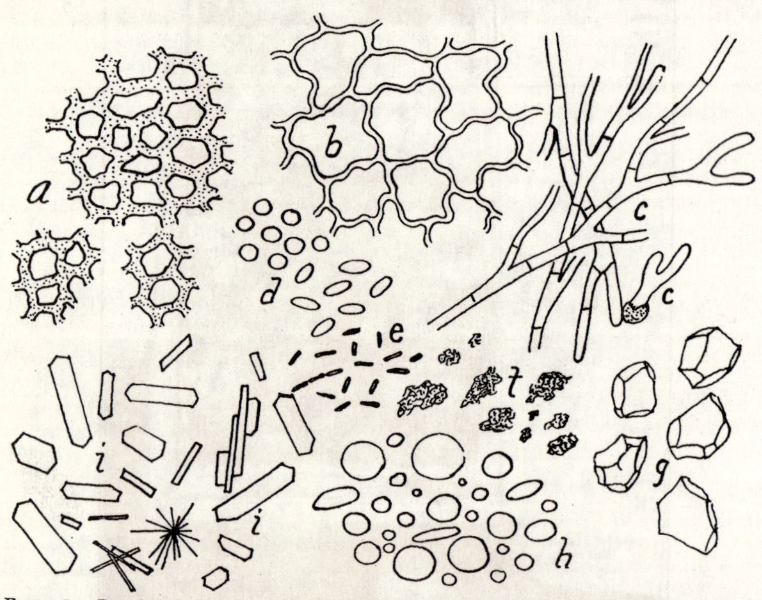

FIG. 98.—Powdered Opium. (*a*) Epidermal fragments of the pericarp are very abundantly present in Turkish opium; (*b*) epidermal cells of the poppy leaf which are likewise abundantly present in gum opium; (*c*) mold hyphæ are usually abundant as are also mold spores (*d*); (*e*) bacteria are abundant; (*f*) dirt particles and (*g*) sand particles are present; (*h*) cereal (wheat) starch is usually present in small amounts; (*i*) crystals of the meconates which are especially abundant in Persian gum opium and constitute the characteristic inclusions of the Chinese smoking opium. It is possible to determine the alkaloidal strength of the Chinese smoking opium by the numerical crystal count. (*Schneider.*)

The term "Druggists Opium" is applied to those sub-varieties of Turkey Opium which are relatively low in moisture content (10 to 25 per cent.) and which are employed in the preparation of granular and powdered opium U.S.P.

"Soft Shipping Opium" is comparatively fresh soft Turkey Opium which averagely contains 30 per cent. or more of moisture.

All of these are covered with remnants of poppy leaves and packed with Rumex fruits. The drug is exported from Constantinople and Smyrna. It yields 10 to 21 per cent. of morphine.

Persian Opium occurs in brick-shaped masses wrapped in red, glossy paper, rarely, in short cylindrical sticks or flat masses, in short truncate cones wrapped in red or white paper, or in flat circular cakes. It is usually of a dark brown color internally, non-granular and homogeneous. It yields 0.38 to 13.5 per cent. of morphine (usually 4–12 per cent.). This variety contains considerable starch.

Indian Opium occurs in spheroidal masses covered on the surface with dried poppy petals and leaves that have been agglutinated with washings and extract of juice and then dried, or in square or brick-shaped masses weighing about 2 pounds and covered with an oiled paper wrapper. It is either dark-brown or black in color, of homogeneous texture and possesses a very bitter taste. It yields from 3 to 15 per cent. of morphine (usually 7.5 to 10 per cent.).

Chinese Opium occurs in flat globular cakes frequently wrapped in white paper. Used entirely by the Chinese. It contains from 4.3 to 11.2 per cent. of morphine.

While the capsules of the Poppy are green they contain the greatest percentage of morphine, but during the ripening process, the amount of this alkaloid decreases while the percentage of other alkaloids like narcotine and codeine increases.

Description.—In rounded or flattened masses of variable size and outline weighing from 4 ounces to 2 pounds; externally grayish-brown, brown or black, covered with fragments of poppy or rumex leaves and at times with some rumex fruits; plastic (tearing apart), when fresh, but becoming hard and brittle through prolonged keeping; internally chestnut brown; odor peculiar, narcotic; taste bitter, characteristic.

Powdered Drug.—Light brown. The characteristic histological elements are yellowish-brown to brownish-red, irregular, granular fragments of hardened latex; fragments of epidermis of poppy capsule consisting of polygonal cells with lignified walls; fragments of epidermal cells of poppy or rumex leaves with elliptical stomata, fragments of rumex fruits with fibrovascular tissue and little or no starch. In addition to these, powdered opium may contain crystals of sugar of milk and fragments of Cacao shells which are used as diluents in order to bring powd. opium of high alkaloidal yield down to the official standard (not less than 10 per cent. nor more than 10.5 per cent. of anhydrous morphine.)

Constituents.—Alkaloids (morphine, codeine, narcotine, narceine, papaverine, thebaine, protopine, laudanine, codamine, cryptopine, gnoscopine, lanthopine, laudanidine, deuteropine, meconine, meconidine, pseudomorphine, etc.), in combination with meconic or sulphuric acid, free meconic acid, glucose, mucilage, pectin, wax, fatty matter, caoutchouc, meconin, odoriferous substances and coloring matter.

Uses.—Opium is used as a somnifacient, analgesic, and calmative.

Substitutes.—Several factitious samples have appeared on the market of blackish-brown color, all deficient in odor and taste and probably representing aqueous extracts of the poppy plant.

Adulterants.—Lead bullets, clay, sand, pebbles, starch, gums, aqueous extract of herbs, pulp of figs, molasses, exhausted opium, extract of poppy capsules, ashes, lead piping, powdered cumin fruits, etc.

PAPAVERIS FRUCTUS (POPPY CAPSULES)

Synonyms.—Poppy Fruits, *Ger.* Mohnkapseln; *Fr.* Capsules de Pavot blanc ou Pavot officinal.

Botanical Origin.—*Papaver somniferum* L.

Part Used.—The dried, fully grown, unripe fruit, to be freed of seeds before making pharmaceutical preparations.

Description.—In globular or oval capsules of variable size, constricted at the base and frequently joined with a short, yellow stalk; crowned at the summit with a 7- to 15-rayed, disk-shaped stigma; outer surface of pericarp smooth, longitudinally furrowed, grayish- to brownish-yellow, often marked with black spots; interior surface bearing thin, brittle placentæ which extend from the sutures for a short distance toward the center and bear numerous tiny, reticulated, reniform, white seeds; odor indistinct; taste bitter.

Constituents.—About 0.2 per cent. of morphine, and minute traces of other alkaloids and meconic acid.

Uses.—Poppy capsules, deprived of their seeds, have been used in the preparation of a sedative syrup. The seeds which abound in a fixed oil are used as a food as well as a source of Poppy oil. Poppy oil is employed by artists as a drying oil and is also used as a salad dressing.

SANGUINARIA N.F. (SANGUINARIA)

Synonyms.—Blood Root, Red Puccoon, Indian Red Paint, Tetterwort, Red Root; *Ger.* Blutwurzel; *Fr.* Sanguinaire.

Botanical Origin.—*Sanguinaria canadensis* L.

Parts Used.—The dried rhizome and roots.

Purity Rubric.—Not more than 2 per cent. of foreign organic matter.

Habitat.—In rich open woods of North America.

Plant.—A low perennial herb, the underground portion of which consists of a horizontally growing, branched rhizome bearing slender rootlets. Both rhizome and rootlets, when freshly broken, emit a red-orange acrid latex. In early spring the rhizome sends up a reniform, palmately 7–9-lobed leaf, with reddish veins, and a scape bearing on its end a large white flower. The flower shows 2 fugacious green sepals, 8–10 white petals, 24 stamens and a fleshy carpel bearing a 2-grooved stigma. The fruit is a 2-valved, 1-celled, many-seeded capsule.

Collection.—The rhizome and roots should be collected in early summer and carefully dried. Rhizomes which are gray internally and devoid of starch should be rejected. The commercial supplies come chiefly from the Southern Appalachian district.

Description.—The drug occurs in entire and broken pieces of rhizome and roots. Rhizome, of horizontal growth, more or less cylindrical, somewhat vertically compressed, simple or branched, 2–10 cm. in length and 5–16 mm. in diameter; externally dark brown, slightly annulate from leaf scars, showing on its upper surface a few stem scars and, on its lower and lateral surfaces, numerous intact or broken filiform roots and also root scars; fracture tough and uneven exhibiting a waxy, brownish-red interior; odor indistinct; taste acrid and bitter.

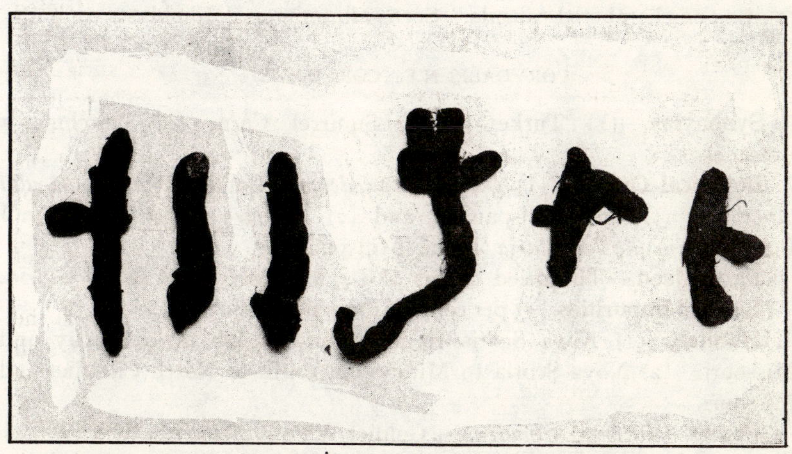

FIG. 99.—Sanguinaria × ½. (*Photograph by Stoneback.*)

Histology.—Transverse sections, when examined microscopically, show the following structures:

1. Epidermis, a layer of thin-walled, outer cells.

2. Cortex consisting of about 10 to 15 rows of parenchyma cells with thin walls, and containing numerous small spheroidal, ovoid, or plano-convex starch grains, and occasionally globules of fixed oil.

3. A comparatively narrow circular zone of numerous small, open collateral, fibrovascular bundles separated from each other by short medullary-rays.

4. A very broad pith of thin-walled parenchyma cells rich in starch.

5. Latex cells, either isolated or arranged in chains and containing an orange-red to red latex, are to be observed scattered among the cells of the cortex, pith and medullary-rays.

Powdered Drug.—Brownish-red, sternutatory; showing numerous fragments of parenchyma and short latex cells with reddish-brown masses, numerous starch grains, mostly single, occasionally 2–3 compound, the individual grains spheroidal, ovoid or plano-convex, and up to 20μ in diameter; few fragments of tracheæ with slit-like pores.

Constituents.—The alkaloids sanguinarine, chelerythrine, protopine, homochelidonine; resin, citric and malic acids, and starch.

Uses.—Blood Root is used as an expectorant and emetic.

FUMARIACEÆ (FUMITORY FAMILY)

Delicate herbs, rarely shrubs, containing milky-watery to watery latex. Leaves more or less compound. Inflorescence a raceme or spike. Flowers irregular, zygomorphic, one or both of the petals of which have a spur. Fruit a one-chambered capsule. Seeds albuminous. Idioblasts common.

CORYDALIS N.F. (CORYDALIS)

Synonyms.—(1) Turkey Corn, Squirrel Corn; (2) Dutchman's Breeches.

Botanical Origin.—(1) *Dicentra canadensis* (Goldie) Walp [*Bicuculla canadensis* (Goldie) Millspaugh], and (2) *Dicentra Cucullaria* (Linné) Bernh. [*Bicuculla Cucullaria* (Linné) Millspaugh].

Parts Used.—The dried tubers of *D. canadensis* or of *D. Cucullaria.*

Limit of Impurities.—3 per cent. of foreign organic matter.

Habitat.—(1) Nova Scotia to Minnesota, south to Kentucky and Missouri. (2) Nova Scotia to Minnesota, south to North Carolina and Missouri.

Plants.—*Dicentra canadensis* (Goldie) Walp is a smooth, delicate herb of rich woodlands whose underground portion consists of branched shoots bearing rootlets and scattered pea-like tubers of yellowish or reddish aspect. Its aerial portion consists of narrow petioled, ternately-compound, glaucous, dissected leaves with linear lobes, and a delicate raceme of heart-shaped flowers having a fragrance resembling hyacinths. The corolla is closed, heart-shaped, flattened and 2-spurred, the spurs being short and rounded. The color is greenish-white, tipped with pink. The fruit is a several-seeded pod.

Dicentra Cucullaria (L.) Bernhardi somewhat resembles the former species in habit but differs mainly from it in bearing underground clusters of tubers, each cluster resembling a scaly bulb, by the flowers being white, tipped with creamy yellow, and in having the spurs of the corolla much longer.

Description.—Tubers spheroidal and often depressed, entire, vertical, up to 15 mm. in diameter and 8 mm. in height, usually single, rarely 2 or more in a cluster; externally nearly smooth; yellowish to reddish to brownish-black, the upper surface concave with a triangular scar, lower surface concave with remains of subterranean shoot; broken or cut surface showing a yellowish, waxy interior; odor indistinct; taste slightly bitter.

The parts of the compound tuber ("bulb") of *D. Cucullaria* are ovoid or triangular-ovoid, up to 12 mm. in length; the larger concave on one surface; with a scar at the apex, and usually attached to the short rootstock in clusters of 3; the smaller grains usually separate, with an acute apex and a scar at the base; externally yellowish-, grayish-, or dark reddish-brown; texture hard and horny; cut surface showing a grayish, waxy interior; odor indistinct; taste slightly bitter.

Constituents.—The alkaloids corydaline and bulbocapnine; fumaric acid, resin, starch, etc.

Uses.—Corydalis has been employed as a bitter tonic, alterative and diuretic.

CRUCIFERÆ (MUSTARD FAMILY)

A family of herbs, rarely shrubs, growing for the most part in temperate regions. The leaves are alternate, simple, rarely compound, exstipulate, entire, or toothed, often more or less hairy. The inflorescence at first is a corymb or shortened raceme, later elongating into a loose raceme. The flowers are regular—rarely irregular (Candytuft), and tetramerous; sepals 4, green, equal, or the 2 laterals may be pouched as nectar receptacles; petals 4, yellow to white, pink or purple and arranged in the form of a cross; stamens tetradynamous, hypogynous; pistil, syncarpous, bicarpellate, superior; carpels lateral; ovary 1-celled but falsely 2-celled by a placental replum and containing several ovules attached to a marginal placenta. The fruit is a capsule (silique) that bursts lengthwise by two valves. The seeds are exalbuminous.

Clear secretory cells containing myrosin are widely distributed and found in all the organs. The stomatal apparatus is characteristic; the pair of guard cells is surrounded by three neighboring cells, one of which is smaller than the other two. The medullary-rays in the xylem are usually prosenchymatous. Crystals of calcium oxalate are wanting. The unicellular non-glandular hairs are found in a variety of shapes. Glandular hairs have been found in comparatively few genera.

SINAPIS ALBA (WHITE MUSTARD)

Synonyms.—Yellow Mustard; *Ger.* Weisser Senfsamen; *Fr.* Moutarde blanche.

Botanical Origin.—*Brassica alba* Hooker filius (*Sinapis alba* L.)

Part Used.—The dried ripe seed.

Standard of Purity.—Not more than 5 per cent. of ash and 1.5 per cent. acid-insoluble ash (S.R.A. No. 22, U.S. Dept. Agric.).

Habitat.—Southern Europe and Asia.

Plant.—An annual herb attaining a height of about 0.6 m. and growing wild in fields throughout the United States. The leaves are all pinnatifid and arranged in alternate fashion along bristly branches. The yellow flowers appear in June and are arranged along racemes. The fruit is a bristly silique with a long sword-shaped beak. The seeds are small, yellow, sub-globular and show a minutely pitted testa.

Production and Commerce.—The drug is obtained from cultivated plants. The seed is sown in fertile soil in April and the plants cultivated in May. The crop is reaped as soon as the fruits have assumed a brown color. It is dried on the ground and then carried in cloths to the thresher, to avoid loss of seeds, and threshed. The quality is largely dependent upon the time of its collection. That collected in dry weather is superior. Most of the commercial supplies have been obtained from plants grown in England, Denmark, Germany, Holland, Roumania and Italy, the product being shipped in bags. The English and Danish varieties are the most highly esteemed.

Description.—The drug occurs in the form of entire, sub-globular seeds of a pale yellowish to yellowish-brown color from 1.5 to 3 mm. in diameter. The testa is minutely pitted and shows on one curved surface a ridge and 2 parallel grooves. Upon removing the testa a greenish-yellow oily embryo is exposed which has a curved hypocotyl and two cotyledons that are folded together lengthwise. Inodorous, unless the seed is moistened, when it is aromatic. Taste strongly pungent.

Histology.—Transverse sections made through the center of the seed show the following peculiarities:

1. Spermoderm, a narrow zone consisting of several regions, viz.: (*a*) Epidermis of large more or less rectangular cells, up to 100μ in diameter, whose walls swell when sections are transferred from alcohol to water, forming numerous layers of mucilage that almost obliterate the cell lumina; (*b*) two layers of large collenchyma cells; (*c*) a row of yellow, slightly lignified, palisade cells, the inner and radial walls of which are considerably thickened. The radial walls show unequal thickening, the upper portions of these taper off to form thin-walls; two or more layers of more or less collapsed parenchymatous cells devoid of pigment.

2. Endosperm, comprising (*a*) an outer layer of thick walled cells, up to 40μ in diameter, which contain numerous oil globules and rounded to polygonal aleurone grains 1–4μ in diameter, and (*b*) several layers of compressed cells without distinct cellular structure.

3. Embryo (filling up the rest of the section) consisting of 2 folded cotyledons and a radicle. The cells bordering the inner sides of the cotyledons are palisade-like. The mesophyll cells of the cotyledons are elongated and contain oil globules and oblong to rounded aleurone grains having numerous globoids. Myrosin cells whose contents take a bright red color on heating sections (previously extracted with ether) with Millon's reagent are scattered through the radicle and cotyledons.

Powdered Drug.—Light yellow to pale brownish-yellow, developing an aromatic odor when moistened. The diagnostic elements are (1) fragments of the outer epidermis of the testa composed of polygonal cells whose walls swell upon contact with water, forming numerous layers of mucilage that almost fill up the lumina; (2) fragments containing palisade-like stone cells "(beaker cells)" which have their inner walls and lower portions of their radial walls considerably thickened; (3) numerous fragments of the embryo containing aleurone grains and globules of oil; (4) fragments containing collenchyma cells.

Constituents.—Fixed oil (20–25 per cent.), sinalbin, a glucoside, myrosin, an enzyme, proteids, mucilage, etc. In the presence of moisture the enzyme, myrosin, acts on the glucoside, sinalbin, breaking it up into acrinyl isothiocyanate (acrinyl sulphocyanide) which is a yellowish, pungent, non-volatile oil, glucose and acid sinapine sulphate.

Uses.—Rubefacient, emetic and condiment.

Adulterants.—Excessive amounts of seeds of allied plants have occasionally been found admixed with the whole mustard. The ground drug has been adulterated with wheat flour, wheat middlings and pea flour, with ground turmeric added to bring up the color and ground capsicum to provide the necessary pungency.

Substitute.—Chinese Colza. The seeds of *Brassica campestris* Linné var. *chinoleifera* Viehoever have recently been imported from China and Japan. They resemble the yellow mustard seeds in color, but are smooth, except for a few slightly reticulated brown seeds, are somewhat smaller, and possess a cabbage-like taste. They yield crotonyl mustard oil, when macerated in water.

SINAPIS NIGRA U.S.P. (BLACK MUSTARD)

Synonyms.—(1) Brown Mustard. Red Mustard; (2) Chinese Mustard; *Ger.* Schwarzer Senf; *Fr.* Moutarde noire.

Botanical Origin.—(1) *Brassica nigra* (L.) Koch., (2) *Brassica juncea* (L.) Cosson and varieties related to these species.

Part Used.—The dried ripe seed.

Limit of Impurities.—5 per cent. of other seeds or other foreign organic matter.

Standard of Assay.—Not less than 0.6 per cent. of volatile oil of mustard (calculated as allyl isothiocyanate).

Habitat.—Southern Europe and Asia, in waste places and along roadsides.

Plant.—*Brassica nigra* is an erect annual herb growing taller than the *Sinapis alba* and having alternate, slender-petioled leaves, the lower of which possess a large irregularly sinuate-dentate terminal lobe and a few small lobes coming off of the mid-rib below it. The fruits (siliques) are short, 4-angled and smooth, on short erect pedicels and appressed to the axis of the raceme. The seeds are mostly reddish-brown and minutely pitted.

Brassica juncea or Chinese Mustard is an annual herb possessing a great variety of forms. It possesses numerous large oval or obovate toothed radical leaves tapering into a narrow petiole with leafy appendages, stem leaves which are sessile, entire and oblong-lanceolate above and petioled toothed below, small, bright yellow flowers and elongated slender rounded silique fruits.

Production and Commerce.—Brown Mustard is cultivated in Italy, Germany, England, Holland, Chili and other countries, the commercial drug being shipped to the United States from Catania, Messina, Triggiano, Palermo and Bari in Italy, from Delhi and Bombay in India, from Coquimbo in Chili and from Lisbon, Portugal. Chinese Mustard is grown in India, Southern Russia and China and is imported chiefly from Tientsin and Yokohama. The seeds of this variety are averagely larger and of a deeper brown color than those of *B. nigra.* The various mustards are shipped in burlap bags.

Description.—Globular, 1 to 1.6 mm. in diameter; externally varying in color from light brown to dark reddish-brown; testa finely pitted or reticulate. When the hull is removed a yellow oily embryo with curved radicle and 2 folded cotyledons are distinguishable; inodorous; taste strongly pungent and acrid.

Histology.—Transverse sections made through the center of the seed and examined under a microscope show a structure somewhat resembling that seen in similar sections of white mustard except for the following:

1. Collenchyma is absent and in place of this will be observed large ("giant") cells directly beneath the epidermis of the spermoderm.
2. The palisade cells are unequal in height.

3. One or two layers of pigment cells containing brownish contents that are colored blue with ferric chloride T. S. are found directly beneath the palisade layer.

Powdered Drug.—Yellowish-brown. The diagnostic elements are (*a*) fragments of the epidermis of the seed coat with mucilaginous walls; (*b*) fragments containing palisade cells of unequal height and pigment cells; (*c*) numerous fragments of embryo and endosperm containing aleurone grains and oil globules.

Constituents.—Fixed oil (30 to 35 per cent.), sinigrin (glucoside), myrosin (enzyme), acid sinapine sulphate, proteids, mucilage, but no starch. In the presence of moisture the glucoside sinigrin is acted upon by the enzyme myrosin forming allyl isothiocyanate or volatile oil of mustard and glucose.

Uses.—Black mustard is employed externally in the form of the ground drug moistened with water as a rubefacient and counter-irritant. It is used internally as a condiment and emetic.

Adulterants.—(1) The seeds of the wild mustard or Charlock (*Brassica arvensis*) which, although of about the same size as Black Mustard, are darker in color (almost black) and not reticulated. The palisade stone cells of this seed become blood red, when ground black mustard adulterated with charlock is heated with a solution of chloral hydrate. (2) Rape seeds (*Brassica Napus*) are larger, bluish-black, and not reticulate. (3) The seeds of *Eruca sativa* are frequently present in Chinese mustard.

DROSERACEÆ (SUNDEW FAMILY)

Herbs (*Drosera*, *Dionaea*, etc.), rarely shrubs (*Roridula* of South Africa), growing in bogs or swamps, or purely aquatic in habit (*Aldrovanda*). Leaves, either rosettes or more or less scattered in alternate fashion over stem, usually glandular-hairy or sensitive-hairy and insectivorous. Inflorescence a loose raceme or cymose umbel. Flowers regular, pentamerous; sepals 5, aposepalous, green; petals apopetalous, varying from white to whitish-pink, pink scarlet, purple to bluish-purple; stamens varying from 15 to 5, hypogynous; pistil syncarpous of 5 to 3, rarely fewer carpels. Fruit a capsule. Seeds albuminous.

DROSERA N.F. (DROSERA)

Synonym.—Sundew, *Ger.* Sonnenthau; *Fr.* Rosée du Soleil.

Botanical Origin.—(1) *Drosera rotundifolia* Linné, (2) *Drosera anglica* Hudson and (3) *Drosera longifolia* Linné.

Part Used.—The air-dried flowering plant.

Purity Rubric.—Not more than 5 per cent. of foreign organic matter and not more than 10 per cent. of acid-insoluble ash.

Habitat.—(1) Europe and Asia, (2) Europe and Asia, (3) Europe and North America.

Plants.—Herbs of small stature with glandular-hairy leaves modified for insect catching purposes. All three species occur in bogs and moist sandy soil in various sections of the United States.

Description.—*Drosera rotundifolia* is a delicate plant of a reddish color throughout, with few fibrous, blackish rootlets; leaves all in a basal rosette, blade sub-orbicular, about 15 mm. in diameter, abruptly contracted into a slender, pubescent petiole, upper surface covered with prominent pinkish-red glandular tentacles; scape filiform, smooth, from 10 to 20 cm. in length, bearing a few, 5-parted, small, white, fugacious flowers in a curved, one-sided raceme.

Drosera anglica is identified by its linear-to obovate-spatulate leaves with blades 1.5–5 cm. long and 3–7 mm. wide or 3 times as long as they are wide and glabrous or sparsely hairy petioles. *Drosera longifolia* is identified by its elongated spatulate leaves with blades 2 to 3 times as long as they are wide, and its slender smooth petioles and scape, declinate at base. Odorless; taste faintly bitter and acidulous.

Constituents.—Resin, peptonizing ferment, tannin, glucose, etc.

Uses.—Drosera has been used as an expectorant in bronchitis and coughs.

SAXIFRAGACEÆ (SAXIFRAGE FAMILY)

Herbs (*Saxifraga*, *Mitella*, *Heuchera*, etc.) or shrubs (*Hydrangea*, *Ribes*, *Philadelphus*, etc.) rich in tannin content, with opposite or alternate leaves usually devoid of stipules, and possessing carpels either separate or partly to completely united. Both stamens and petals are generally inserted on the calyx. Fruit a follicle, capsule, or berry. Seeds with copious albumen.

HYDRANGEA N.F. (HYDRANGEA)

Synonyms.—Seven-barks, Wild Hydrangea Root.

Botanical Origin.—*Hydrangea arborescens* Linné.

Part Used.—The dried rhizome and roots.

Purity Rubric.—Not more than 3 per cent. of foreign organic matter.

Habitat.—United States.

Plant.—A shrub with opposite, petioled, exstipulate, ovate, acute serrate leaves, dark green above, paler beneath. The inflorescence consists of a compound cyme of conspicuous, marginal, neutral, white flowers and inconspicuous, small, central, fertile flowers or all of the flowers may be small and fertile. The fruit is a 15-ribbed capsule.

Production and Commerce.—Hydrangea grows along rocky banks of streams from New York to Florida and west to Iowa and Missouri. The drug is collected in autumn, the commercial supplies coming from Virginia, North Carolina, Michigan and Illinois.

Description.—Rhizome cylindrical, usually cut into pieces from 3 to 10 cm. in length and from 3 to 20 mm. in diameter; externally light brown to yellowish-brown with a pinkish tinge, longitudinally wrinkled, marked

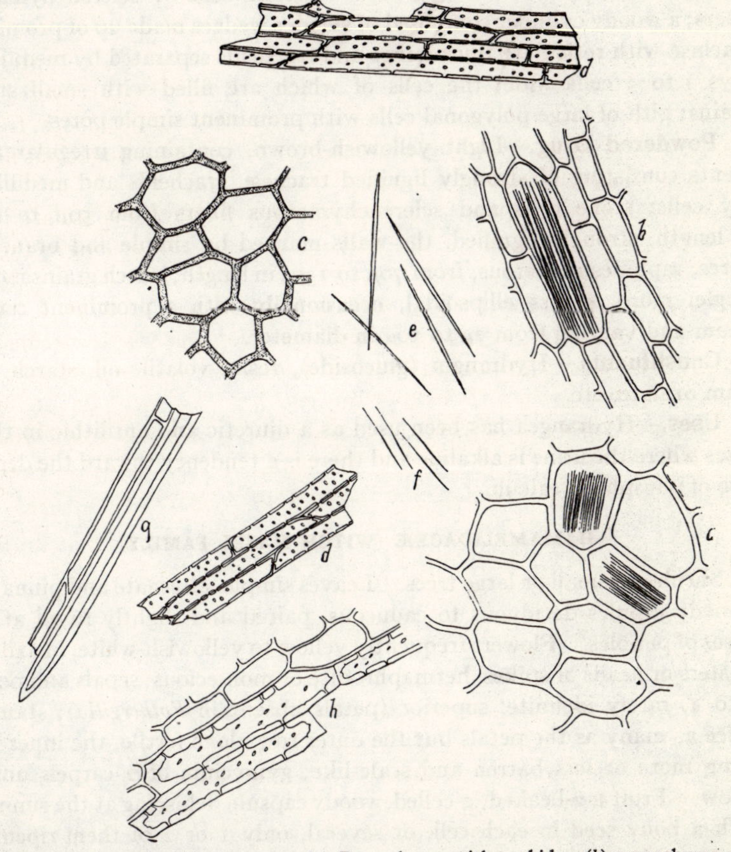

FIG. 100.—Powdered Hydrangea. (*a*) Parenchyma with raphides; (*b*) parenchyma with larger raphides; (*c*) cork tissue; (*d*) tracheids; (*e*), (*f*) acicular crystals; (*g*) bast fibers; (*h*) sclerenchymatous tracheids. (*Schneider.*)

by few elliptical lenticels and occasional prominent buds, short branches or stem scars; from the lower surface arise a few coarse fibrous roots; fracture tough, splintery; internally yellowish-white or light brown, bark thin, easily separable from the distinctly radiate wood which surrounds a prominent whitish pith. Roots attaining a length of 25 cm. and a thickness of 2 mm., irregularly bent and branching, otherwise resembling the rhizome with the exception of the pith being absent. Inodorous; taste sweetish, becoming slightly acrid.

Histology.—Under the microscope, sections of the rhizome of Hydrangea show a gray cork of a few rows of tabular cells, a cortex made up chiefly of parenchyma containing starch, large cells containing raphides and small isolated groups of stone cells or sclerenchymatous fibers; a woody cylinder composed of slender wedges made up of prominent tracheæ with reticulate thickenings and tracheids separated by medullary-rays 1 to 3 cells wide, the cells of which are filled with small starch grains; pith of large polygonal cells with prominent simple pores.

Powdered Drug.—Light yellowish-brown, containing irregular fragments consisting of strongly lignified tracheæ, tracheids and medullary-ray cells; stone cells and sclerenchymatous fibers from 50μ to 200μ in length, strongly lignified, the walls marked by simple and branching pores; raphides numerous, from 70μ to 130μ in length; starch grains mostly single, more or less ellipsoidal, occasionally with a prominent central hilum and varying from 2μ to 10μ in diameter.

Constituents.—Hydrangin (glucoside), resin, volatile oil, starch, calcium oxalate, etc.

Uses.—Hydrangea has been used as a diuretic and antilithic in those cases where the urine is alkaline and there is a tendency toward the deposition of phosphatic calculi.

HAMAMELIDACEÆ (WITCH HAZEL FAMILY)

Shrubs or small or large trees. Leaves simple, alternate and pinnately veined; stipules deciduous to caducous, paired and slightly fused at the bases of petioles. Flowers frequently yellow to yellowish-white, in axillary clusters or heads or spikes, hermaphrodite or monœcious; sepals and petals 5 to 4, rarely idefinite, superior (petals absent in *Fothergilla*); stamens twice as many as the petals but the outer row alone fertile, the inner row being more or less barren and scale-like; gynœcium of 2 carpels united below. Fruit a 2-beaked, 2-celled, woody capsule dehiscing at the summit, with a bony seed in each cell, or several, only 1 or 2 of them ripening.

STYRAX U.S.P. (STORAX)

Synonyms.—Liquid Storax, Sweet Gum; *Ger.* Flussiger Storax; *Fr.* Styrax liquide.

Botanical Origin.—*Liquidambar orientalis* Miller and *Liquidambar Styraciflua* Linné.

Part Used.—Balsam obtained from the trunk.

Habitat.—*L. orientalis* is native to forests of Asia Minor; *L. Styraciflua* to North America, Central America and northern South America.

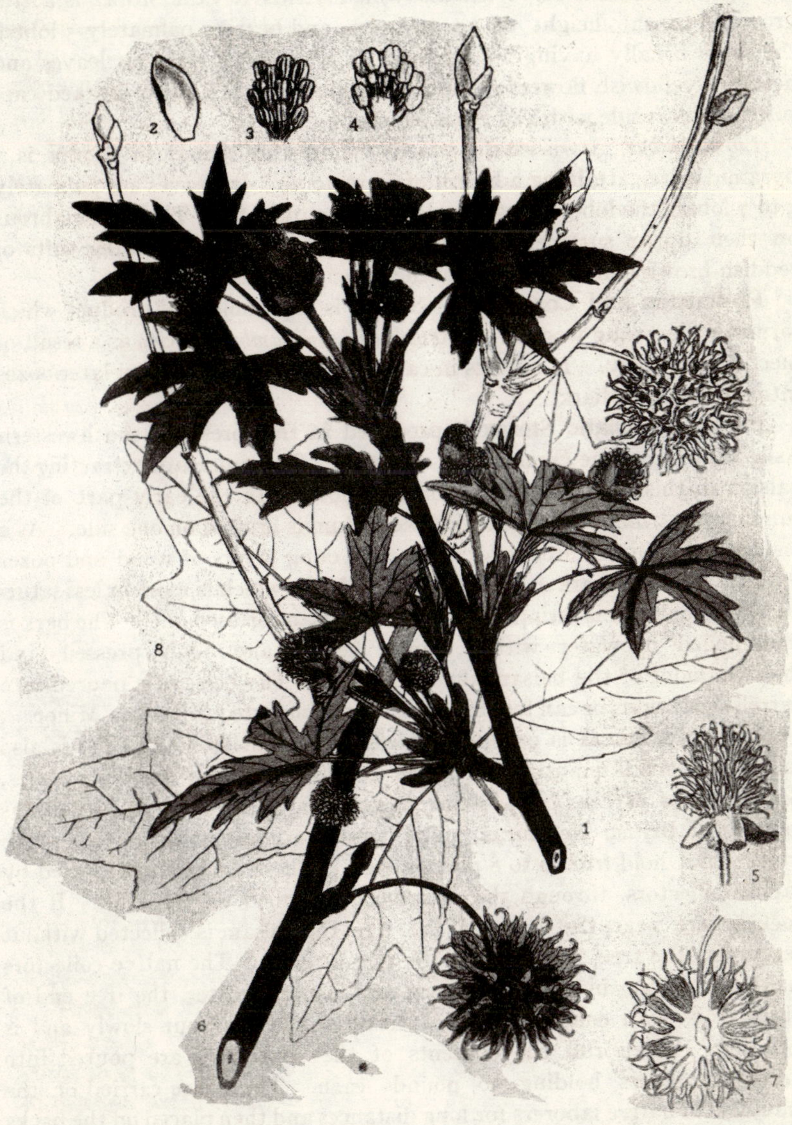

FIG. 101.—*Liquidambar orientalis.* 1. Young shoot with flowers. 2. Bract of male capitulum. 3. Staminate flower. 4. Section of same. 5. Head of pistillate flowers. 6. Branch with fruit. 7. Section of a head of fruit. 8. Mature leaf. (*After Bentley and Trimen.*)

Plant.—*Liquidambar orientalis* which yields Levant Storax is a tree growing to the height of 10 to 15 m. and bearing palmately 5-lobed, the lobes usually having 2 to 4 small lobes, serrate, glabrous leaves and heads of yellowish flowers. The fruit is a spherical head of beaked capsules, each capsule with 1 or 2 winged seeds.

Liquidambar Styraciflua which yields the American Storax is a pyramidal tree attaining a height of 15 to 40 m. Its leaves are palmately 5 to 7 lobed, the lobes being serrulate and acuminate. They are glabrous on their upper surface, their lower surface, however, showing tufts of reddish-brown hairs in the axils of the principal veins.

Production and Commerce.—Storax is a pathological product which forms in the young wood of the trunk of *Liquidambar* species as a result of mechanical injury. It collects in cavities within the wood and later oozes into the wounded bark.

Levant or Asiatic Storax is produced in the forests of southwestern Asia Minor from the *Liquidambar orientalis*. The process of extracting the balsam in this region is carried on as follows: In the early part of the summer the trunk of the Oriental Sweet Gum is bruised on one side. As a result of this injury storax forms in the young layers of wood and oozes into the wounded bark. In autumn, this bark, which is more or less saturated with balsam, is stripped off and the balsam pressed out. The bark is then boiled in water within copper kettles and again pressed, and the remainder of the balsam thus extracted. The balsam is poured into barrels, goat skins or can for shipment. It is imported from Asia Minor.

American Storax is produced chiefly in British Honduras but is also collected in small quantities in North Carolina and other southern states. Great forests of the *Liquidambar Styraciflua* exist in the mountainous country of British Honduras. The balsam exudes into pockets on the trunk which hold from 2 to 8 pounds each. These pockets are located by native collectors, through the excrescences formed on the bark. If the pockets are near the base of the tree, the balsam is collected without destroying the tree, if higher up, the tree is felled. The native collectors make an incision in the excrescence and insert a gutter, the free end of which leads to a container. The thick balsam flows out slowly and is collected. When full the contents of the containers are poured into larger containers holding 50 pounds each. These are carried on the shoulders of native laborers for long distances and then placed on the backs of mules for the balance of the journey to the shipping center. The product is exported from British Honduras in tin cans.

In the Southern United States the method of production is as follows: From March to May shallow cuts are made in the branches. These develop into resin pockets in which from 1 to 4 pounds of balsam accumulates. In some instances the trunk is girdled and after yellowish drops have exuded and hardened, the balsam is collected. Frequently a cut is made in a naturally formed excrescence and the exudation conducted to a container by means of a gutter. The balsam is then placed in cans for shipment.

Description.—A semi-liquid, grayish, sticky, opaque mass which deposits on standing a heavy, dark brown stratum (*Levant Storax*); or a semi solid to solid, yellowish-brown mass, softened by gentle warming (*American Storax*); transparent in thin layers; odor balsamic, characteristic; taste acrid.

It is insoluble in water, but completely soluble, save for accidental impurities, in an equal weight of warm alcohol; almost completely soluble in ether, acetone, benzene and carbon disulphide. When heated on a water-bath, Storax becomes more fluid, and if it is then agitated with warm, purified petroleum benzin, the supernatant liquid, on being decanted and allowed to cool, is not darker than pale yellow and deposits white crystals of cinnamic acid and cinnamic esters. The separated crystals, when heated with diluted sulphuric acid and potassium permanganate, evolve an odor resembling that of oil of bitter almonds.

Constituents. (Levant Storax).—The resin alcohols, α-storesin and β-storesin, which occur partly free and partly combined with cinnamic acid and partly with sodium; ethyl cinnamate, cinnamyl cinnamate (styracin), styrol, phenyl-propyl cinnamate, benzoic acid, vanillin, free cinnamic acid, etc.

American Storax contains styresinol both free and as the cinnamic acid ester, free cinnamic acid, cinnamyl cinnamate, phenyl-propyl cinnamate, styrol, vanillin, etc.

Uses.—Storax is used as a stimulating expectorant in compound tincture of benzoin and other pharmaceutical preparations. It is also employed as a perfume in soaps and toilet preparations.

HAMAMELIDIS FOLIA N.F. (HAMAMELIS LEAVES)

Synonyms.—Witch Hazel Leaves, Striped Alder, Winter Bloom; *Ger.* Zauberhasel; *Fr.* Hamamélis.

Botanical Origin.—*Hamamelis virginiana* Linné.

Part Used.—The dried leaves.

Limit of Impurities.—5 per cent. of stems or other foreign organic matter.

Habitat.—In damp woodlands of North America from Nova Scotia to Florida, west to Minnesota and Texas.

Plant.—A tall shrub or small tree attaining the height of 4.6 m. The leaves are alternate, stipulate, short-petioled, inequilaterally ovate or rhomboid-ovate, with oblique base and sinuate or sinuate-dentate margin. The flowers are yellow and appear in axillary clusters during autumn, as the leaves fall and at about the same time as the ripening of the fruits from blossoms of the previous year. The fruit is a 2-beaked, 2-celled, woody capsule dehiscing loculicidally from the summit, each cell containing a single black seed.

Production and Commerce.—Witch Hazel leaves should be collected in autumn when they contain the most tannin and carefully dried. The commercial supplies used in this country are collected from Virginia to Tennessee and South Carolina.

Description.—Petiole from 1 to 1.5 cm. in length; lamina usually broken, but when entire, broadly ovate or rhomboïd-ovate, inequilateral, from 8 to 12 cm. in length; summit either acute, rounded or acuminate; base oblique; margin sinuate or sinuate-dentate; upper surface brownish-green to dark green, occasionally dark brown with a few stiff hairs; lower surface shiny light green or grayish-green, slightly hairy, with prominent midrib and veins, the latter coursing straight toward the margin; odor slight; taste astringent, slightly aromatic and bitter.

Histology.—Transverse sections of the lamina present the following structures, passing from ventral to dorsal surface.

1. **Upper epidermis** of epidermal cells devoid of stomata and smooth except above the midrib and stronger veins where a few stellate hairs may be discerned.

2. **Palisade parenchyma,** a single layer of columnar cells rich in chloroplasts.

3. **Spongy parenchyma,** a zone of several layers of much-branched chloroplast containing cells and prominent intercellular spaces. Here and there in this region will be seen large idioblasts (colorless stone cells) and small collateral bundles of the delicate veins, adhering to which are sclerenchyma fibers. Some of the cells may contain monoclinic prisms of calcium oxalate, others contain tannin masses.

4. **Lower epidermis,** consisting of a layer of epidermal cells showing stomata and stellate (aggregate) hairs composed of from 4 to 12 straight or bent thick-walled cells, united in their basal portions.

Surface sections of the lower epidermis show numerous small stomatal apparatuses with from 2 to 4 neighboring cells. Characteristic stellate hairs are also visible, the separate hairs being 20μ to 75μ in length.

Transverse sections made through the midrib exhibit collenchyma beneath each epidermis, an arch of open collateral bundles near the upper epidermis and a pith, in the center, surrounded by numerous narrow, radially elongated, open collateral, fibrovascular bundles. Surrounding these is a nearly complete ring of strongly lignified pericyclic fibers. Outside of this area is to be noted a clear parenchyma, some of the cells of which contain monoclinic prisms of calcium oxalate 10μ to 35μ in diameter.

Longitudinal sections through the midrib show the presence of crystal fibers adhering to the sclerenchyma fibers of the pericycle.

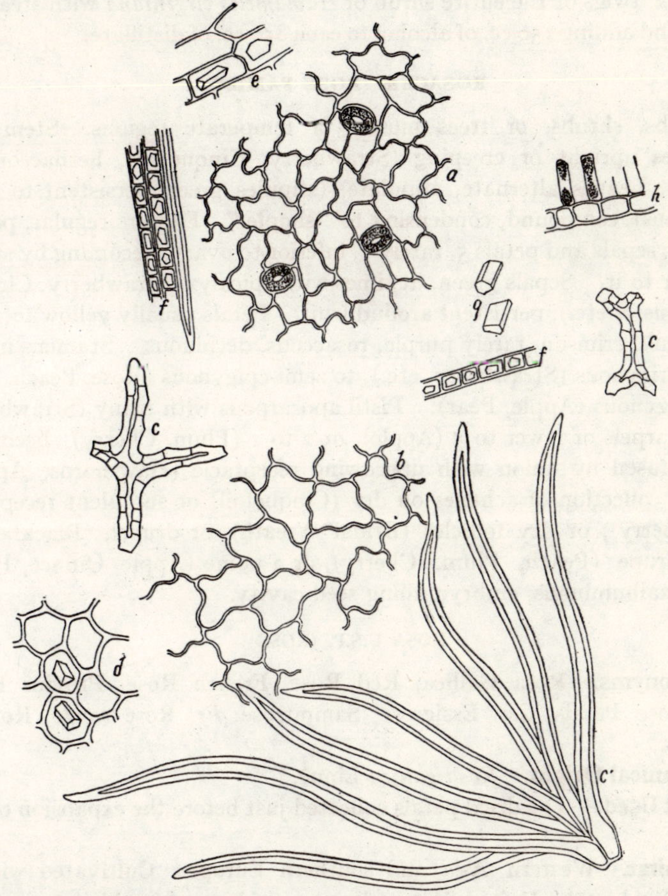

FIG. 102.—Powdered Hamamelis. (*a*) Lower epidermis; (*b*) upper epidermis; (*c*) idioblast from leaf blade; (*c*) stellate trichome; (*d*) parenchyma with crystals; (*e*) parenchyma; (*f*) crystal fibers; (*g*) prismatic crystals; (*h*) epidermis of leaf, upper. (*Schneider.*)

Powdered Drug.—Dull green. Non-glandular hairs unicellular with thick walls and narrow lumina, many bent, arranged in stellate groups; many cells of spongy parenchyma containing tannin masses; sclerenchyma fibers, lignified, thick-walled with adhering crystal fibers; monoclinic prisms of calcium oxalate up to 35μ in diameter; tracheæ mostly spiral and associated with thick-walled wood fibers which take the red color with phloroglucin-hydrochloric acid.

Constituents.—Tannin, a trace of volatile oil, bitter principle, gallic acid, etc.

Uses.—Astringent and hæmostatic.

Note.—Distilled Extract of Witch Hazel U.S.P. is obtained by distilling the bark, twigs or the entire shrub of *Hamamelis virginiana* with steam or water and adding 150 cc. of alcohol to each 850 cc. of distillate.

ROSACEÆ (ROSE FAMILY)

Herbs, shrubs, or trees mostly of temperate regions. Stem and branches upright or creeping (Strawberry, Cinquefoil), herbaceous to woody. Leaves alternate, stipulate, (stipules green, persistent to scaly deciduous), compound, condensing to "simple." Flowers regular, pentamerous; sepals and petals 5, rarely 4, inferior to ovary, becoming by stages superior to it. Sepals green, at times with epicalyx (Strawberry, Cinquefoil, Kousso, etc.), persistent around fruit. Petals usually yellow to white or to pink, crimson, rarely purple, rosaceous, deciduous. Stamens indefinite, perigynous (Strawberry, etc.), to semi-epigynous (Rose, Peach, etc.), and epigynous (Apple, Pear). Pistil apocarpous with many (Strawberry, Rose) carpels or fewer to 5 (Apple), or 2 to 1 (Plum, Cherry), becoming falsely fused by union with upgrowing receptacle (Hawthorns, Apple). Fruit a collection of achenes on dry (Cinquefoil) or succulent receptacle (Strawberry), or dry follicles (Bridal Wreath), or drupel, (Blackberry), or a drupe (Peach, Plum, Cherry), or a pome (Apple, Quince, Pear). Seeds exalbuminous, embryo filling seed cavity.

ROSA U.S.P. (ROSE)

Synonyms.—Rosa Gallica, Red Rose, French Rose, Provins Rose, Red Rose Petals; *Ger.* Essigrose, Sammtrose; *Fr.* Rose rouge, Rose de Provins.

Botanical Origin.—*Rosa gallica* Linnè.

Part Used.—The dried petals collected just before the expansion of the flower.

Habitat.—Western Asia and southern Europe. Cultivated widely. Naturalized in the United States along roadsides and in thickets.

Plant.—A shrub attaining the height of 1 to 1.5 m. It has numerous stems armed with prickles, alternate, imparipinnate leaves, each having 3–5 broadly elliptic leaflets which are obtuse at apex, cordate at base and glandular-serrate along the margin. The flowers are large, usually double, with velvety, purplish-red petals and very fragrant. The fruit is an orange-red, oblong hip containing achenes.

Production and Commerce.—The drug is collected from plants that are cultivated. Just before the flower buds expand, they are cut off with a

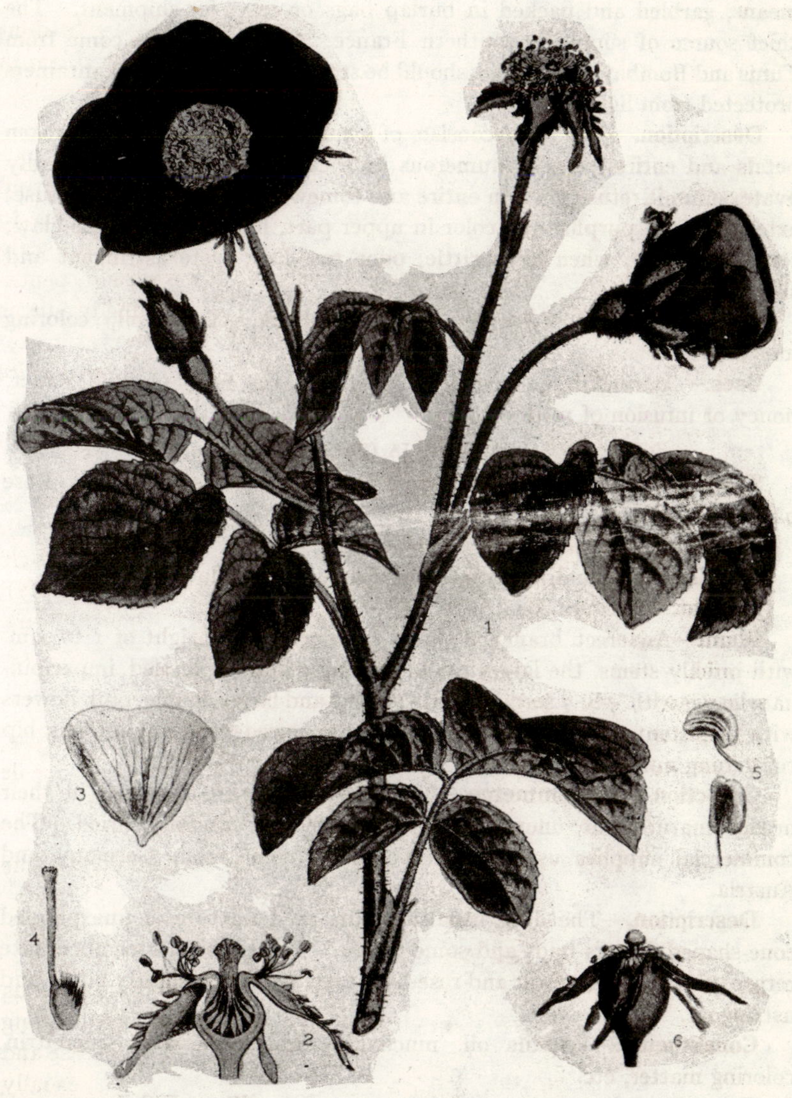

FIG. 103.—*Rosa gallica*. 1. Flowering shoot. 2. Section of flower with petals removed. 3. Petal. 4. A carpel. 5. Anthers. 6. Fruit (A hip). (*After Bentley and Trimen.*)

sharp knife near the base of the corolla, the lower clawed portion being usually left behind. They are carefully but rapidly dried by artificial means, garbled and packed in burlap bags or cases for shipment. The chief source of supply is southern France. Small amounts come from Tunis and Bombay. The drug should be stored in tightly closed containers protected from light.

Description.—The drug consists of a mixture of separate and broken petals and entire cones of numerous imbricated petals. Petals broadly ovate, summit retuse, margin entire and somewhat recurved, base obtuse; externally of a purplish-red color in upper part, light brown in the claw; texture velvety; when dry brittle; odor rose-like; taste astringent and slightly bitter.

Constituents.—Rosa-tannic acid, quercitrin, volatile oil, coloring matter, etc.

Uses.—Astringent and vehicle, chiefly in the form of fluidextract, honey or infusion of rose.

ROSA CENTIFOLIA (PALE ROSE)

Synonyms.—Cabbage Rose, Moss Rose; *Ger.* Blasse Rose; *Fr.* Rose pâle.

Botanical Origin.—*Rosa centifolia* Linnè.

Part Used.—The dried petals and nearly mature flower buds.

Habitat.—Western Asia.

Plant.—An erect branched shrub growing to the height of 1 to 2 m. with prickly stems, the larger prickles being hooked; petioled, imparipinnate leaves with 5 to 7 serrate, acute leaflets and large, double, pink flowers with persistent calyx. The fruit is an orange-red to scarlet, oblong hip containing numerous achenes.

Collection and Commerce.—The flower buds are collected in their nearly mature but unexpanded condition and carefully dried. The commercial supplies used in this country come from Germany and Austria.

Description.—The drug usually occurs as a mixture of unexpanded cone-shaped flowers buds and some petals. Petals obovate or obcordate retuse, pink; odor fragrant and rose-like; taste sweetish, slightly bitter and astringent.

Constituents.—Volatile oil, mucilage, rosa-tannic acid, quercitrin, coloring matter, etc.

Use.—In the manufacture of Stronger Rose Water U.S.P., prepared by distilling the fresh flowers of *Rosa centifolia* with water and separating the clear saturated portion of the distillate.

The official *Oil of Rose* is distilled from the fresh flowers of *Rosa damascena* Mueller or Damascus Rose, a shrub cultivated mainly on the southern side of the Balkan Mountains in Bulgaria, the town of Kizanlik being the main center of production.

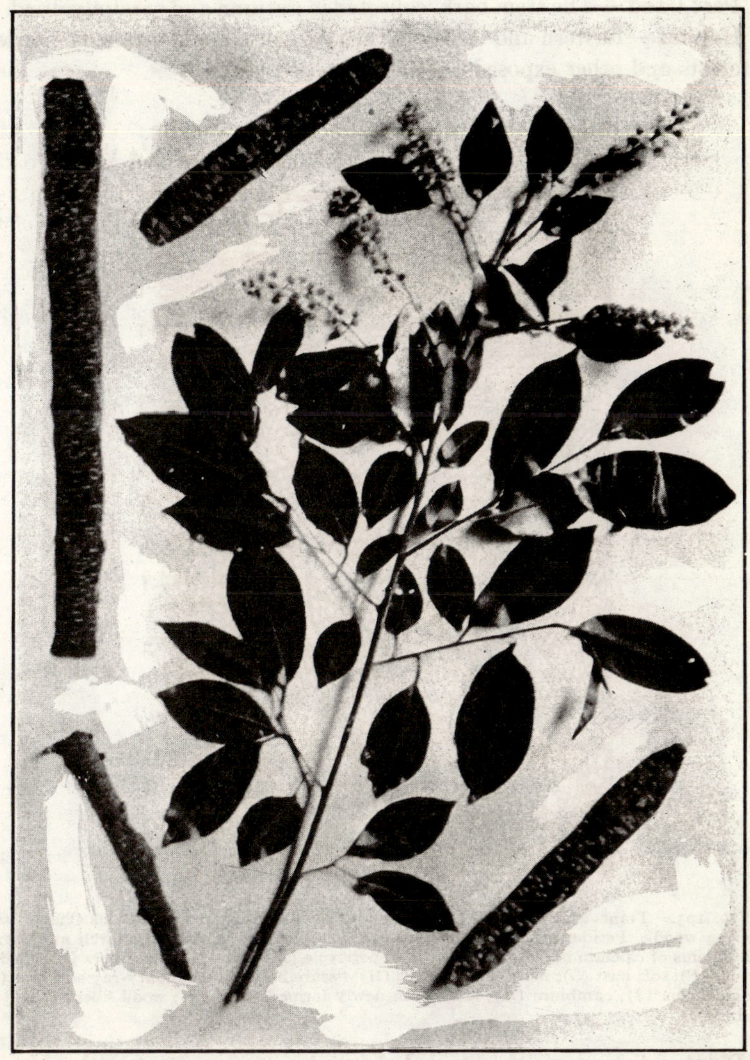

FIG. 104.—*Prunus serotina.* Branch bearing leaves and inflorescences and pieces of bark from same tree.

PRUNUS VIRGINIANA U.S.P. (WILD CHERRY)

Synonyms.—Wild Black Cherry Bark, Wild Cherry Bark, Rum-, Whisky- or Cabinet Cherry; *Ger.* Wildkirchenrinde; *Fr.* Ecorce de cerisier de Virginie.

Botanical Origin.—*Prunus serotina* Ehrhart (*Prunus Virginiana* Miller).

Part Used.—The stem bark, collected in autumn and carefully dried.

Habitat.—Eastern and central North America, along fences, on borders of forests and other exposed or partly exposed places.

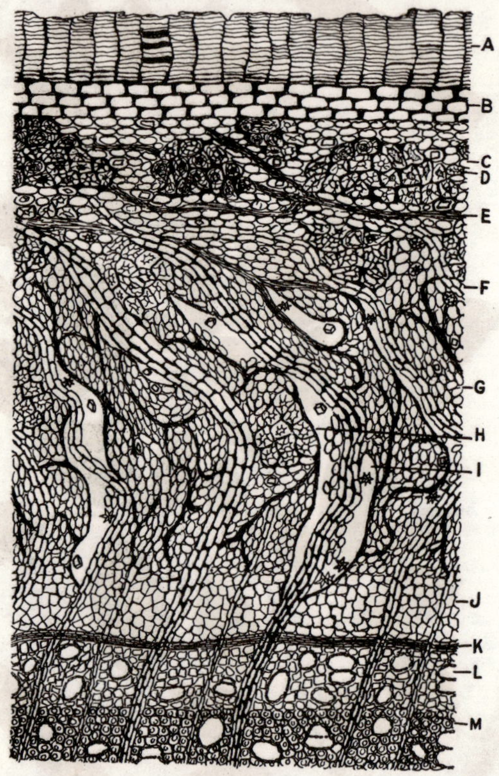

FIG. 105.—Transverse section of bark of *Prunus serotina* Ehrhart (Wild Black Cherry) with adhering wood. Periderm (*A*); collenchyma (*B*); cortex (*C*); containing starch and monoclinic prisms of calcium oxalate; stone cells in pericycle (*D*); sclerenchyma fibers (*E*); medullary-ray (*F*); soft bast (*G*); mass of stone cells (*H*); fissure between medullary-ray and bast (*I*); young phloem (*J*); cambium (*K*); trachea in newly formed wood (*L*); wood fibers in mature wood (*M*).

Plant.—A tree growing to a height of 50 to 110 feet with a trunk diameter of 2 to 5 feet. The bark on young trunks is glossy, smooth, reddish-brown and marked with numerous white, horizontally elongated lenticels; that on young twigs is marked with numerous pale, round lenticels which in time become elongated horizontally. The bark on old trunks is rough, black and scaly. The leaves are alternate, simple, oblong or lanceolate-oblong, 2 to 5 inches long, acuminate at apex, tapering or rounded at base, serrate along margin. The flowers are perfect and white, appearing in May or June on elongated racemes. The fruit is a purplish-black drupe.

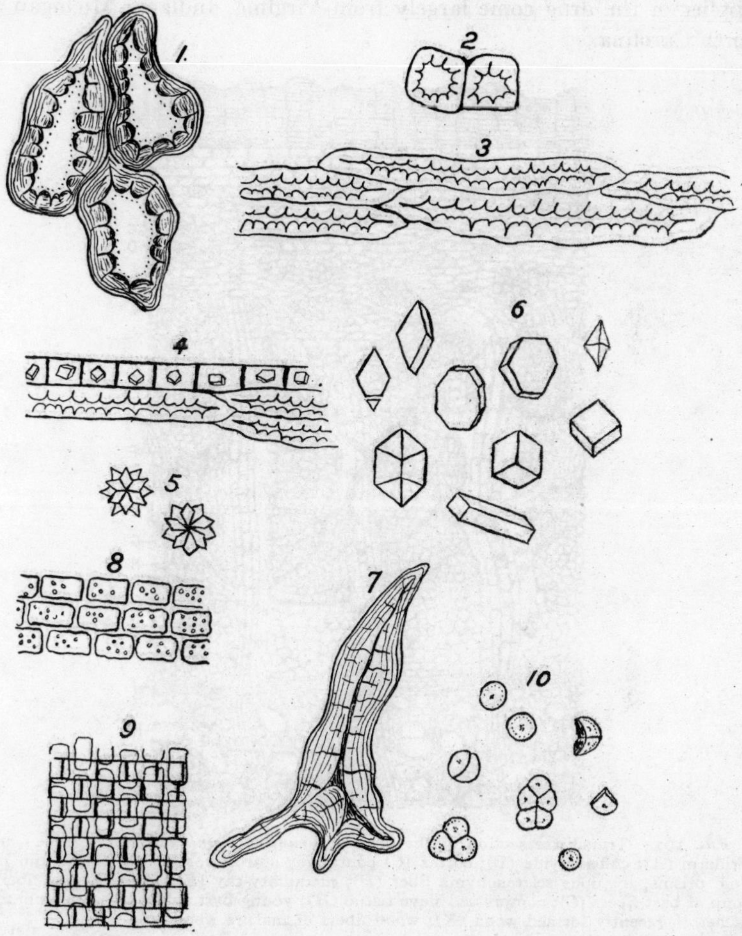

FIG. 106.—Powdered Prunus Virginiana (*Prunus serotina* bark). (1), (2) Stone cells; (3) bast fibers; (4) crystal fiber adhering to bast fibers; (5) rosette aggregates of calcium oxalate; (6) monoolinic prisms of calcium oxalate; (7) typical, heavily lignified, branching, bast fiber; (8) starch parenchyma; (9) medullary-ray cells crossing parenchyma; (10) various types of starch grains found in drug.

Production and Commerce.—The bark is gathered in autumn, carefully dried and stored in closed containers. Two varieties of Wild Cherry bark occur in commerce, the rossed and the unrossed barks. Rossed bark is that which has been deprived of its periderm (corky outer layer). This bark possesses a greenish-brown to light brown outer surface and often scars of ıenticels. Unrossed bark represents the entire bark. The term "borke" has been applied to the thick, rough, blackish outer bark found on older parts of the trunk. This should be removed. The commercial supplies of the drug come largely from Virginia, Indiana, Michigan and North Carolina.

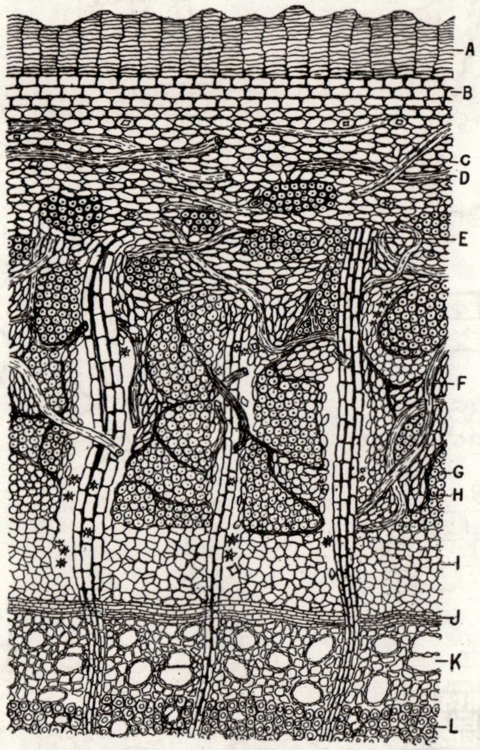

FIG. 107.—Transverse section of the bark of *Prunus Virginiana* Linné (Choke Cherry). Periderm (*A*); collenchyma (*B*); cortex (*C*) containing starch, rosette aggregates and monoclinic prisms; tortuous sclerenchyma fiber (*D*); medullary-ray (*E*); sclerenchyma fiber (*F*); group of bast fibers (*G*); compressed sieve tissue (*H*); young bast (phloem) (*I*); cambium (*J*) trachea in recently formed wood (*K*); wood fibers of mature wood (*L*).

Description.—In transversely curved strips or chips of varible length and breadth and from 0.5 to 8 mm. in thickness; outer surface of rossed bark light-brown or greenish-brown, smooth, except for numerous lenticel-scars; outer surface of unrossed bark, reddish-brown, glossy, smooth, except for numerous lenticels which vary from small and round on bark of young stems to transversely elongated and 3 to 5 mm. in length on bark of older stems, or outer surface roughened and flaky with grayish lichens;

the cork readily peeling off and exposing a greenish middle bark; fracture short, granular and uneven; inner surface light brown, longitudinally striate; odor aromatic, resembling that of bitter almonds, when moistened with cold water; taste astringent, aromatic and bitter.

Histology.—Sections of this bark show the following microscopical features:

1. Cork of varying thickness interrupted by lenticels.
2. Phellogen of meristematic cells.

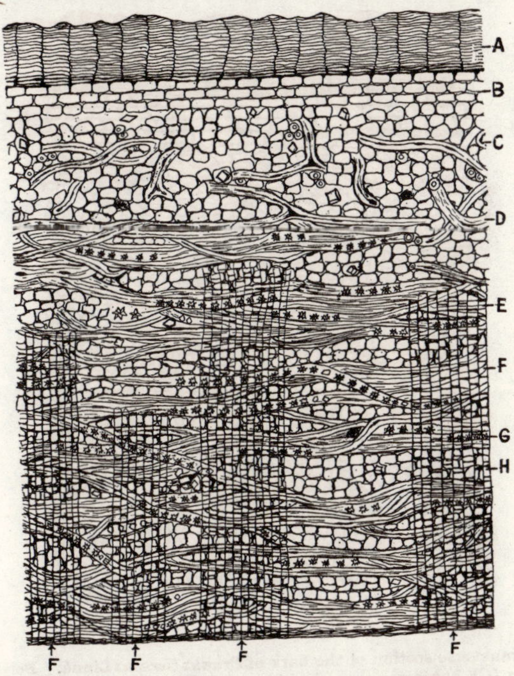

FIG. 108.—Radial-longitudinal section of bark of *Prunus virginiana* Linné (Choke Cherry). Periderm (*A*); Collenchyma (*B*); cortex, containing typical monoclinic prisms of calcium oxalate (*C*); sclerenchyma fiber (*D*); bast fibers and rosette aggregates of calcium oxalate, the latter arranged either singly or in longitudinal rows (*E, G*); soft bast (*H*); medullary-rays (*F*).

3. Phelloderm of tangentially elongated cells, cut off from the phellogen and containing chloroplastids in younger bark.
4. Primary cortex, a narrow zone of tangentially elongated cells containing starch or tannin, occasionally monoclinic prisms of calcium oxalate.
5. Pericycle, containing an interrupted zone of stone cell clusters. Many of these stone cells when isolated by Schulze's maceration process are found to show branching. They all show thick, lignified, porous walls. A few monoclinic prisms may be seen in parenchyma cells of this region, rarely rosette aggregates.

6. Phloem, a broad zone separated by numerous radially running fissures into more or less scythe-shaped masses, each generally consisting of a curved medullary-ray and a phloem patch. The starch-containing medullary rays range from 1 to 6, rarely 8 cells in width, as observed in tangential sections. The phloem patches adhere to the medullary-rays and are composed of a matrix of phloem cells and sieve tissue, the phloem cells containing starch, tannin or crystals. Masses of stone cells and bast fibers accompanied by crystal fibers containing monoclinic prisms occur in

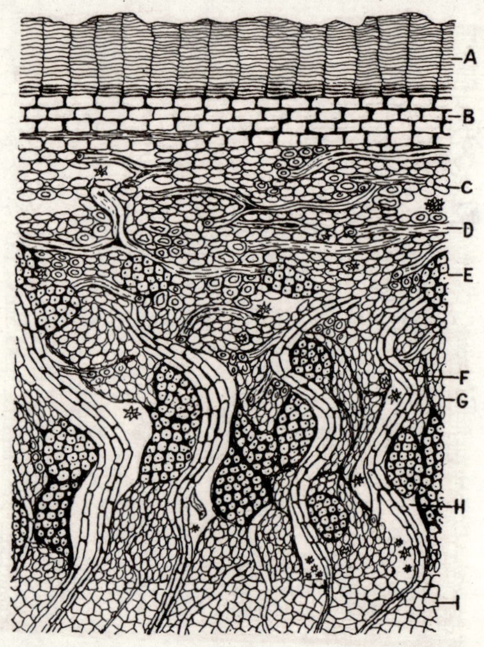

FIG. 109.—Transverse section of the bark of *Prunus Cerasus* Linné. Periderm (*A*); collenchyma (*B*); cortex (*C*), containing starch, few rosette aggregates and no monoclinic prisms of calcium oxalate; tortuous, branching sclerenchyma fibers (*D*); group of bast fibers (*E*); medullary-ray (*F*); soft bast (*G*); fissure between medullary-ray and bast (*H*); young phloem (*I*)

each phloem patch. Rosette aggregates of calcium oxalate occur in groups or singly, mainly in the cells adjoining the medullary-rays or in the fissures between the medullary-rays and bast fibers. In these regions monoclinic prisms also occur. The bast fibers are both simple and branched in character.

Powdered Drug.—Reddish-brown; numerous thick-walled, lignified, simple or branched stone cells and bast fibers, the latter accompanied by crystal fibers containing monoclinic prisms of calcium oxalate; fragments of parenchyma containing tannin and starch; starch grains more or less spheroidal and from 2μ to 15μ in diameter; fragments of cork; rosette crystals of calcium oxalate.

Constituents.—l-mandelonitrile glucoside, a ferment called emulsin, tannin, tri-methyl-gallic acid, l-mandelic acid, dextrose, etc. In the presence of moisture, the ferment emulsin acts upon the lævo-mandelonitrile glucoside hydrolyzing it to hydrocyanic acid, benzaldehyde and glucose.

Uses.—Wild Cherry is employed as an expectorant and simple bitter.

Adulterants and Substitutes.—(1) Bark of *Prunus virginiana* Linné, commonly known as Choke Cherry. This differs from the bark of *Prunus serotina* chiefly by showing no stone cells in pericycle, by having medullary rays which range from 1 to 4 cells in width as observed in tangential-sections, and by showing more rosette aggregates of calcium oxalate in the phloem than monoclinic prisms.

(2) Bark of *Prunus Avium* L., commonly known as Sweet Cherry. This is smoother and lighter colored, being glossy and of a light reddish-brown on twigs and reddish-gray on trunk. The lenticels are fewer and more elongated than those of the 2 previously mentioned species. Microscopically, it shows a very narrow cortex and pericycle in which calcium oxalate occurs mostly as rosette aggregates, rarely as monoclinic prisms. In the phloem occur numerous scattered and tortuous bast fibers giving the bark a more fibrous fracture than that of any species of *Prunus* examined by the writer. The medullary rays are oblique and wavy, when examined in cross sections, and range from 1 to 4 cells in width.

(3) Bark of *Prunus Cerasus* L., commonly known as Sour or Morello Cherry. This bark is smooth, darker than either of the preceeding cherry barks of the same age. The lenticels are fewer and larger than those of the *P. serotina* bark of similar age. It differs microscopically from the official bark by having a broader cortex, shorter and more irregular medullary rays, in possessing smaller and more scattered goups of bast fibers, and in containing very few calcium oxalate crystals which occur as rosette aggregates, never as monoclinic prisms.

(4) The ground drug has been adulterated with wood of the same tree.

RUBUS N.F. (RUBUS)

Synonyms.—Blackberry Bark; *Ger.* Brombeerrinde; *Fr.* Ecorce de Ronce noir.

Botanical Origin.—The section *Eubatus* Focke of the genus *Rubus* Linné.

Part Used.—The dried bark of the rhizome and roots.

Purity Rubric.—Not more than 10 per cent. of adhering wood and not more than 2 per cent. of other foreign matter.

Habitat.—In fields and woodlands of the United States.

Plants.—The section *Eubatus* of the genus *Rubus* comprises a long series of shrubby and usually prickly plants, commonly called "*blackberries*" and "*dewberries*." The blackberries are erect in habit, usually possessing strong, woody, reclining stems together with long, repent stolons. The dewberries are prostrate and trailing in habit with repent or decumbent stems which give rise, at their nodes, to erect flowering canes. Both the blackberries and the dewberries have mostly pinnately 5-foliate leaves on the first year's growth and chiefly pinnately 3-foliate leaves on the flowering canes. Their fruits are etærios, each consisting of a number of drupelets which adhere, when ripe, to the receptacle. Considerable of the Blackberry Bark of commerce has been yielded by the species whose descriptions follow:

Rubus villosus Ait. or Dewberry is a low-growing, nearly prostrate shrub found in dry fields and open places from southern Maine to Virginia and as far west as Kansas. Its stems are woody and bear stout retrorse prickles. Its leaves are imparipinnate, the leaflets rhombic-obovate, finely doubly serrate, smooth or slightly villous beneath. The flowers are white and borne in leafy racemes. The fruit is a short-cylindric or sub-globular etærio.

Rubus nigrobaccus Bailey (*R. allegheniensis* Porter), or the common Blackberry, is found in open woodlands from Nova Scotia to Ontario and southward to North Carolina. It is a shrub attaining a height of 1 to 2 m. Its older stems are reclining, purplish, with prominent stout straightish prickles. Its imparipinnate leaves have serrate leaflets that are appressed-villous above and velvety beneath. Its young branches and pedicels bear numerous glandular hairs. The flowers are white and borne in racemes, only the lower flowers being leafy bracted. The fruit is an etærio of numerous juicy, pleasantly flavored drupelets.

Rubus cuneifolius Pursh, or Sand Blackberry, is an ascending shrub growing in sandy or rocky soil from Connecticut to Florida west to Missouri and Louisiana. It grows to the height of 3 to 12 dm., has reclining stems bearing imparipinnate leaves with cuneate-obovate leaflets, serrate in upper half and white-tomentose beneath. Its inflorescences are 1 to 4 flowered.

Production and Commerce.—The bark is collected in spring or autumn by making a longitudinal incision in the side of the rhizome, when it can readily be removed in quills. It is then carefully dried. The commercial supplies are collected largely in Virginia, North Carolina, Illinois and Michigan.

Description.—In elongated, tough, flexible quills or bands, from 3 to 6 mm. in diameter, the bark up to 2 mm. in thickness; outer surface deep red-brown or dark gray-brown or blackish-brown, somewhat scaly; inner surface yellow or pale brown, strongly and coarsely long straight-striate; fracture tough-fibrous; readily splitting; odor indistinct; taste strongly astringent and bitter.

Powdered Drug.—Light brown. Fragments of thin-walled parenchyma containing either starch, calcium oxalate or tannin; starch grains simple and spheroidal to many-compound, up to 15μ in diameter; numerous bast fibers, thick-walled, porous and lignified; rosette aggregate crystals of calcium oxalate from 15μ to 45μ in diameter; fragments of cork tissue; a few wood fibers and fragments of porous tracheids, from wood adherent to bark.

Constituents.—Tannin; gallic acid; villosin, a glucoside; starch; calcium oxalate.

Use.—Astringent; in the form of fluidextract, syrup or decoction, for diarrhœa.

RUBI FRUCTUS (BLACKBERRIES)

Synonyms.—High Bush Blackberries; *Ger.* Brombeeren; *Fr.* Baies de ronce.

Botanical Origin.—*Rubus nigrobaccus* Bailey and *Rubus villosus* Aiton.

Part Used.—The fresh ripe fruit.

Habitat and Plants.—See Rubus.

Description.—Aggregate fruit, short cylindric or sub-globular, composed of numerous shining black drupelets attached to an esculent receptacle; pericarp externally smooth or with only a few hairs (*R. villosus*); mesocarp fleshy; juice purple-red; endocarps hard, black, surfaces deeply wrinkled; receptacle elongated, fleshy; odor slight; taste sweet, characteristic.

Constituents.—Malic acid, citric acid, tannin, volatile oil, pectin and an invert sugar.

Uses.—In addition to their extensive use as a food, blackberries have been employed as a flavoring agent and astringent in pharmaceutical preparations.

RUBI IDÆI FRUCTUS N.E. (RASPBERRIES)

Synonyms.—Red Raspberries; *Ger.* Himbeeren; *Fr.* Framboises.

Botanical Origin.—Varieties of *Ribus Idœus* L. or *Rubus strigosus* Michaux.

Part Used.—The fresh ripe fruit.

Habitat.—Europe, Asia and North America.

Plants.—*Rubus Idœus* or European Raspberry is a prickly stemmed shrub with upright light colored stems having numerous stiff, straight or slightly hooked prickles, imparipinnate leaves with 3 to 5 oblong-ovate, cut-serrate leaflets which are whitish-hairy beneath, small white flowers with hairy calyx and arranged in racemes, and dark red aggregate fruits. The petioles, midribs, flowering shoots and pedicels exhibit scattered recurved prickles but are not glandular. *Rubus strigosus* or Common Red Raspberry somewhat resembles *R. Idæus* but differs from it in being more slender stemmed, in possessing glandular hairs on the inflorescence axis, and in having a less hairy calyx and a light red fruit.

Description.—Fruit aggregate, hemispherical to subglobular with a deep concavity at its base where it has been separated from the receptacle, consisting of about 20 small rounded-polygonal, succulent drupelets; pericarp externally red with numerous non-glandular hairs up to 640μ long; mesocarp with parenchyma containing a red juice and rosette crystals of calcium oxalate; endocarp wrinkled and stony; odor characteristically aromatic; taste characteristic, sweet and acidulous.

Constituents.—Malic acid, citric acid, invert sugar, volatile oil and pectin.

Uses.—Food and pleasant flavoring agent in pharmaceutical preparations.

Substitute.—Black Raspberries, the fresh ripe fruits of *Rubus occidentalis* Linné are permissible substitutes for pharmaceutical purposes.

BRAYERA N.F. (BRAYERA)

Synonyms.—Kousso, Cusso, Kusso; *Fr.* Cousso: *Ger.* Kosoblüthen.

Botanical Origin.—*Hagenia abyssinica* (Bruce) Gmelin.

Part Used.—The dried panicles of the pistillate flowers.

Limit of Impurities.—10 per cent. of the staminate flowers or other foreign matter. Portions of the stems over 3 mm. in diameter and any binding material must be rejected before the drug is powdered or used.

Ash.—Not more than 5 per cent. acid-insoluble.

Habitat.—Abyssinia.

Plant.—An ornamental, monœcious tree attaining a height of from 6 to 12 m., occurring throughout the tableland of Abyssinia at an elevation of 3000 to 8000 feet above sea-level. The leaves are imparipinnate with 3 to 6 pairs of leaflets below the terminal one, which are sessile and serrate. Both staminate and pistillate flowers occur in broad panicles on the same tree. The fruit is an achene.

Production and Commerce.—The panicles of pistillate flowers are gathered by the natives while in full bloom and dried in the sun. Frequently panicles of staminate flowers are accidentally collected with them. The panicles are compressed into flattened bundles or rolls that are tied in spiral fashion with stems of the same plant. Most of the drug is shipped to Bombay and Aden for reshipment. Small amounts have recently been imported into this country from Marseilles, France.

Description.—This drug formerly came into the market in rolls or flattened bundles of panicles, 25 to 60 cm. long, bound with flattened stems

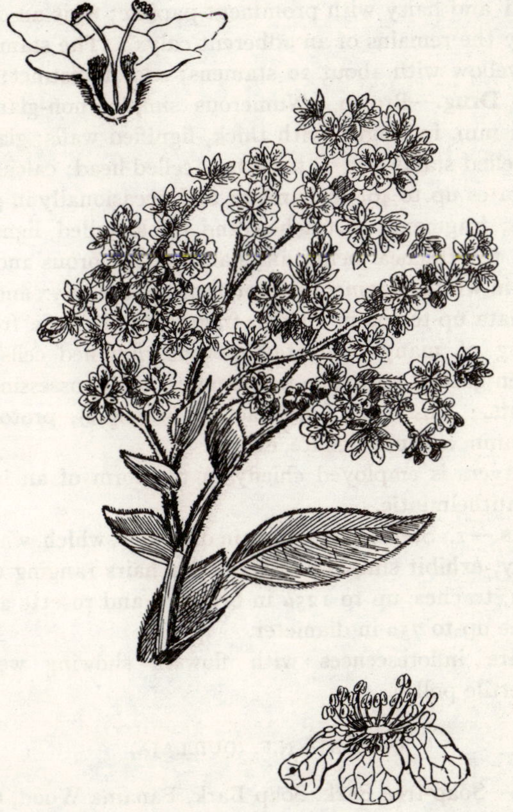

FIG. 110.—*Hagenia abyssinica*—Flowering branch, and male and female flowers. (*Sayre.*)

of *Cyperus articulatus* in spiral fashion. It now occurs in local markets, however, in broken panicles, or more or less stripped from the larger portions of the panicles (loose brayera). Branches cylindrical, somewhat flattened, zigzag, furrowed and wrinkled longitudinally, light brown, hairy and glandular; internally exhibiting a circle of wedge-shaped bundles, the bast and wood fibers of which are yellow, and a large yellowish-brown pith; each node with a scar or branch and subtended by a sheathing bract; internodes generally up to 2 cm. in length; flowers subtended by two ovate, reddish, glandular-pubescent bracts; pedicel short; calyx top-shaped, pubescent beneath, subtended by 5 rigid, spreading, obovate, purple-veined bractlets, persistent and becoming elongated in the fruit. alternating with and larger than the 5 somewhat shriveled, reflexed sepals; petals 5, caducous and usually absent in the drug; carpels 2, styles exserted, stigmas broad and hairy with prominent papillæ; fruit an ovoid achene, surrounded by the remains of an adherent calyx. The staminate flowers are greenish-yellow with about 20 stamens; odor indistinct; taste bitter.

Powdered Drug.—Brown. Numerous simple, non-glandular hairs, up to about 1 mm. in length, with thick, lignified walls; glandular hairs with 1- to 3-celled stalks and 1- to 2- to 4-celled head; calcium oxalate in rosette aggregates up to 40μ in diameter and occasionally in prisms about 15μ in length; fragments of tracheæ and thick-walled, lignified sclerenchyma fibers, the tracheæ being annular, spiral, porous and scalariform and up to 54μ in width, fragments of epidermis of the calyx and bracts with elliptical stomata up to 30μ in length; fragments of tissue from the fruit wall consisting of many elongated, porous, lignified cells; few nearly spherical pollen grains, up to 40μ in diameter, each possessing 3 pores.

Constituents.—Kosotoxin (chief active principle), protokosin, resin, volatile oil, tannin, calcium oxalate, etc.

Uses.—Brayera is employed chiefly in the form of an infusion as a tænifuge and anthelmintic.

Adulterants.—1. Stems over 3 mm. in diameter, which, when examined microscopically, exhibit simple non-glandular hairs ranging up to 4 or 5 mm. in length, tracheæ up to 125μ in breadth, and rosette aggregates of calcium oxalate up to 75μ in diameter.

2. Staminate inflorescences with flowers showing well-developed anthers and fertile pollen.

QUILLAJA N.F. (QUILLAJA)

Synonyms.—Soap-tree Bark, Soap Bark, Panama Wood, Cortex Quillaiæ, China or Murillo Bark; *Fr.* Ecorce de Quillaya; *Ger.* Seifenrinde.

Botanical Origin.—*Quillaja Saponaria* Molina.

Part Used.—The dried inner bark.

Purity Rubric.—Not more than 5 per cent. of outer bark and not more than 1 per cent. of foreign organic matter.

Habitat.—Chile and Peru. Cultivated in Southern California.

Plant.—A glabrous, evergreen, monœcious tree with thick bark containing saponin-glucosides, growing to the height of 18 m. and bearing alternate, ovate, simple, slightly serrate, coriaceous leaves and axillary clusters of white flowers. The fruit consists of 5 leathery follicles cohering at their base and with adherent calyx.

Production and Commerce.—The trees grow wild in Peru and Chile and are cultivated extensively in northern Hindostan. The bark is removed from the trunk and branches, deprived of most of its cork and dried. The commercial supplies to the United States come chiefly from Valparaiso, Chile, and Hamburg, Germany. The bark which comes from

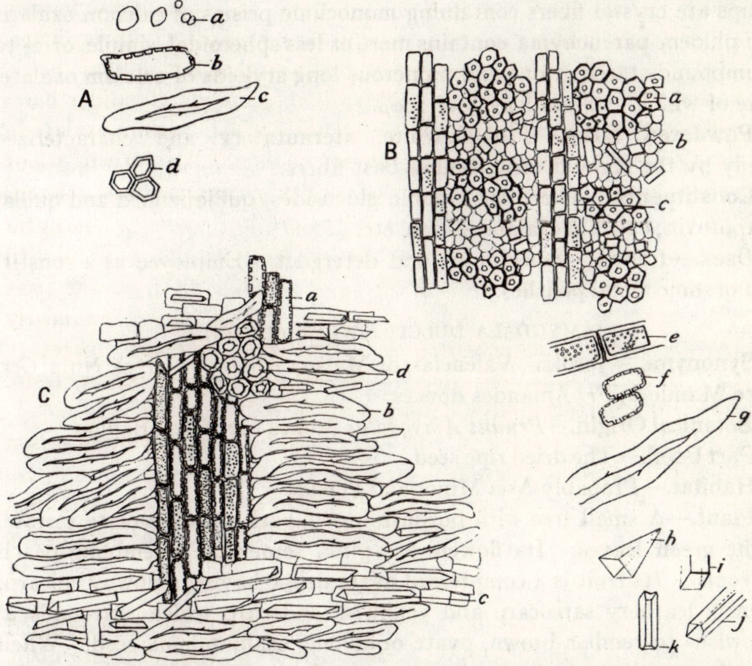

FIG. 111.—Quillaja. *A*, Powdered Quillaja. Starch (*a*); parenchyma cell with simple pores (*f*, *b*); bast fibers (*c*, *g*); parenchyma cells with starch (*e*); portions of styloids (crystals of calcium oxalate (*h*, *i*, *j*, *k*). *B*, Transverse section of Quillaja. Bast fiber (*a*); calcium oxalate (*b*); medullary-ray (*c*). *C*, Longitudinal-radial section of Quillaja. Medullary-ray cells with porous walls (*a*); bast fibers (*b*); styloids (calcium oxalate) (*c*); sclerenchyma cells (*d*).

Chili is the crude inner bark and arrives in burlap bundles. That which is imported from Hamburg is milled and arrives here in two types. One type consists of cut drug (square chips) and the other type is designated as siftings. The latter is usually very high in total ash (up to 20 per cent.), is rich in calcium oxalate and represents the refuse from chip manufacture. Both of the milled products are shipped in bags.

Description.—Soap Bark occurs in flat or partially quilled pieces of variable length, from 3 to 10 mm. in thickness, or in small chips; outer surface brownish-white, often with small brownish patches of cork attached; inner surface yellowish-white or yellowish-gray, nearly smooth, crystalline, with occasional circular depressions and conical projections; fracture uneven, tough and strongly fibrous, exhibiting crystals; odor slight; taste acrid.

Histology.—Sections of Quillaja exhibit mostly phloem, separated into phloem patches by a number of medullary-rays. The bast fibers are thick-walled, strongly lignified, wavy, irregular, and arranged in groups in radial fashion as observed in transverse sections. Surrounding these groups are crystal fibers containing monoclinic prisms of calcium oxalate. The phloem parenchyma contains more or less spheroidal, simple, or 2- to 4-compound starch grains and numerous long styloids of calcium oxalate, some of which attain a length of 200μ.

Powdered Drug.—Pinkish-white, sternutatory and characterized chiefly by the styloids and peculiar bast fibers.

Constituents.—The toxic saponin glucosides, quillajic acid and quillajasapotoxin; calcium oxalate, starch, etc.

Uses.—Irritant, expectorant and detergent. Employed as a constituent of some metal polishes.

AMYGDALA DULCIS (SWEET ALMOND)

Synonyms.—Jordan-, Valencia-, or Malaga Almonds, Greek Nuts; *Ger.* Süsse Mandeln; *Fr.* Amandes douces.

Botanical Origin.—*Prunus Amygdalus* Stokes var. *dulcis* Baillon.

Part Used.—The dried ripe seed.

Habitat.—Probably Asia Minor and Persia.

Plant.—A small tree with purplish-brown bark and lanceolate, serrate, bright green leaves. Its flowers are pink, somewhat resembling peach blossoms. Its fruit is a compressed ovate drupe having a downy epicarp, greenish leathery sarcocarp and yellowish endocarp which surrounds a yellowish- to reddish-brown, ovate or oblong, exalbuminous seed. When ripe the portion of the pericarp external to the endocarp splits into two halves and falls off the stone or "shell."

Production and Commerce.—The almond tree is cultivated in Persia, Turkestan, Mediterranean countries and California. The fruits are gathered when ripe, the hard outer portions of the pericarp removed and the seed with its enveloping papery endocarp collected. The commercial supplies come from Mogador, Morocco, and from Spain, Portugal, France, Sicily and Italy. The chief commercial varieties are Jordan and Valencia almonds. The former comes from Malaga and demands the highest price. Its seeds are long and narrow with a smooth, thin, buff seed coat. Valencia almonds come from Spain and possess broadly ovoid seeds with a thicker, rough, dark brown seed coat.

Description.—The seeds are entire, ovate or oblong-lanceolate, exalbuminous, up to 30 mm. in length, up to 17 mm. in breadth and 9 mm. or less in thickness; spermoderm thin, yellowish- to reddish-brown, coarsely longitudinally furrowed, easily removed on soaking the seed in water; embryo straight, whitish, consisting of two large plano-convex cotyledons, a short conical hypocotyl, and a short plumule at the pointed end of the seed; odor slight; taste bland and sweet. Upon bruising and triturat-

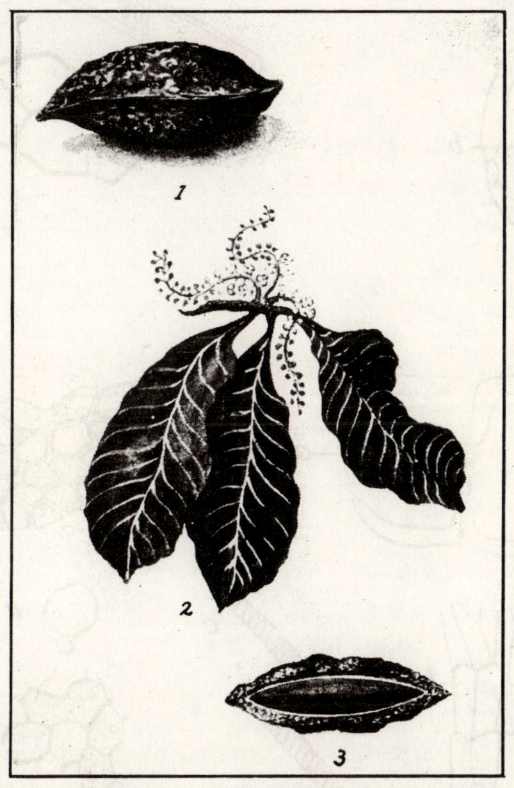

FIG. 112.—*Prunus Amygdalus dulcis.* (1) Fruit; (2) branch bearing leaves and flowers; (3) fruit cut across exposing seed.

ing in water, a milk-white emulsion is produced which is devoid of the odor of benzaldehyde or hydrocyanic acid.

Histology.—Transverse sections of the almond seed show the following microscopic structures:

1. *Seed coat* consisting of (*a*) an *outer epidermis* of erect, rectangular stone cells with rounded angles, the lower half of each of which shows circular pore canals; (*b*) a *hypodermis* of brownish angular cells in 1 or 2

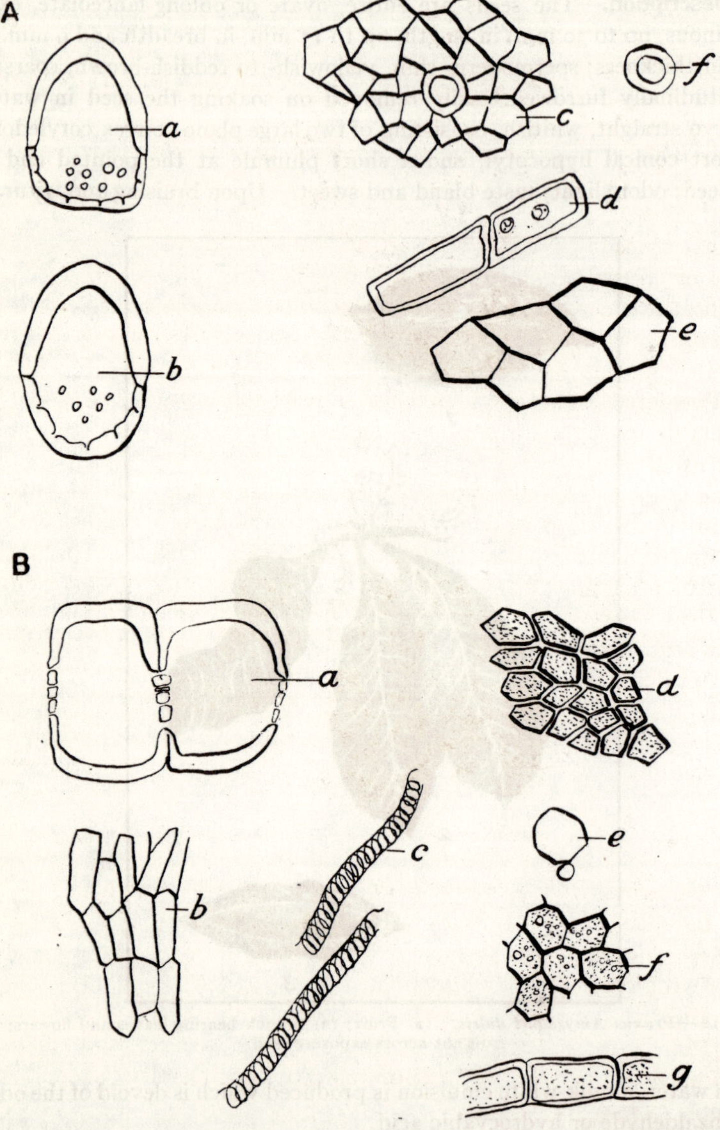

FIG. 113.—*A, Peach kernel meal,* a substitute for almond meal. Stony epidermal cells of seed coat, as seen in transverse view (*a, b*); surface view of hypodermis of seed coat (*c*); the somewhat rounded object near the center is a stone cell; enlarged view of portion of hypodermis (*e*); vertical view of stone cell (*f*); cotyledon cells (*d*). *B, Almond meal.* Transverse view of stone cells (epidermal cells) of seed coat (*a*); epidermal cells of cotyledon (*b*); spiral tracheæ (*c*); cells of a cotyledon containing aleurone (*f*); phytoglobulin and globoid of aleurone grain (*e*); lengthwise view of cells of cotyledon (*g*).

layers that are devoid of intercellular-air-spaces; (*c*) ***spongy parenchyma*** of more or less collapsed cells. Through this region the ***raphe*** courses with its spiral tracheæ. Some of the cells of the parenchyma possess crystals; (*d*) an ***inner epidermis*** of small cells with brown contents.

2. *Perisperm*, a hyaline layer.

3. *Endosperm*, consisting of a layer of small, cubical, aleurone cells with thick walls and a subjacent narrow layer of obliterated cells.

4. *Embryo* of 2 large plano-convex cotyledons and a small hypocotyl. Each cotyledon is covered by an epidermis beneath which is a broad zone of reserve parenchyma containing fixed oil globules and aleurone grains, the latter from 3μ to 15μ in diameter. Some of the aleurone grains contain a phytoglobulin, others globoids, still others a rosette aggregate of calcium oxalate.

Powdered Drug (**Almond Meal**).—Yellowish-white; numerous fragments of reserve parenchyma of endosperm containing aleurone grains and oil globules; fragments of the seed coat with more or less elliptical stone cells having thin, lignified, porous walls; numerous oil globules and aleurone grains, separated globoids and crystals; a few spiral tracheæ.

Constituents.—About 50 per cent. of fixed oil, about 20 per cent. of protein; asparagin, sucrose, gum, etc.

Uses.—Sweet almonds are used as a demulcent and nutritive. Almond meal is used as a detergent.

Adulterant.—The powdered drug has been frequently adulterated with or substituted by Peach Kernel Meal. This is readily detected by the triangular stone cells of the outer epidermis of the seed coat which have rounded angles.

AMYGDALA AMARA (BITTER ALMOND)

Synonyms.—*Ger.* Bittere Mandeln; *Fr.* Amandes amères.

Botanical Origin.—*Prunus Amygdalus* Stokes var. *amara* Baillon (*Amygdalus communis* Linné).

Part Used.—The dried ripe seed.

Habitat.—Probably Asia Minor and Persia.

Plant.—A tree resembling in habit the peach with grayish bark, shining lanceolate, serrate leaves, large, showy pink flowers and compressed ovate drupe fruits.

Production and Commerce.—The bitter almond is cultivated to a less extent than the sweet almond in Mediterranean countries. Our commercial supplies of the seed come from Sicily, Southern France and Morocco.

Description.—Closely resembling the sweet almond in form but averagely smaller and proportionately broader, with a bitter taste, and developing an odor of hydrocyanic acid when made into an aqueous emulsion or when bruised and moistened.

Constituents.—Fixed oil (about 45 per cent.), the glucoside amygdalin, the ferment emulsin, proteids, etc. In the presence of moisture, the ferment emulsin hydrolyzes the amygdalin to form hydrocyanic acid, benzaldehyde and glucose.

Uses.—Bitter almond is used in the production of Oil of Bitter Almond U.S.P. (volatile oil) and with seeds of other varieties of *Amygdalus communis* in the preparation of Expressed Oil of Almond U.S.P. (fixed oil).

PRUNUM N.F. (PRUNE)

Synonyms.—*Fr.* Pruneau noir; *Ger.* Zwetsche, Pflaume.

Botanical Origin.—*Prunus domestica* Linné.

Part Used.—The partially dried ripe fruit.

Habitat.—Southwestern Asia.

Plant.—This plant is the freestone variety of *Amygdalus Persica* which is closely allied to the almond in its general characters—coarsely serrate, broad leaves which appear after the solitary, pink flowers, and a soft-fleshed fruit, at maturity, with a deeply pitted stone.

Production and Commerce.—The trees are cultivated for their fruit in California, France, Germany and Asia Minor. The fruits are gathered when ripe, passed through a dilute solution of lye, rinsed in water, partially dried in the sun or by dehydration methods and graded as to weight and size. The chief source of the drug used in this country is California.

Description.—The fruits occur as ellipsoidal or oblong, brownish-black, somewhat compressed drupes more or less shriveled externally; the sarcocarp is sweet and acidulous; the putamen or stone is brown, flattened, ellipsoidal, smooth, irregularly ridged; the seed is almond-shaped and possesses a taste resembling that of bitter almond.

Constituents.—Sugar, tartaric, malic and other organic acids, etc.

Uses.—Laxative and nutrient. When used in the preparation of confection of senna and for other pharmaceutical purposes it should contain from 30 to 35 per cent. of its natural moisture.

LEGUMINOSÆ (PEA AND BEAN FAMILY)

Herbs, shrubs or trees of all regions, with tubercled roots, the tubercles containing bacteria (*Pseudomonas radicicola*). Stem usually erect, rarely creeping (*Trifolium repens*). Leaves alternate, compound—rarely simple—stipulate, sometimes tendriliform (Pea, etc.), or reduced to phylloid petioles (*Acacia sp.*). Inflorescence a raceme (*Cytisus*, etc.) or spike (*Glycyrrhiza*), at times condensed almost to a head or capitulum (Sp. of clover, *Mimosa*, etc.). Flowers pentamerous (rarely 4), regular (sub. fam. *Mimosaceæ*), to irregular (sub. fam. *Cæsalpinaceæ, Papilionaceæ*). Sepals 5 united, green; petals 5 (rarely 4) variously related, in *Papilionaceæ* one superior, external, posterior—standard or vexillum, 2 lateral form wings or alæ, 2 inferior, internal and anterior, slightly adherent, form keel. Stamens 10 to 4, free, or in *Papilionaceæ* united by filaments into a monadelphous (10) or a diadelphous (9 to 1) tube, inserted perigynously. Pistil monccarpellary, ovary with sutural placentation, style simple. Fruit a legume or loment. Seeds exalbuminous.

To this family belong important forage plants like clovers, alfalfa, vetches, cowpeas, economic food-yielding plants such as peas, beans and lentils, and timber trees as Kentucky-coffee, honey locust, black locust, etc. The histological characters vary for the most part in the different sub-families and genera. Those common to all the Leguminosæ, according to Solereder, are simple perforations in the tracheæ and simple-pitted wood prosenchyma.

GLYCYRRHIZA U.S.P. (GLYCYRRHIZA)

Synonyms.—Licorice Root, Liquorice Root, Sweet Wood, *Ger.* Lakritzenholz, Süssholz; *Fr.* Réglisse, Bois doux.

Botanical Origin.—*Glycyrrhiza glabra* Linné var. *typica* Regel et Herder and *Glycyrrhiza glabra* Linné var. *glandulifera* Regel et Herder or other varieties of *Glycyrrhiza glabra* Linné having a yellow and sweet wood.

Parts Used.—The dried rhizome and roots.

Ash.—Not more than 2.5 per cent. acid-insoluble.

Habitat.—Southern Europe, Western and Central Asia.

Plants.—*Glycyrrhiza glabra typica* which yields the commercial variety known as Spanish Licorice, is a perennial herb cultivated on a large scale in southern Europe. Its underground portion consists of a spreading slender rhizome bearing fibrous roots. Its aerial portion consists of a branched stem attaining a height of 1 to 1.5 m. bearing alternate imparipinnate leaves with petioled, pale green, ovate, entire leaflets and axillary spikes of violet-colored papilionaceous flowers. The fruit is a compressed legume containing kidney-shaped seeds.

Glycyrrhiza glabra glandulifera, the source of Russian Licorice, somewhat resembles the former species, differing from it mainly by its underground portion consisting of a large rhizome which gives off long, thick, fusiform roots and by its aerial portion being glandular-hairy.

Production and Commerce.—The plants grow wild and are cultivated in southern Europe, Russia, Syria and Persia. About 95 per cent. of the licorice entering American commerce is collected from wild plants and most of it comes from Asia Minor. The commercial supplies of the root come chiefly from Barcelona, Alicante and Seville, Spain, from

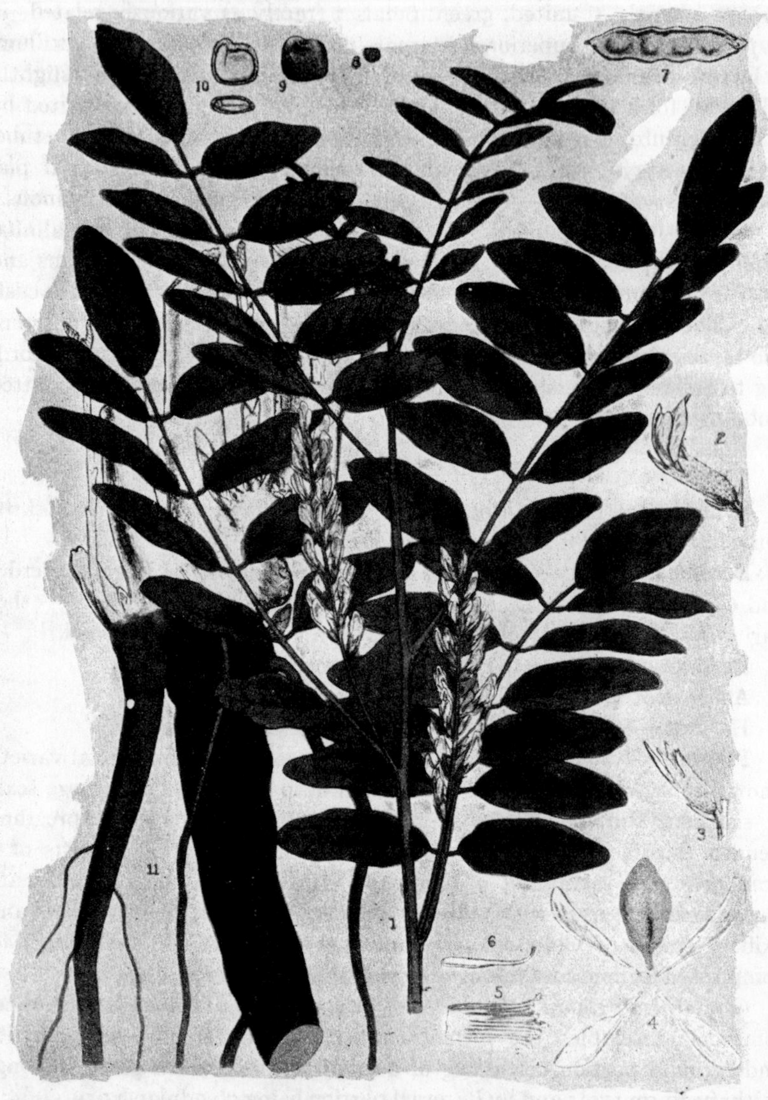

FIG. 114.—*Glycyrrhiza glabra.* 1. Upper part of flowering plant. 2. Flower. 3. Calyx. 4. Petals. 5. Stamens. 6. Pistil. 7. Legume. 8, 9. Seeds. 10. Sections of same. 11. Portion of root and base of stem. (*After Bentley and Trimen.*)

Marseilles, France, from Leghorn, Italy, from Smyrna, Alexandretta and Haifa, Syria, from Greece, and from Constantinople, Turkey and are generally named after the country in which they were grown. Russian licorice root (peeled and unpeeled) is imported from Hamburg and London. Persian licorice is exported from Bussorah, Persia. Licorice root is shipped in covered and uncovered bales. The cut root is shipped in bags. The chief causes of inferiority are poorly dried and moldy roots. Licorice extract occurs chiefly in two commercial varieties, viz: Italian and Spanish. The Spanish is the better and is made in large quantities at Seville, Spain. The Italian is made extensively at Catairia, Italy. Licorice extract is also made in large quantities in Philadelphia, Pa. Stick licorice (extract) comes packed in bay leaves.

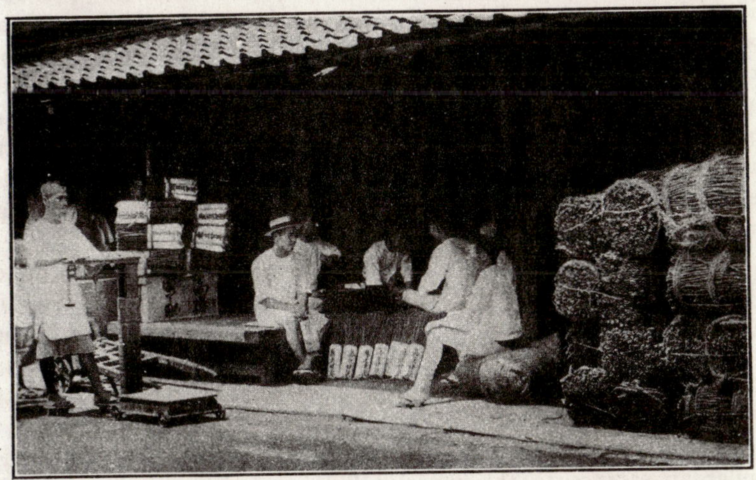

FIG. 115.—Wholesale dealer in licorice root. On the right of the illustration are piled up the bales of licorice root as imported from China. These roots are cut into a certain length and packed in paper bags as seen on the left hand side of the picture. (*After a photograph by Parke, Davis and Company.*)

A very good Licorice Root is yielded by *Glycyrrhiza malensis*. This drug is now imported from China.

Spain is the largest producer of cultivated licorice.

There are four general types of Spanish root now produced. These are the Toledo, Seville, Zaragosa and Alicante. The Toledo is the best root and is usually a cent and a half higher than the other Spanish grades. Next comes the Seville root which is from one-half to one cent higher than either the Zaragosa or Alicante, which are regarded as being of about the same quality. Spanish root is harvested from the same ground every third year and in harvesting a furrow of approximately four feet in width is turned with the plow and the roots are then collected and transferred to large drying sheds with open ends toward the prevailing wind. The roots are spread on the floor of this drying shed to a depth of about six feet and are frequently worked over with large forks until they are so dry that they break with a snap. The roots are then ready for baling. This drying process takes from four to six months. In the drying the root shrivels and any adhering dirt falls off in the forking. All other grades or types of root are dried in very much the same manner. Grecian licorice requires usually from six to eight months before it is sufficiently dried for shipping.

Description.—**Spanish (or Italian, Turkish, Levant) Licorice** usually occurs on the market in bundles of nearly cylindrical segments of the rhizomes and roots bound with wire, but occasionally, as small pieces, known as "cut licorice," rarely in the entire form, segments of variable length and 5 to 20 mm. in diameter; externally yellowish-brown or purplish-brown, longitudinally wrinkled with patches of cork adhering, the upper portion of the rhizome showing a knotty crown, the thinner rhizomes showing alternate buds, the roots small and emanating from the rhizome near the buds; fracture coarsely fibrous; internally greenish-yellow or lemon yellow, bark and wood radiate, the rhizome having a small pith; odor distinct; taste sweetish and slightly acrid.

Russian Licorice usually occurs as broken or longitudinally cut segments of peeled roots, rarely as roots, in the unpeeled condition; segments of variable length and from 1–5 cm. in diameter; when deprived of cork, externally pale yellow, otherwise brownish-red; fracture coarsely fibrous internally lemon-yellow, cortex and wood radially cleft and radiate; odor distinct; taste sweetish.

Persian Licorice occurs in large thick segments which have a strikingly similar appearance to the unpeeled Russian variety. It is yielded by *Glycyrrhiza glabra* Linné var. *β. violacea.*

Histology.—Transverse sections of the older parts of the rhizome of Spanish Licorice exhibit the following microscopical structure:

1. *Cork,* of many layers of cork cells with reddish-brown contents.
2. *Cork cambium,* of somewhat collapsed meristematic cells.
3. *Secondary cortex,* of one or more layers of collenchymatic cells some containing monoclinic prisms of calcium oxalate.
4. *Primary cortex,* a very narrow zone of cortical parenchyma, some of the cells containing ellipsoidal or oval starch grains, others monoclinic prisms of calcium ovalate.
5. *Phloem,* a broad zone of elongated, radially arranged phloem patches separated from one another by prominent medullary rays of the phloem. Each phloem patch consists of a matrix of soft bast in which

are found groups of thick walled bast fibers, adhering to which are cells of crystal fibers containing monoclinic prisms of calcium oxalate.

6. *Cambium*, a zone of several layers of meristematic cells.

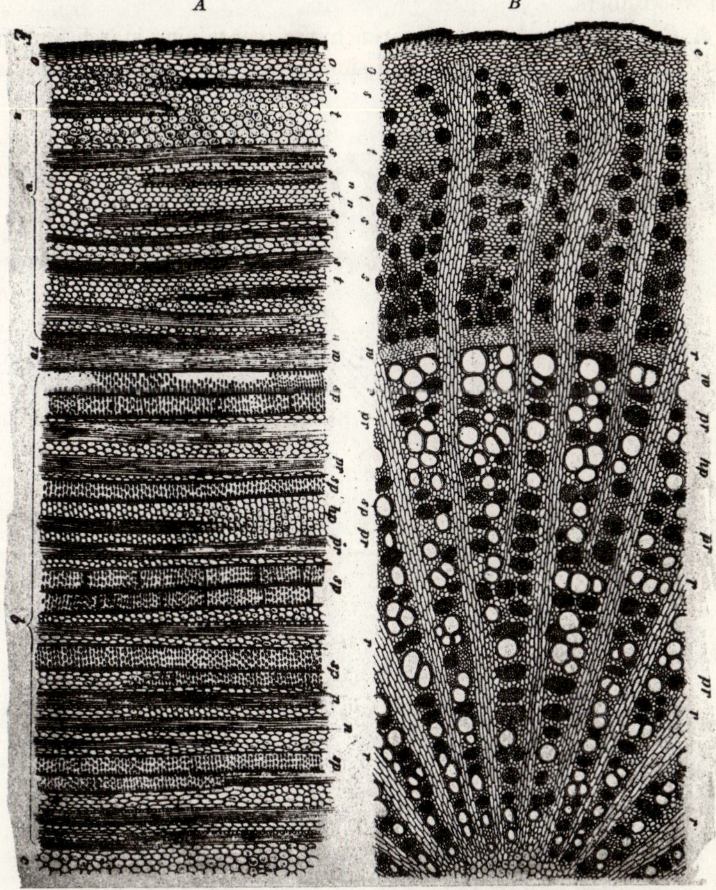

FIG. 116.—Glycyrrhiza. *B*, Representative portion of a transverse section of *G. glabra* rhizome, deprived of starch by maceration in weak alkali, × 65. *A*, Radial-longitudinal section of same, × 65. *a*, bark; *b*, wood; *c*, pith; *e*, cork; *o*, cortex; *r*, medullary rays; *s*, bast fibers; *t*, soft bast; *n*, crystal fibers; *w*, cambium; *hp*, wood parenchyma; *pr*, wood fibers; *sp*, tracheæ. (*After Berg.*)

7. *Xylem*, a broad zone of numerous, elongated, radially arranged xylem patches, separated from each other by medullary rays which are continuous, through the cambium, with those of the phloem. Each xylem patch consists of a matrix of starch and crystal containing wood parenchyma imbedded in which are broad tracheae with yellowish walls

and compact groups of thick, yellow-walled wood fibers that are partially surrounded by the cells of crystal fibers containing monoclinic prisms of calcium oxalate. Each trachea is surrounded by a ring of yellow tracheids and wood fibers.

8. *Pith*, a central zone of parenchyma, containing starch and monoclinic prisms of calcium oxalate of similar character to those found in the cortex.

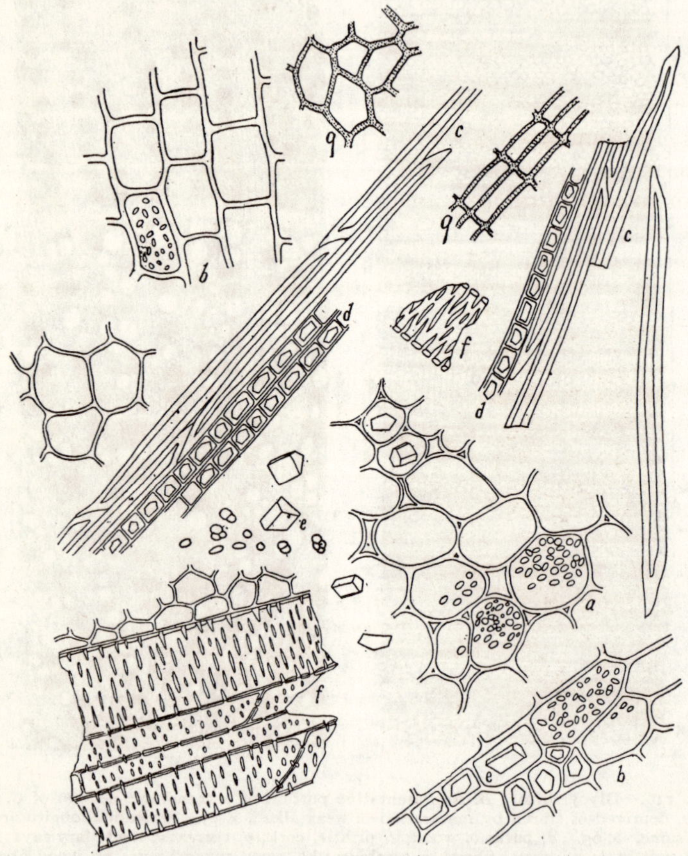

FIG. 117.—Powdered Glycyrrhiza. (*a*) Parenchyma; (*b*) parenchyma with crystals and starch; (*c*) bast; (*d*) crystal bearing fibers; (*e*) crystals; (*f*) ducts and tracheids; (*g*) cork tissue. (***Schneider.***)

Longitudinal sections, cleared by warming in chloral solution, show bands of bast fibers in the phloem and of wood fibers in the xylem, their ends tapered and spliced over each other. Adhering to the outside of a group of these fibers will be noted long rows of superimposed cells, each containing a monoclinic prism of calcium oxalate. These are the crystal fibers. The tracheae will be found to be rather short with thick yellow walls, the broader usually marked by compactly arranged oval shaped bordered pores, the narrower with ovate pits or reticulations. The medullary rays, as determined in tangential sections, are 1 to 8 cells wide.

Powdered Drug.—Brownish-yellow (Spanish or Persian Licorice) or pale yellow (Peeled Russian Licorice); starch grains numerous, mostly single, oval or elliptical, with an elongated ovate or linear or crescentic cleft, the majority varying from 3 to 12μ in length, but attaining in some instances a length of 20μ; numerous fragments of bast and wood fibers, adhering to which are crystal fibers, the cells of which contain monoclinic prisms of calcium oxalate up to 20μ in diameter; fragments of parenchyma with clear walls, and frequently with monoclinic crystals or starch; fragments of mostly porous and few reticulate tracheae often with accompanying tracheids, fragments of reddish-brown cork tissue in unpeeled drug.

Constituents.—5 to 7 per cent. of glycyrrhizin (an intensely sweet, water-soluble principle); glycyramarin (a bitter principle); mannit, yellow-coloring matter, volatile oil, resin, starch, sucrose, glucose, calcium oxalate, etc.

Uses.—Demulcent, expectorant and flavoring agent. The powdered root is extensively employed as a pill excipient and the fluidextract to disguise the taste of nauseous preparations

Most of the licorice imported is used by the tobacco manufacturers in the flavoring of tobacco. The candy industry consumes a fair quantity. Small quantities of licorice paste are employed in the manufacture of shoe polish.

Allied Drugs.—American or Wild Licorice is the root of *Glycyrrhiza lepidota* (Nutt.) Pursh, which grows wild in the western part of the United States and lower Canada. It contains up to 6 per cent. of glycyrrhizin.

Manchurian Licorice is the root of *G. uralensis* Fischer indigenous to Siberia. It resembles unpeeled Russian licorice differing chiefly from the latter by its wavy medullary-rays, softer wood with lacunæ, more readily separable cork and less sweet taste.

COPAIBA U.S.P. (COPAIBA)

Synonyms.—Balsam of Copaiba, Copaiva, Balsam of Copaiva; *Fr.* Copahu; *Ger.* Copaiva balsam.

Botanical Origin.—South American species of *Copaiba* Miller.

Part Used.—An oleoresin.

Habitat.—Tropical regions of South America, notably Brazil, Venezuela and Colombia.

Plants.—Trees considerably branched, the branches having smooth bark and bearing alternate paripinnate leaves, each with 6 to 10 entire, ovate, coriaceous, pellucid-punctate leaflets. The flowers are small and white, each consisting of a receptacle bearing 5 sepals, 10 stamens and a monocarpellary pistil. The fruit is a one-seeded legume.

Production and Commerce.—The drug is thought to represent a morbid product of the cell walls of the wood parenchyma which accumulates in cavities within the trunk of the tree. These cavities enlarge and join with each other to form huge reservoirs that hold frequently several gallons of oleoresin. The oleoresin is obtained commercially by cutting large inward and downward sloping cavities in the wood of the trunk near its base. Into these the oleoresin flows. It is transferred from the cavities to barrels or other containers. Copaiba is imported from Para, Brazil and Maracaibo, Venezuela.

Description.—A more or less viscid liquid of pale yellow to brownish-yellow color, with or without greenish fluorescence and having a characteristic aromatic odor and persistent, bitter and acrid taste. It is insoluble in water and partly soluble in 95 per cent. alcohol. It is soluble in dehydrated alcohol, carbon disulphide, chloroform and ether, in fixed and volatile oils. When heated on a water bath, no odor of turpentine is evolved.

Adulterants.—(1) Gurjun Balsam is yielded by several trees of the genus *Dipterocarpus* (Fam. *Dipterocarpaceæ*) native to India, Siam and other countries of Southern Asia. Like Copaiba it is a thick and viscid liquid with an odor resembling it but weaker, and a bitter aromatic taste; but it lacks the persistent acridity of Copaiba. Its presence as an admixture may be ascertained by the following test: Dissolve several drops (3 or 4) of the volatile oil separated by steam distillation from the suspected sample in 3 cc. of glacial acetic acid. Mix the solution with 1 drop of a freshly prepared 1–10 aqueous solution of sodium nitrite, and carefully underlay this with 2 cc. of concentrated sulphuric acid. If Gurjun Balsam be present, the acetic layer will assume a pink coloration.

(2) Paraffin Oils. These may be detected by shaking 5 cc. of the sample with 15 cc. of alcohol, heating the mixture to boiling for one minute, cooling and allowing it to stand for one hour. If oil separates, the presence of paraffine oils is indicated.

(3) Oil of Turpentine. Detected by its characteristic odor, upon heating the sample.

(4) African Copaiba is obtained from an unidentified tree growing near the western coast of Africa. It is dark yellow with a peppery odor and dextrorotatory, forming a crystalline deposit on standing.

(5) Castor Oil.

(6) Olive Oil.

Constituents.—40 to 90 per cent. of a laevo-rotatory volatile oil (highest in the Para variety) containing caryophyllene; 35 to 40 per cent. of resin acids, copaivic acid, bitter principle, etc.

Uses.—Copaiba is employed as a stimulant and disinfectant to the genito-urinary tract and as a stimulating expectorant.

BALSAMUM PERUVIANUM U.S.P. (BALSAM OF PERU)

Synonyms.—Peru Balsam, Black Balsam; *Ger.* Perubalsam; *Fr.* Baume de Sansonate.

Botanical Origin.—*Toluifera Pereiræ* (Royle) Baillon (*Myroxylon Pereiræ* Klotzsch).

Part Used.—A balsam.

Habitat.—Central America. Naturalized in Ceylon and Florida.

Plant.—A evergreen tree branching 2 to 3 m. from the ground, attaining a height of 25 m., and found growing in dense forests near the coast of San Salvador. It bears alternate, imparipinnate, hairy leaves each with 9–13 ovate and emarginate leaflets. Its flowers are white, each with a cup-shaped calyx and arranged in loose racemes. Its fruit is a 1-seeded, yellowish-brown legume, narrowed towards the stalk end.

Production and Commerce.—The balsam is a pathological product formed by mechanical injury to the trees. During November and December or after the rainy season, the native Indians beat the stems of the balsam trees with a blunt instrument on 4 sides, leaving alternate similar areas of bark unbruised so as not to kill the trees. The injured bark soon cracks and is readily pulled off in long strips. A small quantity of balsam exudes from this bark but insufficient to be worth while collecting it. About 5 days after the beating of the stems, torches are applied to the bruised bark and the latter is charred. About a week later the bark drops off or is removed and the balsam freely exudes from the stem. It is collected by covering the denuded wood with rags, which, after becoming soaked with the exudation, are thrown into water and boiled. The balsam separates and sinks to the bottom. The water is decanted and the balsam poured into tin containers. The commercial supply of this drug is imported into United States from San Julian, San Salvador.

Description.—A thick, viscid, dark-brown liquid; free from stringiness or stickiness; transparent and reddish-brown in thin layers; odor aromatic, vanilla like; taste bitter, acrid, with a persistent after taste, producing a burning sensation when swallowed. It is soluble in alcohol, glacial acetic acid and chloroform with not more than a slight opalescence. Its specific gravity is 1.130 to 1.160 at 25°C.

Adulterants.—(1) Turpentine. This may be detected by warming 1 Gm. of the suspected sample with 5 cc. of purified petroleum benzin on a water bath for about 10 minutes, and evaporaing 2 cc. of this benzin solution, which will give off vapor having the characteristic odor of turpentine, if same be present.

(2) Colophony. If the residue left after following the method indicated above be treated with several drops of nitric acid, a greenish or bluish color would indicate the presence of rosin.

(3) Fixed oils. The presence of fixed oils as added adulterants may be determined by shaking 1 Gm. of the suspected material with a solution of 3 Gms. of chloral hydrate and 2 cc. of distilled water. Cloudiness would indicate fixed oil admixture.

Constituents.—About 63 per cent. of Cinnamein (a volatile oil containing benzyl benzoate, benzyl cinnamate, etc.), resin esters, cinnamic acid peruviol, dihydro-cinnamic acid, vanillin, etc. The more cinnamein or oil of Peru balsam, the higher the value of the drug.

Uses.—Balsam of Peru is employed externally in the form of an ointment as a parasiticide in scabies, ring-worm and pediculosis, also in the form of a solution for sluggish granulations. It is used internally as a stimulating expectorant.

TOLU U.S.P. (TOLU)

Synonyms.—Balsamum Tolutanum, Tolu Balsam; *Fr.* Baume de Tolu; *Ger.* Tolubalsam.

Botanical Origin.—*Toluifera Balsamum* Linné. (*Myroxylon Toluifera* H.B.K.)

Part Used.—A balsam.

Habitat.—South America (Colombia, Venezuela, New Granada).

Plant.—A tree with spreading crown somewhat like *Toluifera Pereiræ*, differing from it mainly by its habit of branching about 14–16 m. above ground, in having leaves with 7–11 leaflets and these with acuminate summits, and in bearing dense racemes of flowers, each with a tubular calyx.

Production and Commerce.—Most of the drug is produced in the province of Tolu along the Magdalena river, in Colombia. It is obtained by making V-shaped incisions in the trunk, extending into the wood. As many as 20 to 30 of these are made in one tree. Below each V-shaped cut, the bark and wood are hollowed out and a calabash is fixed by the collector to catch the flow of balsam. From time to time the balsam collector goes round the trees and empties the exudate from the calabashes into bags of hide which are slung over the back of a donkey. In these bags the balsam is shipped to Cartagena and Savanilla where it is transferred to cylindrical tin cans, containing from 10 to 25 pounds and exported.

Description.—A yellowish-brown or brown plastic mass, becoming brittle when old, dried, or exposed to cold; transparent in thin layers;

soluble in alcohol, chloroform and ether; odor vanilla-like; taste aromatic and slightly pungent.

Adulterant.—Rosin. This may be detected by dissolving 1 Gm. of the sample in 25 cc. of carbon disulphide, filtering the liquid and evaporating 15 cc. of the filtrate to dryness. The residue, thus obtained, is dissolved in glacial acetic acid and a few drops of concentrated sulphuric acid are added. A green color results if rosin be present.

Constituents.—Volatile oil (about 7 per cent.), containing benzyl benzoate and benzyl cinnamate, resin, cinnamic acid, benzoic acid, vanillin, etc.

Uses.—Stimulating expectorant, antiseptic and flavoring agent in cough syrups.

GALEGA N.F. (GALEGA)

Synonyms.—Goat's Rue, European Goat's Rue; *Ger.* Pestilenzkraut, Geisraute; *Fr.* Rue de Chèvre.

Botanical Origin.—*Galega officinalis* Linnè.

Part Used.—The dried flowering herb.

Purity Rubric.—Not more than 3 per cent. of foreign organic matter. None of its stems should be over 4 mm. in diameter.

Habitat.—Southern Europe and W. Asia. Naturalized in the United States.

Plant.—A hardy perennial herb growing to the height of 2 to 3 feet and possessing odd-pinnate leaves and papilionaceous flowers which, while purplish-blue in the pure species, vary from white, lilac to rose colored in the several varieties.

Production and Commerce.—Galega is gathered in Italy and France when the plants are in flower, carefully dried and packed in burlap bags and bundles. The commercial supplies are imported chiefly from Leghorn and Marseilles.

Description.—The drug generally occurs as cut and broken portions of the flowering tops. Stem smooth and branched; leaves imparipinnate with six to eight pairs of leaflets; stipules lanceolate, sagittate on one side; leaflets bright green, smooth or slightly hairy, short petioled, lanceolate or ovate lanceolate, obtuse, slightly mucronate, from 2 to 5 cm. in length and from 2 to 6 mm. in breadth; flowers small, white to purplish-blue, papilionaceous, in axillary racemes; fruit a slender legume containing 4 to 6 brownish black seeds; odor indistinct; taste mucilaginous, slightly bitter and astringent, the saliva being colored a yellowish-green.

Constituents.—Tannin, bitter principle, etc.

Uses.—Galega has been employed as a galactagogue, diuretic and stimulant.

TRIFOLIUM N.F. (TRIFOLIUM)

Synonym.—Red Clover Blossoms.

Botanical Origin.—*Trifolium pratense* Linné.

Part Used.—The dried inflorescence.

Purity Rubric.—Not more than 2 per cent. of foreign organic matter.

Habitat.—Europe. Naturalized and extensively cultivated in the United States.

Plant.—A low growing, common, perennial herb with ascending slender hairy stems bearing trifoliate leaves with broad, bristle-pointed stipules, the leaflets varying from ovate to obovate in outline, frequently notched at the apex, and showing a pale spot on their upper surface. The small butterfly-shaped flowers are borne in ovoid heads that are long or short peduncled, their color varying from magenta to whitish.

Description.—Heads ovoid with rounded summit from 1.2 to 2.6 cm. in length, shrivelled, purplish-red and more or less brown from drying, consisting of numerous, small, closely set, papilionaceous flowers arranged on a receptacle. Each flower exhibits a hairy calyx with subulate teeth, a corolla whose petals are united below, the standard longer than the wings but when recurved appearing shorter, diadelphous stamens (9 and 1) and a slender, simple style; odor fragrant and characteristic; taste sweetish, then slightly bitter.

Constituents.—Volatile oil, coumaric acid, salicylic acid, sitosterol, myricyl alcohol, isorhamnetin, glucosides, sugar, etc.

Uses.—Red Clover Blossoms are employed in the form of fluidextract, compound fluidextract, compound syrup and infusion as an alterative, and as sedative in whooping cough.

MELILOTUS N.F. (MELILOT)

Synonyms.—Yellow Melilot, Yellow Sweet Clover.

Botanical Origin.—*Melilotus officinalis* (Linné) Lamarck.

Part Used.—The dried leaf and flowering top.

Purity Rubric.—Not more than 3 per cent. of its stems over 3 mm. in diameter or other foreign matter.

Habitat.—Europe. Naturalized in the United States.

Plant.—A tall, much branched herb frequently found on waste grounds and in fields. The leaves are alternate, trifoliate, with obovate-oblong, closely serrate leaflets. The flowers are small and yellow and occur on short spike-like racemes. The fruit is a cross-ribbed, smooth, one seeded, ovoid legume.

Description.—Stems pale olive green, mostly less than 3 dm. in length and up to 5 mm. in thickness, slender, terminating in small spike-like racemes, the younger portions very slightly pubescent; leaves glabrous or glabrate, petiolate, trifoliate, with subulate stipules, the leaflets obovate-oblong, rounded, truncate, or slightly notched at the apex, closely serrate along the margin; racemes 1 dm. or less on length, many flowered, the flowers having a 5-lobed, bell-shaped calyx, a yellowish papilionaceous corolla that is free from the stamen tube; legumes 2.5 to 3.5 mm. long obovate, cross ribbed and containing a single seed; odor aromatic, coumarin-like; taste sweetish, slightly pungent and bitter.

Constituents.—Coumarin, coumarin-splitting enzyme, volatile oil, melilotic acid, etc.

Use.—Yellow Melilot is used as one of the ingredients in Species Emollientes N.F.

HÆMATOXYLON N F. (HEMATOXYLON)

Synonyms.—Logwood, Campeachy Wood, Blackwood; *Fr.* Bois de Sang, Bois de Campêche; *Ger.* Blutholz, Campecheholz.

Botanical Origin.—*Hæmatoxylon campechianum* Linné.

Part Used.—The heartwood.

Purity Rubric.—Not more than 2 per cent. of foreign organic matter.

Habitat.—Central America.

Plant.—A tree averagely 7 m. in height but attaining a height of about 15 m. under favorable environment. Its trunk is crooked and covered with rough bark. This bears crooked branches showing numerous white lenticels and numerous sharp spines. The leaves are alternate, paripinnate, with 3 or 4 pairs of sessile, obcordate leaflets. The sweet smelling flowers are arranged on axillary racemes near the ends of the branches and are characterized by the brownish-purple calyx and yellow corolla. The fruit is a slender, membranous, lanceolate, compressed pod, 1- or 2-seeded, dehiscent down the center of each valve.

Production and Commerce.—While native to Central America, the logwood tree has been naturalized in the West Indies. The trees are felled when about 10 years old. The bark and sapwood are removed and the heartwood remaining is cut into logs or billets about 13 feet long and sent into commerce. These vary from a purplish-red to blackish-brown color externally, are hard and heavy and have a reddish-brown internal color. For pharmaceutical purposes it is subsequently cut into chips which have a reddish-brown aspect. On long exposure to the air, logwood chips develop a metallic lustre, due to a violet colored substance with a greenish metallic luster, haematin ($C_{10}H_{12}O_6$), being formed by oxidation, through the action of a ferment on haematoxylin. Such chips are of little or no value pharmaceutically and should be rejected. The market supply comes from Campeachy, Honduras, St. Domingo and Jamaica. Campeachy Logwood is considered the best. About 400,000,000 pounds of logwood are annually consumed. The chief use of the article is as a dye-wood.

Description.—The drug usually occurs as small chips of variable size of a reddish-brown color externally, or occasionally as a coarse reddish powder. The fracture of the thinner chips is tough-fibrous, the freshly fractured or cut surface exhibiting a dark yellowish-red aspect; odor indistinct; taste sweetish and astringent.

Haematoxylon imparts a yellowish color to slightly acidified water, the color being changed to purple or violet-red by alkaline solutions.

Histology.—Transverse sections show many irregular concentric zones of wood fibers and crystal fibers alternating with wood parenchyma, the latter surrounding tracheæ, arranged either singly or in groups of 2 or 3. Parallel medullary rays traverse the transverse section. In tangential sections the medullary-rays range in width from 1 to 7 rows of cells.

Powdered Drug.—Reddish-brown. Numerous elongated, deep brown wood fibers with thickened walls, adhering to which are frequently found crystal fibers containing monoclinic prisms of calcium oxalate, the latter up to 30μ in length; tracheæ with simple pits or bordered pores; medullary ray cells; fragments of tissue containing resin cells with reddish-brown resin masses; cells containing tannin.

Constituents.—Haematoxylin ($C_{16}H_{14}O_6+3H_2O$), volatile oil, tannin, resin, quercetin and calcium oxalate.

Uses.—Unfermented logwood is employed as an astringent. The partly fermented article is widely used in the arts in the preparation of a dye and an ink.

BAPTISIA N.F. (BAPTISIA)

Synonyms.—Wild Indigo, False Indigo, *Ger.* Baptisie; *Fr.* Indigo sauvage.

Botanical Origin.—*Baptisia tinctoria* (Linné) R. Brown.

Part Used.—The dried root.

Limit of Impurities.—10 per cent. of its stem bases, overground parts or 2 per cent. of other foreign organic matter.

Habitat.—Eastern United States.

Plant.—A smooth, slender, somewhat glaucous, branched herb, 3 to 9 dm. in height, growing in dry woods and fields and emitting a disagreeable odor when bruised. The leaves are trifoliate and sessile with cuneate-obovate leaflets. The inflorescence is a short, loose raceme of yellow flowers. The fruit is a sub-cylindric, bladdery, many seeded legume.

Description.—Fleshy, up to 4 cm. in thickness, usually cut into elongated cylindrical segments; the crown from 5 to 8 cm. in thickness, more or less warty and marked by stem scars; outer surface dark brown; usually longitudinally wrinkled, transversely warty, or the thicker pieces covered with a soft corky layer, bearing few branching rootlets; fracture tough, the fractured surface whitish; bark section radially striate, wood section inconspicuously radiate, porous; odor indistinct; the bark bitter and acrid, the wood nearly tasteless.

Powdered Drug.—Light grayish to Grayish-brown. Starch grains numerous, simple or 2- to 4-compound, the individual grains spheroidal or plano convex up to 16μ in diameter, the larger grains occasionally showing a central cleft; fragments of parenchyma the cells of which are filled with

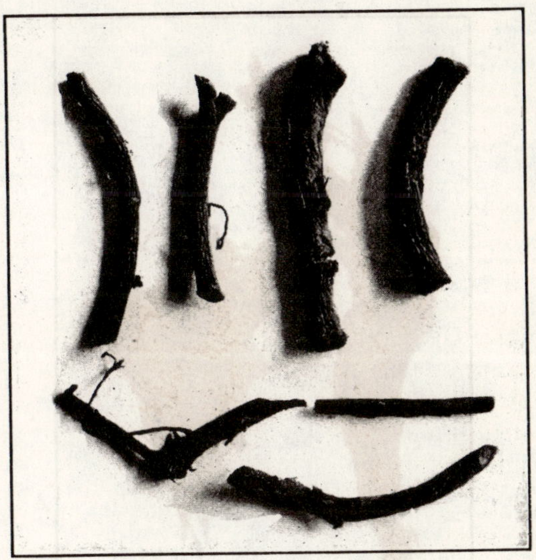

FIG. 118.—Wild indigo root (Baptisia). × ⅜.

tarch; relatively few fragments of slightly lignified cork tissue with cells having yellowish-brown walls; tracheæ with slit-like or bordered pores associated with fragments of sclerenchyma fibers that are long, thick-walled; fragments of medullary rays with cells having thick, lignified and porous walls and containing starch.

Constituents.—Cytisine (an alkaloid), baptin, baptisin (glucosides), etc.

Uses.—Antiseptic and stimulant.

KRAMERIA U.S.P. (KRAMERIA)

Synonyms.—Rhatany; *Ger.* Ratanhiawurzel, *Fr.* Ratanhia.

Botanical Origin.—(1) *Krameria triandra* Ruiz et Pavon and (2) *Krameria argentea* Martius.

Part Used.—The dried root.

Habitat.—(1) Peru and Bolivia; (2) Brazil.

Plants.—Shrubs of low stature with spreading branches and grayish-brown bark. The leaves are simple, entire, obovate and silvery-gray hairy. The inflorescences are racemes of red flowers, each possessing a cruciform calyx of 4 scarlet-red sepals, 4 red petals, 4 monadelphous stamens and a monocarpellary pistil with a one-celled ovary. The fruit is an indehiscent 1 to 2 seeded pod.

Production and Commerce.—*Krameria triandra* grows on the sand slopes of the Cordilleras range in Bolivia and Peru. Its root is known in commerce as Peruvian Krameria or Knotty Krameria and is shipped to this country mainly from Peru.

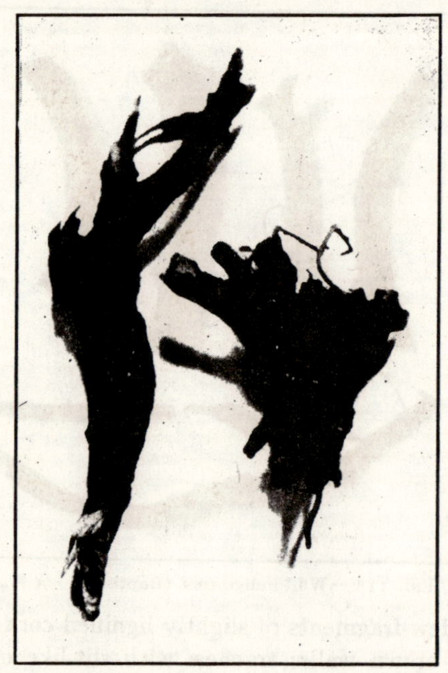

FIG. 119.—Peruvian or "knotty" krameria. × ½.

Krameria Ixina grows in United States of Colombia, the provinces of Pernambuco and Goyaz of Brazil and in British Guiana. Its root is commercially known as Savanilla Krameria and has been imported from United States of Colombia.

Krameria argentea grows in northeastern Brazil. Its root is known in commerce as Para or Brazilian Krameria and is exported from Para and Rio de Janeiro, Brazil.

Description.—Peruvian Rhatany (Knotty Krameria) consists of a knotty, several headed crown with numerous branching roots of variable length and usually less than 1 cm. in thickness, cylindrical, somewhat tapering, externally light reddish-brown or brownish-red, the crown with rough, scaly cork, the roots smooth or slightly longitudinally wrinkled and devoid of transverse fissures; fracture of bark slightly fibrous, of wood tough and splintery; internally bark pinkish-brown and less

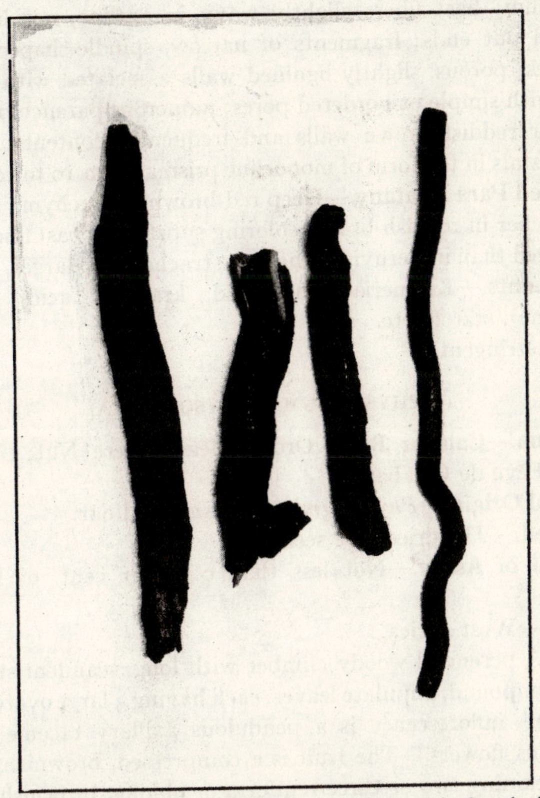

FIG. 120.—Savanilla Krameria, × ½. (*Photograph by Stoneback.*)

than ⅓ the radius of the root, readily separable in young roots from the yellowish, pinkish-white and finely radiate wood; odor indistinct; wood nearly tasteless, bark astringent.

Para Rhatany usually consist of separate roots less flexuous and tapering than those of Peruvian Rhatany and usually not exceeding 15 mm. in thickness; externally dark purplish-brown or chocolate-brown and marked with many transverse fissures; fracture of bark slightly fibrous, of wood less tough than Peruvian Rhatany; internally bark about two-fifth or more of the radius. both bark and wood darker than Peruvian Rhatany, the bark reddish-brown and the wood reddish; odor indistinct; taste of bark strongly astringent, coloring saliva red. The wood is nearly tasteless.

Powdered Peruvian Rhatany.—Reddish-brown. Starch grains simple or 2- to 4-compound, the individual grains spheroidal, ellipsoidal or plano-convex, up to 35μ in diameter and sometimes with a central radial or stellate hilum; bast fibers slightly wavy in outline, non-lignified, with long drawn out ends; fragments of narrow, spindle-shaped wood fibers having thick, porous, slightly lignified walls associated with tracheæ and tracheids with simple or bordered pores; numerous parenchyma cells with yellowish or reddish-brown walls and frequently contents; few calcium oxalate crystals in the form of monoclinc prisms, from 10 to 100μ in length.

Powdered Para Rhatany.—Deep red-brown parenchyma and suberous elements richer in reddish-brown coloring substance; bast fibers larger and thicker walled than in Peruvian Rhatany; tracheæ also larger.

Constituents.—Krameria-tannic acid, krameric acid, krameria-red (phlobaphene), starch, etc.

Use.—Astringent.

PHYSOSTIGMA (PHYSOSTIGMA)

Synonyms.—Calabar Bean, Ordeal Bean, Esere Nut; *Ger.* Kalabarbohne; *Fr.* Fève de Calabar.

Botanical Origin.—*Physostigma venenosum* Balfour.

Part Used.—The dried ripe seed.

Standard of Assay.—Not less than 0.15 per cent. of Physostigma alkaloids.

Habitat.—West Africa.

Plant.—A perennial woody climber with long, scandent stems bearing pinnately-compound, stipulate leaves, each having 3 large ovate, acuminate leaflets. The inflorescence is a pendulous axillary raceme of purplish papilionaceous flowers. The fruit is a compressed, brownish, reticulated legume, containing two or three reniform or oblong, brownish seeds.

Production and Commerce.—The plant grows wild in the vicinity of the Gulf of Guinea in western Africa. The seeds are collected when the fruits are mature. The commercial supplies are imported through London.

Description.—The drug occurs as entire, oblong, ellipsoidal, more or less reniform, anatropous seeds, from 16 to 30 mm. long and from 10–15 mm. in thickness; externally reddish or chocolate brown, smooth except near the groove where it is somewhat wrinkled; groove about 2 mm. broad and extending nearly the whole length of the convex edge and in

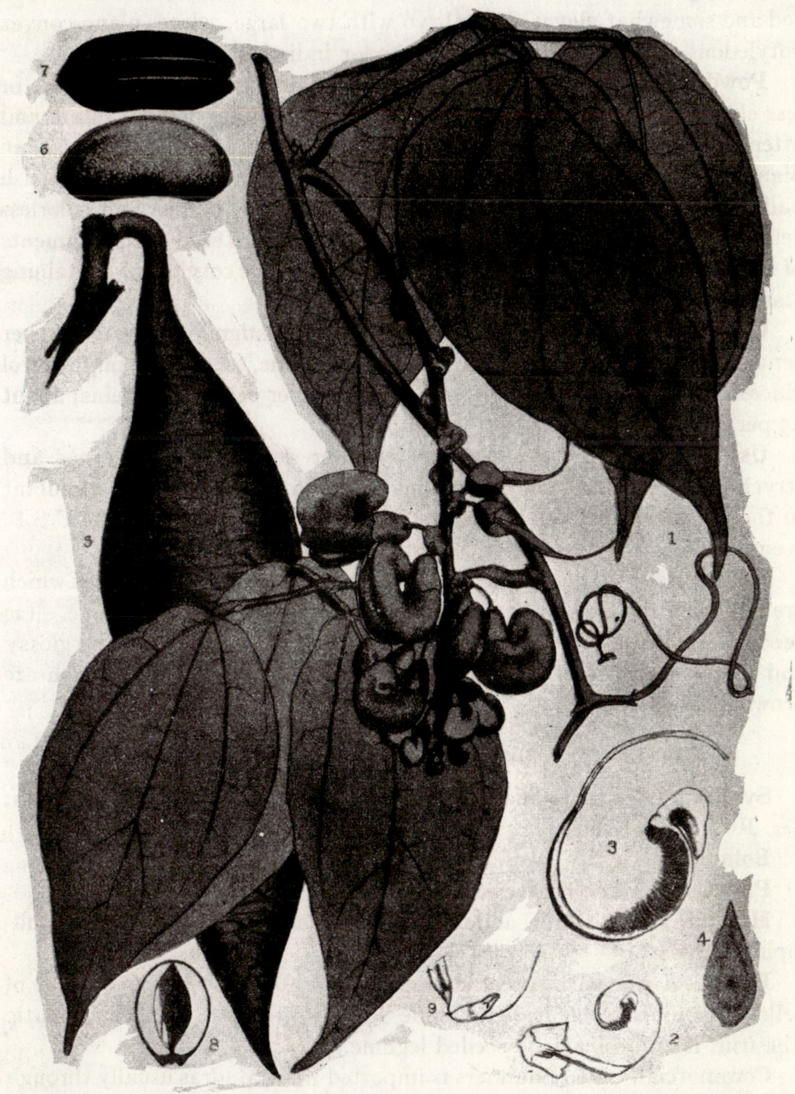

FIG. 121.—*Physostigma venenosum.* 1 Flowering branch. 2. Pistil. 3. Terminal part of style and appendage. 4. Transverse section through appendage. 5. Legume. 6, 7. Seeds. 8. Cross section of dry seed. 9. Portion of embryo showing base of one cotyledon, the plumule and the hypocotyl. (*After Bentley and Trimen.*)

which are sometimes found the remains of a white funiculus; margins of the hard spermoderm on both sides of the groove yellowish-red or brownish-red and somewhat elevated; embryo with two large, white, plano-convex cotyledons and a small hypocotyl; odor indistinct; taste starchy.

Powdered Drug.—Grayish-white in color, showing numerous more or less ellipsoidal to reniform starch grains usually with a distinct hilum and often with radiating or irregular fissures, the grains from 5 to 150μ in diameter or length; fragments of thick walled, non-lignified, brownish palisade cells with brownish contents and irregular, porous and colorless cells containing a red colored substance from the hard seed coat; fragments of large, polygonal, thin, colorless walled cells of the cotyledons containing starch and fixed oil; reticulate tracheæ.

Constituents.—The alkaloids (eserine) physostigmine (0.1 to .25 per cent.), eseridine, calabarine (liquid), physovenine, eseramine; phytosterol glucosides; stigmasterol, sistosterol; about 20 per cent. of proteins; about 45 per cent. of starch; etc.

Uses.—Physostigma is used as a motor depressant in tetanus and strychnine poisoning and, in combination with cathartics, as a stimulant to the unstriped muscle of the intestine. Physostigmine salicylate U.S.P. is employed as a myotic and as an antidote for atropine.

Substitutes.—(1) Seeds of *Physostigma cylindrospermum* Holmes which are subcylindrical, about 4 cm. long and possess a shorter groove. (2) Seeds of *Entada scandens* Benth. that are lenticular, flat, brown and glossy and about 5 cm. in width. (3) Seeds of *Mucuna urens* DC. which are brownish and rounded.

SANTALUM RUBRUM U.S.P. (RED SAUNDERS)

Synonyms.—Red Sandal Wood, Red Santal, Ruby Wood, Chandam; *Ger.* Rothes Santelholz; *Fr.* Santal Rouge.

Botanical Origin.—*Pterocarpus santalinus* Linné filius.

Part Used.—The heartwood.

Habitat.—Indo-China and Southern India. Cultivated in the Philippine Islands.

Plant.—A tree with spreading branches, trifoliate leaves and spikes of yellow papilionaceous flowers. The leaflets are oval and emarginate. The fruit is an orbicular, 2-seeded legume.

Commercial.—Red Saunders is imported from Madras usually through Hamburg.

Description.—In the form of a coarse powder or very small chips, of a brownish-red or purplish-red color; odor indistinct, taste slightly astringent. It imparts a red color to alcohol and chloral hydrate solution but no color to water.

Powdered Drug.—Purplish- to brownish-red. Numerous wood fibers with sharply pointed and occasionally forked ends, with thick, porous, yellowish, lignified walls and the lumina containing fine granules; few tracheæ containing pale lemon yellow, resinous masses; few crystal fibers with monoclinic prisms of calcium oxalate up to 20μ long; occasional medullary rays 1 cell wide and 3 to 6 cells deep.

Constituents.—Santalin (coloring principle) tannin, etc.

Use.—Coloring agent in Tinct. Lavender Co.

ACACIA U.S.P. (ACACIA)

Synonyms.—Gum Arabic, Gum Senegal, Gum Acacia, Galam Gum, Egyptian Thorn; *Fr.* Gummic arabique vraie; *Ger.* Arabisches Gummi.

Botanical Origin.—*Acacia Senegal* Willdenow (*A. Verek* Guill. et Perr.) or some other species of *Acacia.*

Part Used.—The dried gummy exudation from the stems and branches.

Limit of Impurities.—One per cent. of water-insoluble residue and 15 per cent. of moisture.

Habitat.—Africa.

Plant.—*Acacia Senegal* is a tree, with grayish bark, growing to the height of about 6 m. and forming open forests in the Anglo-Egyptian Sudan, Sennaar and Gedaref. It is called "Verek" by the natives of Senegambia and "Hashab" by those of Kordofan. Its leaves are bipinnate. Its inflorescence is a spike of yellow regular flowers. Its fruit is a broad legume containing 5 or 6 seeds.

Production and Commerce.—Most of the official gum, representing the variety known as "Kordofan Gum," is yielded by cultivated trees of *Acacia Senegal* which form forests known as "geneinas" that are owned by Arab sheiks. Only a very small amount is collected from wild untapped trees. These trees are usually tapped from February to May when the fruits called "Arad" are ripe. Tapping is accomplished by making a transverse incision with a small axe and tearing off a thin strip of bark from 2 to 3 ft. long and 1 to 3 in. broad, care being exercised to leave a thin layer of inner bark covering the wood. The gum slowly exudes as a viscous liquid, collects in a tear at the base of the wound and gradually hardens. In from 3 weeks to 2 months, depending upon the time of the year, the tears are ready to be collected. The natives pick the tears and place them in leather bags which, when full, are emptied on a heap. The gum is subsequently bleached by the sun's rays and garbled by native girls, who remove pieces of bark and sieve out the sand. In the cleaned state the Kordofan Gum is packed into sacks, carried on the backs of camels to Khartoum, El Obeid and Omduram and consigned to Port Sudan and Cairo from whence it enters the world's commerce, or, it may be reshipped

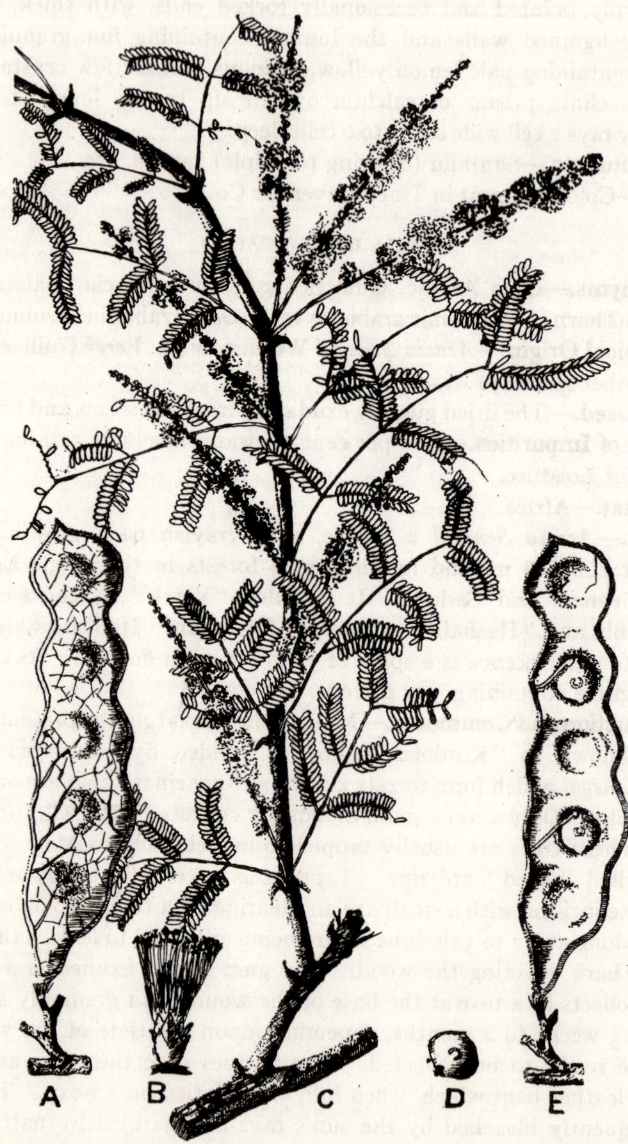

FIG. 122.—*Acacia Senegal.* Fruit viewed externally (*A*); flower (*B*); branch of plant (*C*) showing short, sharp, curved thorns, bipinnate leaves and inflorescences; seed (*D*); internal aspect of leguminous fruit (*E*).

to Smyrna, Trieste or other Mediterranean ports for further consignment. Senegal Gum is exported from the Senegal river to Bordeaux and Marseilles. This variety usually occurs in larger tears which are less fissured and more colored than the Kordofan gum. It generally contains some vermiform tears.

The two chief commercial varieties of Gum Arabic are (1) Kordofan Gum and (2) Senegal or West African Gum. The former is considered the best variety.

The commercial supplies of Kordofan Gum are chiefly imported into the U. S. A. from Cairo and indirectly through London. Senegal Gum is imported from Bordeaux and Marseilles.

Description.—Acacia occurs in ovoid, somewhat spheroidal tears, or in broken, angular fragments from 2 to 30 mm. in diameter, varying in color from white to yellowish-white to light amber-colored; translucent; very brittle; fractured surface glass-like, sometimes iridescent; nearly inodorous; taste mucilaginous.

It is insoluble in alcohol but slowly soluble in twice its weight of cold water, forming a mucilaginous liquid, which is acid to litmus. Acacia is precipitated from solutions containing it by alcohol, basic lead acetate test solution, saturated solution of sodium borate and ferric chloride test solution.

Powdered Drug.—Whitish. It contains few or no vegetable tissues or starch grains.

Constituents.—Arabic acid in combination with calcium, magnesium and potassium, an oxydase enzyme, water, and ash.

Uses.—Acacia is employed medicinally as a demulcent; pharmaceutically it is used as an emulsifying agent and also to impart viscosity to mixtures containing insoluble and heavy powders. The bulk of the acacia imported is used in the textile, confectionery, mucilage, paste and polish industries.

Adulterants.—(1) Mesquite Gum is obtained from *Prosopis juliflora*, a leguminous plant indigenous to Mexico. It occurs in brownish tears of variable size. It differs from Acacia in being usually darker in color and in not precipitating from its solution when solutions of ferric chloride, sodium borate or lead sub-acetate are added. (2) Artificial Gums made from starch or dextrin. (3) The powdered drug has been admixed with starch and white dextrin.

Allied Drug.—Gummi Indicum, also called "Ghatti Gum" or "Indian Gum" is an exudation from the stems of *Anogeissus latifolia* Wall (Fam. *Combretaceæ*), a tree indigenous to India and Ceylon. It occurs in vermiform or rounded, transparent, brittle tears of pale yellow-color. It may be distinguished from Acacia by its dull surface, uniform glassy fracture

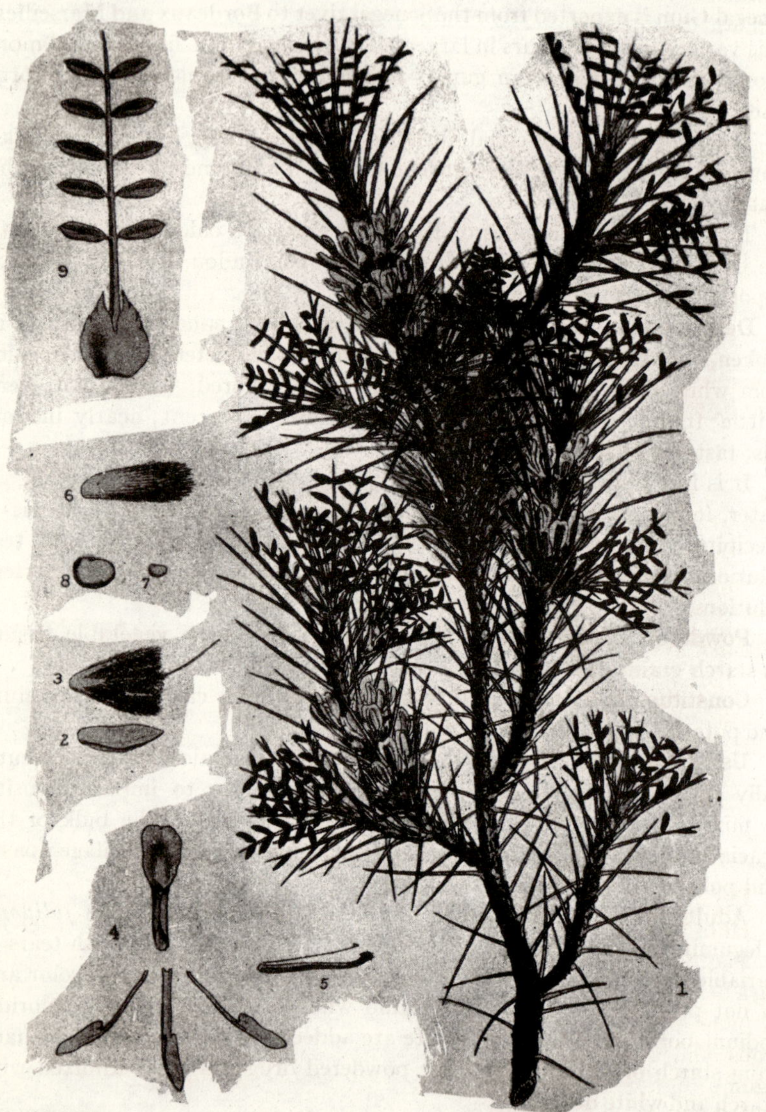

FIG. 123.—*Astragalus gummifer*. 1. Branch with flowers. 2. Bract. 3. Calyx. 4. Petals. 5. Stamens. 6. Legume. 7, 8. Seed. 9. A leaf. (*After Bentley and Trimen.*)

devoid of cracks, and the presence of many vermiform tears. It contains arabic acid and its salts.

TRAGACANTHA U.S.P. (TRAGACANTH)

Synonyms.—Gum Tragacanth, Hog Gum, Goat's Thorn; *Ger.* Traganth; *Fr.* Gomme Adragant.

Botanical Origin.—*Astragalus gummifer* Labillardiere or other Asiatic species of Astragalus.

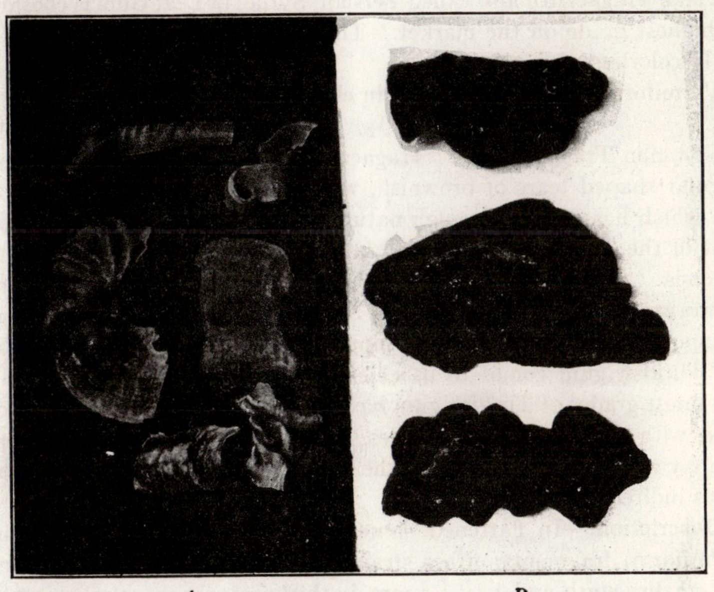

A B

FIG. 124.—*A*, Tragacanth; *B*, Indian Gum, × 45/67. (*Photograph by Stoneback.*)

Part Used.—The dried gummy exudation.

Habitat.—Western Asia and Southeastern Europe.

Plants.—Thorny, much branched shrubs with reddish-gray bark attaining a height of about 1 m. Their leaves are pinnately compound with 10 to 15 pairs of obovate, grayish-green leaflets. Their flowers are papilionaceous, yellow, with 10 diadelphous stamens. Their fruit is a small hairy legume containing a single, brown, kidney-shaped seed.

Production and Commerce.—A number of species of *Astragalus* grow wild in the mountainous districts of Kurdistan, Persia, Syria, Asia Minor, Armenia and Greece. The gum is the result of the transformation of some of the walls of the pith and medullary-ray cells to mucilage. It exudes spontaneously to the surface of the bark, but is obtained on a large scale by punctures or transverse incisions made in the main stem and older branches. The gum is allowed to dry on the bark before it is collected. The nature of the incision governs the shape of the product. The length of time consumed in drying influences the color of the product. The whiter and more translucent, the shorter the time involved in drying. It is carried to Bagdad, Smyrna, Constantinople and Persian Gulf ports where it is garbled and assorted into three varieties, viz: Flake, Vermiform and Common Tragacanths.

Flake Tragacanth also called Persian, Syrian or Leaf Gum is considered the highest grade on the market. This occurs in ribbon-like, lamellated nearly colorless pieces.

Vermiform Tragacanth occurs in elongated, narrow, twisted strings or coils.

Common Tragacanth or "Tragacanth in sorts" occurs in rounded or irregular shaped tears of brownish, waxy aspect. This grade represents gum which has exuded through naturally produced ruptures in the bark. Most of the Tragacanth imported into this country recently is produced in Persia. Great quantities are gathered in Shiraz, Persia. It is carried by caravan from Teheran, Ispahan, Sultanabad and Hamadan to Bagdad for export. The finer grades are shipped in cases, the poorer in burlap bags. The Turkish gum comes to us chiefly from Constantinople. Even the very finest grades of Turkish gum have a distinctly yellow cast when combined with the fine Persian grades. Small lots occasionally come from Bombay and Aleppo. Much of the fine Persian gum reaches the United States indirectly through London.

Description.—In flattened, lamellated, ribbon-like (Syrian) or linear (Vermiform) fragments, either straight or spirally twisted, and from 0.5 to 3 cm. in length and 1 to 2.5 mm. in thickness; nearly colorless, whitish, or light-brown, translucent, and horny; fracture short; odor indistinct; taste mucilaginous. If 1 Gm. of the gum be added to 50 cc. of water, it swells and forms a smooth, nearly uniform, stiff, opalescent mucilage devoid of cellular fragments, that does not change in consistency on standing 2 or 3 days. This mucilage slowly darkens when even a small percentage of sodium borate is dissolved in it.

Microscopical Characteristics.—Sections of Tragacanth, previously softened in water, and mounted in glycerin, exhibit lamellæ of mucilaginous walls and a few mostly spherical simple or 2- to 4-compound starch grains, the individual grains being from 3 to 25μ in diameter.

Powdered Drug.—Whitish; starch grains for the most part simple, spheroidal or ellipsoidal, a few being 2- to 4-compound, the separate grains from 3 to 25μ in diameter. Few or no fragments of lignified vegetable tissue should be present.

Constituents.—About 60 to 70 per cent. of bassorin, a substance which swells but does not dissolve in water; about 10 per cent. of polyarabian-trigalactan-geddic acid, soluble in water; starch, etc.

Uses.—Tragacanth is used pharmaceutically as an adhesive agent in pill masses and troches and as an agent for the supsension of insoluble powders in mixtures. It has been used medicinally as a demulcent.

Substitutes.—(1) **Indian Gum,** occasionally termed Karaya or Kadaya Gum, is yielded by *Cochlospermum gossypium*, a member of the *Bixaceæ* family, growing in India and adjacent countries. This article is largely used by the paste, cigar and ice cream industries. Upwards of 2,000,000 pounds are imported annually into the United States, the bulk being shipped from Bombay in bags. The U. S. Dept. of Agriculture requires that it contain not more than 0.7 per cent. of crude fiber. It is found in rounded or vermiform tears with a rough surface and glassy fracture. When softened in water and mounted in glycerin and examined under the microscope, it shows threads of a granular substance, a few rosette aggregates of calcium oxalate up to 30μ in diameter, starch grains of spheroidal outline up to 7μ in diameter, occasionally chains of bacteria, fungal hyphæ, and sometimes yellowish-brown to reddish-brown fragments, containing lignified sclerenchyma fibers.

When 1 Gm. of Indian Gum is added to 50 cc. of water, an uneven mucilage is formed which contains a few reddish-brown to yellowish-brown fragments. On stirring it separates in the form of coarse, uneven strings, (*distinction from Tragacanth*). When 1 Gm. of Indian Gum is boiled with 20 cc. of water until a mucilage results and 5 cc. of hydrochloric acid is added, and the mixture again boiled for five minutes, a pinkish or reddish color develops (*distinction from Tragacanth*).

(2) **Gum Kuteera** obtained from *Sterculia urens* (Fam. *Sterculiaceæ*) somewhat resembles Tragacanth. This gum comes from a tree growing in Persia and is frequently mixed with Tragacanth. It is naturally in the form of yellowish-brown tears or irregular masses, swelling with water, but has not infrequently been whitened with carbonate of lead in order to disguise its presence.

SENNA U.S.P. (SENNA)

Synonyms.—(1) Alexandria or Nubia Senna; *Ger.* Alexandrinische Senna; *Fr.* Séné d' Alexandrie. (2) Indian or Tinnevelly Senna; *Ger.* Indische Senna, Sennesblätter; *Fr.* Séné de Tinnevelly.

Botanical Origin.—(1) *Cassia Senna* Linné. (*Cassia acutifolia* Delile) and (2) *Cassia angustifolia* Vahl.

Part Used.—The dried leaflets.

Limit of Impurities.—Not more than 10 per cent. of its stems and not more than 2 per cent. of its pods or other foreign organic matter.

Ash.—Not more than 3 per cent. acid-insoluble.

Habitat.—(1) The middle and upper Nile districts of Africa. (2) Arabia and Africa.

Plants.—*Cassia Senna* is a low growing shrub with branched whitish stems, paripinnate, stipulate leaves with pale green leaflets, and large yellow flowers borne in axillary racemes. Its fruit is a broadly elliptical, somewhat reniform, flattened, membranous legume containing 6 or 7 seeds. *Cassia angustifolia* resembles the former species in habit, but is leaflets are yellowish-green, frequently broader, and usually more abruptly pointed; its pods are more narrowly elliptical or reniform and 8 seeded.

Production and Commerce.—Alexandria Senna is the product of wild plants of *Cassia acutifolia*, growing in El Hejaz (a country bordering the Red Sea opposite Egypt and below Syria) and in the Anglo-Egyptian Sudan, and to a lesser extent of plants which have recently been cultivated in India. The Sudan Senna is claimed to be worthless and only employed to adulterate the good supply from El Hejaz. The leaves are now usually gathered by the natives of El Hejaz and the Sudan during the winter months. They either take hold of the bushes with both hands and pull them off, allowing them to drop to the ground or cut down the bushes allow them to dry in the sun and later strip off the leaves. The latter practice is followed by the Bedouins in the country between Suakin and Kassala. After being completely dried, they are placed in hampers made of palm leaves. Each hamper holds 2¼ Kentars or 225 pounds. Three of those are placed on each camel's back and carried to Port Sudan whence it is conveyed either to Port Said, Cairo, or Alexandria. Here it is cleaned and graded into whole leaf, half leaf and siftings. Cairo is the leading market for Alexandria Senna. Thence about 75 per cent. of that reaching this country is shipped direct, the other 25 per cent. comes indirectly through London. Alexandria Senna is received in large bales packed loosely.

Indian Senna is the product of cultivated plants of *Cassia angustifolia* grown in southern India (Tinnevelly Senna) or of plants growing in Northern India and the Anglo-Egyptian Sudan. The leaves are collected, dried in the sun and packed in bags for shipment. The Tinnevelly Senna is the best grade of Indian Senna. It is carefully collected from cultivated plants and consists of leaflets of excellent green color, free from admixture with stems or pods or other extraneous matter. This is exported from Tuticorin, Madras and Calcutta. Inferior grades of Indian Senna have been offered on the market. These are collected dried and garbled with less care and contain discolored leaflets, legumes, etc. About 75 per cent.

of the commercial supply imported by this country comes direct from India. The remaining 25 per cent. comes through London. Tinnevelly Senna is shipped to United States direct from Tuticorin, Madras and Calcutta, India and indirectly through London. The product arrives in bales packed under pressure and burlap covered.

Arabian Senna, is collected from wild plants of C. *angustifolia* which thrive in Southern Arabia. This drug is shipped in the crude state from Hodeida to Port Sudan and thence carried by rail to Cario where it is garbled and graded. At Cairo it is sometimes mixed with Alexandria Senna and exported under the latter name. Some of this mixture has occurred frequently on the American market under the name of "Alexandria Senna."

Senna Pods, representing the dried ripe fruits of the C. *Senna* and C. *angustifolia* are also imported as a separate article as are also Senna Siftings. The latter frequently contain an excess of sand.

Description.—**Alexandria Senna** occurs as a mixture of entire and broken leaflets, pods and frequently stalks of the compound leaves. Leaflets short petiolate, with petiole up to 1 mm. in length; lamina inequilaterally lanceolate or lance-ovate, from 2 to 2.5 cm. rarely up to 4 cm. in length and from 6 to 10 mm. in breadth, its apex acute or mucronate, margin entire, base unequal, upper surface pale green nearly smooth; under surface grayish-green, with appressed hairs and showing prominent midrib; odor characteristic taste mucilaginous and bitter. Pods few, broadly elliptical, somewhat reniform, thin and membraneous and containing 6 to 7 seeds.

Indian Senna occurs as entire leaflets or as a mixture of entire and broken leaflets occasionally admixed with portions of compound leaves and pods. Leaflets short petiolate, with petiole up to 2 mm. long; lamina inequilaterally lance ovate, from 2 to 5 cm. in length and from 6 to 15 mm. in breadth, its apex broadly acute, margin entire, base unequal, upper surface yellowish green and glabrous, lower surface pale yellowish-green, slightly hairy, midrib and veins elevated; odor and taste resembling Alexandria Senna. Pods few, more narrowly elliptical and reinform than those of Alexandria Senna and usually containing 8 seeds.

Histology.—Transverse sections made through the **lamina** of an Indian Senna leaflet **outside of the midrib** show the following structural peculiarities. (Note: Leaflets should be kept in a moist chamber until supple before sectioning. Sections should be mounted in chloral hydrate for examination.)

1. Upper epidermis with prominent cuticle and possessing stomata that are sunken below its surface level.

2. Palisade Parenchyma of a single layer of elongated, narrow, columnar cells containing chloroplastids.

3. Spongy Parenchyma consisting of rather loosely arranged rounded cells, some of which contain rosette aggregates or 4–6 sided prisms of calcium oxalate, others, chloroplastids. Through this region course the bundles of the smaller veins.

4. Palisade Parenchyma of a single layer of columnar cells which differ from the upper palisade layer in being shorter and wavy walled.

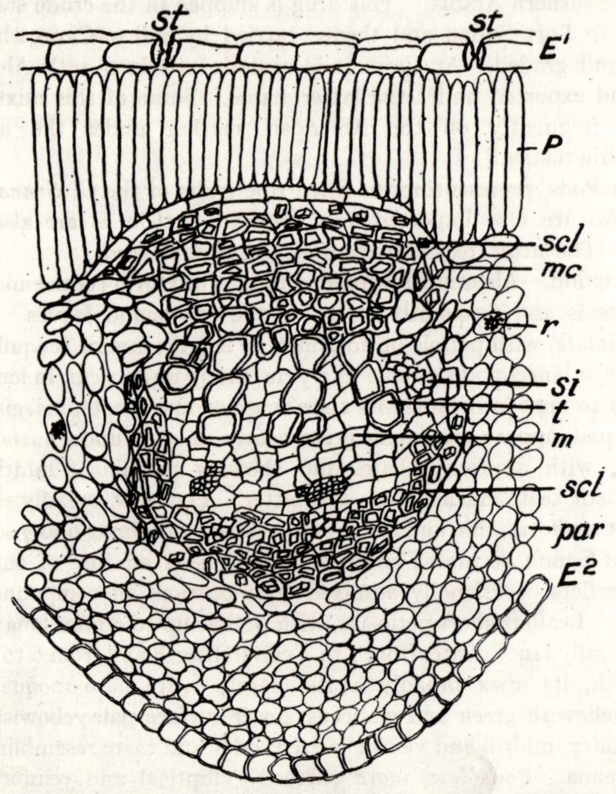

FIG. 125.—Indian Senna. Transverse section through midrib of leaflet, showing upper epidermis (E^1); lower epidermis (E^2); sunken stomata (*st*); palisade parenchyma (*P*); parenchyma (*par*); sclerenchyma fibers in pericycle (*scl*); tracheæ (*t*); sieve tissue (*si*); monoclinic prisms (*mc*) and rosette aggregates (*r*) of calcium oxalate.

5. Lower epidermis with prominent cuticle and possessing sunken stomata. Both epidermises show a few outgrowths in the form of one-celled, papillose, straight to slightly curved, non-glandular hairs. Each of these, when observed, has its base wedged between adjacent epidermal cells.

Transverse sections cut through the **midrib of the lamina** show a fan shaped group of collateral bundles in the center, xylem being uppermost, phloem beneath. Both above and below the group of bundles occurs an arc of thick walled pericyclic fibers, somewhat ovate in shape above and crescent shaped below. On the outer surface of each arc of fibers is a layer of cells, most of which contain prisms of calcium oxalate. These are found to be the cells of crystal fibers when longitudinal sections are examined. Separating the upper layer of crystal fibers from the upper epidermis is a layer of small cells and finally a layer of palisade cells.

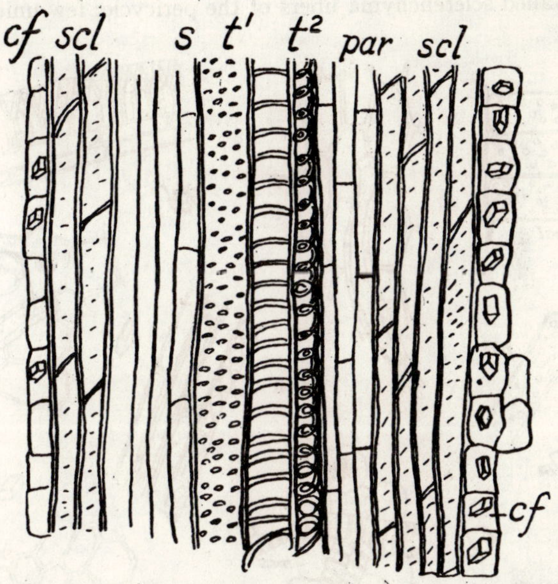

FIG. 126.—Indian Senna. Longitudinal-radial section through center of midrib. Crystal fibers (*cf*); pericyclic fibers (*scl*); parenchyma (*par*); pitted trachea (t^1); spiral trachea (t^2); sieve (*s*).

Between the lower arc of crystal fibers and the lower epidermis occur several layers of parenchyma shading off into collenchyma.

Longitudinal sections cut through the centre of the midrib show the lengthwise aspect of the elements. The tracheæ are spiral, annular and pitted. The pericyclic fibers are elongated, narrow, thick-walled with tapered ends spliced over each other and showing oblique slit-like pores. A crystal fiber is just outside of each group of these. The upper epidermis is readily distinguished from the lower by locating the layer of palisade cells directly beneath it.

Surface sections of both upper and lower epidermis exhibit polygonal epidermal cells amongst which will be noted broadly elliptical stomata, each of which has 2 unequal neighboring cells parallel to its longer axis; occasionally a third neighboring cell at the end of the stoma is present.

Unicellular, papillose, pointed, non-glandular hairs and the rounded scars of the bases of these will also be observed.

Fragments of Senna show a red coloration when mounted in alkaline solutions.

Powdered Drug.—Powdered Indian Senna is light yellowish-green. Calcium oxalate in rosette aggregates, from 9 to 10μ in diameter, and in prisms 12 to 15μ in length, usually in crystal fibers that adhere to groups of thick-walled sclerenchyma fibers of the pericycle; few unicellular, non-

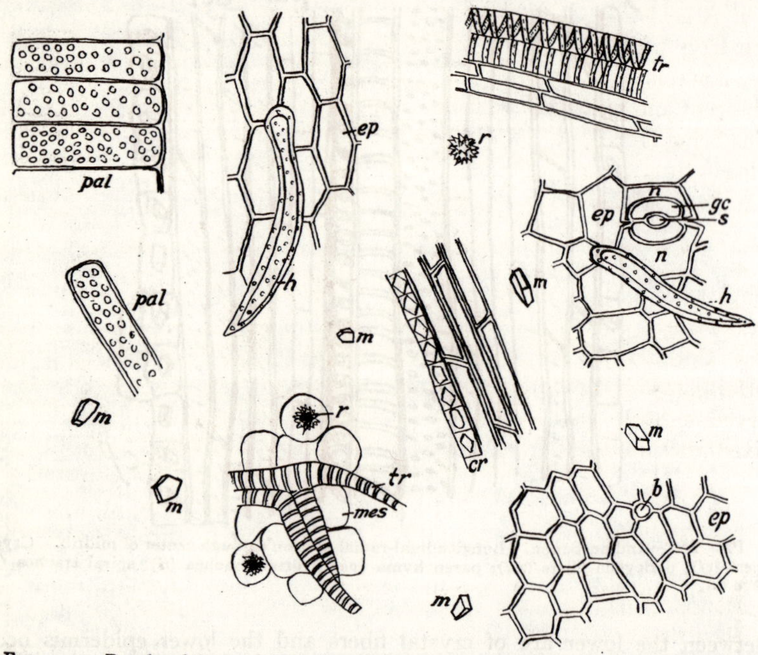

FIG. 127.—Powdered Senna. Palisade parenchyma (*pal*); epidermis (*ep*); unicellular, non-glandular, papillose hairs (*h*); stoma (*s*); guard cells (*gc*); neighboring cells (*n*); spiral tracheæ (*tr*); base of non-glandular hair (*b*); rosette crystals of calcium oxalate (*r*); monoclinic prisms of calcium oxalate (*m*); spongy parenchyma (*mes*); crystal fiber (*cr*) containing monoclinic prisms of calcium oxalate.

glandular, straight or curved hairs or fragments thereof; fragments of epidermis, some of which show elliptical stomata with two unequal, parallel neighboring cells; spiral, annular and pitted tracheæ.

Powdered Alexandria Senna is light green and differs from powdered Indian Senna mainly by showing more numerous hairs and more stomatal apparatuses accompanied by 3 neighboring cells.

Constituents.—Aloe-emodin, rhein, kaempferin, isorhamnetin all occurring free and in the form of glucosides; kaempferol, a phytosterol glucoside, myricyl-alcohol, mucilage, resin, starch, calcium oxalate, etc.

Use.—Senna leaflets and pods are extensively used as a purgative.

Adulterants.—1. The leaflets and pods of *Tephrosia appolinea* (Fam. *Leguminosæ*) a plant indigenous to Egypt. The leaflets of this plant are obovate or obcordate in outline, have parallel veins of the first order, frequently show emarginate apex and are smaller than the average Senna leaflet. The pods are cylindrical up to 3 cm. long and about 3 mm. in breadth. Occasionally found in Alexandria Senna.

2. Argel Leaves. The leaves of *Solenostemma Argel* (Fam. *Asclepiadaceæ*) have been admixed with Alexandria Senna. They are short petiolate, lanceolate, coriaceous, with entire margin, equal base, acute apex, pubescent and pinnately veined. The midrib alone is distinct, the lateral veins being indistinct. The non-glandular hairs are uniseriate and 3 to 4 celled.

3. Dog Senna. The leaflets of *Cassia obovata* are broadly obovate, mucronate, from 12 to 22 mm. in length and about half as broad.

4. Arabian or Bombay Senna. (See p. 325.) These leaflets are elongate lanceolate in outline, averagely longer and narrower than those of Alexandria Senna and are often partly discolored.

5. Coriaria Leaves. The leaves of *Coriaria myrtifolia* Linné (Fam. *Coriariaceæ*), a Mediterranean shrub, are ovate to ovate-lanceolate, 3 nerved, coriaceous and glabrous. They have been cut into segments and mixed with cut Alexandria Senna. For details of histology see p. 517.

SCOPARIUS N.F. (SCOPARIUS)

Synonyms.—Broom Tops, Irish or Scotch Broom, Broom; *Ger.* Besenginster; *Fr.* Genêt à balais.

Botanical Origin.—*Cytisus scoparius* (Linné) Link.

Part Used.—The dried tops.

Purity Rubric.—Not more than 5 per cent. of stems over 3 mm. in diameter and not more than 2 per cent. of other foreign organic matter.

Habitat.—Europe and Western Asia. Naturalized in the United States.

Plant.—A shrub growing to the height of 1 to 2.4 m., with numerous 5-angled, green, flexible branches bearing trifoliate leaves with sessile upper leaflets. The inflorescences appear from May to June as racemes of bright yellow papilionaceous flowers. The fruit is a compressed legume containing numerous seeds.

Production and Commerce.—The younger green, flexible tops are gathered before the flowering of the plant and dried. While small amounts of the drug are gathered in the Pacific Northwest and in the

Cape Cod district, most of the commercial article is collected in Great Britain and Southern Europe. The imported article is largely shipped to the U. S. A. from London and Marseilles in burlap bags or bundles.

Description.—The drug occurs either in the form of thin, flexible, branched, pentangular twigs, 2 to 3 mm. in thickness or as cut segments of these; externally dark-green, nearly smooth, with numerous reddish-brown cork patches; fracture short-fibrous, that of thicker pieces being tough and splintery; internally yellowish; upper leaves sessile, often absent in the drug; odor slight, peculiar on bruising; taste bitter and disagreeable.

Histology.—Transverse sections made through the young portion of the twig exhibit an angular outline and the following peculiarities:

1. Epidermis of oblong and square cells with thick outer cuticle.

2. Cortex of several layers of cortical parenchyma cells, at intervals extending into the wings. It will be observed that 2 groups of thick walled sclerenchyma fibers occur in each wing region of cortex. Between the group nearest the epidermis and the epidermis itself occur one or two layers of collenchyma cells.

3. Pericycle, containing an interrupted band of thick-walled, lignified pericyclic fibers.

4. A circle of compactly arranged open-collateral bundles, separated by narrow medullary rays. Each bundle exhibits a narrow phloem consisting of soft bast, a cambium, and a comparatively broad xylem of numerous wood fibers and spiral tracheæ.

5. Pith, a central zone of large, more or less polygonal, thin walled cells.

Powdered Drug.—Dark green to brownish-green. Fragments of epidermis in surface view showing polygonal cells and small broadly elliptical stomata, each surrounded by small neighboring cells; non-glandular trichomes, thick walled, unicellular and papillated; fragments containing annular, but mostly spiral or double spiral tracheæ and tracheids; fragments of sclerenchyma fibers with simple pores; pollen grains football-shaped; fragments of parenchyma of pith and cortex; few starch grains up to 20μ in diameter.

Constituents.—The liquid alkaloid, sparteine; the yellow flavone, scoparin; the volatile alkaloid, genisteine, tannin, etc.

Uses.—Scoparius is employed as a diuretic in dropsy in the form of the infusion and fluidextract.

Adulterant.—The tops of *Osyris alba* Linne. (Fam. *Santalaceæ*) which have a many striated stem and white wood.

KINO U.S.P. (KINO)

Synonyms.—Gum Kino, Malabar-, East India-, Madras-, or Cochin-Kino; *Fr.* Kino de l'Inde; *Ger.* Kino.

Botanical Origin.—*Pterocarpus Marsupium* Roxburgh.

Part Used.—The dried juice, obtained from the trunk.

Purity Rubric.—Not less than 45 per cent. of alcohol-soluble extractive and not less than 80 per cent. of water-soluble extractive.

Habitat.—Forests of Eastern India.

Plant.—A large timber tree with alternate, imparipinnate leaves having 5–7 emarginate leaflets, pale yellow flowers and an orbicular indehiscent legume containing a single seed.

Production and Commerce.—The phloem region of the bark of this tree has been found to contain a large number of tubular cells arranged in axial rows. These cells contain a red astringent fluid which exudes to the surface when the bark is wounded. Kino is collected by the natives who make vertical incisions in the bark of the trunk with oblique lateral ones running into them. The red juice that flows is collected in cups or other receptacles, evaporated to the consistency of a hard mass in the sun, and broken up into small fragments. It is packed in wooden boxes and shipped to the U. S. A. either direct from Bombay, India or through London.

Description.—In small, brittle, angular fragments, usually less than 10 mm. in diameter, varying in color from dark reddish-brown to reddish-black; when crushed upon a slide and examined under the microscope the angular fragments are more or less translucent with a glass-like, conchoidal surface, the thinner pieces having a yellowish-red or deep brownish-red color, the pieces often being marked by nearly parallel, curved and straight lines; inodorous; taste very astringent; when masticated it colors the saliva somewhat pink.

Constituents.—About 75 per cent. of kinotannic acid which gives a greenish color with ferric salts, kinoin, kino red, pyrocatechin, gallic acid, gum, etc.

Use.—Astringent.

CATECHU (CATECHU)

Synonyms.—Black Catechu, Cutch, Terra Japonica; *Ger.* Catechu; *Fr.* Cachu.

Botanical Origin.—*Acacia Catechu* Willd.

Part Used.—An extract prepared from the heartwood.

Habitat.—India and Burmah.

Plant.—A tree with crooked trunk, spiny branches, brown bark, and reddish-black heartwood, attaining a height of about 12 m. Its leaves are bipinnate, each showing from 10 to 20 pairs of pinnæ. Each pinna or lobe of the bipinnate leaf possesses from 20 to 30 pairs of leaflets. The flowers are yellow and borne on elongated dense racemes. The fruit is a brownish, flattened legume containing several brown shining seeds.

Production and Commerce.—The Catechu trees are quite common in India and Burmah where the astringent bark is used for tanning and the wood for fuel, charcoal and posts, the drug catechu, being chewed by the natives as a masticatory. Catechu trees also abound in Ceylon and in Eastern Africa.

When the trunk has attained a diameter of about a foot, the tree is cut down and the trunk and thicker branches deprived of their bark and

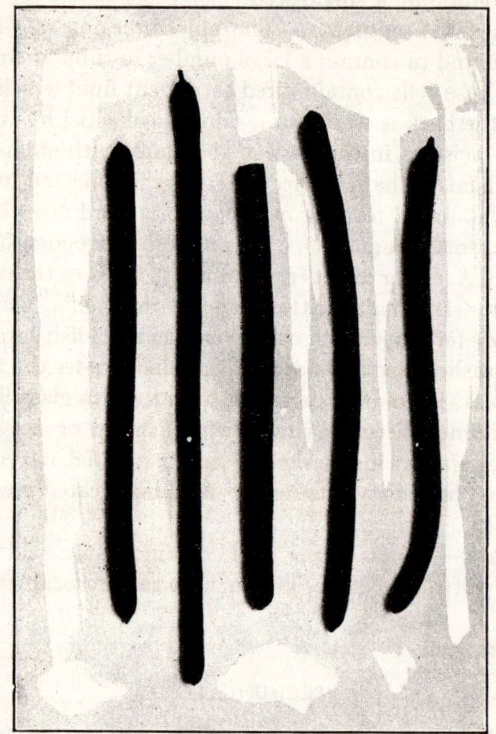

FIG. 128.—Cassia Fistula. × ⅕. (*Photograph by Stoneback.*)

sapwood. The reddish-black heartwood is then cut into chips and boiled in water, contained in an earthern pot, over a fire place. When the liquid begins to thicken, it is decanted into an iron pot and boiled down until the aqueous extract is sufficiently hardened (of the nature of a thick syrup), when it is poured into clay molds, or large leaves made into cups, or on mats, where it is allowed to completely harden through the agency of the sun and air. It is then broken into smaller masses for the market.

Description.—In blackish masses which are easily broken, frequently showing fragments of mats or leaves on the lower surface, the fractured surface dull glossy, internally with numerous small cavities; almost completely soluble in boiling water; inodorous; taste astringent and sweet.

Constituents.—About 25 per cent. of catechutannic acid; acaciatechin, catechu-red, quercetin, etc.

Uses.—Catechu was formerly extensively employed as an astringent but is now replaced largely by Gambir or Pale Catechu. It is used in the tanning and dyeing industries.

CASSIA FISTULA N.F. (CASSIA FISTULA)

Synonyms.—Purging Cassia, Cassia Pods, Indian Laburnum, Cassia Stick Tree; *Fr.* Casse officinale; *Ger.* Purgiercassie.

Botanical Origin.—*Cathartocarpus Fistula* (Linné) Persoon.

Part Used.—The dried fruit.

Purity Rubric.—Not more than 2 per cent. of foreign organic matter.

Habitat.—India. Naturalized in Africa, West Indies and South America.

Plant.—A tree attaining a height of about 15 m. with gray bark and paripinnate leaves with 3 to 7 pairs of ovate leaflets and racemes of yellow flowers that appear from May to June. The fruit is an elongated, reddish-brown to black, cylindrical loment with numerous compartments, each containing a flattened, ovoid, shiny, reddish-brown seed embedded in a brownish, hardened pulp.

Production and Commerce.—The fruits are gathered in India, the East Indies, West Indies and South America, packed in burlap bundles or bags (East Indian and Indian) or in cylindrical baskets made of plaited cane (West Indian). The drug is imported from Calcutta, Karachi, London, Rotterdam and Hamburg, the West Indies and South America. The fruits should be collected when ripe and carefully dried. The best fruits are those which do not rattle when shaken. These possess the most pulp.

Description.—Purging Cassia occurs as entire cylindrical or broken loments, from 25 to 65 cm. in length and 18 to 25 mm. in diameter; externally reddish-brown to nearly black, showing a constriction at the base and frequently an attached portion of the pedicel, also a longitudinal groove on one side and a smooth line or slight ridge on the other which indicate the sutures; internally the cavity is divided into numerous compartments, each containing a reddish-brown, shiny, flattened, ovoid seed embedded in a blackish-brown sweet pulp; odor prune like.

Constituents.—From 25 to 30 per cent. of pulp which contains up to 60 per cent. of sugar, also mucilage, proteins, volatile oil, etc.

Uses.—As a laxative and in the preparation of confection of senna.

TAMARINDUS N.F. (TAMARIND)

Synonyms.—Tamarind Pulp; *Ger.* Tamarinden; *Fr.* Tamarinier.

Botanical Origin.—*Tamarindus indica* Linné.

Part Used.—The partially dried ripe fruit, deprived of the brittle outer portion of the pericarp and preserved in sugar or hot syrup.

Purity Rubric.—Not more than 2 per cent. of foreign organic matter.

Habitat.—Africa. Cultivated in India and the East Indies.

Plant.—A large spreading tree with alternate paripinnate leaves, each with 8 to 10 pairs of leaflets, and lateral racemes of yellow flowers. The fruit is a flattened indehiscent legume with a brownish brittle endocarp, succulent, acid and stringy mesocarp and leathery endocarp enclosing a few seeds.

Production and Commerce.—The plants are grown in the West Indies, East Indies and Egypt. There are two important commercial varieties, West Indian and East Indian. West Indian Tamarind is prepared by first separating the epicarp and then packing the fruits in barrels with hot syrup as a preservative. It occurs as light reddish-brown to dark brown or black brown masses of preserved pulp containing seeds. East Indian or Black Tamarind occurs in black masses or cakes which are prepared by pressing together pulp, shells and seeds and sometimes preserving with salt. It is more acid in taste than the West Indian article.

Description.—A pulpy mass of a light reddish-brown color, changing with age to a dark brown; or black (E. Indian); containing some branching fibers and numerous reddish-brown, smooth, oblong or quadrangular, compressed seeds, each enclosed in a tough membrane. Odor distinct; taste sweet and agreeably acid.

Constituents.—Tartaric acid, citric acid, potassium bitartrate, pectin, tannin, invert sugar, etc.

Uses.—Laxative and refrigerant and in preparation of confection of senna.

GERANIACEÆ (GERANIUM FAMILY)

Herbaceous, rarely semi-succulent, sub-shrubby plants. Stems cylindrical, often hairy or glandular hairy. Leaves alternate to opposite, stipulate; venation from pinnate to palmate, so leaf shape from ovate to pinnatifid to pinnatipartite to subpalmatifid to palmatipartite to compound palmate. Inflorescence either a dichesial or scorpioid cyme. Flowers regular pentamerous (*Geranium*) to irregular pentamerous (*Pelargonium*); sepals five, aposepalous; petals five, apopetalous, varying in color from greenish-white or pink-red to scarlet, scarlet-crimson to crimson-purple; anthers ten or five, hypogynous or inserted into slightly developed hypognous disc; pistil pentacarpellary, ovary five-celled with two, rarely one ovule in each cell, styles elongate, fused round a stylar column of receptacle, then continued as a stylar tip which splits into five stigmatic surfaces. Fruit a regma, rarely a simple capsule. Regma splits into five recurved carpels, each then dehiscing to set free two or one seeds. Seeds exalbuminous.

GERANIUM N.F. (GERANIUM)

Synonyms.—Cranesbill, Wild Geranium, Spotted Geranium, American Kino; *Ger.* Felckstorchschnabelwurzel; *Fr.* Racine de Bec-de-Grue tacheté.

Botanical Origin.—*Geranium maculatum* Linné.

Part Used.—The dried rhizome.

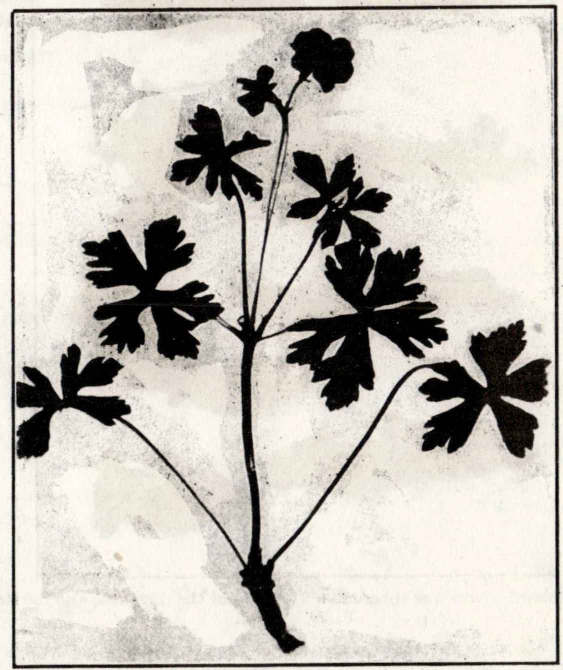

FIG. 129.—*Geranium maculatum.*

Purity Rubric.—Not more than 2 per cent. of foreign organic matter.

Habitat.—In rich woods of Canada and the United States.

Plant.—A perennial herb with long petioled, nearly orbicular, reniform or cordate, deeply 3 to 5 parted radical leaves. Its stem leaves are shorter, 2 in number and opposite. The inflorescence is an umbellate cluster of rose-purple flowers with 1–5 long peduncles usually bearing a pair of leaves at the base of the pedicels. The sepals are 5 and awn pointed.

The petals are 5, hypogynous, and hairy at the base. The stamens are 10. The pistil is compound and shows a 5-lobed, 5-celled ovary which is terminated by a 5-cleft style. The fruit is a regma.

Production and Commerce.—The rhizome is collected in autumn, washed, deprived of most of its stem bases and roots and dried. The commercial supplies come from Virginia, North Carolina, Michigan and Indiana.

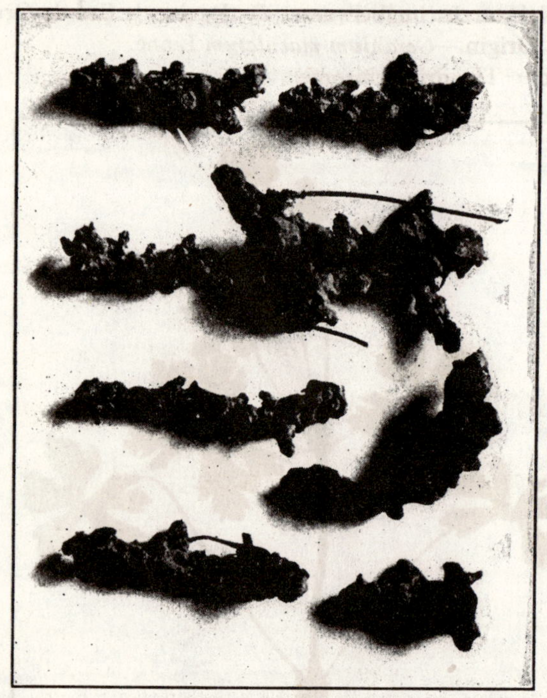

FIG. 130.—Geranium. Note the tuberculated surface of the rhizomes, also the stem scars and bases. × ½.

Description.—Usually simple, occasionally branched, horizontal, tuberculated rhizomes up to 10 cm. long and 3 to 15 mm. broad; externally dark purple or reddish-brown, the upper surface with circular stem scars and buds, the lateral surfaces and lower surface nodulated and annulated; fracture short and nearly even; internally showing a thin bark, a distinct cambium and a large grayish-purple pith; odor indistinct, taste very astringent.

Histology.—Transverse sections of the rhizome exhibit the following internal structure.

1. *Cork* of about 10 rows of tangentially elongated cells, the outer layers with brownish walls and a brownish amorphous content, the inner layers with colorless walls.

2. *Cork cambium* of thin-walled more or less collapsed cells.

3. *Cortex* composed of an outer zone of about 5 layers of tangentially elongated oval cells and a broad inner zone of nearly isodiametric cortical parenchyma containing either starch grains, rosette aggregates of calcium oxalate or tannin masses.

4. A circle of few small *fibrovascular bundles* whose intrafascicular cambia are joined by interfacicular cambia into a closed cambium ring. In the medullary-ray regions, on the outside of each interfacicular cambium, a patch of soft bast (sieve tubes and phloem cells) is developed, but no accompanying xylem on the inner face of the interfacicular cambium is present.

5. Pith, a large central cone of nearly isodiametric cells containing either starch, rosette aggregates of calcium oxalate or tannin masses.

Powdered Drug.—Purplish-brown. Numerous fragments of starch, crystal- and tannin-parenchyma; starch grains numerous, ovoid or ellipsoidal up to 35μ in length with excentric hilum; numerous rosette aggregate crystals of calcium oxalate up to 145μ in diameter (usually 60 to 120μ); numerous fragments colored bluish-black with ammonio-ferric alum T.S.; small spiral and reticulate tracheæ associated with porous and reticulate tracheids; fragments of cork tissue.

Constituents.—Tannin, starch and calcium oxalate.

Use.—Astringent.

LINACEÆ (FLAX FAMILY)

Herbs with slender stems and alternate, simple, narrow leaves. Inflorescence cymose with regular pentamerous flowers; pistil five-carpelled with a five-celled ovary containing two ovules in each cavity and having a single style with knob-like stigma. While the flower is still in bud condition or soon after, there commences an ingrowth of the mid-rib of each carpel which proceeds until, when plant is in fruit, there are formed 10 cavities each enclosing a seed. Seeds, anatropous, mucilaginous, flattened, containing a large embryo and slight albumen.

LINUM U.S.P. (LINSEED)

Synonyms.—Flaxseed; *Ger.* Flachssamen; *Fr.* Grains de Lin.

Botanical Origin.—*Linum usitatissimum* Linné.

Part Used.—The dried ripe seed.

Standard of Assay.—Not less than 30 per cent. of non-volatile, ether-soluble extractive of which at least 98 per cent. is saponifiable.

Limit of Impurities.—2 per cent. of other seeds or foreign organic matter.

Habitat.—Unknown. It is cultivated chiefly in the temperate regions of the Eastern and Western Hemispheres.

Plant.—An annual herb having an erect, smooth stem attaining a height of .7 m. and branching at the summit. The leaves are alternate, small, linear-lanceolate and sessile. The flowers are pale-blue and terminal. The fruit is a small globular capsule with persistent basal calyx and containing 10 exalbuminous seeds, one in each cell.

Production and Commerce.—Flax is grown for its seed and fiber in nearly all countries within the temperate zones as well as in some tropical regions. The countries yielding most of the world's supply of flaxseed are United States, Canada, Russia, Argentina, India and Holland. The seeds are sown in early spring on clean moist land with a grain drill, at a depth of about an inch. The plants are cut when the fruits are fully matured, bound and shocked, and the seeds separated by thrashing. The seed is then cleaned and stored in dry places until marketed. The two principal flaxseed markets in the United States are Minneapolis and Duluth. In 1924, the United States produced 30,173,000 bushels of flaxseed. The states yielding this quota in the order of their production were North Dakota, Minnesota, South Dakota, Montana, Kansas, Wisconsin, Iowa, Nebraska, Missouri and Wyoming.

Description.—The seed is exalbuminous, of compressed ovate or ovate-lanceolate outline, pointed at one end, rounded at the other and from 4 to 6 mm. in length; externally glabrous and shiny, chestnut-brown, with a pale-yellow, linear raphe along one edge; internally exhibiting a brown seed coat and yellowish-green endosperm and cotyledons; odor slight, becoming very characteristic in the ground or crushed drug; taste mucilaginous and oily.

Histology.—Transverse sections of this seed can readily be made by fixing in cork preparatory to cutting them. Upon mounting in chloral hydrate solution and examining under the microscope the following structures are apparent:

1. **Seed coat** consisting of the following regions: (*a*) Epidermis of a single layer of large cells with cutinized outer walls and containing mucilage that shows stratification upon coming in contact with water; (*b*) two layers of more or less collapsed parenchyma cells with intercellular-air-spaces (in the region of the raphe, but one layer of these cells is evident and a bundle here traverses this tissue); (*c*) a layer of yellowish-brown, radially elongated and lignified stone cells with large central lumina; (*d*) a hyaline layer of narrow colorless cells; (*e*) a layer of pigment cells with reddish-brown amorphous contents.

2. **Endosperm** of from 6 to 10 layers of parenchymatic cells with moderately thickened walls and containing small aleurone grains and globules of fixed oil.

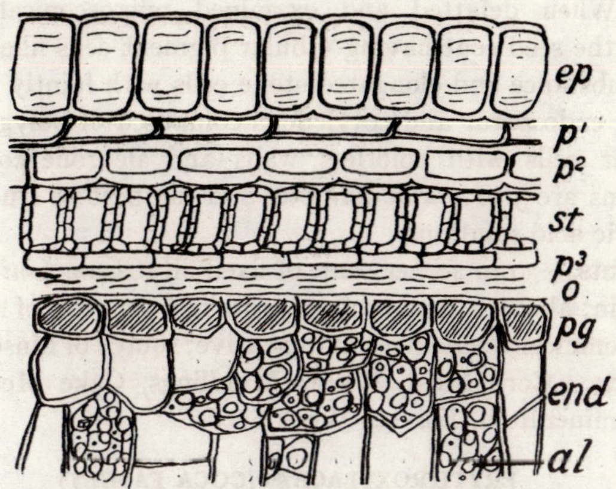

FIG. 131.—Transverse section through a representative portion of the seed of *Linum usitatissimum* showing epidermis (*ep*) with mucilage contents; parenchyma cells (p^1, p^2); stone cells (*st*); parenchyma (p^3); cells with obliterated walls (*o*); pigment cells with brownish contents (*pg*); endosperm (*end*); aleurone grains (*al*).

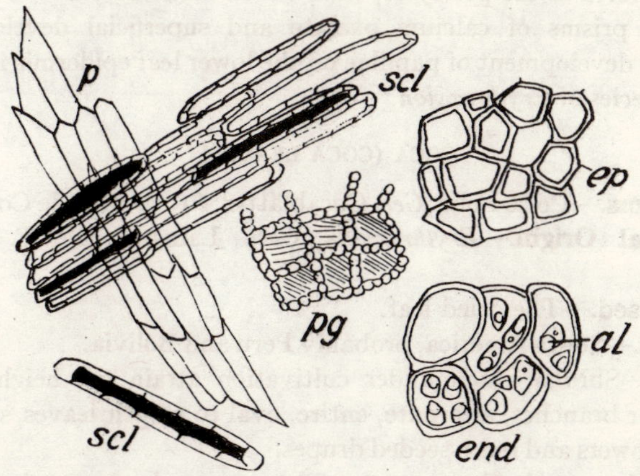

FIG. 132.—Ground flaxseed. Stone cells (*scl*) and parenchyma (*p*) of seed coat; pigment cells with porous walls and brownish contents (*pg*); epidermis of seed coat (*ep*); endosperm (*end*) the cells of which contain aleurone grains (*al*) and fixed oil.

3. **Two large planoconvex Cotyledons,** each consisting of a covering outer epidermis of polygonal cells enclosing numerous radially elongated cells that contain abundant aleurone and oil. The aleurone grains are from 3μ to 20μ (averagely 10 to 15μ) in length and can best be studied in mounts stained with dilute iodine or picric acid solution. In such

mounts each will be seen to consist of a protein matrix containing one or two more or less angular phytoglobulins and large rounded globoids.

Ground Drug.—Dark gray (Powdered drug-yellowish-brown), greatly oleaginous. When defatted and examined microscopically it shows fragments of the seed coat having tabular pigment cells filled with a reddish-brown substance and elongated stone cells with faintly yellow walls, fragments of endosperm and cotyledons composed of polygonal or elongated angular cells with colorless walls and aleurone contents. The aleurone grains are 3 to 20μ in diameter and can best be studied in dilute iodine or picric acid solutions.

Constituents.—30 to 40 per cent. of fixed oil (*Oleum Lini U.S.P.*) containing linolein; about 25 per cent. of protein, 6 per cent. of mucilage, etc.

Uses.—Demulcent, emollient and laxative; source of Linseed oil U.S.P.

Adulterants.—Corn Meal, Wheat Middlings, Cake Meal sometimes containing a mineral oil, Foreign Weed Seeds.

ERYTHROXYLACEÆ (COCA FAMILY)

A small family of tropical plants, mostly shrubs, closely allied anatomically to the *Linaceæ*, with pentamerous flowers and drupe fruits. The outstanding histological characteristics are the presence of sclerenchyma fibers in the pericycle, thin-walled cork cells, rosette crystals or monoclinic prisms of calcium oxalate and superficial development of cork. The development of papillae on the lower leaf epidermis is recorded for most species of *Erythroxylon*.

COCA (COCA LEAVES)

Synonyms.—Cocæ Folia; *Ger.* Cocablätter; *Fr.* Feuilles de Coca.

Botanical Origin.—*Erythroxylon Coca* Lamarck and *E. truxillense* Rusby.

Part Used.—The dried leaf.

Habitat.—South America, probably Peru and Bolivia.

Plants.—Shrubs which under cultivation attain the height of 6 ft., with slender branches, alternate, entire, oval to elliptic leaves, small white or yellow flowers and red 1-seeded drupes.

Production and Commerce.—The coca shrubs are extensively cultivated in Bolivia and Peru where they grow on the slopes of valleys in the Andes at an elevation of from 1500 to 6000 ft. and in a moist atmosphere. They are also cultivated in Java and Formosa. Peru produces the largest amount of drug—although the province of La Paz in Bolivia yields the largest crops of any district. The seeds are planted in nurseries and when the seedlings are sufficiently strong these are transplanted to long terraces called "humachas" built up above one another like the steps of a staircase, each being supported by a little rampart of earth reinforced by stones. The plants begin to yield in about 18 months but it takes from 3 to 5 years for the coca shrub to be in full bearing. There are three pickings a year, occasionally a fourth. The mature leaves are plucked by the Andean Indians and dried, first in a closed drying chamber where the leaves are spread on a floor of beaten earth and afterwards on a paved open drying floor. They are then stored in dry buildings and subsequently packed in bales. Although produced in large quantities, comparatively little of the crude drug is shipped out of South America. Most of it is consumed by the natives while considerable is employed in the manufacture of cocaine.

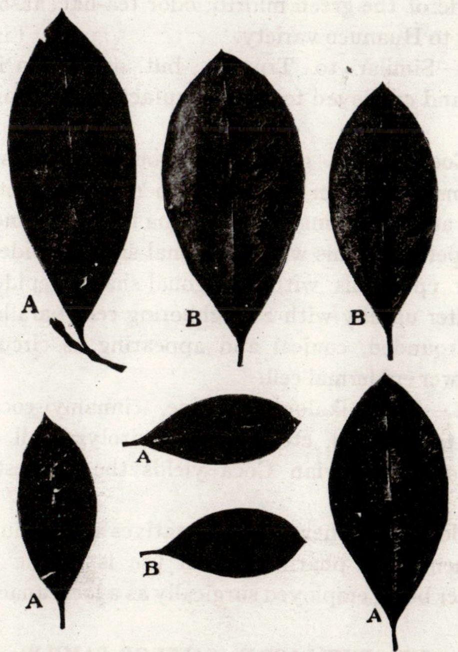

FIG. 133.—Coca Leaves. *A*, Upper side. *B*. Lower side. Natural size. (*After Sayre.*)

The commercial varieties of Coca leaves are the Huanuco or Bolivian Coca yielded by *Erythroxylon Coca*, the Peruvian or Truxillo Coca, yielded by *E. truxillense* and the Java Coca yielded by *E. truxillense*.

Description.—*Huanuco Coca.*—Brownish-green, mostly entire, shortly and stoutly petioled; the blade elliptical, thick, slightly coriaceous, averagely from 3.5 to 8 cm. in length and from 2.5 to 4 cm. in breadth, glabrous, apex acute, base tapering, margin entire; midrib reddish-brown, traversed on the upper surface by a slight ridge, very prominent on lower surface, the remaining venation somewhat obscure, especially above; on lower surface, 2 conspicuous curved lines of collenchyma tissue run longitudinally, one on either side of the midrib and about ⅓ of the distance between it and the margin; odor slightly tea-like; taste bitter and slightly aromatic followed by a sensation of numbness.

Truxillo Coca.—Pale green, brittle and usually considerably broken, shortly and stoutly petioled; the blade obovate to oblanceolate, 1.6 to 5 cm. in length and ⅓ to ½ as broad, glabrous, much thinner than the Huanuco variety, apex acute, narrowed from near the middle to the petiole, margin entire; on lower surface 2 curved lines of collenchyma tissue, usually incomplete or obscure (frequently absent) run longitudinally one on either side of the green midrib; odor tea-like; taste and numbing sensation similar to Huanuco variety.

Java Cocoa.—Similar to Truxillo, but only seen in commerce in powdered form and employed for the manufacture of cocaine in Germany and Holland.

Powdered Coca.—Dark green; numerous fragments of mesophyll; monoclinic prisms of calcium oxalate up to 15μ in diameter or in crystal fibers, the latter accompanying sclerenchyma fibers; fragments of tracheæ; fragments of upper epidermis with polygonal-shaped epidermal cells; fragments of lower epidermis with polygonal-shaped epidermal cells and stomata, the latter usually with 2 neighboring cells parallel to the stoma; papillae short, rounded, conical and appearing as circular markings in center of each lower epidermal cell.

Constituents.—The alkaloids cocaine, cinnamyl-cocaine, α and β truxilline; coca-tannic acid, etc. When hydrolyzed all the alkaloids of coca yield ecgonine. Bolivian Coca yields the greatest percentage of cocaine.

Uses.—The leaves are chewed by the natives as a stimulant, restorative and tonic. Their chief pharmaceutical use is in the manufacture of cocaine, the latter being employed surgically as a local anaesthetic.

ZYGOPHYLLACEÆ (CALTROP FAMILY)

Zygophyllaceæ or Caltrop Family.—Herbs, shrubs or trees (*Guaiacum*) having jointed, often divaricate branches. Leaves usually opposite, stipulate and compound. Flowers regular or irregular, pentamerous, white, yellow, red or blue (*G. officinale*). Fruit a capsule.

GUAIACI LIGNUM (GUAIAC WOOD)

Synonyms.—Lignum Vitae, Lignum Benedictum, Rockwood; *Ger.* Guajakholz; *Fr.* Bois de Gayac.

Botanical Origin.—(1) *Guajacum officinale* Linné and (2) *Guajacum sanctum* Linné.

Part Used.—The heartwood.

Habitat.—(1) West Indies and South America. (2) West Indies.

Plants.—Evergreen trees with ash-gray bark, knotty branches, resinous wood and paripinnate leaves. The flowers are large, of blue to purple color, and occur in axillary clusters. The fruit is a capsule.

Production and Commerce.—The bark and sapwood are removed from the trunk and thicker branches, after first peeling the trees. The central heartwood is then collected and used mainly for the manufacture of implements. The waste heartwood from turners in the shape of shavings or raspings is usually alone used in pharmacy and medicine. The commercial supplies are obtained from Azua, Dominican Republic and from Gonaives, Hayti.

Description.—Usually in the form of shavings, chips or raspings of a greenish-brown color, heavier than water, entirely free from adhering bark and containing only a few chips or shavings of a whitish color (*sap wood*). Almost odorless except when heated; taste bitter and acrid when chewed for some time.

Powdered Drug.—The powder, when examined under the microscope, exhibits numerous fragments of more or less lignified, thick-walled wood fibers up to 28μ in width, some with simple, oblique pores; tracheæ from 90 to 160μ in width, some filled with resin; numerous small masses of resin; wood parenchyma and medullary ray cells up to 20μ in width, with lignified, porous walls and usually containing resin; occasionally tangential views of the medullary rays show an elliptical group of from three to six cells; the resin masses and resinous tissue become bluish-green on the addition of iodine T.S.

If powdered Guaiac Wood be placed in a solution of sodium chloride (1 in 3); the blackish-brown part only will sink and this does not exceed in amount the portion which floats.

Constituents.—From 20 to 25 per cent. of resin consisting of guaiaretic, guaiaconic, and guaiacic acids, guaiacsaponin, vanillin, etc. Guaiaconic acid is readily converted by oxidizing agents, such as H_2O_2 and Fe_2Cl_6, into guaiac-blue.

Use.—Guaiac wood is now chiefly used as a source of the official resin.

GUAIACUM N.F. (GUAIAC)

Synonyms.—Guaiac Resin, Gum Guaiac; *Fr.* Résine de Gayac; *Ger.* Guajakharz.

Botanical Origin.—*Guajacum officinale* L. and *Guajacum sanctum* L.

Part Used.—The resin of the wood.

Purity Rubric.—Not more than 15 per cent. of matter insoluble in alcohol.

Habitat.—South America and West Indies.

Plants.—See under *Guaiaci Lignum.*

Production and Commerce.—Resin of Guaiac naturally exudes from the Guaiac trees but the commercial article is obtained largely by cutting incisions in the bark of the trees or by heating the ends of logs that have first been scarified in the middle and suspended horizontally in the air by appropriate supports. The resin runs out from the scarified area and is collected in calabash cups. The commercial supplies are chiefly obtained from Azua, Dominican Republic and from Gonaives, Hayti, and arrive in bags packed within cases.

Description.—In irregular pieces or somewhat globular masses of a deep greenish-brown or dark olive color on surfaces exposed to the air and reddish-brown on freshly fractured surfaces; brittle, the freshly fractured surface having a glassy lustre; odor balsamic; taste slightly acrid. Not more than 15 per cent. is insoluble in alcohol.

An alcoholic solution on the addition of ferric chloride solution becomes blue changing rapidly to green.

Powdered Drug.—Grayish becoming green on exposure to the air.

Constituents.—Guaiaconic, guaiaretic, guaiacinic, guaiacresinic and guaiacic acids, guaiacsaponin, vanillin, a gutta percha like substance called guaiaguttin, guaiac yellow, etc.

Uses.—Stimulant, diaphoretic, expectorant, laxative, alterative and astringent.

RUTACEÆ (RUE AND CITRUS FAMILY)

Herbs (*Ruta*, *Diosma*, *Barosma*) or shrubs (*Xanthoxylum*) or trees (*Citrus*). Stems upright, often wiry xerophytic, in sub-family *Ruteæ*, elongated and spiny in sub-family *Zanthoxyleæ*, woody and green in sub-family *Aurantieæ*. Leaves alternate or oppostite, simple (*Ruta*), rarely whorled (*Pilocarpus*), or pinnatifid, as in *Ruta graveolens*, or pinnate, as lower parts of *Ruta graveolens*, becoming reduced pinnate in *Citrus Aurantium*. Leaves extipulate or with spiny stipules (*Zanthoxylum*). Stems and leaves abound in more or less sunken glands. Flowers pentamerous, varying in color from yellow in *Ruta* to white in *Citrus* to pink (*Barosma betulina*) or pink crimson as in some *Barsoma* and *Diosma* species, rarely to pinkish-purple (*Pilocarpus*); sepals five, aposepalous, becoming in *Citrus* more or less synsepalous; petals five, apopetalous, becoming more or less synpetalous and tubular (*Correa grandiflora*); stamens five, simple or with expanded bases, lobed, or lobes developed as staminal stipules and more or less split (*Citrus*); pistil of ten, five, three or two carpels, ovary as many-celled. Fruit a capsule (*Dittany*, *Zanthoxylum*), hesperidium (*Citrus*) or rarely a samara (*Ptelea*). Seeds albuminous or exalbuminous. Many of the plants contain volatile oils in their secretory cavities. Membrane crystals and hesperidin are common to the Citrus spp. Pericyclic fibers occur usually in isolated groups within the plant axis.

BUCHU U.S.P. (BUCHU)

Synonyms.—Bookoo, Buku, Bucco, Diosma; *Fr.* Feuilles de Bucco; *Ger.* Buccoblätter.

Botanical Origin.—*Barosma betulina* (Thunberg) Bartling and Wendland, *Barosma crenulata* (Linné) Hooker, and *Barosma serratifolia* (Curtis) Willdenow.

Part Used.—The dried leaf.

Limit of Impurities.—8 per cent. of its stems and 2 per cent. of other foreign matter.

Habitat.—South Africa.

Plants.—Low shrubs with glandular-punctate twigs and angled branches. The leaves are small, opposite, coriaceous and pellucid-punctate. The leaves are obovate or rhomboidally obovate (*B. betulina*) or linear-lanceolate (*B. serratifolia*) with more or less serrulate margins. The flowers are pink to white. The fruit consists of 5 follicles.

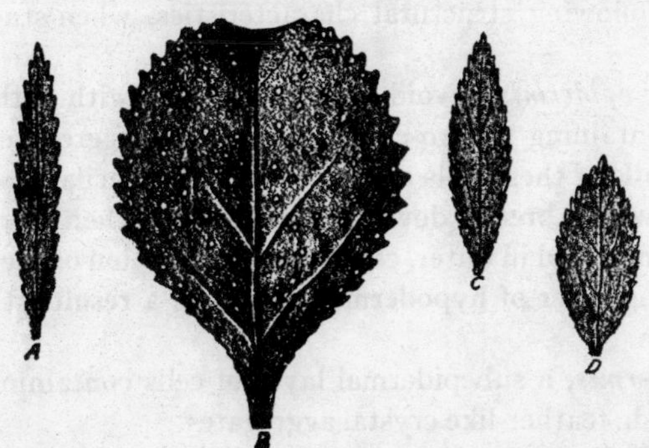

FIG. 134.—Buchu leaves and adulterant. (*A*) Leaf of *Empleurum ensatum;* (*B*) leaf of *Barosma betulina* (enlarged); (*C*) leaf of *Barosma serratifolia;* (*D*) leaf of *Barosma crenulata.* (*From Sayre.*)

Production and Commerce.—The leaves are gathered in the Cape Colony district of South Africa by the natives who cut off the branches when the shrubs are in flower or fruit, allow them to dry and then beat off the leaves. About 90 per cent. of the supply used by this country comes from Cape Town, South Africa. The other 10 per cent. comes through London. Buchu is shipped in large bales. Short Buchu represents the leaves of *B. betulina* and *B. crenulata* whereas Long Buchu consists of the leaves of *B. serratifolia*.

Distinctions between the Commercial Varieties of Buchu.—

	Barosma Betulina (Short Buchu)	Barosma Serratifolia (Long Buchu)
Outline of Blade:	Obovate to rhomboid obovate.	Linear lanceolate.
Apex:	Obtuse, and recurved.	Rounded or truncate.
Base:	Cuneate.	Acute
Margin:	Serrulate to denticulate with an oil-gland at base of each tooth.	Serrulate with an oil-gland at the base of each tooth.
Up. Surface:	Yellowish-green, papillose.	Dark-green to yellowish-green.
L. Surface:	Yellowish-green, pellucid-punctate, and wrinkled.	Grayish-green, pellucid-punctate.
Size:	9–25 mm. long × 6–20 mm. broad.	12–40 mm. long × 4–10 mm. broad.
Texture:	Brittle and coriaceous.	Coriaceous.
Odor:	Aromatic, mint-like.	Aromatic, mint-like.
Taste:	Pungent.	Pungent.

The leaves of *Barosma crenulata*, also known commercially as Short Buchu, somewhat resemble both of these other species, differing chiefly in their outline which is oblong-ovate to lanceolate (broader than long buchu) and in their apex which is obtuse like *B. betulina* but not recurved.

Histology.—Transverse and surface sections of either of the varieties exhibit the following structural characteristics, when studied microscopically:

1. *Upper epidermis* devoid of stomata, but with a thick cuticle and with cells containing sphero-crystals or crystal aggregates of hesperidin. The inner walls of these cells are composed of a mucilaginous modification of cellulose which breaks down into mucilage, when dry cut transverse sections are mounted in water, causing the separation of the epidermis from the underlying layer of hypodermal cells with a resultant elongated rent in the section.

2. *Hypodermis*, a subepidermal layer of cells containing mucilage and often brownish, feather-like crystal aggregates.

3. *Palisade Parenchyma*, a single row of columnar cells rich in chloroplastids, a few containing rosette aggregates of calcium oxalate.

4. *Spongy Parenchyma*, a zone of loosely arranged mesophyll cells and air-spaces, the cells mostly containing chloroplastids, a few rosette aggregates of calcium oxalate. Fibrovascular bundles of the open collateral type course through this region. In the midrib and larger vein regions they are arranged in crescent-shaped groups and separated from the lower epidermis by collenchyma.

5. *Lower epidermis* with thick cuticle and numerous stomata, the latter surrounded by from 4 to 6 neighboring cells.

A few unicellular, non-glandular hairs occur on both upper and lower epidermis. Spherical-shaped internal glands containing oil globules occur in the mesophyll near the margins of the leaf.

Powdered Drug.—Light-green. Characteristic elements: Epidermal cells with straight vertical walls and containing sphaero-crystals or crystal

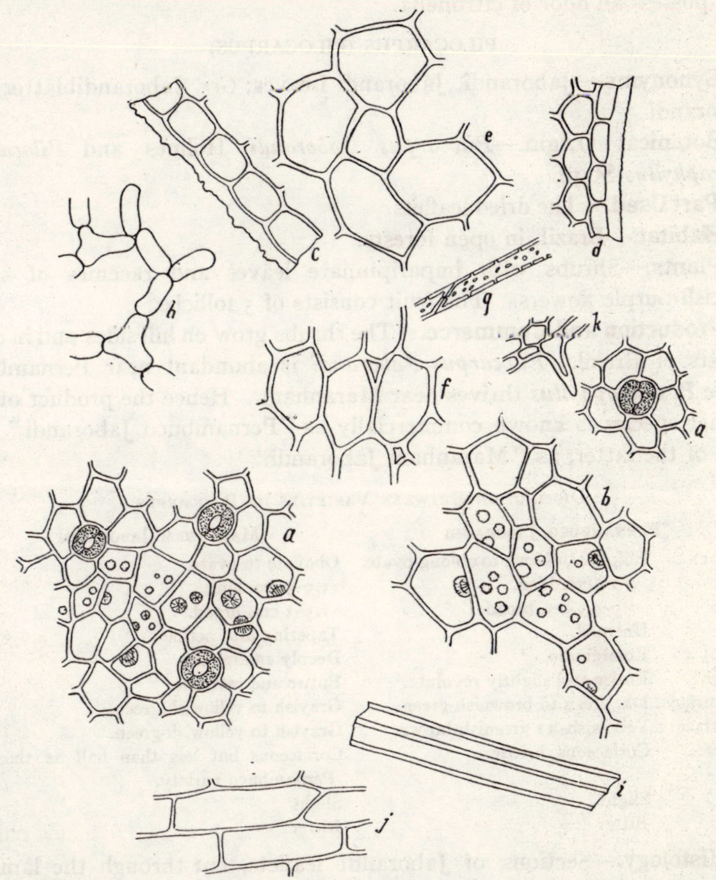

FIG. 135.—Powdered Short Buchu. (*a*) Lower epidermis; (*b*) upper epidermis; (*c*) lower epidermis, lateral view; (*d*) upper epidermis, lateral view; (*e, f*) parenchyma; (*g*) tracheids; (*h*) spongy tissue cells; (*i*) bast cells; (*j*) parenchyma, longitudinal view; (*k*) trichome. (*Schneider*.)

aggregates of hesperidin, 30 to 50μ in diameter; numerous oil globules; numerous elliptical stomata with 4 to 6 neighboring cells in lower epidermis; rosette crystals of CaO, 15 to 30μ in diameter.

Constituents.—Volatile oil containing diosphenol; diosmin, hesperidin, mucilage, occurring in the subepidermal layer of cells of the leaves, etc.

Adulterants and Substitutes.—The leaves of *Empleurum ensatum* (*Rutaceæ*) have been substituted for long buchu. These are narrower, have a bitter taste, an acute apex and are without an oil-gland at the base of each tooth.

The leaves of *Barosma pulchella* are smaller than the official Buchus and possess an odor of citronella.

PILOCARPUS (PILOCARPUS)

Synonyms.—Jaborandi, Jaborandi Leaves; *Ger.* Jaborandiblätter; *Fr.* Jaborandi.

Botanical Origin.—*Pilocarpus Jaborandi* Holmes and *Pilocarpus microphyllus* Stapf.

Part Used.—The dried leaflets.

Habitat.—Brazil, in open forests.

Plants.—Shrubs with imparipinnate leaves and racemes of small pinkish-purple flowers. The fruit consists of 5 follicles.

Production and Commerce.—The shrubs grow on hill sides and in open forests of Brazil. *Pilocarpus Jaborandi* is abundant near Pernambuco while *P. microphyllus* thrives near Maranham. Hence the product of the former species is known commercially as "Pernambuco Jaborandi" and that of the latter, as "Maranham Jaborandi."

Distinction Between Varieties of Pilocarpus

	Pernambuco Jaborandi	Maranham Jaborandi
Outline:	Elliptical, oblong to oblong-ovate. 4–10 cm. long. 1.5–4.5 cm. broad.	Obovate to ovate. 1.5–5 cm. long. 1.5–3 cm. broad.
Base:	Unequal.	Tapering into petiole.
Apex:	Emarginate.	Deeply emarginate.
Margin:	Entire and slightly revolute.	Entire and revolute.
Up. Surface:	Dk. green to brownish-green.	Grayish to yellowish-green.
L. Surface:	Yellowish- or greenish-brown.	Grayish to yellowish-green.
Texture:	Coriaceous, brittle.	Coriaceous but less than half as thick as Pernambuco variety.
Odor:	Slight	Slight
Taste:	Bitter	Bitter

Histology.—Sections of Jaborandi leaflets, cut through the lamina, present the following structures for examination:

1. *Upper epidermis* of more or less tangentially elongated cells, as observed in cross section, with a thick, yellow outer cuticle and frequently showing outgrowths in the form of long, yellowish, thick-walled, unicellular, non-glandular, bent or curved hairs.

2. *Palisade parenchyma* consisting of from 1 to 3 layers of columnar cells mostly possessing chloroplasts, some, rosette aggregates of calcium oxalate. Scattered amongst these cells are large, more or less spheriodal internal glands containing oil globules.

3. *Spongy parenchyma*, a broad zone of irregularly shaped cells and prominent intercellular spaces. Many of the cells in this region possess a rosette aggregate of calcium oxalate.

4. *Lower epidermis* of more or less tangentially-elongated epidermal cells and stomatal apparatuses. The outer walls of the epidermal cells are covered by a thick yellow cuticle. Hairs similar to those which occur on the upper epidermis are present but more numerous. In surface view the stomata appear more or less rounded and usually surrounded by 4 narrow neighboring cells.

Constituents.—The alkaloids pilocarpine, isopilocarpine and pilosine; volatile oil, resin, etc.

Uses.—Pilocarpus is employed as a diaphoretic and sialagogue. Both the hydrochloride and nitrate of its alkaloid pilocarpine are used as a myotic and physiological antidote for atropine or belladonna poisoning.

Adulterants.—Leaflets of other species of *Pilocarpus* and of species of *Swartzia*.

XANTHOXYLUM N.F. (XANTHOXYLUM)

Synonyms.—Prickly Ash Bark, Toothache-Bark or Tree, Yellow Wood; *Fr.* Clavalier; *Ger.* Zahnwehrinde.

Botanical Origin.—(1) *Zanthoxylum americanum* Miller and (2) *Zanthoxylum Clava-Herculis* Linné.

Part Used.—The dried bark.

Purity Rubric.—Not more than 2 per cent. of foreign organic matter.

Habitat.—(1) In rocky woods and along streams, Quebec to Minnesota, south to Virginia, Kentucky, Missouri and Kansas. (2) In dry soil along the sandy coast from Virginia to Florida and west to Texas.

Plants.—*Zanthoxylum americanum* Miller, commercially known as Northern Prickly Ash, but also as Toothache Tree, Angelica Tree and Yellow- or Pepper Wood, is a shrub growing to the height of about 4 m. with grayish pungent bark covered with numerous white lenticels and scattered prickles. Its leaves are alternate, imparipinnate with 5 to 6 ovate-oblong leaflets that are downy when young. Its yellowish-green flowers appear before the leaves in sessile, axillary, umbellate clusters. Its fruit is a 2-valved capsule containing a single black seed.

Zanthoxylum Clava-Herculis L. known as Southern Prickly Ash, Sea-Ash or Prickly Yellow Wood, is a small tree attaining a height of 12 m. purple-gray, whose aromatic and pungent bark shows numerous corky cones through which prickles protrude. Its leaves are alternate, imparipinnate and prickly with 7 to 17 ovate-oblong leaflets that are shiny on the upper surface. Its flowers appear after the leaves in terminal cymes.

Description.—**Northern Prickly Ash Bark.**—In transversely curved fragments or quills, from 2 to 15 cm. in length; bark from 0.5 to 2 mm.

in thickness; outer surface light gray to brownish-gray with grayish patches of foliaceous lichens bearing numerous small black apothecia; longitudinally wrinkled and with numerous whitish lenticles; the cork occasionally abraded, showing the yellowish or orange inner bark; inner surface yellowish-white, finely longitudinally striate and usually with numerous, bright, shining crystals; fracture short, uneven; odor slight; taste bitter, acrid, becoming pungent.

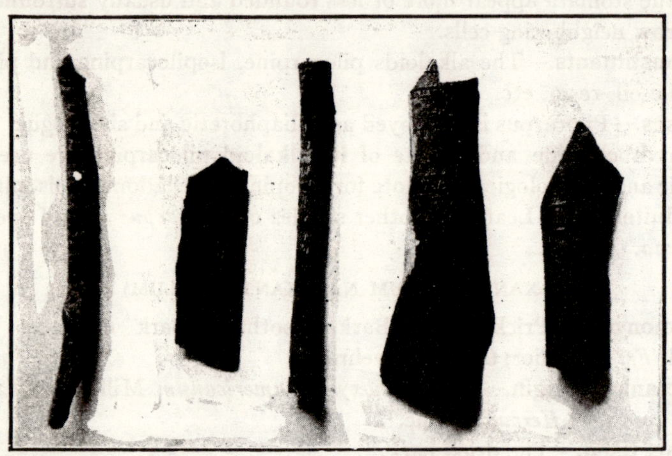

Fig. 136.—Northern prickly ash bark.

Histology of Northern Prickly Ash Bark.—Under the microscope transverse sections of Northern Prickly Ash Bark show an outer corky layer consisting of from 4 to 20 rows of cells, the tangential walls being more or less thickened and lignified; a wide stratum of collenchyma inside of the cork cambium composed of from 8 to 10 rows of tangentially elongated cells, with very thick walls and containing plastids; a more or less indistinct row of endodermal cells beneath which occur small groups of sclerenchyma fibers; the phloem consists of numerous parenchyma cells among which are included large oil-secretion reservoirs and occasionally a few stone cells, separated into phloem patches by medullary rays which are mostly one cell in width; the parenchyma cells as well as the oil-secretion reservoirs contain numerous colorless oily globules. Scrapings from either the inner or outer surface show numerous rod-shaped crystals and flat prisms, from 15μ to 240μ in length.

Southern Prickly Ash Bark.—In transversely curved or irregular, oblong, flattened pieces, or in quills from 2 to 40 cm. in length, bark from 1 to 4 mm. in thickness; outer surface light gray to brownish-gray, marked by numerous large, barnacle-shaped projections of cork, from 0.5 to 3.5 cm. in thickness, otherwise with numerous grayish patches of foliaceous lichens, bearing blackish apothecia, and numerous, elliptical lenticels; inner surface light yellowish-brown to olive brown, obscurely longitudinally striate and free from crystals; odor and taste as in Northern Prickly Ash Bark.

Histology of Southern Prickly Ash Bark.—Under the microscope, transverse sections of Southern Prickly Ash Bark show a strong development of lignified cork occurring in the form of rings, the successive layers being separated by several rows of narrow tabular cells strongly thickened on the tangential walls; beneath the cork cambium occurs a thin layer of

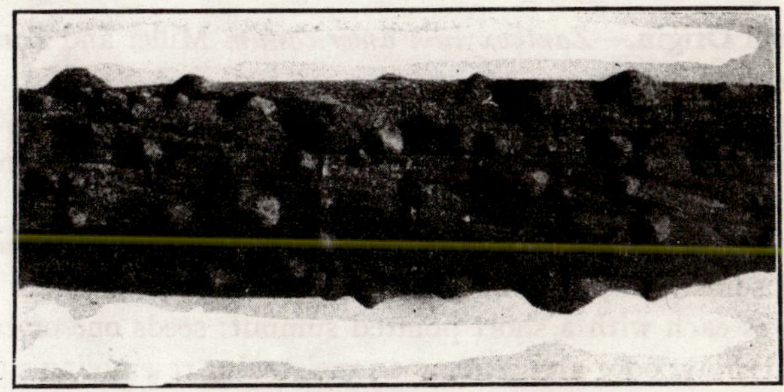

FIG. 137.—Southern prickly ash bark.

collenchyma followed by the outer tissues of the primary cortex and consisting of small groups of rather large stone cells and occasional, scattered groups of sclerenchyma fibers and parenchyma; the inner bark consists of parenchyma, a more or less indistinct sieve tissue among which are numerous, large, light yellowish oil-secretion reservoirs, medullary rays from 1 to 2 cells in width and occasional groups of stone cells and bast-fibers; starch grains numerous, nearly spherical, from 2μ to 10μ in diameter, and occurring in the parenchyma cells and medullary rays; calcium oxalate chiefly in monoclinic prisms from 10μ to 25μ in diameter, occurring in crystal fibers and in parenchyma cells of the primary cortex.

Powdered Southern Prickly Ash.—Grayish-brown; numerous cork cells, nearly colorless and strongly lignified, fragments of parenchyma containing either small starch grains, oily globules or monoclinic prisms of calcium oxalate; stone cells in small groups with thick, colorless walls and containing frequently a reddish-brown substance; bast-fibers few and non-lignified.

Powdered Northern Prickly Ash.—Similar to the preceeding but stone cells are comparatively few and there are fewer cork cells.

Constituents.—Two resins, an acrid volatile oil, an alkaloid, a phenolic compound termed zanthoxylin, etc.

Uses.—Stimulant, sialogogue, alterative. The bark is chewed for the relief of toothache.

Adulterant.—Southern Prickly Ash bark has been both adulterated with and substituted by the bark of *Aralia spinosa*, commonly known as Hercules Club. This can readly be detected by the presence of numerous sharp spines on its outer surface that are not mounted on corky cones.

XANTHOXYLI FRUCTUS N.F. (PRICKLY ASH BERRY)

Synonyms.—Toothache Tree Berries; *Fr.* Clavalier; *Ger.* Zahnwehbeeren.

Botanical Origin.—*Zanthoxylum americanum* Miller and *Zanthoxylum Clava-Herculis* Linné.

Part Used.—The dried fully grown fruit.

Purity Rubric.—Not more than 2 per cent. of foreign organic matter.

Habitat and Plant.—*See Xanthoxylum.*

Description.—Capsules with or without (*Z. Clava-Herculis*) short stalks, ellipsoidal, grayish-brown and dehiscent, when dry, into 2 convex carpel valves each with a short pointed summit; seeds one or two black, oblong, and shiny; odor aromatic, upon moistening resembling citral; taste warmly aromatic and pungent and followed by a tingling sensation upon chewing.

Constituents.—Volatile oil, resin, etc.

Use.—Prickly Ash Berry is employed as an ingredient in compound fluidextract of stillingia and compound syrup of stillingia N.F.

AURANTII DULCIS CORTEX U.S.P. (SWEET ORANGE PEEL)

Synonyms.—Orange Peel; *Fr.* Ecorce d'Oranges douces; *Ger.* Apfelsinenschalen.

Botanical Origin.—*Citrus Aurantium* var. *sinensis* Linné.

Part Used.—The fresh outer rind of the ripe fruit.

Habitat.—Northern India. Cultivated in Florida and California.

Plant.—*Citrus Aurantium* is a blunt spiny tree of medium height with leaves varying through the lighter shades of green, having an acuminate apex and a broadly-winged petiole. Flowers are fragrant, white, axillary, with 20–24 stamens and a globose ovary. Fruit is from 2¾–3¼ inches in diameter with hollow core, acid pulp and tight skin.

C. Aurantium var. sinensis Linné is the Sweet Orange (*C. sinensis* Osbeck). A solid core and sweet pulp characterizes the fruit.

Description.—The outer, orange yellow layer recently separated by grating or paring and consisting of epidermal cells, parenchyma cells of the sarcocarp with chromoplastids, oil reservoirs, globules of volatile oil and prismatic membrane crystals of calcium oxalate; odor fragrant; taste pungently aromatic.

Constituents.—Volatile oil, hesperidin, etc.

Uses.—Flavoring agent and source of oil of orange U.S.P.

AURANTII AMARI CORTEX U.S.P. (BITTER ORANGE PEEL)

Synonyms.—Seville Orange Peel, Wild Orange Peel, Curaçao Orange Peel; *Fr.* Ecorce d'Oranges amère; *Ger.* Pomeranzenschale.

Botanical Origin.—*Citrus Aurantium* Linné (*Citrus vulgaris* Risso).

Part Used.—The dried rind of the unripe fruit.

Habitat.—Northern India. Cultivated widely in the subtropics.

Plant.—A small tree attaining a height of about 10 or 15 feet and possessing greenish-brown bark, fragrant, evergreen, ovate, pellucid punctate, leaves and white flowers. The fruit is round, rough skinned, from 2 to 4 in. in diameter and contains a bitter, acid pulp.

Description.—In irregular bands (ribbons) or elliptical, somewhat curved, acutely pointed pieces (quarters), from 3 to 6 cm. in length and with recurved edges; outer surface yellowish or reddish or greenish-brown, roughened from fine reticulate ridges and numerous, minute pits, inner surface whitish, with many slight, conical projections and linear, anastomosing fibro-vascular bundles; fracture hard, short; odor fragrant and aromatic; taste aromatic and bitter.

Histology.—1. Outer epidermis (epicarp) of small angular cells.

2. Mesocarp, composed of (1) outer region of thick walled cells, some containing chloroplastids or chromoplastids, others membrane crystals of calcium oxalate, the latter up to 45μ in length. Arranged in two irregular rows within this zone are large oil reservoirs; (2) a broader inner region of branching cells surrounding large intercellular-air-spaces. Through this region course anastomosing fibrovascular bundles.

Constituents.—Volatile oil, the glucosides aurantiin and aurantiamarin; hesperidin, aurantiamaric acid, etc.

Uses.—Aromatic bitter and flavoring agent.

LIMONIS CORTEX U.S.P. (LEMON PEEL)

Synonyms.—*Fr.* Écorce de Limon; *Ger.* Limonenschale.

Botanical Origin.—*Citrus medica* var. *Limonum* (Risso) Hooker filius.

Part Used.—The outer yellow rind of the fresh ripe fruit.

Habitat.—Northern India. Cultivated in Italy, Sicily, Spain, Portugal, etc.

Plant.—A small, unevenly branched tree with stiff, short thorns and ovate, serrate, green leaves whose wingless petioles may have narrow margins. Flowers solitary or in clusters. The petals are white above and reddish-purple below. The stamens are from 20 to 40. The fruit is oval or oval-oblong, yellow, and has an acid pulp. An apical papilla is prominent. Seeds small and smooth.

Description.—The outer, lemon yellow or dark yellow layer, recently separated by grating or paring, and consisting of the epidermis, numerous parenchyma cells containing yellow chromoplastids, and large oil reservoirs with globules of the volatile oil; odor fragrant, distinctive; taste pungent, aromatic.

Histology.—The epidermis is composed of small tabular cells. The hypoderm contains numerous chromoplasts. The mesocarp has colorless, thin-walled parenchyma and large elliptical oil reservoirs; parenchyma cells contain a layer of granular protoplasm adhering to the walls and occasionally membrane crystals of calcium oxalate which are irregularly polygonal, 15 to 25μ in diameter.

Constituents.—Volatile oil, hesperidin, etc.

Use.—Flavoring agent.

SIMARUBACEÆ (AILANTHUS FAMILY)

A family of chiefly tropical shrubs or trees containing bitter principles. The leaves are alternate and pinnate. The flowers are diœcious or polygamous and arranged in axillary panicles (*Picrasma excelsa*) or racemes (*Quassia amara*). The plants are distinguished from those of the *Rutaceæ* by the absence of secretory cavities.

QUASSIA U.S.P. (QUASSIA)

Synonyms.—Bitter Wood, Bitter Ash, Lofty Quassia; *Fr.* Bois de Quassie; *Ger.* Lignum Quassiæ, Quassienholz.

Botanical Origin.—(1) *Picrasma excelsa* (Swartz) Planchon and (2) *Quassia amara* L.

Part Used.—Wood.

Habitat.—(1) West Indies; (2) Northern South America.

Plants.—*Picrasma excelsa* is a tree attaining the height of 24 m. with a trunk diameter of from .5 to 1 m. with grayish-brown, wrinkled bark and spreading branches. The leaves are imparipinnate with 9–17 ovate petiolate leaflets. The flowers are small, yellowish-green and borne in axillary panicles. The fruit is a small black drupe. *Quassia amara* varies from a shrub to a tree with spreading branches that bear 4–5 narrow obovate leaflets. The flowers are bright red and borne in terminal racemes. The fruit is a 5 chambered pod.

Production and Commerce.—There are two commercial varieties viz.: Jamaica from *Picrasma excelsa* and Surinam from *Quassia amara*. Jamaica Quassia is imported from Kingston and St. Ann's Bay, Jamaica

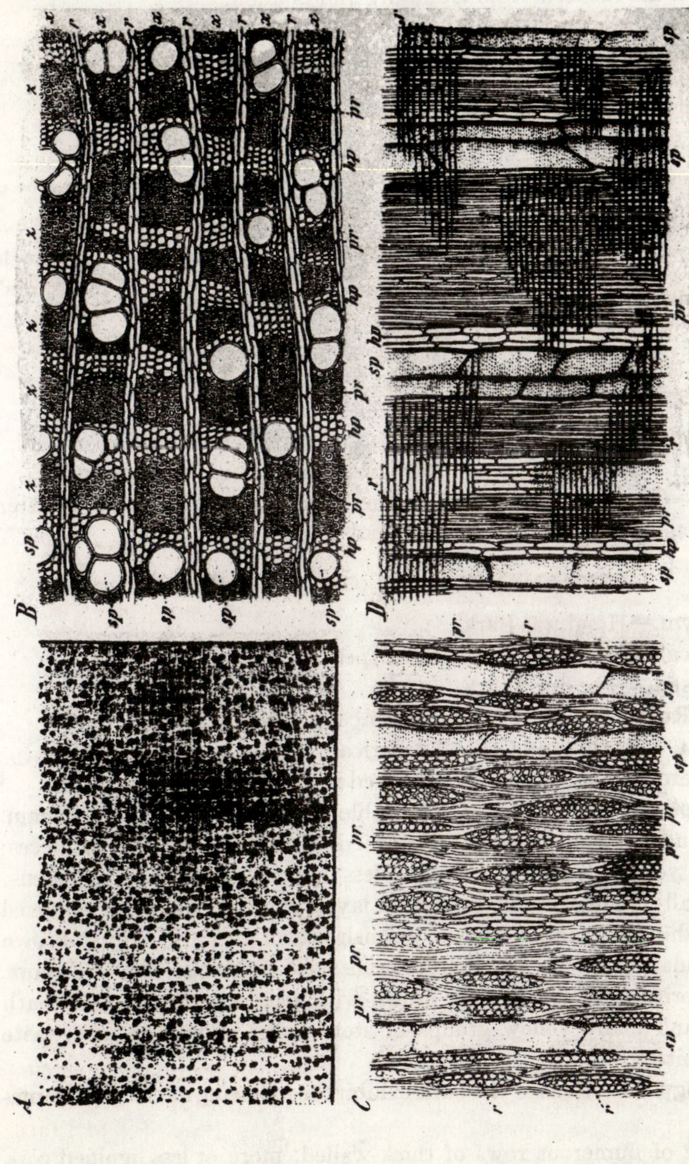

FIG. 138.—Jamaica Quassia. *A*, cross section of wood × 3. *B*, cross section of wood, × 65. *C*, tangential-longitudinal section of wood, × 65. *D*, radial-longitudinal section of wood, × 65. Wood parenchyma, *hp*; wood fibers, *pr*; tracheæ, *sp*; medullary rays, *r*, separating xylem patches, *x*. (*After Berg.*)

in the form of logs sawed from the trunk and thicker branches. It is also imported in the cut form from Hamburg and London.

Jamaica	Surinam
Usually in yellow chips, shavings or raspings, occasionally in billets.	Occurs similarly but billets usually thinner.

Microscopical Characteristics

Jamaica	Surinam
Tracheæ comparatively broad, usually in groups of 2–6, occasionally single and surrounded by numerous wood fibers.	Tracheæ narrower, single or in pairs, occasionally in groups of 3 or 4.
Medullary rays lignified, 1–5 cells wide and 10–20 rows deep.	Medullary rays lignified, 1–4 cells wide (mostly 1–2 cells wide) and 10–30 rows deep.
Calcuim oxalate in tetragonal or hexagonal prisms or micro-crystals, abundant in medullary rays.	Calcuim oxalate crystals absent.
Parenchyma lignified and in interrupted tangential bands.	Parenchyma similar.

Constituents.—Jamaica Quassia contains the bitter principles α-picrasmin and β-picrasmin, etc. Surinam Quassia contains quassins.

Uses.—Quassia is employed in the form of an infusion as a bitter tonic and as a rectal injection for thread worms in children.

CASCARA AMARGA N.F. (CASCARA AMARGA)

Synonym.—Honduras Bark.

Botanical Origin.—An unidentified species of *Picramnia* (?).

Part Used.—The dried bark.

Purity Rubric.—Not more than 2 per cent. of foreign organic matter.

Habitat.—Mexico and Central America.

Commercial.—The drug comes packed in matting from Honduras.

Description.—In long quills of variable diameter the bark up to 8 mm. thick, often in broken, irregular, flattened or transversely curved pieces; externally yellowish-brown, more or less covered with grayish-lichens, longitudinally fissured, with rough cork layers or with cork partly removed and reddish-brown; inner surface grayish-brown to dark reddish-brown with irregular striations and minute transverse markings; fracture short, hard and brittle; internally dark brown with a light yellow zone beneath the cork and many yellow groups of stone cells; odor indistinct; taste intensely bitter.

Histology.—Sections of the bark exhibit the following microscopic structure:

1. *Cork* of numerous rows of thick-walled, more or less lignified cork cells many containing a reddish or yellowish coloring material.
2. *Cork cambium* of meristematic cells.
3. *Cortex* composed of starch-parenchyma and isolated stone cells.

4. *Pericycle* composed of a nearly continuous ring of stone cells and scattered groups of sclerenchyma fibers associated with crystal fibers beneath which is a narrow zone of starch-parenchyma.

5. *Phloem*, separated into a number of phloem patches by starch-containing medullary rays mostly 1 to 4 cells wide and arranged in regular rows. Scattered about in the phloem will be noted groups of bast fibers adhering to which are crystal fibers containing monoclinic prisms of calcium oxalate. Numerous large groups of thick-walled stone cells are also scattered through this region. Sieve tubes and starchy-parenchyma occur between the lignified elements of each phloem patch.

Powdered Drug.—Light brown; numerous groups of sclerenchyma fibers adhering to which are crystal fibers containing monoclinic prisms of calcium oxalate, the latter up to 40μ in length; numerous stone cells isolated or in groups, fragments of medullary-rays and parenchyma containing single or 2- to 4-compound starch grains; fragments of cork tissue.

Constituents.—Bitter principle, starch, calcium oxalate, etc.

Uses.—Bitter tonic and employed as an ingredient of Compound Fluidextract of Trifolium N.F. and Compound Syrup of Trifolium N.F.

BURSERACEÆ (MYRRH FAMILY)

Shrubs and trees of tropical climes having schizogenous secretion reservoirs in their bark which contain gum, resin, and oil. Leaves alternate and compound. Flowers small, regular and hermaphrodite, arranged in racemes or panicles. Fruit a drupe.

MYRRHA U.S.P. (MYRRH)

Synonyms.—Gum Myrrh; *Fr.* Myrrhe; *Ger.* Myrrhe.

Botanical Origin.—*Commiphora Myrrha* (Nees) Baillon or other species of *Commiphora*.

Part Used.—A gum-resin.

Purity Rubric.—Not less than 30 per cent. of alcohol-soluble extractive and not more than 4 per cent. of acid-insoluble ash.

Habitat.—Northeastern Africa and Arabia.

Plants.—The genus *Commiphora* contains over 60 species. One of these, *Commiphora Myrrha* (Ness) Baillon, is a small tree which is claimed by Holmes to yield Myrrh. It has whitish-gray bark and rough, stunted, spiny branches, trifoliate leaves, dioecious flowers and oval-lanceolate, brown, drupaceous fruits.

Production and Commerce.—The trees grow in forests in the Red Sea districts of northeast Africa (Somaliland) and western Arabia. The gum-olea-resin, which is at first yellow, is formed in schizogenous secretion reservoirs in the bark and pith. It exudes spontaneously through natural fissures in the bark and through induced incisions. After hardening it becomes brownish-yellow to reddish-brown and is collected. There are three commercial varieties—African or Somali Myrrh, Arabian or Fadhli Myrrh and Yemen Myrrh. *African Myrrh* is considered the best variety. It is the most aromatic, and exhibits an unctuous, granular surface, often with whitish striae or spots, when fractured. It is sent from Somaliland to Aden for shipment to the world's markets. *Arabian Myrrh* is less aromatic and has a less dusty appearance than the African variety and is devoid of whitish markings internally. *Yemen Myrrh* is the least aromatic.

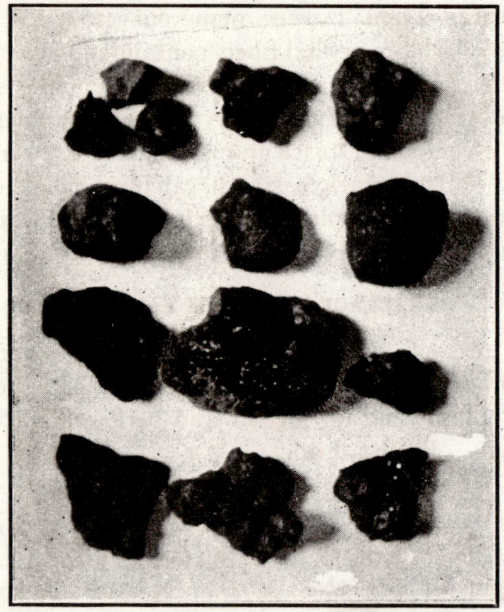

FIG. 139.—Myrrh. Note the masses and tears of variable size.

It occurs in large masses of a dark reddish-brown color which, when fractured, are devoid of an oily surface and whitish markings. It is shipped from Makullah, Arabia to Aden and Bombay. The commercial supplies of Myrrh are shipped chiefly from Aden, Arabia and from Bombay, India to Europe and America.

Description.—It occurs in brownish-yellow or reddish-brown rounded or irregular masses or tears covered with a brownish-yellow dust; fracture waxy, the internal surface occasionally marked with white lines; odor aromatic, characteristic; taste aromatic, bitter and acrid. Myrrh gives a purplish color with nitric acid. It yields a yellowish emulsion when triturated with water.

Constituents.—From 2.5 to 6.5 per cent. of a yellow volatile oil, from 25 to 35 per cent. of resin, gum, bitter principle, etc.

Uses.—Myrrh is used as an antiseptic mouthwash, emmenagogue, stimulant tonic and as an application to sore gums.

Adulterants.—(1) Gum resins from other species of *Commiphora*, notably the Bdelliums. These do not take a purple color with nitric acid. (2) Gums. (3) Sand. (4) Vegetable fragments.

MELIACEÆ (MAHOGANY FAMILY)

Tropical trees or shrubs with wood often hard, colored and odoriferous. Leaves alternate, exstipulate, pinnately compound, rarely simple and entire. Inflorescence a terminal or axillary raceme. Flowers hermaphrodite or rarely polygamo-diœcious, regular; sepals five to four, small; petals usually five to four, hypogynous; stamens generally ten to eight rarely five, very rarely twenty to sixteen, inserted outside the base of the hypogynous disc; filaments united into a tube; carpels usually five to three; style simple; ovary free, usually five- to three-celled. Fruit a drupe (*Melia*), berry (*Vavaea*), or capsule (*Cedrella*). Seeds exalbuminous or with fleshy albumen.

COCILLANA N.F. (COCILLANA)

Synonym.—Cocillana Bark, Guapi Bark.

Botanical Origin.—*Guarea Rusbyi* (Britton) Rusby.

Part Used.—The dried bark.

Purity Rubric.—Not more than 5 per cent. of wood or other foreign organic matter.

Habitat.—Bolivia, along the eastern slope of the Andes Mts.

Plant.—A tree.

Description.—In flat or curved pieces up to 2 cm. thick and of variable length and width; outer surface fissured, grayish-brown or gray from adherent lichens, frequently abraded in spots and then orange-brown; inner surface brown, coarsely and irregularly longitudinally striate; fracture of outer bark short, of inner bark splintery-fibrous and soft; odor characteristic; taste astringent and slightly nauseous.

Histology.—The outer bark exhibits one or more zones of cork alternating with parenchyma and isolated stone cells. The middle bark shows a matrix of starch-parenchyma scattered within which are groups of thick-walled stone cells and bundles of sclerenchyma fibers with accompanying crystal fibers. The inner bark shows large groups of bast fibers surrounded by crystal fibers which contain monoclinic prisms of calcium oxalate and separated tangentially by phloem parenchyma and sieve tissue and radially by wavy medullary rays, 1 to 3 cells in width. The medullary ray cells are often lignified and contain either starch or reddish amorphous masses. Secretory cells with a yellowish-white, granular, caoutchouc-like content occur in the parenchymatous regions.

Powdered Drug.—Light brown; numerous groups of lignified sclerenchyma fibers having pointed ends, some showing accompanying crystal fibers containing monoclinic prisms of calcium oxalate, the latter up to 25μ in length; fragments of parenchyma and medullary-rays with reddish-brown contents on starch grains; numerous angular or irregular stone cells

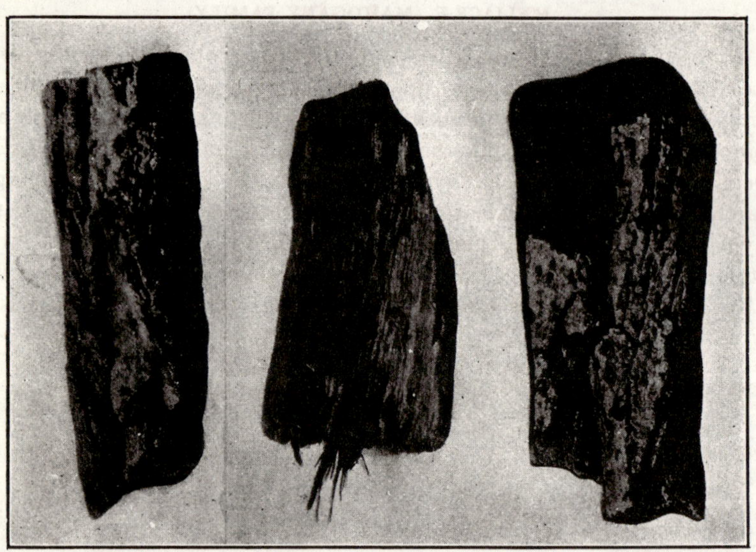

FIG. 140.—Cocillana bark. Outer surface of two pieces is shown on right and left, while inner surface aspect appears in central piece.

with thick, yellowish, lamellated and porous walls, up to 150μ in length; numerous single, spheroidal or 2- to 4-compound starch grains, the individual grains up to 20μ in diameter; fragments of dark brown cork.

Constituents.—The alkaloid rusbyine, resins, a caoutchouc-like substance, fixed oil, tannin, etc.

Use.—Cocillana is used as an expectorant.

POLYGALACEÆ (MILKWORT FAMILY)

Herbs or shrubs with upright, herbaceous or woody stems often branching profusely, the branches occasionally becoming geotropic or subterranean and bearing cleistogamous flowers. Leaves simple, often lanceolate or linear, exstipulate, alternate. Inflorescence a raceme, spike (*Polygala Senega*) or head (*P. lutea*). Flowers irregular, hermaphroditic with commonly eight stamens. Fruit a two-celled capsule (*P. Senega*), rarely a drupe or samara. Pollen grains barrel-shaped.

SENEGA U.S.P. (SENEGA)

Synonyms.—Seneca Snakeroot, Senega Snakeroot, Rattlesnake Root Mountain Flax; *Ger.* Senegawurzel; *Fr.* Polygala de Virginie.

Botanical Origin.—*Polygala Senega* Linné.

Part Used.—The dried root.

Limit of Impurities.— Five per cent. of stems or other foreign organic matter.

Habitat.—In woods and rocky soil of Southern Canada and Eastern United States as far south as South Carolina and west to Wisconsin, Minnesota and Missouri.

Plant.—A perennial herb whose underground portion consists of a conical, twisted, branched root with a knotty crown. The aerial portion consists of several erect or ascending, smooth stems arising to the height of 1.5 to 3 dm. and bearing alternate, sessile, lanceolate or oblong-lanceolate bright green leaves with rough margins. The inflorescence consists of a close spike of small, white flowers that differ from some of the Polygalas in being chasmogamous. The fruit is a small, loculicidally dehiscent, 2-celled capsule containing 2 black seeds, each of which has a caruncle of about the same length as the seed.

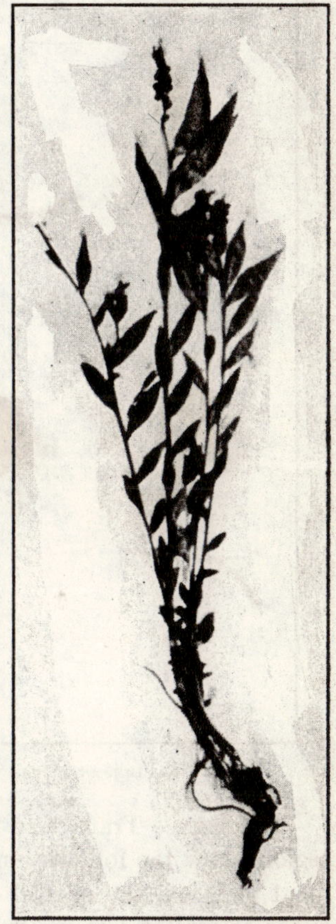

FIG. 141.—Polygala Senega.

Production and Commerce.—There are two commercial varieties of this drug *e.g.*, Northern and Southern Senega. The Northern Senega is collected mainly in the province of Manitoba and in Minnesota; the Southern, mainly from Virginia to Texas. The root should be dug in autumn, cleaned and carefully dried. The commercial supplies used in the United States come mainly from Saskatchewan, Canada, Minnesota, Georgia and South Carolina.

Description.—This drug occurs as a mixture of entire, conical, more or less tortuous and branched roots and broken pieces thereof together with detached rootlets; when entire the roots are up to 8 cm. (Southern Senega) or 15 cm. (Northern Senega) in length and up to 7 mm. (Southern Senega) or 12 mm. (Northern Senega) in thickness; externally brownish-yellow or dark brown purplish near crown (Northern Senega), the crown being rose tinted with numerous buds and short stem bases, the rest of the root longitudinally wrinkled and frequently marked by a keel; fracture short, wood pale yellow, usually eccentrically developed; odor peculiar, methyl salicylate like, taste sweetish, afterwards acrid.

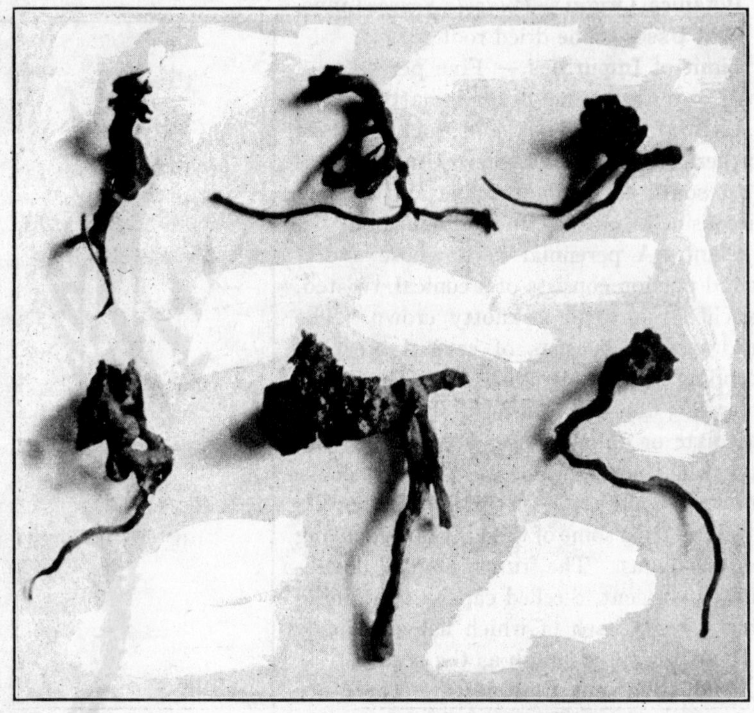

FIG. 142.—Senega. Note the multiple crown and keel. × ½.

Histology.—Transverse sections of the root, cut through the keel region, show the following microscopic peculiarities: An eccentric development of wood, the central cylinder varying in outline from elliptical or ovate or reniform to irregularly fan-shaped or even separated by broad wood parenchyma rays into 2 or more masses and being surrounded by an unevenly developed cortex and phloem which is thickest next to the broadest strands of wood, and where the wood-wedges are shorter or absent and the parenchyma rays very broad, the cortex and phloem occupy a proportionately narrower zone of the cross-section; in older roots a corky layer of from 4 to 5 rows of tangentially elongated, light yellowish or yellowish-brown cells; outer bark of about 20 rows of cells on one side of the root and only 10 or less on the other, the cells having slightly thickened walls and containing a colorless or pale yellow, amorphous substance, which is liberated in the form of large globules on the addition of a drop of potassium hydroxide T.S.; inner bark, the cells in radial rows, consisting of parenchyma, small groups of sieve tissue and medullary rays, the latter from 1

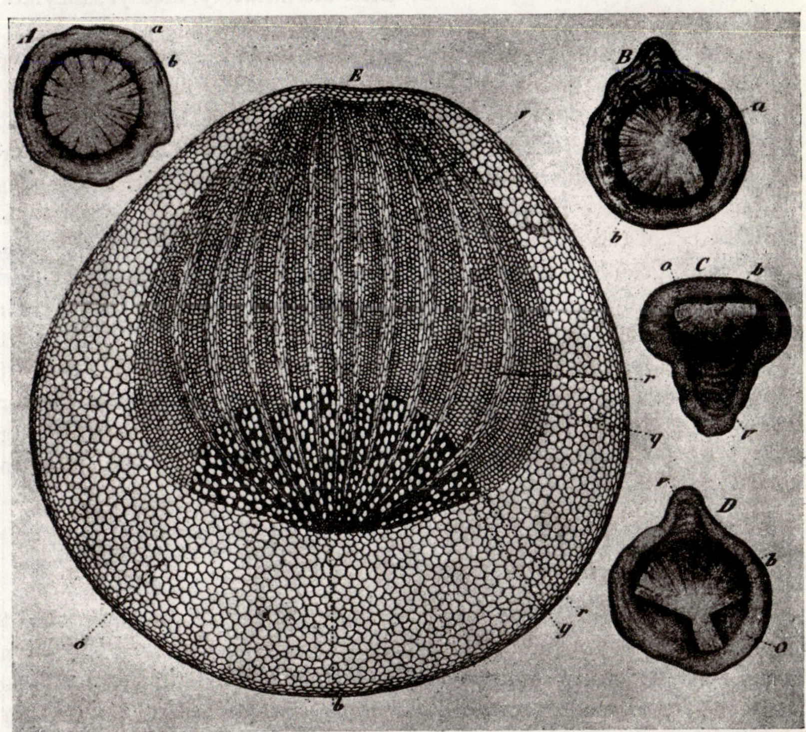

FIG. 143.—*Senega.* *A, B, C, D,* Transverse sections through Senega root at different levels showing the characteristic variation of the cortex, phloem and wood. *E,* Transverse section through the keel portion of a root approaching that of Fig. *C.* in conformation, × 60. The phloem, extending out from the half circle of xylem, has pressed as a blunt cone into the keel and has crowded out the cortex which is alone completely developed on the opposite side. *a,* bark; *b,* wood; *o,* cortex; *r,* medullary rays; *sp,* tracheæ; *t,* phloem; *w,* cambium; *y,* xylem. (*After Berg.*)

to 3 cells wide; all the cells in this zone show a collenchymatous thickening of the walls and contain an amorphous substance similar to that found in cells of the outer bark; woody layer of tracheæ with bordered pores, wood-fibers with oblique simple pores, tracheids, and medullary rays, the latter being rather indistinct and resembling the wood-fibers; tissues of the central region of wood colored yellowish- or reddish-brown on the addition of a drop of potassium hydroxide T.S.

Powdered Drug.—Brownish-yellow and consisting of fragments of lignified simple and bordered pored tracheæ, non-lignified, thick walled wood fibers, parenchyma containing a pale yellow amorphous substance and collenchymatic medullary-ray cells.

Constituents.—The glucosides senegin and polygalic acid, the former being of the nature of a saponin, the latter sternutatory, methyl salicylate, pectin, resin, sugar, etc.

Methyl salicylate occurs in greatest quantities in the recently gathered drug as well as in the dried drug that has been carefully prepared and stored. Its presence may be determined by the following test:

Extract 10 Gm. of the powdered drug with the aid of a Soxhlet apparatus, using 50 cc. of ether and 2 drops of hydrochloric acid, continuing the extraction for 4 hours and replacing any ether lost by evaporation. Take 25 cc. of this solution and evaporate on the water bath to dryness. Dissolve the residue in 10 cc. of chloroform, transfer to a test tube and pour 5 cc. of sulphuric acid beneath the solution. A reddish-brown color should be produced at the zone of contact between the liquids. If 10 cc. of the original ether solution be placed in a beaker in which 10 cc. of water has been previously placed and the mixture warmed on the water bath until the ether has evaporated, the aqueous solution, upon filtering and adding a few drops of ferric chloride solution, should take on a pinkish purple color.

Use.—Stimulating expectorant in sub-acute and chronic bronchitis.

EUPHORBIACEÆ (SPURGE FAMILY)

Often herbaceous, more rarely shrubby, rather seldom arborescent plants. Stem, leaves and other parts in several genera traversed by latex canals that are either ramifying cells (*Euphorbia*) or laticiferous vessels (*Manihot*, *Hevea*, etc.) or rows of laticiferous sacs (*Micrandra*) and contain a white latex with acrid, often poisonous contents or alkaloid or hydrocarbon, at times, rubber contents. Leaves alternate, exstipulate to stipulate, simple to pinnate or palmate. Inflorescence cymose. Flowers usually, as in *Ricinus*, etc., pentamerous, diclinous; sepals five, green, aposepalous, becoming rudimentary or absent in *Anthostema* and *Euphorbia*. Petals none or five, more or less petaloid; stamens numerous to ten to five or one (*Euphorbia*); pistillate flowers rarely of twenty to ten apocarpous or loosely syncarpous carpels (Sandbox tree), commonly of three syncarpous carpels with distinct radiate styles; ovary as many-celled as carpels with two to one ovules in each cell. Fruit a tricoccoid regma or capsule, rarely winged, indehiscent, nut-like. Seeds with oily endosperm. Flowers at times surrounded and subtended by more or less petaloid and expanded bracts and bracteoles.

RICINUS (CASTOR OIL SEED)

Synonyms.—Castor Bean, Castor-oil Plant, Palma Christi; *Ger.* Ricinussamen; Fr. Semences de ricin.

Botanical Origin.—*Ricinus communis* Linné.

Part Used.—The dried ripe seed.

Habitat.—India. Widely naturalized and cultivated.

Plant.—The castor-oil plant is either found under cultivation or growing wild in most tropical and warm temperate countries. It varies from an annual, monoecious herb in temperate regions to a tree attaining the height of 40 feet in the tropics. There are hundreds of forms of the plant which vary in size, color of stem and leaves, leaf markings, branching, size,

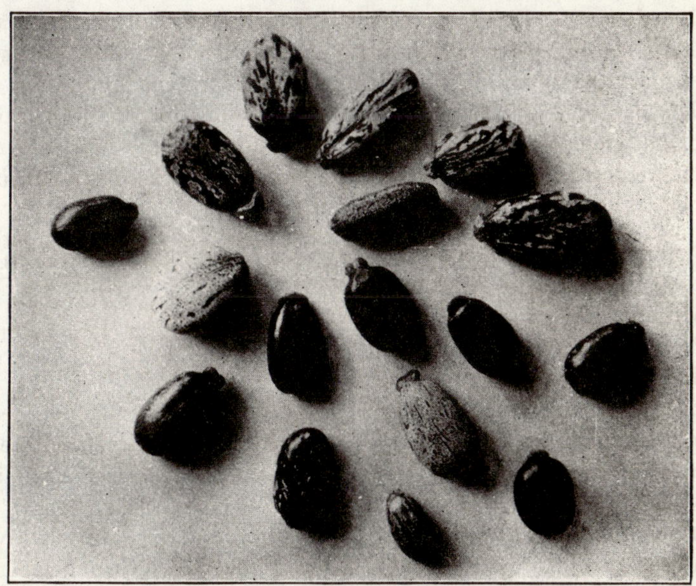

FIG. 144.—Castor Oil seeds (*Ricinus communis*).

color and markings of seeds, etc. The leaves are large, alternate, peltate, palmately 5–12 lobed, the lobes serrate or dentate. The inflorescence is a raceme of staminate and pistillate flowers, the staminate flowers occurring above the pistillate on the floral axis. The fruit is a 3-celled capsule covered generally with soft spines and dehiscing into 3 cocci, each containing an ovoid albuminous seed.

Production and Commerce.—Most of the commercial castor seed is produced in India and South America, although Italy and Oklahoma have been furnishing fair sized lots. The castor oil is obtained from the seed chiefly by the "cold press" method, castor oil cake or pomace being a by-product.

Description.—Seed ovate-oblong, from 8 to 18 mm. in length and up to about 8 mm. in breadth, flattened on the ventral surface, the dorsal surface convex; at one end is a wart-like caruncle covering the micropyle from which a line-like raphe extends to the chalaza at the other end of the seed; testa smooth, glossy and brittle, grayish or gray-brown and marbled with reddish-brown to black spots and lines; tegmen white, membranous adhering to the large, yellowish-white, oily endosperm which surrounds a straight embryo; embryo extending lengthwise between the halves of endosperm and consisting of 2 papery cotyledons and a conical hypocotyl; nearly inodorous; taste oily and acrid.

Constituents.—Fixed oil (Oleum Ricini U.S.P.) (45 to 50 per cent.) consisting of the glycerides of ricinoleic, isoricinoleic, dihydroxystearic acids, etc.; a toxalbumose called ricin, lipase and protein.

Uses.—Castor-oil seeds are employed mainly for the preparation of castor oil which is extensively used as a purgative and lubricant. The cake representing the residue after extracting the oil is used as a fertilizer.

TIGLIUM (CROTON SEED)

Synonyms.—Croton-oil Seed, Physic Nut, Purging Croton; *Ger.* Kroton; *Fr.* Graines de Tilly.

Botanical Origin.—*Croton Tiglium* Linné.

Part Used.—The dried ripe seed.

Habitat.—Southeastern Asia.

Plant.—A small tree growing to the height of 15 to 20 ft. and bearing alternate, acuminate, petiolate leaves which vary in color from metallic green to bronze and orange, 3-celled capsular fruits and ovoid albuminous seeds.

Production and Commerce.—The Croton trees are cultivated extensively in India and Ceylon for the seed from which the official croton oil is obtained. The commercial supplies of seed are shipped chiefly from Columbo, Ceylon and Bombay, India in bags. Occasional lots come indirectly through London.

Description.—Seed albuminous, ovate-oblong, slightly quadrangular, convex on the dorsal and somewhat flattened on the ventral surface; from 10 to 15 mm. in length; externally dull grayish-brown, often mottled with black due to abrasion of the testa; caruncle readily detached and usually absent in the drug of commerce; in other features resembling castor seed.

Constituents.—About 50 per cent. of fixed oil (Oleum Tiglii U.S.P.) containing croton-resin to which its active properties are ascribed; the toxic albumoses termed croton-albumin and croton-globulin; proteids, a lipase, etc.

Uses.—The seeds are used for the production of croton oil, the latter being used as a vesicant, counter-irritant and drastic purgative.

Allied Drug.—The Purging Nut, *Jatropa Curcas* Linné (Fam. *Euphorbiaceæ*) indigenous to Tropical America, yields Curcas seed, from which a yellowish, purgative oil is obtained. The seeds somewhat resemble croton seeds but their testa is dull black and marked with wrinkles and white patches. They contain the toxalbumose, curcin.

STILLINGIA N.F. (STILLINGIA)

Synonyms.—Queen's Root, Queen's Delight, Silver Leaf; *Fr.* and *Ger.* Stillingie.

Botanical Origin.—*Stillingia sylvatica* Linné.

Part Used.—The dried root.

Purity Rubric.—Not more than 3 per cent. of foreign organic matter. "Stillingia which has been stored for more than 2 years must not be used." N.F.

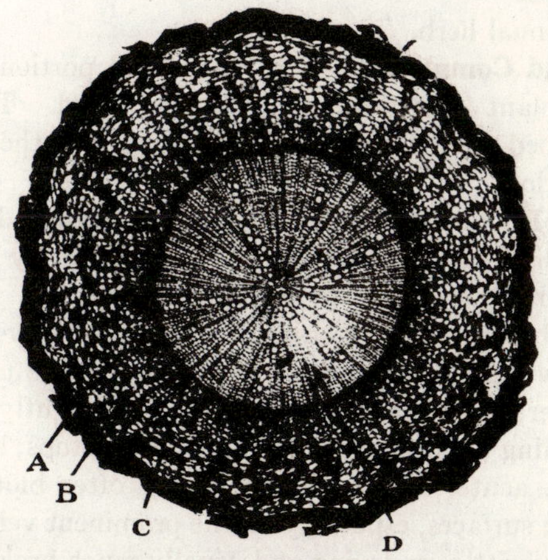

FIG. 145.—Stillingia—Cross-section of root. (17 diam.) (*A*) Cork; (*B*) parenchyma of cortex; (*C*) medullary ray; (*D*) xylem. (*From Sayre.*)

Habitat.—Southeastern United States, from Virginia to Florida.

Plant.—A perennial monoecious herb containing milk juice. From an underground, branched, slenderly fusiform root arises a smooth, erect stem which bears sessile, lanceolate, serrate leaves and yellow terminal spikes of flowers. The fruit is a rough, greenish-brown, 3-celled capsule, each cell containing a single seed.

Description.—When entire, terete, unequally tapering, rarely branched, usually in pieces attaining a length of 40 cm. and from 0.5 to 3 cm. in diameter, externally reddish-brown, longitudinally wrinkled; fracture very fibrous; internally the bark is light reddish-brown, thick, spongy, finely fibrous, with numerous resin cells and easily separable from the porous, radiate wood; odor distinct; taste bitter, acrid and pungent.

Constituents.—Volatile oil, acrid fixed oil, acrid resin termed sylvacrol, tannin, starch, calcium oxalate, etc.

Uses.—Stillingia is used as an alterative and antiluetic, frequently in combination with other drugs.

EUPHORBIA N.F. (EUPHORBIA)

Synonym.—Euphorbia Pilulifera, Pill Bearing Spurge, Snake Weed, Cat's Hair.

Botanical Origin.—*Euphorbia hirta* Linné.

Part Used.—The dried herb.

Purity Rubric.—Not more than 5 per cent. of foreign organic matter and not more than 3 per cent. of acid-insoluble ash.

Habitat.—India.

Plant.—An annual herb.

Production and Commerce.—The overground portion is collected in India when the plant is in flower or fruit and dried. The commercial supplies are shipped from India, those imported into the United States coming from London.

Description.—Roots usually present, small, branched, and reddish; stems slender, cylindrical, obliquely erect, dichotomously branched from near the base, branches recurved at apices; branches and stem only sparsely leafed at base, pale greenish-brown, rough or hairy; stems coarsely pilose with yellow hairs which are rather dense on the upper parts but sparse on the lower; pubescence consisting of short, slightly curved, unicellular hairs, becoming almost hispid at the flowering tops; leaves opposite, oblong-lanceolate, acute, serrulate, dark green, often blotched with red, pubescent on both surfaces, especially on the prominent veins on the lower surface, becoming brittle on drying and usually much broken in the drug; flowers small, numerous, in short peduncled axillary cymes; fruits about 1 mm. in diameter, yellow 3-celled capsules; seeds about 0.9 mm. in diameter, tetragonal, pale brown. Odor aromatic and characteristic; taste faintly bitter, aromatic and acrid.

Constituents.—Resins, caoutchouc, glucoside, tannin, gum, etc.

Use.—Euphorbia is employed as a constituent of certain asthma preparations, including Antiasthmatic Elixir N.F.

CASCARILLA (CASCARILLA)

Synonyms.—Sweetwood Bark, Sweet Bark. *Fr.* Ecorce éluthérienne; *Ger.* Kaskarillrinde.

Botanical Origin.—*Croton Eluteria* (Linné) Bennett.

Part Used.—The dried bark.

Habitat.—West Indies.

Plant.—A shrub.

Commercial Source.—Nassau, on island of New Providence, West Indies.

Description.—In quills or curved pieces from 0.5 to 2.5 mm. in thickness, externally gray, somewhat fissured; the corky layer easily detached, more or less coated with a white lichen; the uncoated surface dull-brown, inner surface smooth; fracture short, the fractured surface having a resinous and radially striate appearance. Odor characteristic, strong and musk-like when the bark is burned; taste warm, aromatic and very bitter.

Powdered Drug.—The powdered drug is pale-brown and has an odor resembling that of clove. When examined under the microscope, it exhibits simple starch grains up to 13μ in diameter and occasionally two- to three-compound; calcium oxalate in monoclinic crystals or rosette aggregates up to 25μ in diameter; fragments of parenchyma tissue, some of the cells containing starch, calcium oxalate or tannin; cells filled with reddish-brown resin or yellow oil; somewhat lignified cork cells, polygonal in outline with evenly thickened, lamellated walls and irregular lumina; non-porous bast fibers, some with lignified walls, up to 16μ in diameter; tracheæ with bordered pores very few or absent.

Constituents.—Volatile oil containing eugenol; resin, a crystalline bitter principle (cascarillin), vanillin, tannin, starch, etc.

Use.—Aromatic bitter.

KAMALA (KAMALA)

Synonyms.—Rottlera, Kameela, Glandulæ Rottleræ.

Botanical Origin.—*Mallotus philippinensis* Müller Argoviensis.

Part Used.—The hairs of the capsules.

Habitat.—Southeastern Asia.

Plant.—A shrub with evergreen leaves and glandular-hairy, 3-celled capsules.

Production and Commerce.—The plants abound in Indo-China and India where the capsules are gathered by the natives who remove the hairs by rolling the capsules in baskets and rubbing the surface of the fruits. The hairs form a red powder, which is then passed through a sieve to remove sand and other impurities. The drug is shipped from Indo-China and India to the various markets of the world.

Description.—A brick-red, granular, inodorous and tasteless powder which when examined under the microscope shows numerous more or less spheroidal glandular hairs with a one-celled stalk and a glandular head of

20 to 40 or more radiately elongated cells, more or less separated, and an upraised or depressed cuticle. Amongst these glandular hairs will be found stellate aggregate hairs which are generally curved or hooked at their ends. Particles of sand and fragments of epidermis of capsule may also be seen in the field.

Constituents.—An active taenifuge principle called rottlerin, a red resin, a yellow resin, wax, coloring matter, etc.

Use.—Kamala is used as a taenifuge and a dye-stuff.

Adulterants.—Ferric oxide, sand, colored starch, etc.

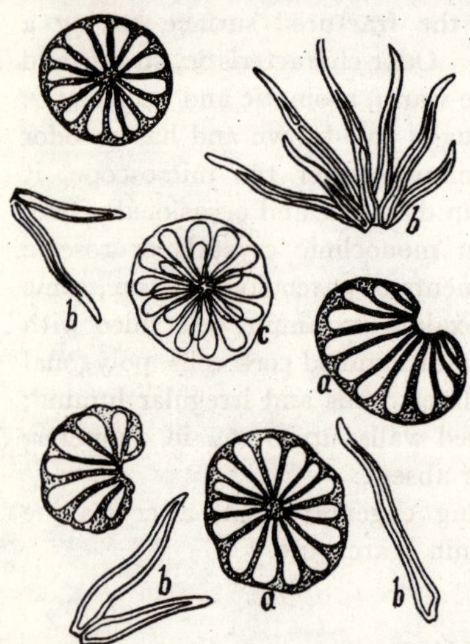

FIG. 146.—Kamala. (*a*) Deep reddish brown glandular trichomes; (*b*) aggregate simple trichomes; (*c*) gland decolorized with a weak solution of potassium hydrate. (*Schneider*.)

Substitute.—Wars or wurus, consisting of the hairs of the fruits of *Flemingia congesta* Roxb. (Fam. *Leguminosæ*). This material has a dull purple color and is distinguished microscopically by its somewhat ellipsoidal shaped glandular hairs and simple, 2-celled, non-glandular hairs, the basal cell of which is short, the terminal elongate and pointed.

ANACARDIACEÆ (SUMAC FAMILY)

Shrubs or trees producing in stems and leaves secretion contents that are either acrid watery or acrid opalescent or white viscid, viscid acrid and poisonous. Leaves alternate, rarely opposite, simple (*Rhus Cotinus*), three-foliate (*Rhus toxicodendron*) or pinnate (*Rhus glabra*, *R. venenata*, etc.). Inflorescence frequently terminal and composed of racemes or cymes, often reduced to a simple raceme. Flowers small, clustered, green, greenish-white to greenish-yellow; sepals five, rarely six or four, green, small; petals five, smaller than sepals; stamens equal in number to the petals and alternate, rarely fewer, sometimes double in number, rarely indefinite, inserted hypogynously or upon an enlarged disc that surrounds or swells up between stamens and pistil; pistil monocarpellary, more rarely bicarpellary, very rarely, as in *Spondieæ*, of ten to five carpels, ovary one-celled with single ovule. Fruit a drupe. Seeds exalbuminous with large embryo filling seed cavity.

RHUS GLABRA U.S.P. (RHUS GLABRA)

Synonyms.—Sumac Berries, Scarlet Sumac Fruit, Sleek; *Fr.* Sumac; *Ger.* Sumach.

Botanical Origin.—*Rhus glabra* Linné.

Part Used.—The dried ripe fruit.

Limit of Impurities.—5 per cent. of stems or other foreign organic matter.

Habitat.—In old waste fields and along fences in Canada and United States.

Plant.—*Rhus glabra* commonly know as Smooth Upland Sumac and Scarlet-, White- or Sleek Sumac varies from a shrub to rarely a tree, growing to the height of 1 to 6 m. The stems are smooth and somewhat glaucous. The leaves are alternate, exstipulate, imparipinnate with from 11 to 31 lanceolate or oblong-lanceolate leaflets. Each leaflet is dark green above,

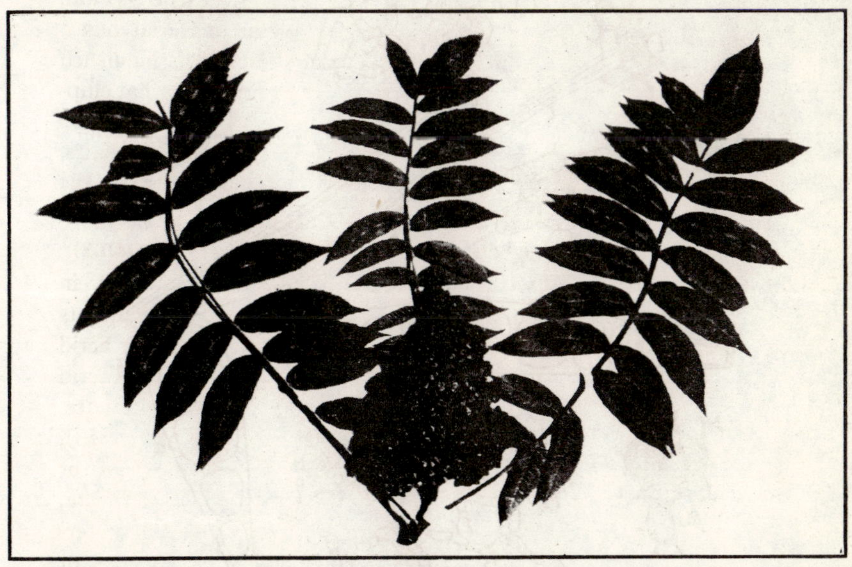

FIG. 147.—*Rhus glabra*. Branch with three imparipinnate leaves and a pyramidal cluster of drupes. The latter alone are official.

whitish beneath, acuminate at the summit, rounded or oblique at the base and sharply serrate along the margin. Their color changes to red in autumn. The flowers are small, green and polygamous and arranged on erect terminal thyrses. The fruit is a crimson drupe containing a single exalbuminous seed. The bark and leaves of this plant are employed in the tanning and dyeing industries.

Description.—The drug occurs in the forms of entire drupes. Each is subglobular, somewhat compressed, 3.5 to 5.5 mm. in length and 2 to 4 mm. in diameter; externally dark-red, velvety with short hairs, summit with remnants of short style, base occasionally with a five-cleft calyx and slender pedicel; epicarp and mesocarp, thin; endocarp smooth and shiny, reddish; seed dark brown, very hard, exalbuminous; odorless, taste sour and astringent.

Powdered Drug.—Brownish-red. Non-glandular hairs numerous, elliptical, spatulate or ovoid, uniseriate, up to 300μ in length, containing a

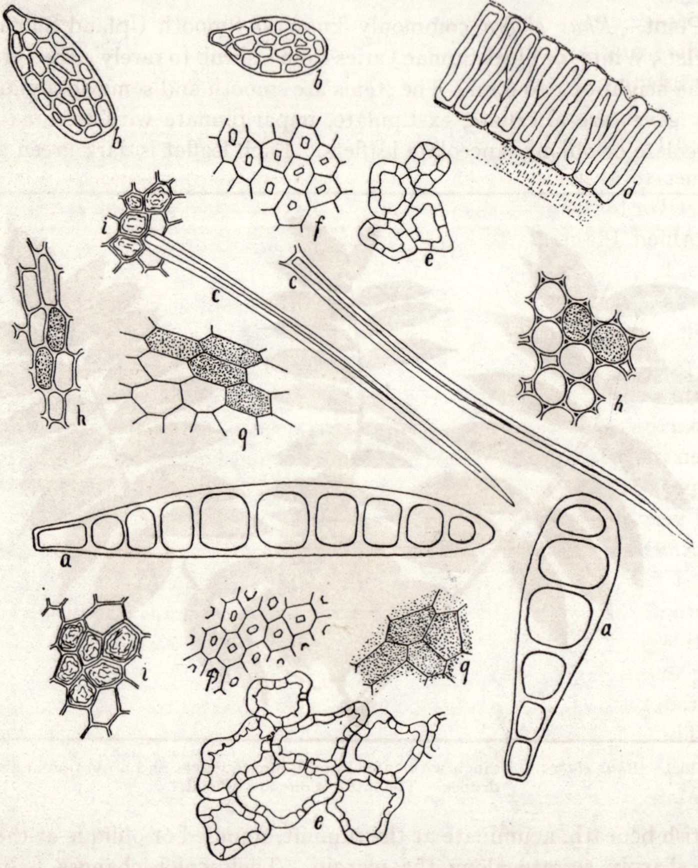

FIG. 148.—Powdered Rhus Glabra. (*a*) Deep red, uniseriate non-glandular trichomes; (*b*) brownish-red or brown glandular trichomes; (*c*) colorless unicellular trichomes; (*d*) outer layer of seed coat, lateral view; (*e*) thick-walled porous cells of testa; (*f*) colorless crystal-bearing layer of testa; (*g*) endosperm cells; (*h*) parenchyma of pericarp; (*i*) epidermal cells of pericarp. (*After Schneider.*)

pink or red cell-sap and often rod-shaped crystals; glandular hairs brownish or brownish-red, numerous, with a short, unicellular stalk and multicellular head; numerous fragments of endosperm; fragments of endocarp containing small stone cells with irregularly thickened walls and taking a red color with phloroglucin and hydrochloric acid; fragments of embryo with small angular cells containing aleurone and fixed oil; occasional fragments of reddish epicarp, with adhering mesocarp containing spiral tracheæ.

Constituents.—Tannin, gallic acid, acid calcium and potassium malates, fixed oil, coloring matter, etc.

Uses.—Rhus Glabra is employed as an astringent in gargles and as a refrigerant.

Substitute.—The fruits of *Rhus typhina* L. Staghorn Sumac, a small tree or shrub growing in lower Canada and the United States, are recognized by many to be superior to the official article on account of their higher total acidity. These fruits may be distinguished from those of *R. glabra* by being densely covered with long, linear, crimson hairs.

Allied Plants.—*Rhus toxicodendron* of American authors (*Rhus radicans* L.), commonly known as Poison Ivy, Three-leaved Ivy or Poison Oak is a woody vine, climbing by aerial rootlets, or an erect bushy plant, having several races that differ in habit and shape of leaves. The leaves are petioled, 3-foliate, each leaflet being short petioled, ovate or rhombic, entire or slightly sinuate or dentate, acuminate, inequilateral, rounded or narrowed at the base. The inflorescence is an axillary panicle of small green flowers. The fruit is a glabrous or slightly pubescent, grayish drupe. It is abundant throughout the greater part of the United States and very poisonous.

Rhus toxicodendron was official in the sixth and seventh editions of the U.S.P. The fresh leaflets made into a fluidextract are employed internally in the treatment of nervous disorders and in dermatötherapy, particularly in the treatment of poisoning by the same plant. Rost and Gilg make mention of it as having been used in the treatment of cancer (Ber. d. Deut. Pharm. Gesellsch. vol. 22, pp. 300, 332, 1912).

There are probably no other plants in existence which cause as much human distress and suffering as *Rhus toxicodendron* and *Rhus venenata.*

Many substances are referred to in the literature as causing the dermatitis produced by these plants. They include a vapor, gas, volatile alkaloid, volatile acid, infection by bacteria, glucoside, non-volatile acid, resin, polyhydric phenol and a non-volatile oil.

That the poisonous substance was a non-volatile oil, which resinifies on exposure to the atmosphere, was discovered by Pfaff (Merck's Report, vol. 19, p. 95, 1910) who found it to exist in all parts of the plant.

As to how this non-volatile oil comes in contact with individuals, the consensus of opinion seems to be that the winds and domestic animals carry the pollen grains and hairs. Pfaff and Schwalbe found the pollen grains and hairs to contain the poisonous substance. On the other hand, Rost and Gilg, in a very extensive work (Ber. d. Deut. Pharm. Gesellsch.

vol. 22, pp. 300–332, 1912) were unable to find the poison in the hairs and pollen from these plants.

Rhus venenata De Candolle is commonly known as swamp-sumac, poison sumac, poison elder and poison dogwood. The latter synonym must not be confused with the flowering dogwood, which is a member of the *Cornaceæ* family.

It is a shrub possessing a slender clustered stem, which sometimes takes a tree-like form, reaching to a considerable height. The stem is brittle, showing for the most part a pithy region internally. The leaves are 7–13 foliate, with slender reddish green petioles. The leaflets are obovate, oblong, dark green and glossy on the ventral surface, paler on the dorsal side, and without marginal teeth. The midrib and veins are prominent. The flowers are diœcious and are in narrow axillary panicles, yellowish green to white in color. The petals are slightly reflexed. The stamens appear nearly twice as long as the petals. The fruit is a smooth, white drupe, often remaining on the branches until spring. The leaf scars are prominent, alternate and of a somewhat crescent shape. The bark on young stems is mottled with conspicuous lenticels.

HISTOLOGY OF STEM

We find the epidermis to be composed of a single layer of epidermal cells with a thick outer cuticle. The subepidermal region shows a couple of layers of cork cells, more or less tangentially elongated. The cortex region is compact in nature and consists for the most part of sclerosed parenchyma. Numerous rosette aggregate crystals of calcium oxalate are found in this region. Resin canals are present in the primary cortex, which, according to Solereder, is common in the *Rhus venenata*. The structure of the pericycle varies according to the age of the plant. In the older stems isolated groups of sclerenchyma fibers occur usually in the form of adjacent arcs. The convex side of each of these is directed towards the exterior. The inner concave side of each arches over a dome-shaped phloem in the centre of which is a single resin canal. In younger stems the arcs (strands) of sclerenchyma fibers are joined with each other by means of sclerosed parenchyma. In this way the pericycle consitutes a continuous ring of stereomatic structure, which covers the phloem-containing resin canals as a single band. A zone of cambium cells, more or less collapsed, is found separating the phloem region from the xylem. The prosenchyma forming the structure of the wood has simple and bordered pores. The medullary-rays are usually one and two cells wide, with four cells as the maximum width. As stated by Solereder (Syst. Anat. of Dicotyledons vol. 1, p. 245) the resin canals, which are characteristic for the plants of *Anacardiaceæ*, often extend from the bast region and penetrate into the medullary region, where they end blindly. The canals are narrow-branching vessels filled with a dark reddish brown substance of a resinous nature. This substance responded to the cyanin test for resin. On treatment with alcoholic potash solution the resinous material combines with it to form a nigrescent compound. This reaction is characteristic of the poisonous substance causing the dermatitis produced by poisonous species of *Rhus* plants. The pith consists of thin-walled parenchyma cells with an occasional duct.

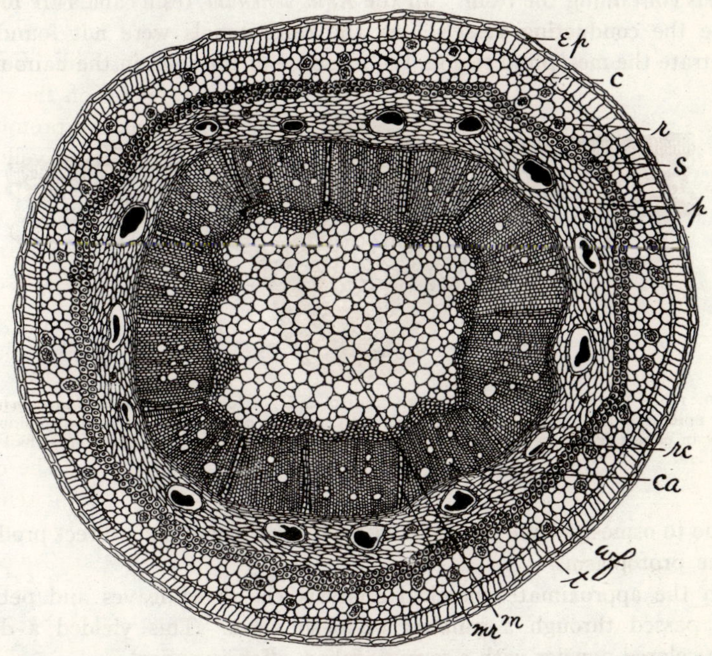

FIG. 149.—Transverse section of young stem of *Rhus venenata* DC. Epidermis (*ep*); cortex (*c*); rosette crystal of calcium oxalate (*r*); continuous ring of stereomatic tissue in pericycle (*s*); phlœm (*p*); resin canals (*rc*); cambium (*ca*); wood fibers (*wf*); trachea of xylem (*t*); medullary-ray (*mr*); and pith (*m*).

HISTOLOGY OF LEAF

The lamina is of dorsoventral structure. A layer of thin-walled cells forms the epidermis of the ventral surface. In the mesophyll region there is a ventral stratum of palisade tissue and a dorsal pneumatic tissue of large roundish cells, which often contain rosette crystals of calcium oxalate. Stomata lacking subsidiary cells and raised a little above the adjoining epidermis are present in the dorsal epidermal region. The resin canals, which were present in the fibrovascular bundles of the stem, also accompany the vascular bundles of the leaf in both the larger and smaller veins. Collenchyma tissue is present in the dorsal region of the midrib. Non-glandular unicellular and uniserate hairs are found in the dorsal region. They are present in greater number along the veins. Many contain the "resinous substance" of Schwalbe, which responds to the nigrescent reaction when treated with alcoholic potash solution. Schwalbe accounts for the presence of this resinous material in the hairs of *Rhus toxicodendron* as a product of osmosis from the neighboring lacticiferous vessels containing the resin. In the *Rhus venenata*, resin canals are found to be the conducting vessels. As the resin canals were not found to penetrate the mesophyll region, the presence of the resin in the hairs may

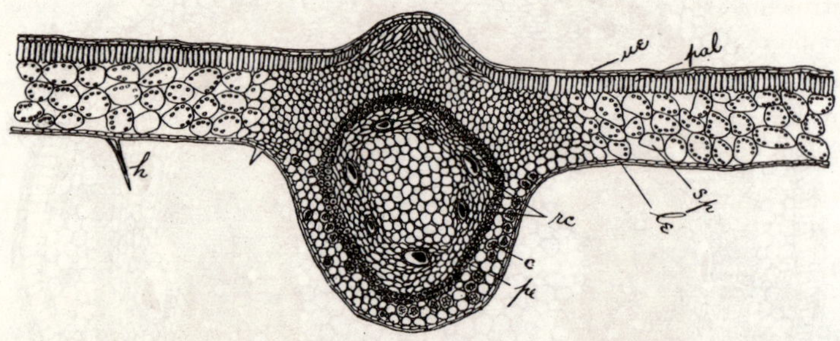

FIG. 150.—Transverse section through midrib and portion of lamina of *Rhus venenata*. Upper epidermis (*ue*); palisade parenchyma (*pal*); spongy parenchyma (*sp*); lower epidermis (*le*); resin canals (*rc*); rosette crystal of calcium oxalate (*c*); pericyclic fibers (*pe*); hair (*h*). Magnified.

be due to osmosis. We are inclined to believe it may be a direct product of the protoplasm.

In the approximate chemical analysis the dried leaves and petiole were passed through a number 60-mesh sieve. This yielded a dark green-colored powder with a very peculiar, offensive odor.

The sample being in a dry state, oxidation and change of character of some constituents most likely took place, which must be considered.

On ignition the powder yielded 6.5 per cent. ash content. The residue was grayish brown and had an alkaline reaction. Traces of potassium, chlorides, phosphates and sulphates were found in the ash. Nitrogen was determined by the Kjeldahl method. Thc presence of nitrates and nitrites could not be found.

Four extractions were carried out by the Soxhlet continuous extraction method. Each extraction extended over a period of 3 days, allowing the solvent to macerate the sample during the nights.

A good grade of low-boiling petroleum ether was used in the first extraction. In this solvent ethereal and non-volatile fixed oil was obtained, as well as a great amount of chlorophyll. On standing a white waxy-like substance separated out of the petroleum extract.

By spontaneous evaporation of a portion of the petroleum extract a yellowish brown, oily residue was obtained. This residue, when taken up with neutral alcohol, is neutral in reaction.

The alcoholic solution of the residue was optically inactive, which Pfaff states is true of the non-volatile oil causing the dermatitis.

The residue from the petroleum ether extract, when taken up with alcholic potash solution, can be saponified. No glycerin is liberated.

To confirm, practically, that the poisonous principle was obtained in the petroleum ether extract, the same was applied to the inner forearm with a piece of cotton and allowed to remain. In twenty-four hours inflammation with violent itching occurred and in thirty hours vesication had taken place.

An alcoholic solution of the residue, when treated with a solution of lead acetate, will cause precipitation of the lead salt of the oil to take place. By treatment of this lead compound with hydrogen sulphide. Stevens was able to isolate the oil from the *Rhus toxicodendron*.

FIG. 151.—Surface view of dorsal epidermis of *R. venenata* lamina, showing hairs (*h*), wavy walled epidermal cells (*e*), and stomata (*s*). Magnified.

As irritation is often due to precipitation of proteins, experiments were made to precipitate egg and blood albumen from 0.5 per cent.

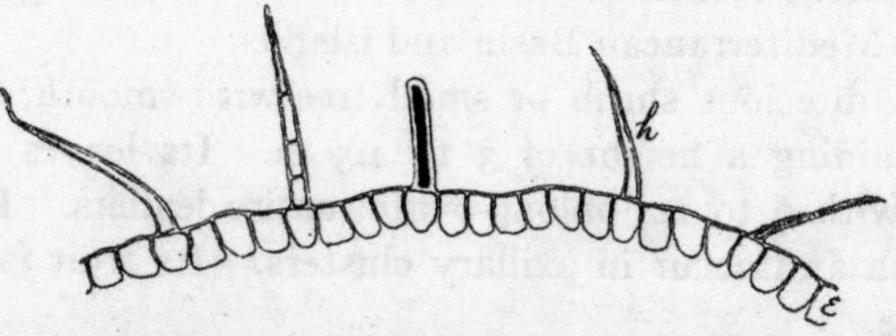

FIG. 152.—Lateral view of portion of dorsal epidermis of *Rhus venenata* lamina. Epidermal cells (*e*); non-glandular hair (*h*).

solutions, by treatment with an alcoholic solution of the residue from the petroleum ether extract. Negative results were obtained.

In the presence of fixed oil, alkaloids are often extracted simultaneously by petroleum ether, but no alkaloids could be extracted from the stems or leaves of this plant.

The second extraction was with ether. This was not carried out until all the petroleum ether had evaporated from the marc.

The ether extract was dark red-brown in color, which yielded a residue of the same color. When taken up with neutral alcohol the reaction was unchanged. Precipitation took place when the ether extract was treated with lead acetate solution. An alcoholic solution of the ether residue will precipitate a resin out of solution when poured into water. No poisonous principle was found in the ether extract when applied to the inner forearm.

The alcoholic extraction which was carried out after all the ether evaporated yielded a yellowish-brown solution in which tests for tannin were positive. No poisonous constituent was found in the alcohol extract.

The water extract gave tests for mucilaginous substances when mixed with alcohol by precipitating them out of solution. Fehling's solution was reduced by the aqueous extract.

Cases of *Rhus* poisoning in the winter months are frequently met with, and are accounted for by the presence of the hairs on the stems and branches throughout the entire year.

Generally the hairs penetrate into the sudoriferous and sebaceous glands. This observation is corroborated by the fact that parts of the skin perspiring easily are affected most frequently by the poisonous principle-(Youngken and Slothower, A.J.P. vol. 92, pp. 695–701, 1920).

MASTICHE N.F. (MASTIC)

Synonyms.—Pistacia Galls, Lentisk, Mastich, Resina Mastiche; *Ger.* Mastix; *Fr.* Mastic.

Botanical Origin.—*Pistacia Lentiscus* Linné.

Part Used.—A concrete resinous exudation.

Purity Rubric.—Not more than 1 per cent. of foreign organic matter.

Habitat.—Mediterranean Basin and islands.

Plant.—A diœcious shrub or small tree with smooth, brownish-gray bark and attaining a height of 3 to 4.5 m. Its leaves are alternate, paripinnate, with 6 to 10, oblong-ovate, entire leaflets. Its flowers are small, greenish and occur in axillary clusters. Its fruit is an orange-red obovate drupe.

Production and Commerce.—The mastic tree is cultivated on the island of Chios in the Grecian Archipelago but is found growing in Cyprus and other islands of this group. It is chiefly collected on the island of Chios from which the entire commercial supply is alone shipped to the markets of the world. The inner bark contains oleoresin reservoirs in which the drug is formed. Longitudinal incisions are made into this region of the stem at close intervals extending from the branches to the ground and the oleoresin induced to run. It collects as small tears on the outside of the wounds which, after hardening, are collected. Some tears are also collected from the branches, these having been formed through spontaneous exudation.

Description.—In sub-globular, lenticular, ovoid or pyriform tears, 3 to 7 mm. in length, pale yellow or greenish-yellow, transparent having a glassy luster, the surface occasionally dusty; brittle, becoming plastic when chewed; odor slight, balsamic; taste mildly terebinthinate. Not less than 97 per cent. of the drug is soluble in ether and not less than 80 per cent. is soluble in alcohol. Its acid number is not less than 50.

Constituents.—α- and β-Masticonic acid, α- and β-Masticoresene, α- and β-Masticinic acid; volatile oil consisting chiefly of *d*-pinene, bitter principle, etc.

Uses.—Mastic is used as filling for carious teeth and in the manufacture of paints and varnishes.

Adulterants.—Resins from allied species of *Pistacia*, notably *P. mutica* and *P. Khinjuk* (Bombay Mastic) and *P. Terebinthinus* (Chios Turpentine), Sandarac and Olibanum.

CELASTRACEÆ (STAFF TREE FAMILY)

Shrubs (*Evonymus*), or shrubby climbers (*Celastrus*). Leaves alternate, rarely opposite, simple, entire or toothed. Inflorescence of axillary cymes or terminal racemes. Flowers perfect (*Evonymus, Pachistima*) or polygamo-diœcious (*Cleastrus*), greenish (*Celastrus*), greenish or yellowish-white (*Evonymus Europæus*), greenish-purple (*Evonymus americanus*) to dark-purple (*Evonymus atropurpureus*); calyx four- to five-lobed; corolla of four to five petals; stamens four to five, perigynous, inserted on a disc, which fills the base of the calyx and sometimes covers the ovary; ovary three- to five-celled. Fruit a two- to five-celled capsule. Seeds albuminous with fleshy, succulent, reddish aril (*Evonymus, Celastrus*) or white membranous aril (*Pachistima*).

EUONYMUS N.F. (EUONYMUS)

Synonyms.—Wahoo Bark, Burning Bush; *Ger.* Spillbaumrinde; *Fr.* Ecorce de fusain.

Botanical Origin.—*Evonymus atropurpureus* Jacquin.

Part Used.—The dried bark of the root.

Limit of Impurities.—5 per cent. of adherent wood or 2 per cent. of other foreign organic matter.

Ash.—Not more than 4 per cent. acid insoluble.

Habitat.—Eastern and Central United States and lower Canada.

Plant.—A shrub growing to the height of six to ten feet or, rarely, (frequently west of the Mississippi) a slender tree twenty to twenty-five feet high, with a trunk six or seven inches in diameter and covered with ash gray fluted bark. It is found growing in rich soil generally along the edge of woods, from Ontario to northern Florida and west to Montana, Arkansas and the Indian Territory. The branchlets (twigs) are obtusely four- angled and bear simple, opposite, elliptical to ovate, acuminate, serrulate and membranous leaves, two to five inches long and one to two inches broad. The dark purple flowers appear on seven to fifteen flowered cymes from May until the middle of June. The fruit is a three to four deeply lobed capsule from one-half to two-thirds inch in diameter, with

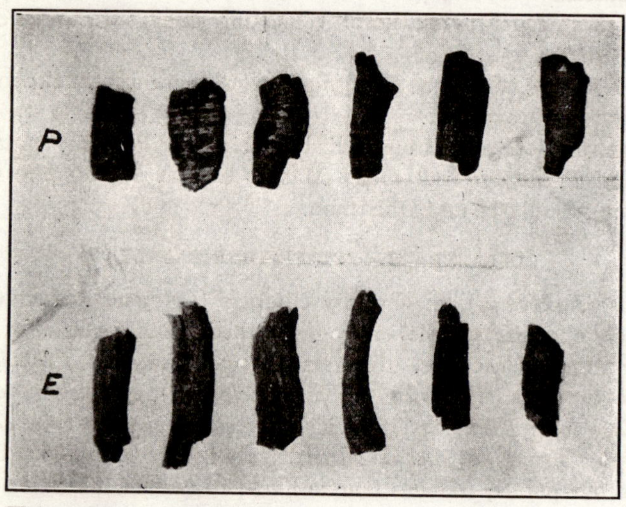

FIG. 153.—Wahoo (*Evonymus atropurpureus*) bark (*E*); Wafer ash (*Ptelea trifoliata*) bark (*P*).

light purple valves. It ripens in October, dehisces to expose its seeds, and remains on the cyme during the early winter months. The seeds are characterized by being covered with a thin scarlet aril.

Description.—It occurs in transversely curved pieces or single quills of variable size and 1 to 4 mm. thick. Its outer surface is grayish to grayish-brown, irregularly furrowed and ridged and showing occasional transverse lenticels. Its inner surface is light brown or light buff. Its fracture is short, exhibiting silky projecting caoutchouc threads in the inner phloem region. Its odor is characteristic and its taste, bitter and acrid.

Histology.—Under the microscope, passing from outer to inner surface, this bark presents the following peculiarities:

1. An irregular cork zone showing lenticels and many layers of tangentially elongated cork cells whose walls may be either suberized or slightly lignified.

2. A cork cambium of meristematic cells.

3. A narrow cortex of cortical parenchyma cells, some of which contain more or less spheroidal starch grains while others contain rosette aggregates of calcium oxalate.

4. A very broad phloem, occupying most of the width of the section and consisting of cone-shaped phloem masses, in cross section, traversed by wavy, secondary medullary-rays. Primary medullary-rays separate the cone-shaped phloem masses one from the other. These are one-cell

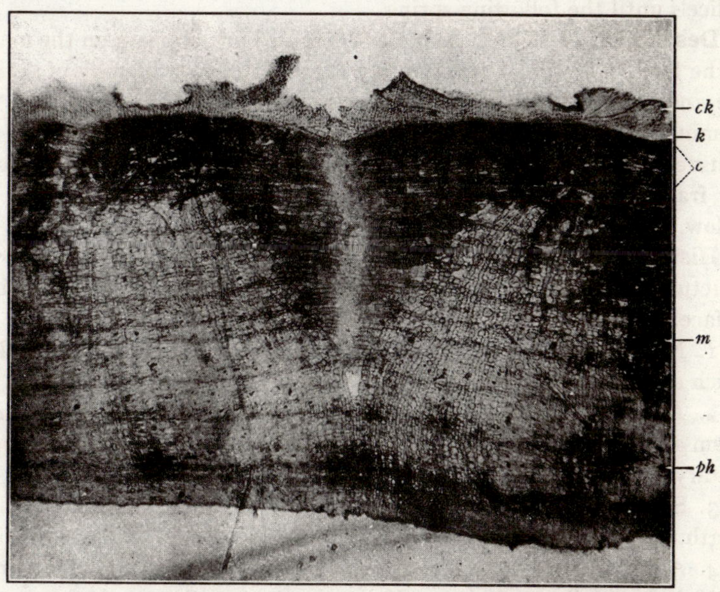

FIG. 154.—Cross-section through root-bark of *Evonymus atropurpureus*. Note the two broad dome-shaped phloem patches, one on either side of a wedge-shaped, primary medullary-ray. Cork (*ck*); cork cambium (*k*); cortex (*c*); portion of medullary ray (*m*); phloem (*ph*).

wide in the inner phloem but broaden out into fan-shaped wedges farther out. Some of the phloem cells and medullary ray cells contain starch grains while others possess rosette aggregates of calcium oxalate. Secretory cells containing a caoutchouc-like substance which dissolves in chloroform and carbon disulphide are found scattered about amidst other cells of the phloem region.

Adulterant.—The bark of *Ptelea trifoliata* Linné, commonly known as Wafer Ash, a small Rutaceous tree, attaining the height of from twenty to twenty-five feet with a straight trunk six to twelve inches in diameter. It grows in rich moist soil from Lake Ontario to northern Florida and west to Minnesota and Colorado. Its branchlets bear alternate, rarely opposite trifoliate leaves, each of which consists of a fairly stout petiole two and one-half to three inches long bearing upon its extremity three sub-sessile, ovate to oblong, serrate leaflets. The terminal leaflet is generally larger than the other two. The greenish-white flowers appear from March to June in terminal compound cymes and possess a rather disagreeable odor. The fruits are orbicular samaras two-thirds to three-fourths of an inch in diameter, the wing portion of each being membranous, reticulate and emarginate. They ripen in the southern latitude in early summer but not until late in autumn in the northern states and persist on the long slender pedicels until the following spring.

Description of Wafer Ash Bark.—This bark appears on the market in the form of irregular transversely curved pieces or in quills of variable size and three to four mm. thick. Its outer surface is light brown with prominent broad, irregular, transverse, grayish-white lenticels and transverse ridges. Its inner surface is brownish-yellow and smooth. Its fracture is short, the broken surfaces appearing waxy and pale yellow. The odor is faint and the taste bitter and acrid.

Histology of Wafer Ash Bark.—Under the microscope the following structural characteristics may be observed, passing from outer to inner surface:

1. Numerous layers of tangentially elongated cork cells, the walls of which are more or less lignified.

2. A cork cambium (phellogen) of delicate walled cells, rich in protoplasm and exhibiting cross walls. Many of the cells of this region possess solitary rhombohedral crystals of calcium oxalate.

3. Several layers of stone cells forming a continuous sclerenchyma sheath.

4. A broad cortex zone consisting of tangentially-elongated cortical parenchyma cells and intercellular-air-spaces. Some of the cortical parenchyma cells contain numerous spheroidal or ovate starch grains while others contain rosette aggregates of calcium oxalate. The starch grains are simple or two to four compound. Scattered about in the cortical and outer phloem regions will be seen sclerenchyma fibers either isolated or in small groups.

5. A broad phloem consisting of numerous phloem patches separated from each other by wavy medullary rays which are one to five cells wide as seen in tangential section. Secretion sacs containing oil are found scattered in both cortex and phloem. Some of the intercellular-air-spaces show rows of calcium oxalate crystals.

Constituents of Euonymus.—The crystalline alcohols, eunonymol, euonysterol, atropurol and homoeuonysterol; tannin, phytosterol glucoside, calcium oxalate, starch, etc.

Use.—Cholagogue cathartic in torpid liver, constipation and dropsy.

SAPINDACEÆ (SOAPBERRY FAMILY)

Trees, shrubs, undershrubs or rarely herbs of tropical climes containing the glucoside saponin. Stem erect or climbing (*Paullinia*) often provided with tendrils. Leaves commonly alternate and compound. Flowers in racemes or panicles (*Paullinia*), perfect or polygamo-diœcious, yellowish in *Paullinia Cupana.* Fruit a capsule (*P. Cupana*), samara, drupe or berry. Seeds exalbuminous.

GUARANA N.F. (GUARANA)

Synonyms.—Guarana Paste, Brazilian Cocoa, Guarana Bread; *Ger.* and *Fr.* Guarana.

Botanical Origin.—*Paullinia Cupana* Kunth.

Part Used.—Paste made from crushed seed.

Standard of Assay.—Not less than 4 per cent. of caffeine.

Habitat.—Brazil.

Plant.—A climbing shrub. The leaves are alternate, imparipinnate, long petioled, with 5 oblong-ovate, roughly sinuate-serrate and acuminate leaflets. The inflorescences consists of axillary spicate panicles of yellow flowers. The fruit is an ovoid or pear-shaped capsule with a short beak and six-ribbed. The seeds are brownish black, about the size of a grape, and resemble small horse-chestnuts, each being invested with a flesh-colored aril.

Production and Commerce.—Guarana is prepared almost exclusively by the Guaranis, a tribe of South American Indians, from the seeds of plants which are cultivated in the valley of the lower Madeira. Here the seeds are removed from the capsules, washed, roasted for about 6 hours, and their coats removed by placing them in bags and beating them with clubs. The kernels are then broken in a mortar, mixed with water and made into a doughy paste. Tapioca is sometimes added to increase plasticity. The paste is then moulded into cylindrical rolls and slowly dried by fire. The commercial supplies are obtained from Brazil.

Description.—Usually in cylindrical sticks, about 3 to 5 cm. in diameter, externally dark reddish-brown; hard and heavy; fracture uneven, often fissured in the center; internally pale reddish-brown, showing more or less coarse fragments of seeds and occasionally their blackish-brown integuments; odor slight; taste slightly astringent and bitter.

Powdered Drug.—Pinkish-brown, consisting for the most part of irregular masses of altered starch grains; unaltered starch grains occasional, of varying shapes 25μ in diameter; occasional fragments with narrow, elongated sclerenchymatous cells, the walls being thick, yellowish and non-lignified.

Micro-chemic test: Place on a slide a drop of hydrochloric acid, add about 0.001 Gm. of powdered Guarana, then add a drop of gold chloride T.S. and allow the mixture to stand for a few minutes; beginning at the edge of the mount, crystals of caffeine gold chloride separate in the form of orthorhombic plates and needles, the latter usually occurring in spheroidal aggregates and finally forming branching groups.

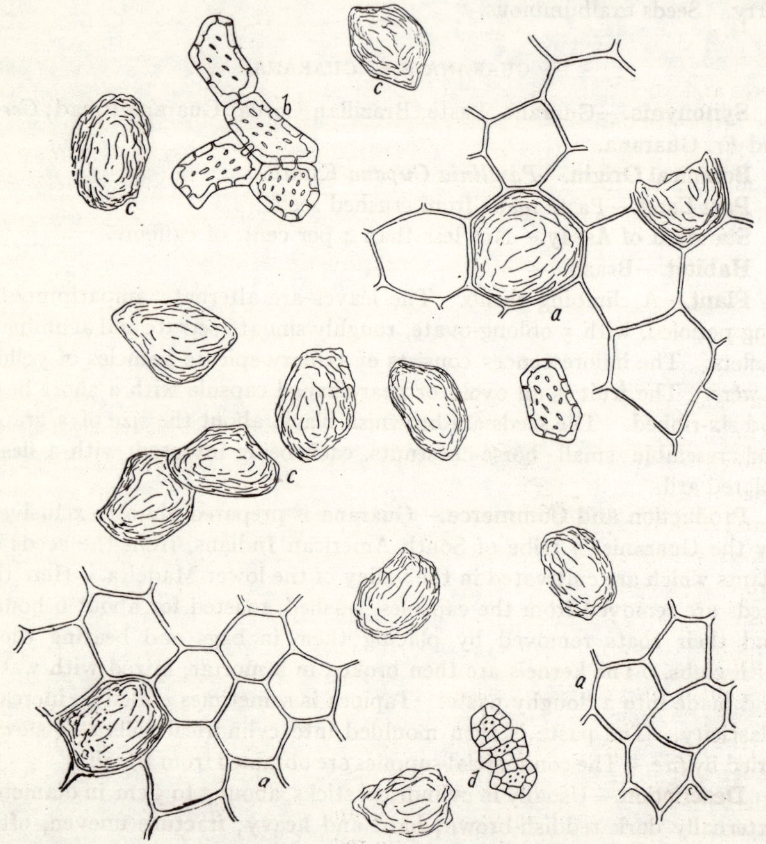

FIG. 155.—Powdered Guarana. (*a*) Parenchyma with pasty starch; (*b*) stone cells; (*c*) masses of pasty starch; (*d*) small stone cells. (*After Schneider.*)

Constituents.—Up to 4.5 per cent. of Guaranine (caffeine); guaranatin; tannin, catechin, volatile oil, fixed oil, saponin and starch.

Use.—Guarana is used as a stimulant in nervous headache.

ACERACEÆ (MAPLE FAMILY)

Chiefly trees, occasionally shrubs, of temperature regions with watery sap. Leaves opposite, simple and palmately-lobed, cleft (*Acer*) or pinnate

(*Negundo*). Inflorescence a raceme, condensing in some species to a capitulum of cymes. Flowers small, regular, polygamous or diœcious; sepals five to four, green; petals none or five, variously colored; stamens usually eight, hypogynous or perigynous; nectar disc around stamens or between them and pistil; pistil bicarpellary with two-celled ovary. Fruit a samara. Seeds green, exalbuminous, with coiled or folded embryo and long thin cotyledons.

Histologically, the plant axis is characterized by the presence of sclerenchyma elements in the pericycle, narrow tracheæ with simple pores and wood fibers with simple pores. Calcium oxalate occurs in either the form of monoclinic prisms or rosette aggregates.

The bark of *Acer spicatum* or Mountain Maple has been employed as a substitute for Viburnum Opulus. This contains astringent, but no nervine and uterine tonic principles.

RHAMNACEÆ (BUCKTHORN FAMILY)

Shrubs or low trees usually of branching or spreading habit. Branches either cylindric or long, green or hardened, checked back and spinescent, occasionally, especially flowering branches, developing tendrils for support. Leaves simple, usually alternate. Flowers hermaphrodite or more or less diclinous, pentamerous to tetramerous, greenish to greenish-yellow to yellowish-white; sepals five to four; petals five to four alternating with sepals; stamens five, opposite the petals, perigynous; pistil either free in center of a receptacular cup or more or less fused with it and so semi-inferior; ovary typically three-celled becoming rarely four-celled with two to one atropous ovules in each cavity. Fruit of three indehiscent cocci, each enclosing a single albuminous seed with straight embryo imbedded in albumen.

This family is characterized histologically as follows:

(1) The frequency of mucilage cells or lysigenous mucilage receptacles; (2) the presence in many plants of anthraquinone derivatives that give an orange to red color with alkaline solutions; (3) the frequence of glandular differentiation of the leaf teeth; (4) absence of glandular hairs; (5) non-glandular hairs either unicellular, uniseriate or stellate; (6) calcium oxalate in rosette aggregates and solitary crystals; (7) tracheæ with simple pores, or bordered pits (when in contact with medullary rays); (8) subepidermal development of cork; (9) mucilaginous modification of the epidermal cell walls of the leaf.

CASCARA SAGRADA U. S. P. (CASCARA SAGRADA)

Synonyms.—Rhamnus Purshiana, Sacred Bark, Chittem Bark, Bear Wood; *Ger.* Amerikanische Faulbaumrinde; *Fr.* Ecorce sacrée.

Botanical Origin.—*Rhamnus Purshiana* De Candolle.

Part Used.—The dried bark.

Habitat.—Southwestern Canada, Washington, Oregon and northern California.

Plant.—A tree with reddish-brown bark and hairy twigs growing to the height of 4.5 to 10 m. The leaves are petiolate, elliptical, acuminate, serrulate, dull green above and pubescent beneath. The inflorescence is an axillary umbellate cyme of small greenish flowers. The fruit is a black drupe composed of 3 indehiscent cocci.

Production and Commerce.—The Cascara trees grow abundantly in northern California, Oregon, Washington and southwest British Columbia,

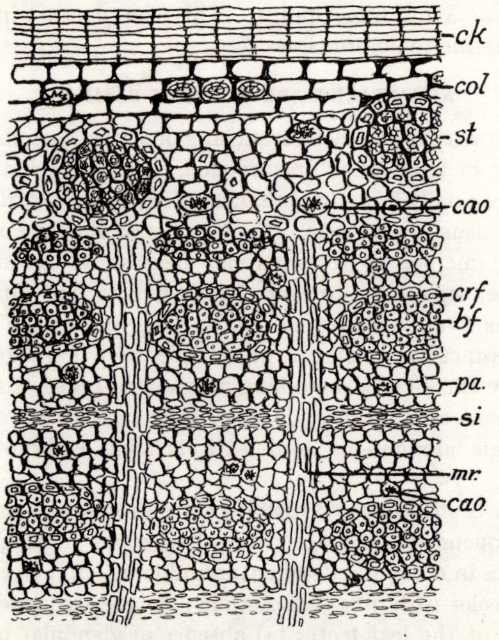

FIG. 156.—Transverse section of Cascara Sagrada (*Rhamnus Purshiana*). Diagrammatic. Cork (*ck*); collenchyma (*col*); mass of stone cells (*st*) surrounded by crystal fibers; rosette crystals of calcium oxalate (*cao*); crystal fibers (*crf*) adhering to bast fibers (*bf*); phloem parenchyma (*pa*); sieve tubes (*si*); medullary-ray (*mr*).

from which districts the drug of commerce is obtained. The bark of the trunk and branches is usually gathered from April to September chiefly by Indians and ranchers who peel the bark off in long strips. In peeling, longitudinal incisions two to four inches apart are made along the trunk, generally before the tree is felled. The bark is then peeled off in strips to within one foot of the ground. The tree is next cut down and the bark removed from the branches in strips. Trees four inches or less in diameter are not employed, the bark on these being too thin. Foreign matter such as sand and moss is generally removed by scraping. The bark is then placed on racks or hung over galvanized wire, with sap side downward, stretched tight and allowed to dry. It is subsequently broken into pieces and put into sacks holding from 50 to 100 pounds. The annual yield has been estimated as from 3 to 4 million pounds. The fresh bark contains a principle which acts as a gastro-intestinal irritant and emetic. It should be collected at least one year before being used medicinally.

Description.—It occurs in flattened or transversely curved pieces or quills, of variable length and up to 5 mm. thick; outer surface dark-brown or brownish-red, longitudinally ridged, frequently more or less covered with grayish or whitish lichens bearing small blackish apothecia, sometimes with numerous lenticels and occasionally with mosses; inner surface light-yellow to reddish-brown, or dark brown in old mature bark, longitudinally striate, becoming red when moistened with alkaline solutions; fracture short with projections of bast fibers in the inner bark; odor distinct; taste bitter and slightly acrid.

Histology.—*In transverse section* passing from outer to inner surface, the following structural characteristics are evident:

1. **Cork,** or outer bark, composed of several layers of rectangular cork cells. The most external layers are dead and appear black because they are filled with air. The inner layers of this region are living and have brownish contents.

2. **Cork cambium** (phellogen), a layer of delicate cells, with protoplasmic contents, in the process of division.

3. **Cortex, or middle bark,** consisting of two regions, viz.: an outer zone of two or three rows of brownish collenchyma cells, and an inner broader zone of tangentially elongated cortical parenchyma cells. Imbedded within this zone will be noted numerous groups of stone cells.

4. **Phloem, or inner bark,** a very broad zone composed of irregular-shaped, elongated, phloem masses separated from each other by medullary rays which converge in the outer phloem region. Each phloem mass consists of numerous sieve tubes and phloem cells, some of which latter contain spheroidal starch grains while others contain monoclinic prisms or rosette aggregates of calcium oxalate. Embedded within the phloem masses, in tier-like fashion, will be noted groups of bast fibers, each group of which is surrounded by a row of crystal fibers, individual cells of which can only be made out in this kind of a section. Each of these contains a monoclinic prism of calcium oxalate. The medullary rays possess brownish contents which take a red color with an alkaline solution.

In radial longitudinal section, a lengthwise view of the tissues will be seen. The medullary rays appear 15 to 25 cells in height and crossing at right angles to the other elements. The crystal fibers here will be seen to be composed of vertical rows of superimposed thin-walled cells, each of which contains a monoclinic prism of calcium oxalate. The bast fibers appear elongated and taper ended and are associated with crystal fibers.

In a tangential longitudinal section which has been cut through the phloem, the exact range in width of the medullary rays may be ascertained.

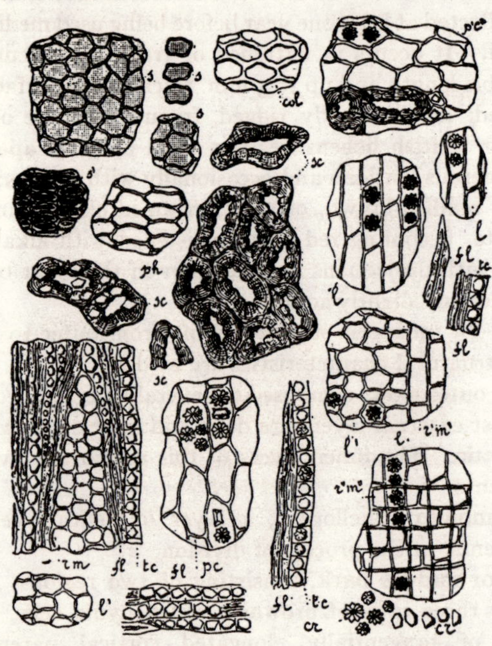

FIG. 157.—Powdered Cascara Sagrada Bark, × 210. *col*, Collenchyma of the cortex *cr*, Rosette aggregates and monoclinic prisms of calcium oxalate. *fl*, Bast fibers. *l*, *l'*, Phloem fragments as seen in longitudinal and transverse sections. *pc*, *p'c'*, Cortex fragments as viewed in longitudinal and transverse sections. *ph*, Phelloderm. *rm*, portion of medullary ray, tangential section. *r'm'*, medullary ray, transverse section. *r''m''*, the same, radial section. *s*, *s'*, Cork in surface view and section. *Sc*, stone cells. *tc*, crystal fibers. (*After Sayre, from Greenish and Collin.*)

In this bark the medullary rays are spindle-shaped in tangential view and one to four cells in width.

Powdered Drug.—Brown. Numerous broken bundles of bast fibers adhering to which are crystal fibers containing monoclinic prisms of calcium oxalate; isolated monoclinic prisms or rosette aggregates of calcium oxalate, up to 20μ in diameter; masses of stone cells with thick, lamellated and porous walls; fragments of reddish-brown cork; masses of parenchyma and medullary-ray tissue colored red upon addition of an alkaline solution; numerous spheroidal starch grains up to 8μ in diameter.

Constituents.—Anthraquinone derivatives including **emodin** and isoemodin; resin, bitter principle, an enzyme, tannin, etc.

Use.—Cascara sagrada is extensively used as a tonic-laxative.

Adulterant.—Bark of *Rhamnus Californica*. The bark of this tree is invariably present in "Cascara Bark" collected in lower parts of California. It is best distinguished from the genuine article by its medullary-rays which range from 1 to 7 cells in width, as observed in tangential sections.

FRANGULA N.F. (FRANGULA)

Synonyms.—Buckthorn Bark, Alder Buckthorn; *Fr.* Ecorce de Bourdaine; *Ger.* Faulbaumrinde.

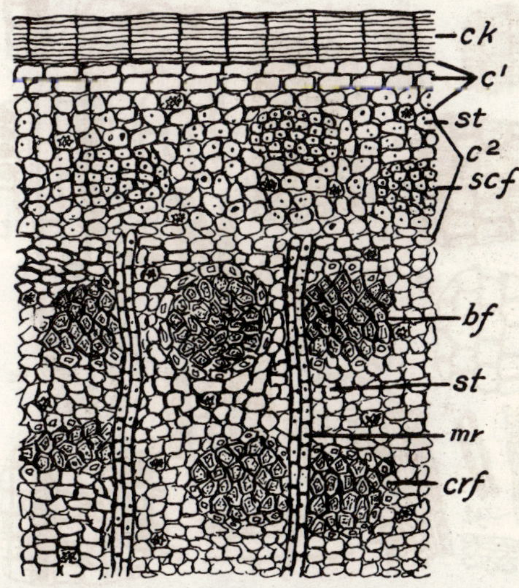

FIG. 158.—*Rhamnus Frangula.* Transverse section of bark showing cork (*ck*); secondary cortex (c^1); primary cortex (c^2); starch grains (*st*); sclerenchyma fibers (*scf*) in cortex; bast fibers (*bf*); medullary-rays (*mr*); crystal fibers (*crf*) adhering to bast fibers. Note rosette aggregates of CaŌ in various cells of the phloem and cortex.

Botanical Origin.—*Rhamnus Frangula* Linné.

Part Used.—The dried bark.

Purity Rubric.—Not more than 2 per cent. of foreign organic matter.

Habitat.—Europe and Western Asia.

Plant.—A smooth, thornless arborescent shrub growing to the height of 4.6 m. and frequently found growing in hedges. The leaves are broadly ovate in outline, obtuse at apex and entire or slightly sinuate along the margin. The flowers are hermaphrodite, pentamerous and arranged in axillary clusters of 2 or 3. The fruit is a dark purple juicy drupe with 2 nutlets.

Production and Commerce.—Frangula is collected in Russia, Germany and other European countries by stripping the bark from the stem and branches and drying it slowly. Like Cascara Sagrada, it contains in its fresh condition an emetic principle. The bark is kept for a year or longer before being marketed for medicinal use. During this time its glucoside frangulin is said to be developed and its emetic principle disappears. The commercial supplies of this bark are imported into the United States in bales or large bags from Hamburg and Trieste.

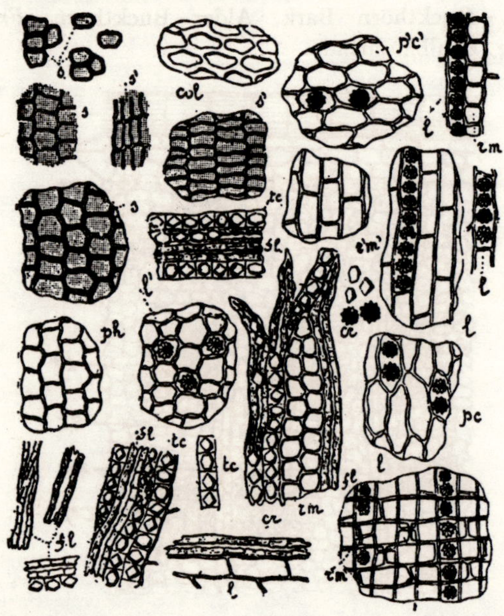

FIG. 159.—Powdered Frangula Bark (*Rhamnus Frangula*), × 210. *col*, Collenchyma of the cortex. *cr*, monoclinic prisms and rosette aggregates of calcium oxalate. *fl*, bast fibers with pitted walls. *l*, *l'*, fragments of phloem in longitudinal and transverse section. *pc*, *p'c'*, Cortical parenchyma, in longitudinal and transverse section. *ph*, Phelloderm. *rm*, *r'm'*, medullary ray in tangential and radial-longitudinal section. *s*, *s'*, Cork in tangential and transverse section. *tc*, crystal fibers. (*After Sayre, from Greenish and Collin.*)

Description.—The drug occurs in quills or flattened pieces of variable length and breadth and from 0.5 to 2 mm. in thickness; outer surface varying from light gray to purplish-brown to purplish-black, with numerous rounded or transversely elongated whitish lenticels and occasional irregular patches of foliaceous lichens, some of which display small, blackish apothecia; inner surface smooth, orange brown or dark brown, finely longitudinally striate, becoming red when moistened with alkaline solutions; fracture short, slightly fibrous in the inner layer; odor distinct; taste slightly bitter.

Histology.—Transverse sections exhibit the following microscopical structures:

1. Cork, of numerous layers of purplish-brown, to reddish-brown, tabular cork cells, containing a purple to purple-crimson coloring matter.

2. Cork cambium of meristematic cells, mostly collapsed.

3. Cortex of several layers of thin walled cells, some of which contain a brownish amorphous substance, others minute starch grains, still others rosette aggregates of calcium oxalate up to 25μ in diameter.

4. Phloem, a broad region traversed by starch and active principle containing medullary-rays that tend to converge in groups. The phloem patches between the medullary-rays contain tangentially elongated groups of bast fibers having thick, strongly lignified, yellowish walls and narrow lumina. Each group of bast fibers is more or less surrounded by a layer of crystal fibers, the cells of which contain monoclinic prisms of calcium oxalate up to 15μ in diameter. The medullary-rays are 1 to 3 cells in width.

Powdered Drug.—Yellowish-brown and distinguished from that of Cascara Sagrada chiefly by its absence of stone cells. (See Fig. 159.)

Constituents.—The yellow crystalline glucoside frangulin; frangula-emodin, chrysophanic acid, isoemodin, tannin, rhamnol, the sugars rhamnose and xylose, coloring matter, etc.

Use.—Tonic-laxative.

Substitute.—The bark of *Rhamnus carniolica* Kerner, distinguished from Frangula by its medullary-rays being 1 to 7 cells wide, by its cortex containing groups of stone cells and by its cork cells being devoid of purplish or crimson coloring matter.

STERCULIACEÆ (COLA FAMILY)

Rarely herbs, usually shrubs or tall, often heavy trees with soft wood and broad annual rings. The cambium, in developing bast, produces one, two, three, four or five alternating layers of hard and soft bast which, in some species of this as well as the *Tiliaceæ* family, form long finger-like processes pushing out into the cortex. Leaves alternate, sometimes simple and pinnately veined (*Theobroma*) or passing to palmately veined or palmately compound. Flowers hermaphrodite; sepals five, sometimes surrounded by bracteoles forming an epicalyx; petals usually five; stamens typically five, hypogynous, opposite petals, distinct or slightly fused in monadelphous fashion (*Melochia*, *Waltheria*) or, stamens subdivided above into few or numerous staminal leaflets, anthers two-celled; pistil many to ten- to five- or four-carpelled; carpels apocarpous or more usually partially or completely united. Fruit either follicles, or fused to form a capsule of ten or more, frequently five dehiscent carpels or, carpels splitting asunder into cocci or, becoming a woody capsular nut (*Theobroma*) or, rarely, the fruit may become succulent. Seeds globose or subglobose and often provided with wings, arils or similar appendages; embryo straight, large and surrounded by scanty albumen.

SEMEN THEOBROMATIS (COCOA SEED)

Synonyms.—Cocoa Bean, Cacao Seed; *Fr.* Féves du Mexique; *Ger.* Kakaobohnen.

Botanical Origin.—*Theobroma Cacao* Linné.

Part Used.—The prepared dried ripe seed.

Habitat.—West Indies, South America, Central America and Mexico.

Plant.—A small tree growing to the height of 9 to 12 m. and bearing pink flowers which spring directly from its trunk and thicker branches. The fruit is a large, red, woody, melon-like, capsular nut containing about 50 to 70 seeds embedded in a mucilaginous pulp.

Production and Commerce.—The fruits are broken open by the natives who remove the seeds and place them in boxes or in holes, in the ground, where they are allowed to undergo a fermentation (sweating process) whereby certain bitter and acrid principles are destroyed. They are then dried. The commercial supplies come largely from Venezuela, Guiana, Brazil, Ecuador, Trinidad, Mexico, West Indies and the Gold Coast.

Cacao represents the roasted kernels of the ripe seeds. After roasting Cocoa seed, the shell, representing the inner layers of the pericarp, spermoderm and perisperm, is readily removed. This is marketed as *cocoa shells*. The roasted embryo is then broken up and constitutes *cocoa nibs* or *cracked cocoa*.

Chocolate, also known as plain chocolate, bitter chocolate, chocolate liquor or chocolate coatings, is a solid or plastic mass prepared by grinding cocoa nibs without the removal of fat or other constituents.

Sweet Chocolate or sweet chocolate coatings represents chocolate mixed with sucrose and frequently with cocoa butter, spices and flavoring materials. *Milk Chocolate* is prepared by mixing powdered milk with sweet chocolate.

Description.—Seed with adherent inner layers of pericarp ellipsoidal or oblong-ovate, somewhat flattened, obtuse, 15 to 25 mm. in length; externally reddish-brown to dark brown, with hilum at broader end, connected with chalaza at the narrower end by a raphe which runs along one of the narrow sides; the thin brittle shell separable from the embryo; embryo, oily, reddish-brown to chocolate-brown and consisting of 2 fleshy peculiarly folded cotyledons and a short hypocotyl, the latter at the hilum end; odor agreeable, characteristic; taste oily, aromatic and bitter.

Constituents.—The alkaloid theobromine, about 50 per cent. of fixed oil, 15 per cent. of starch, 15 per cent. of proteins, cacao-red and small amounts of coffeine and tannin.

OLEUM THEOBROMATIS U.S.P. (OIL OF THEOBROMA)

Synonyms.—Cacao Butter, Butter of Cacao; *Fr.* Oleum Concretum e Semine Theobromæ Cacao, Beurre de Cacao; *Ger.* Kakaobutter.

Botanical Origin.—*Theobroma Cacao* Linné.

Part Used.—The fixed oil obtained from the roasted seeds.

Description.—Cacao butter is a yellowish-white solid, having an agreeable odor and a bland, chocolate-like taste. It is brittle at temperatures below 25°C. and melts between 30° and 35°C. It is freely soluble in ether, chloroform and benzene, soluble in boiling dehydrated alcohol and slightly soluble in 95 per cent. alcohol. Its saponification value is not less than 188 nor more than 195. Its iodine value is not less than 33 nor more than 38.

Preparation.—The seeds of the Chocolate plant are roasted and the seed coats or cocoa shells separated by winnowing. The oil is then expressed by subjecting the kernels to hydraulic pressure between hot iron plates and run into moulds, where it congeals.

Constituents.—The glycerides of oleic, palmitic and stearic acids.

Uses.—Cacao butter is used in the making of suppositories, as an excipient for certain pills, and as an emollient.

Adulterants.—Wax, stearin and tallow have been occasionally found in Cacao butter. Either of these may be detected by the following test: Dissolve 1 Gm. of the suspected substance in 3 cc. of ether in a test tube at a temperature of 17°C. (63°F.), plunge the tube into melting ice. If either of these substances be present, the liquid will become turbid or deposit white flakes in less than 3 minutes and will not clarify at 15°C.

CACAO PRÆPARATUM N.F. (COCOA)

Synonym.—Prepared Cacao.

Botanical Origin.—*Theobroma Cacao* Linné.

Part Used.—The powder prepared from the roasted, cured kernel of the ripe seed, deprived of a portion of its fat.

Limit of Impurities.—Three per cent. of cocoa shells, 6 per cent. of crude fiber and 15 per cent. of starch.

Standard of Assay.—Ether extract yields less than 18 per cent. or more than 25 per cent. of fat, and the fatty residue does not have a spicy odor and taste.

Description.—A reddish-brown powder, devoid of sweetness, and having a chocolate like odor and taste. The diagnostic histological elements are: numerous small, simple, spherical or 2- to 4-compound starch

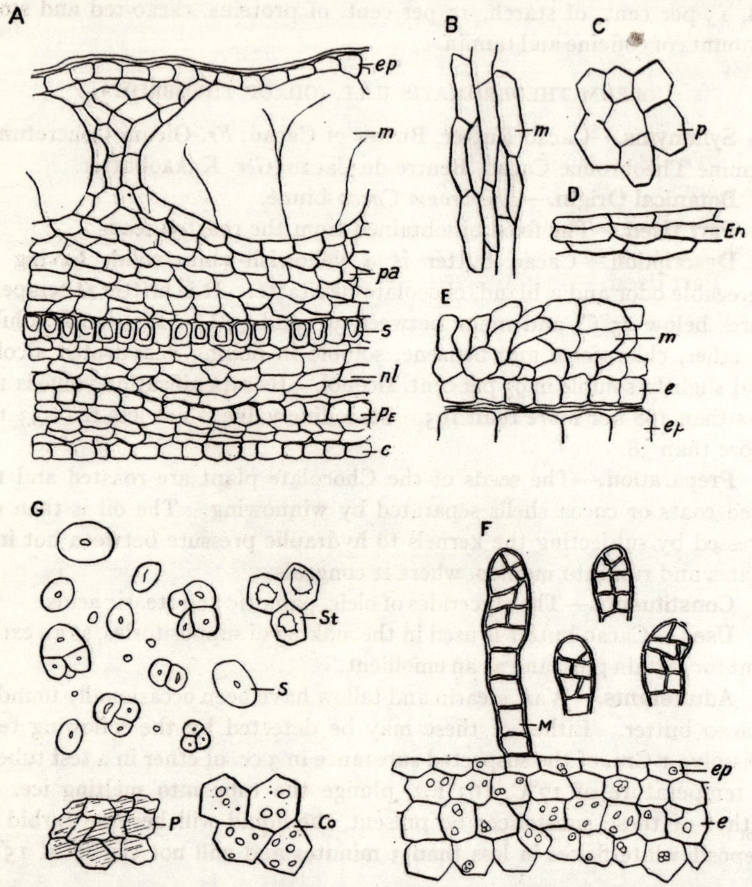

FIG. 160.—Chocolate (*Theobroma Cacao*) seed. *A*, Transverse section through outer region of seed. Epidermis of spermoderm (*ep*); mucilage cell (*m*); spongy parenchyma (*pa*); stone cell layer (*s*); nutritive layer (*nl*); perisperm (*Pe*); parenchyma (*c*). *B*, Surface view of mesocarp parenchyma. *C*, Epidermis of spermoderm in surface view. *D*, Surface view of endocarp. *E*, Cross-section through outer part of bean. Mesocarp (*m*); endocarp (*e*); outer epidermis of spermoderm (*ep*). *F*, cross-section through outer portion of cotyledon. Mitscherlichian body (hair); epidermis of cotyledon (*ep*); starch and oil parenchyma (*e*). *G*, Powdered Cocoa. Stone cells (*st*); cells of cotyledon (*co*); starch (*s*); pigment cells (*p*).

grains up to 12μ in diameter, some of which have become altered during the curing and roasting processes and appear swollen and resembling in size and outline the starch grains of wheat and corn; needle and prismatic shaped crystals of fat, numerous aleurone grains, numerous fragments of parenchyma of cotyledons with thin-walled cells, some containing brownish, reddish-brown or purplish-brown cacao-red; fragments of epidermis of cotyledons with polygonal cells and reddish-brown granular contents.

Uses.—Cocoa is used medicinally to mask the taste of bitter substances like quinine. Its chief use is as a nutrient beverage.

KOLA N.F. (KOLA)

Synonyms.—Cola, Kola Nut, Gooroo Nuts, Bichy Nuts; *Ger.* Kolanuss; *Fr.* Noix de Gourou.

Botanical Origin.—*Cola nitida* (Ventenat) Schott and Endlicher, or other species of *Cola*.

Part Used.—The dried cotyledon.

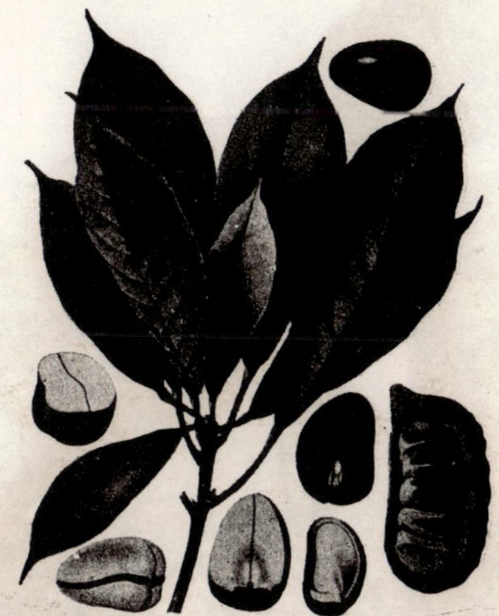

FIG. 161.—Cola (Kola Nut). Showing longitudinal section of fruit × ⅙; cross-section of red seed × ⅙; longitudinal section of red seed showing embryo × ⅙; cross-section of red seed × ⅙; longitudinal section of white seed. (*Sayre after Kohler.*)

Purity Rubric.—Not less than 1 per cent. of caffeine and not more than 1 per cent. of foreign organic matter.

Habitat.—Africa. Cultivated in South America and West Indies.

Plants.—Large trees with smooth bark. The leaves are alternate, lance-ovate, acuminate. The flowers are yellow or purple of two kinds, staminate and pistillate and arranged in small axillary clusters. The fruit of *Cola acuminata* consists of 5 yellowish-brown woody follicles, each containing 1 to 3 white or red seeds.

Production and Commerce.—The trees are cultivated for the drug chiefly in the British West Indies.

Our present commercial supplies are chiefly shipped to the U. S. A. in bags from Grenada, Kingston, St. Lucia, Port of Spain and Spaulding in the British West Indies. Kola is also obtained from the west coast of Africa where the trees grow wild.

Description.—The drug occurs as entire or broken cotyledons, of irregularly plano-convex, broadly oval, or polygonal outline, up to 40 mm. in length and up to 22 mm. in diameter; heavy, hard and tough; externally brown, the outer surfaces slightly wrinkled, the inner surfaces lighter and smoother; edges slightly incurved and sharp; odor indistinct; taste slightly astringent.

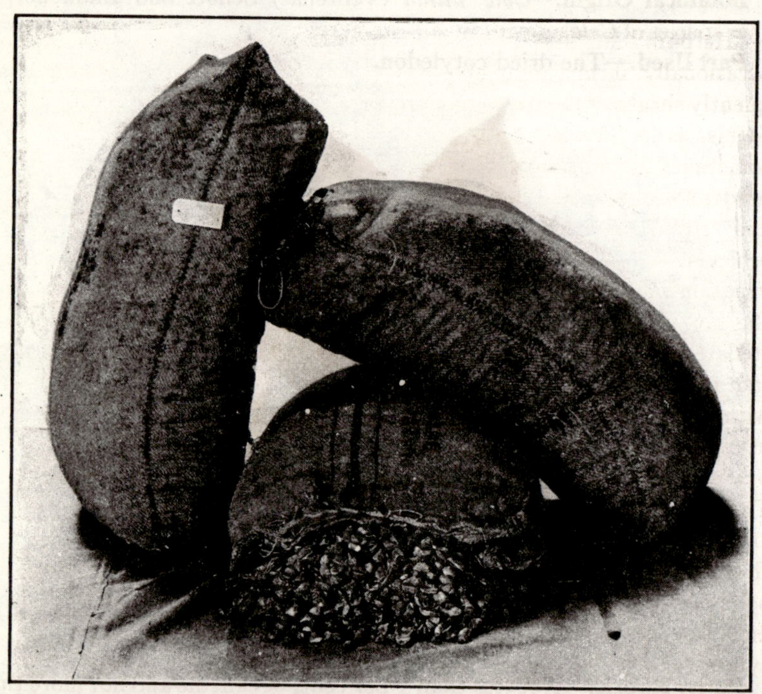

FIG. 162.—Original burlap bags of Kola Nuts. (*Courtesy of Parke, Davis and Company.*)

Powdered Drug.—Reddish-brown. Starch grains numerous, some unaltered, others altered, the unaltered grains up to 45μ in diameter, ellipsoidal, spherical, or irregularly oblong and occasionally with a protuberance on one side, the larger grains frequently exhibiting a circular central hilum or a fissure and showing a distinct polarization cross when examined under a petrographic microscope.

Uses.—Kola is used medicinally as a cerebral, cardiac and nerve stimulant. Large quantities are employed in the manufacture of summer beverages.

Constituents.—1 to 2.5 per cent. of Caffeine (up to 2.5 per cent.) a glucoside called kolatin (which on oxidation yields kola red), kolatein. theobromine, starch, fat, tannin and a lipase.

Adulterants.—*False Kola Nuts*, representing the seeds of *Heritiera litoralis* Dryand (Fam. *Sterculiaceæ*). These are sub-orbicular and flattened with purplish-brown cotyledons, one of which being about one-half the size of the other. They contain no caffeine.

The seeds of *Lucuma mammosa* Griesbach (Fam. *Sapotaceæ*) which possess a strong odor of hydrocyanic acid and are devoid of caffeine.

MALVACEÆ (MALLOW FAMILY)

Herbs in temperate regions (*Malva rotundifolia, Althæa officinalis*, etc.), occasionally shrubs in temperate regions (*Hibiscus Syriacus*, etc.), frequently shrubs or tall trees in the tropics. Stems, as in *Sterculiaceæ* and *Tiliaceæ*, sometimes forming numerous layers of hard and soft bast. Leaves alternate and stipulate, ovate, ovate-cordate, orbicular or palmately compound, with venation pinnate or palmate, often hairy, the non-glandular hairs being usually stellate. Stems, roots and leaves contain mucilage cells. Secretory cavities with brown contents have been observed in the axis and leaves of species of *Gossypium*, *Fugosia* and *Thespesia*. The phloem patches are cone-shaped and the primary medullary rays between these are wedge-shaped in their outer portion, as observed in cross section. Inflorescence a raceme or fascicle of cymes. Flowers regular, pentamerous; calyx green, of five aposepalous sepals, but frequently surrounded outside by an epicalyx. Both calyx and epicalyx are persistent. Corolla of five petals, varying in color, which are more or less fused with stamens at their bases; stamens monadelphous and forming an upright column enclosing the styles; anthers one-celled, dehiscing transversely; pollen grains echinate; pistil loosely or strongly syncarpous, rarely sub-apocarpous of thirty to five carpels. Fruit either a set of cocci united into a ring (*Althaea*, *Malva*) follicles, or a capsule (*Gossypium*). Seeds albuminous with oily and mucilaginous albumen.

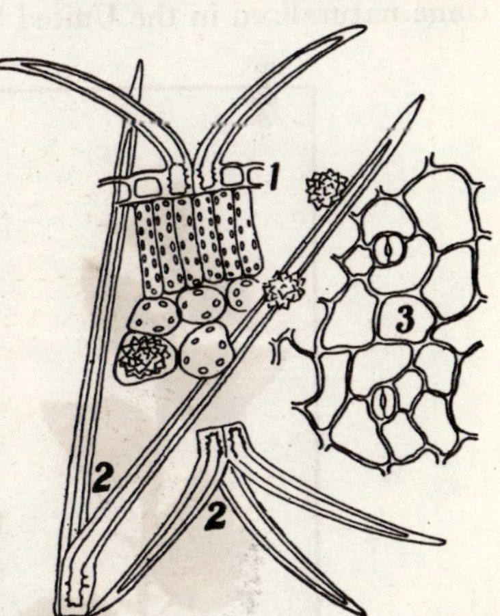

FIG. 163.—Histology of Mallow leaf. (1) Transverse section of leaf showing stellate trichome, epidermal, palisade and spongy tissue cells. Aggregate crystals of calcium oxalate are present. (2) Stellate or aggregate trichomes; (3) epidermal cells (lower) showing stomata. Mallow leaves have been extensively employed for adulterating leafy spices and drugs. (*After Schneider.*)

ALTHÆA U.S.P. (ALTHÆA)

Synonyms.—Marsh Mallow Root, Mortification Root, White Mallow; *Ger.* Eibischwurzel; *Fr.* Racine de Guimauve.

Botanical Origin.—*Althaea officinalis* Linné.

Part Used.—The dried root deprived of the brown, corky layer and small roots.

Habitat.—Europe.

Plant.—A perennial herb with erect wooly stems, 6 to 12 cm. high, alternate, ovate to slightly cordate, occasionally 3-lobed, serrate, velvety leaves and large, pale, rose-colored, axillary flowers, the calyx of each of which is surrounded by a 6 to 9 cleft involucel. The fruit is a set of cocci united into a ring.

Production and Commerce.—Althæa is native to Europe but has become naturalized in the United States where it grows wild in salt marshes

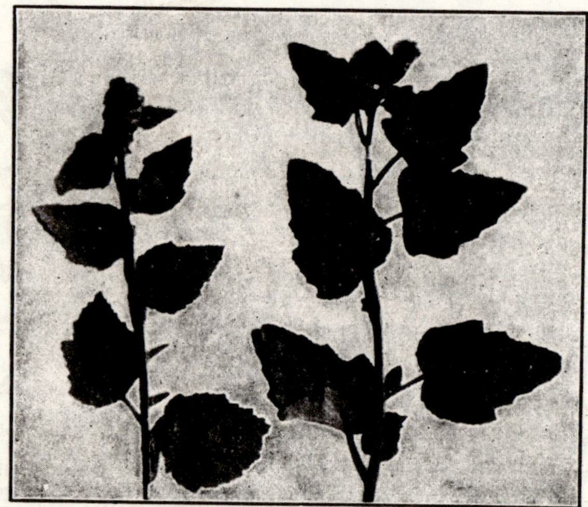

FIG. 164.—*Althæa officinalis.* Both leaves and root are official.

near the coast of New England and along tidal rivers in New York and Pennsylvania. The roots which are rich in mucilaginous principles are collected in autumn from plants of the second year's growth, washed, peeled cut into segments, or cubes and carefully dried. Most of the article of commerce is obtained from plants cultivated in France, Germany, Italy, Spain and Holland.

Description.—Marshmallow root occurs for the most part in small, more or less cubical shaped pieces of grayish-white color about 5 mm. in diameter, seldom as nearly entire roots or long segments thereof, when nearly entire, externally whitish, longitudinally furrowed, often spirally twisted and covered with somewhat loosened, hairy-like bast fibers; fracture of bark fibrous, of wood short and granular; internally yellowish-white; bark 1 to 2 mm. thick, porous, and separated from the slightly radiate wood by a distinct cambium zone; odor slight; taste sweet and mucilaginous.

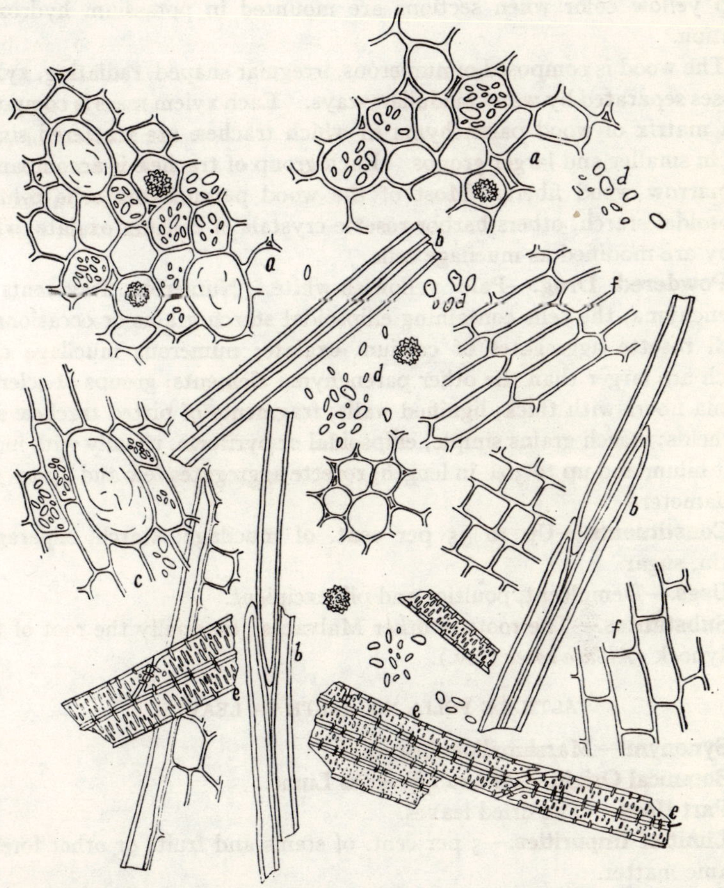

FIG. 165.—Powdered Althæa. (*a*) Parenchyma with mucilage cells, starch and rosette aggregate crystals; (*b*) bast fibers; (*c*) parenchyma, longitudinal view; (*d*) starch granules and crystals; (*e*) tracheids; (*f*) parenchyma, longitudinal view. (*Schneider.*)

Histology.—Transverse sections of the peeled root exhibit a comparatively narrow bark and broad wood zone separated from each other by a prominent cambium. The bark shows a little cortical parenchyma adhering here and there to the outside, the cells of which contain either ellipsoidal starch grains or rosette aggregates of calcium oxalate. The greater portion of the bark, however, consists of phloem patches separated by phloem medullary-rays. Each phloem patch shows alternating horizontally arranged layers of hard and soft bast. The former contain groups of thick walled, more or less lignified and angular bast fibers, the latter, groups of sieve tubes, phloem cells with starchy or rosette crystal contents and mucilage cells. The contents of the mucilage cells take on a deep yellow color when sections are mounted in potassium hydroxide solution.

The wood is composed of numerous, irregular shaped, radiating, xylem masses separated by wavy medullary-rays. Each xylem mass is composed of a matrix of wood parenchyma in which tracheæ are scattered singly and in smaller and larger groups. Each group of tracheæ is accompanied by narrow wood fibers. Most of the wood parenchyma cells contain ellipsoidal starch, others harbor rosette crystals of calcium oxalate, while many are modified as mucilage cells.

Powdered Drug.—Pale yellowish-white. Numerous fragments of parenchyma, the cells containing ellipsoidal starch grains or occasionally small rosette aggregates of calcium oxalate; numerous mucilage cells which are larger than the other parenchyma elements; groups of sclerenchyma fibers with thick, lignified walls; fragments of pitted tracheæ and tracheids; starch grains simple, ellipsoidal or pyriform, usually with indistinct hilum and up to 30μ in length; rosette aggregates few and up to 35μ in diameter.

Constituents.—Up to 35 per cent. of mucilage; starch, asparagin, pectin, sugar.

Uses.—Demulcent, poultice and pill excipient.

Substitutes.—The roots of other Malvaceæ, especially the root of the Hollyhock (*Althæa rosea* Cav.).

ALTHÆÆ FOLIA N.F. (ALTHÆA LEAVES)

Synonym.—Marshmallow Leaves.

Botanical Origin.—*Althæa officinalis* Linné.

Part Used.—The dried leaves.

Limit of Impurities.—5 per cent. of stems and fruits or other foreign organic matter.

Description.—Leaf thin, but thick-looking because of its hairy covering, gray-green or yellowish gray-green and densely tomentose; petioles one-sixth to one-fifth as long as the blades; blades varying from 5 to 15 cm. in length and from 3 to 10 cm. in breadth, broadly ovate or cordate in outline, rounded or nearly truncate at the base, acute at apex; margin doubly serrate-dentate, the principal teeth from one to three pairs, the lowest almost large enough to be regarded as lobes. the secondary very irregular, triangulate, acute, broader than long, the sinuses acute; two to six principal veins originating with the midrib in the petiole, prominent on lower surface; branches of midrib ending in marginal teeth; odor indistinct; taste mucilaginous.

Powdered Drug.—Grayish-green. Numerous unicellular non-lignified, stellate hairs up to 600μ long, and in clusters of two to six; few short-stalked glandular hairs with multicellular heads; fragments of epidermal tissue with stomata; fragments of mesophyll, some cells of which contain mucilage, others rosette aggregates of calcium oxalate up to 30μ in diameter, still others chloroplasts; a few echinate pollen grains up to 125μ in diameter.

Constituents.—Mucilage, calcium oxalate, etc.

Uses.—Demulcent and poultice.

GOSSYPIUM PURIFICATUM U.S.P. (PURIFIED COTTON)

Synonyms.—Absorbent Cotton, Cotton Wool; *Gr.* Baumwolle; *Fr.* Coton absorbant.

Botanical Origin.—Cultivated varieties of *Gossypium herbaceum* Linné and other species of *Gossypium.*

Part Used.—The hairs of the seed, freed from adhering impurities and linters and deprived of fatty matter.

Habitat.—Africa and Asia. Cultivated in the United States and in many other countries to the 40° latitude on either side of the equator.

Plants.—Annual or biennial herbs with long, branching tap root and branching stems, about 2 to 4 feet high under cultivation, pubescent; leaves palmately 3 to 4 lobed; flowers large, showy and yellow with a purple red blotch at the base of each petal (*G. barbadense*) or white, turning red on the second day of blooming (*G. hirsutum*) flowers. Each flower is subtended by an involucre of generally 3 bracts united at the base. The fruit is a 3- to 5-celled capsule which when mature dehisces, exposing a loose mass of white hairs, the outgrowth of numerous seeds.

Production and Commerce.—The absorbent cotton used in the United States is prepared chiefly, if not entirely, from the hairs of the seed of cultivated varieties of *Gossypium hirsutum* or American Upland Cotton and *G. Barbadense* or Sea Island Cotton. Both of these cottons are cultivated in the cotton belt of the South, although the culture of Sea Island Cotton is mostly confined to a small area along the coast of South Carolina, Georgia and Florida. It is estimated that 99 per cent. of the cotton crop in the United States is Upland Cotton.

The mature fruit of the cotton plant is a 3- to 5-celled, leathery capsule called a "boll." It splits open by 3 to 5 valves exposing a white fluffy mass, which consists of numerous seeds, each concealed within a dense covering of its hairs. The hairs are outgrowths or elongations of epidermal cells of the seed coat. There are generally 2 kinds of hairs on the seed, viz.: long hairs known as "fiber" or "staple" and short hairs or "fuzz." Cotton is picked when the bolls split and the fibers project in a twisted mass. It is placed in baskets which are emptied into wagons which carry it to the gin house. Here the cotton is ginned, a process whereby the raw cotton is separated from the seed and linters. Raw cotton is composed of a mass of hairs, each of which has oil globules and often other impurities adhering to it. Moreover, each raw cotton hair is covered with a waxy cuticle which is impermeable to water. In order to be of service as an absorbent in surgery it must be deprived of the oily

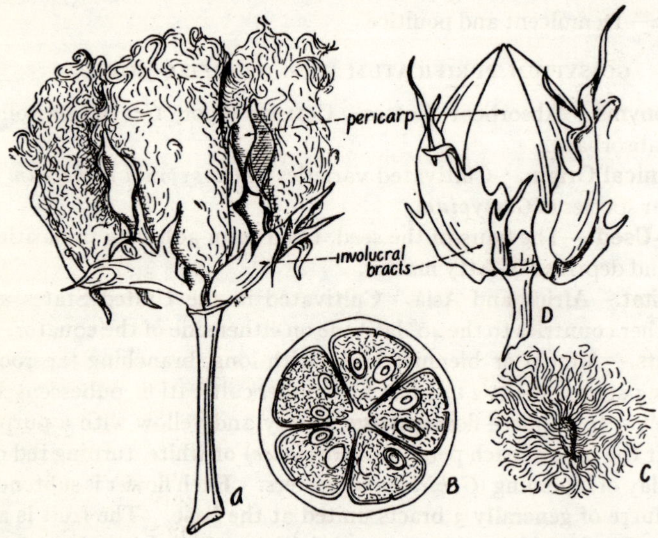

FIG. 166.—Upland cotton (*Gossypium hirsutum*). *A*, mature boll opened out; *B*, cross-section of young boll; *C*, single seed with hairs; *D*, young boll. (*From Robbins "Botany of Crop Plants."*)

material as well as its waxy cuticle and purified. This is accomplished by boiling the raw cotton under pressure with a dilute solution of caustic soda, washing in water to remove alkali, bleaching with chlorinated lime and hydrochloric acid, again washing and drying. The fibers are then loosened by a machine, and made into a light fluffy mass by further separating them with currents of air.

Description.—A soft, white mass of fine filamentous hairs without odor or taste. Under the microscope each purified cotton hair appears as a hollow, flattened and twisted band with a thickened wall of cellulose and a broad lumen. With careful focusing with a high power objective, the wall shows spiral striations. Absorbent cotton is soluble in ammoniated cupric oxide test solution but insoluble in the ordinary solvents. Iodine solution imparts to cotton a yellow color which is changed to blue upon the addition of sulphuric acid.

Constituent.—Cellulose in its purest form.

Uses.—Absorbent cotton is employed as an absorbent and protective dressing in surgery and as a filtering medium in pharmacy.

GOSSYPII CORTEX N.F. (COTTON ROOT BARK)

Synonyms.—Gossypii Radicis Cortex; *Ger.* Baumwollwurzelrinde; *Fr.* Ecorce de la Racine Cotonnier.

Botanical Origin.—Cultivated varieties of *Gossypium herbaceum* Linné, *Gossypium Barbadense* Linné, or *Gossypium hirsutum* Linné.

Part Used.—The recently-gathered air-dried bark of the root.

Limit of Impurities.—5 per cent. of wood or other foreign organic matter.

Habitat.—Asia and Africa. Cultivated in United States and many other countries.

Production and Commerce.—The drug should be made into fluid extract as soon after it is gathered as possible, for its yellow resin soon changes into an inert, brownish to reddish oxidized substance. The commercial supplies are obtained from Virginia, the Carolinas and other Cotton growing states of the south.

Description.—In flexible bands or quilled pieces attaining a length of about 30 cm. and a thickness of about 1 mm.; outer surface orange-brown, slightly longitudinally wrinkled with small circular lenticels, the cork and cortex frequently exfoliated and exposing the fibrous inner bark; inner surface light-brown, striated longitudinally; fracture tough, fibrous, the inner bark separating readily into fibrous layers; odor indistinct taste slightly acrid.

Histology.—Passing from outer to inner surface, transverse sections reveal the following peculiarities:

1. Cork consisting of many layers of large brick-shaped yellowish-brown cells with thin walls.

2. Cortex of several layers of parenchyma containing mostly simple or 2–4 compound starch grains, the individual grains being more or less spheroidal and up to 20μ in diameter. Some cells in this region possess tannin contents others rosette crystals of calcium oxalate while here and there a few secretion reservoirs lined with epithelium and containing yellowish-brown masses may be observed.

3. Phloem, a broad zone of large, conical phloem patches, each of which is separated from its neighbor by a large, wedge-shaped primary, starch-

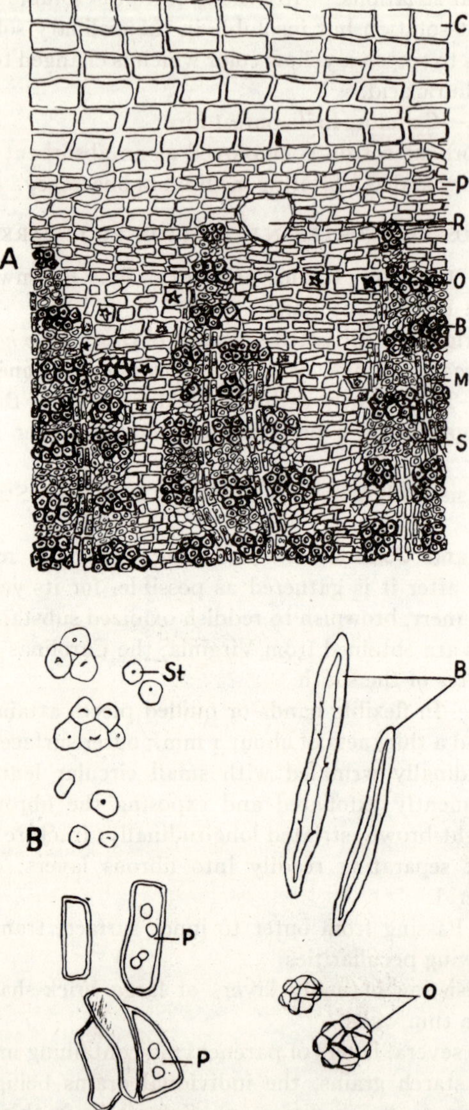

FIG. 167.—*A*, Transverse section of Gossypii Cortex (cotton root bark). Cork (*C*); cortical parenchyma, many of the cells containing tannin (*P*); secretory cavity (*R*) lined with epithelium and containing, in the freshly gathered bark, a pale yellow resin which darkens with age; rosette aggregate of calcium oxalate (*O*); bast fibers (*B*); soft bast (*S*); medullary-ray (*M*). *B*, Powdered cotton root bark. Starch grains (*St*); parenchyma containing starch (*P*); rosette aggregates of calcium oxalate (*O*).

containing, medullary ray which broadens out toward the cortex. Each phloem patch is traversed by narrow, secondary phloem medullary rays and shows alternating, tangentially arranged groups of strongly lignified bast fibers and soft bast. Some of the phloem cells in the soft bast regions contain rosette aggregates of calcium oxalate, others starch grains.

Constituents.—A yellow resin, tannin, etc.

Uses.—Emmenagogue and oxytocic.

THEACEÆ (TERNSTRŒMIACEÆ, CAMELLIACEÆ OR TEA FAMILY)

Evergreen shrubs or low branching or tall, often heavy trees with watery juice. Leaves for the most part alternate, evergreen, often leathery, sometimes membranous; stipules either bud scales and caducous or often absent; leaf margins sinuate or serrate (*Thea*). Inflorescence a raceme becoming by condensation terminal, one-flowered. Flowers regular, perfect, pentamerous; sepals five, rarely four to three, deciduous, occasionally subtended by bracteolar scales; petals five, brittle and succulent, varying from greenish-white or greenish-yellow through yellow to white or, from whitish-pink to pink, scarlet, crimson, very rarely a tendency toward purple; stamens typically five but, as they grow, they subdivide into staminal leaflets so that in their mature condition they are apparently indefinite and mono- to polyadelphous; stamens inserted hypogynously or perigynously and opposite the petals; pistil of typically five syncarpous carpels but reduced in some species to four to three or two. Fruit usually a capsule (*Thea*), five- to three-celled, dehiscing longitudinally, more rarely a fleshy, semi-baceate, semi-drupacous indehiscent fruit. Seeds with scanty or no albumen and often attached to inner angle of cells by projecting spongy placentæ.

THEA (TEA)

Synonyms.—Tea Leaves; *Fr.* Thé; *Ger.* Thee.

Botanical Origin.—*Thea sinensis* L. and its varieties (*Bohea*, *viridis*, *stricta*).

Part Used.—The prepared leaves and leaf buds.

Habitat.—Southern Asia, probably India.

Plants.—Evergreen shrubs, 3 to 5 feet high with alternate, elliptical or oblong-lanceolate, shiny, coriaceous, short petiolate, serrate leaves, white axillary flowers, and capsular fruits.

Production and Commerce.—The plants are extensively cultivated for the leaves in China, Japan, India, Ceylon, Java and Brazil. The leaves and leaf buds are gathered and either roasted in pans over a fire, cooled, rolled into balls, allowed to ferment and dried rapidly, producing the class of teas known as "green teas," on account of the dull green color of the product, or they are placed on trays, allowed to wither, rolled under pressure, allowed to ferment on mats, then dried and graded by sifting, producing the class of teas termed "black teas." Some grades are mixed with the sweet scented flowers of jessamine, orange, gardenia, etc. or placed in contact with these. There are numerous varieties and blends of teas on the market. The commercial supplies are chiefly obtained from China, Japan, India and Ceylon.

Description.—Usually in rolls or balls or crumpled masses, when entire nearly elliptical or oblong-lanceolate, short petiolate, summit acute or emarginate, base nearly spatulate tapering into a short petiole; margin serrate or nearly entire; color greenish or blackish green. Upper surface glabrous, lower surface smooth or hairy; more or less leathery; odor agreeably aromatic; taste bitter and astringent.

Histology.—The diagnostic histological elements found in tea are large, elongated, irregular, colorless idioblasts, numerous elongated unicellular, thick-walled, non-glandular hairs 10μ wide and about 1 mm. long. rosette aggregates of Ca$\bar{O}$, and stomata with 3–4 neighboring cells.

Adulterants.—1. *Camellia leaves:* Lower epidermis thick walled and more or less papillose. Idioblasts same as in tea.

2. *Acer Negundo Leaves.*—Non-glandular hairs and glandular hairs, the glandular hairs with a 2–3 celled stalk and large 1-celled head.

3. *Cherry Leaves* (*P. avium*).—Possess numerous small rosette aggregates of Ca$\bar{O}$ in lower epidermal cells.

4. *Gromwell leaves* (*Lithospermum officinale*) have stiff, scythe shaped hairs.

5. *Ash leaves* (*Fraxinus* spp.) have horned stomata, due to increased thickenings of the cuticle at the opening of the stomata. Epidermal cells very wavy in outline.

6. *Mulberry leaves* (*Morus alba* and *Morus nigra*) have cystoliths in the epidermal cells, non-glandular and glandular hairs, the latter with a unicellular stalk and a 5–9 celled glandular head.

7. *Strawberry leaves* (*Fragaria vesca*) exhibit long, unicellular, non-glandular hairs, the basal portions of which have thick walls with simple pores. Glandular hairs with 3-celled stalk and large head.

8. Leaves of *Willow Herb* (*Epilobium angustifolium*) contain numerous raphides and the non-glandular hairs are slightly wavy, rather broad and with rounded ends. Water stomata occur beneath teeth.

9. *Willow leaves* (*Salix*) exhibit small stomata with 2 accompaning cells; the hairs are crooked and with thin walls. Ca$\bar{O}$ in rosettes and monoclinic prisms.

10. *Wistaria* (*Kraunhia floribunda*) leaflets have non-glandular hairs with 2 short basal cells and a long, thin, pointed, distal cell.

11. Exhausted tea leaves and stems.

Constituents.—Caffeine (theine), gallotannic acid, gallic acid, resin, volatile oil, traces of theobromine, theophylline, adenine, etc.

Uses.—Tea is used as a cerebral and cardiac stimulant and as a source of caffeine. Much of the caffeine of commerce is made from tea siftings.

GUTTIFERÆ (GAMBOGE FAMILY)

Tropical trees (*Garcinia*), rarely shrubs, containing resinous principles in schizogenous resin canals found in cortex and pith. Leaves opposite, coriaceous. Flowers diœcious, generally pentamerous or tetramerous with usually five stamens which are subdivided. Fruit a berry (*Garcinia Hanburyi*), drupe or capsule. Seeds generally large; embryo large to huge, often with enlarged radicle and reduced or absorbed cotyledons.

CAMBOGIA U.S.P. (GAMBOGE)

Synonyms.—Pipe Gamboge, Gutta Gamba, Cambodia; *Ger.* Gummigutt; *Fr.* Gommegutte.

Part Used.—A gum resin.

Botanical Origin.—*Garcinia Hanburyi* Hooker filius.

Purity Rubric.—Not less than 65 per cent. of alcohol-soluble extractive, not more than 1 per cent. of acid insoluble ash and not more than 1 per cent. of foreign organic matter.

Habitat.—Siam, Cochin China and Annam.

Plant.—A spreading tree with orange-brown bark, opposite, ovate, leathery leaves and small, yellow, axillary clusters of diœcious flowers. The fruit is an orange-green, oily berry about the size of a crab apple that has 4 locules, each containing a seed.

Production and Commerce.—The gum resin constituting the drug occurs as a yellowish juice in schizogenous resin canals which are found in cortex, pith, leaves, flowers and fruit. It is collected mainly in Cochin China and Siam by making spiral incisions into the bark of the trunk from the ground upward. The juice exudes and is collected in hollow bamboo stems, allowed to harden, and the bamboo stem then stripped off. Most of the drug is exported from Singapore in the form of "pipes" packed in cases. Smaller amounts come from Bangkok and London.

Description.—In hard, cylindrical, brittle sticks, from 2 to 5 cm. in diameter, and of variable length; externally grayish-orange-brown, longitudinally striate; fracture conchoidal, smooth, orange red; odorless; taste very acrid. When triturated in a mortar with water it yields a yellow emulsion which darkens and becomes almost transparent upon the addition of ammonia water.

Powdered Drug.—Bright yellow. Chloral mounts exhibit scattered fragments of vegetable tissues. Few or no starch grains should be evident. Most of the powdered drug dissolves in chloral hydrate solution.

Constituents.—A resin called cambogic acid, gum, an oxidase enzyme, volatile oil, etc.

Uses.—Gamboge is employed medicinally as a hydragogue cathartic. It is also used by violin makers in preparing a stain for their wood.

Adulterants.—Cereal flours particularly wheat and rice, sand, and vegetable fragments.

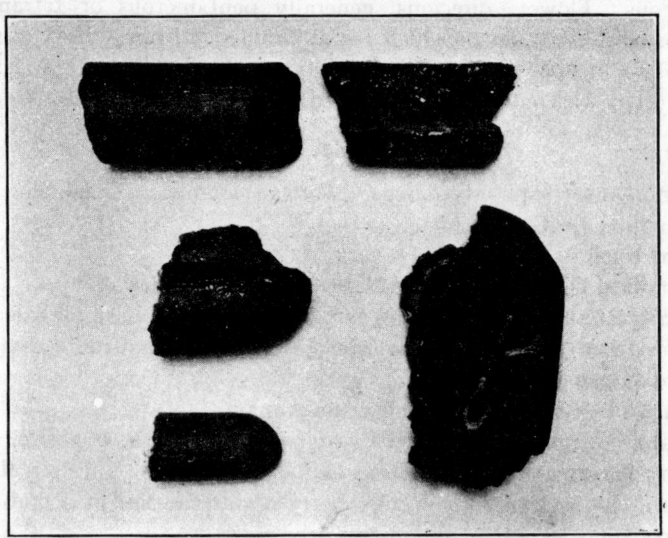

FIG. 168.—Gamboge, in broken pipes, × 16/35. (*Photograph by Stoneback.*)

CANELLACEÆ (CANELLA FAMILY)

Trees, the bark of which contains aromatic principles. Leaves alternate, pellucid-punctate. Flowers regular, golden-yellow, or white, and arranged in terminal or axillary cymes. Fruit a berry containing two to many seeds with oily and fleshy albumen.

CANELLA N. F. (CANELLA)

Synonyms.—White Cinnamon. *Fr.* Canelle blanche; *Ger.* Weisser Zimmt.

Botanical Origin.—*Canella Winterana* Linné (Gaertner).

Part Used.—The dried rossed bark.

Purity Rubric.—Not more than 2 per cent. of foreign organic matter.

Habitat.—West Indies.

Commercial Source.—Nassau, on island of New Providence, West Indies.

Plant.—A tree of medium height with ash-gray bark, alternate, coriaceous, pellucid-punctate leaves and white flowers.

Description.—In quills usually from 1 to 3 cm. in length and from 1 to 4 cm. in thickness, occasionally two or three times this size, or in irregular fragments of quills, from 1.5 to 5 mm. in thickness and 2 to 3 cm. in width, the outer periderm mostly removed; outer surface light brownish-yellow or pale orange-brown, more or less scaly, with a few very shallow fissures, often more or less reticulate with slight ridges; inner surface paler, somewhat smooth, but showing coarse, longitudinal striæ; fracture short and granular, pale yellow, with an irregular, slightly darker band just inside of the center. Odor slight unless the bark is heated, then aromatic, resembling that of cinnamon; taste aromatic, warm, somewhat bitter and mucilaginous.

Powdered Drug.—Light brown to brownish-red; numerous, isodiametric, thick-walled stone cells, the walls with simple or branching pores; calcium oxalate in rosette aggregates up to 50μ in diameter; starch grains simple or two- to three-compound up to 20μ in diameter; oil cells with suberized walls numerous.

Constituents.—Resin, bitter principle, volatile oil containing engenol, cineol and terpenes; mucilage, starch, etc. No tannin.

Uses.—Aromatic bitter and condiment; a constituent of Hiera Picra N. F.

CISTACEÆ (ROCK ROSE FAMILY)

Herbs or shrubs whose stem and branches are often glandular, pubescent or tomentose, with simple or stellate trichomes. Leaves simple, entire, the lower ones opposite, upper alternate. Flowers perfect, regular, terminal and solitary, or in cymes or unilateral racemes; sepals five, the external ones often bractiform or wanting; petals five (*Helianthemum* and *Hudsonia*) rarely three or none (*Lechea*); stamens hypogynous, indefinite; carpels three to five; ovary free, one-celled. Fruit a one-celled, three- to five-valved capsule.

HELIANTHEMUM (HELIANTHEMUM)

Synonyms.—Rock-rose, Frost-weed.

Botanical Origin.—*Helianthemum canadensē* Michx.

Part Used.—The dried herb.

Habitat.—Eastern United States in sandy soil as far south as North Carolina.

Plant.—A low shrub having erect, branching, reddish, hairy stems attaining a height of 5 dm. The leaves lanceolate or oblanceolate, green on upper surface, pale on lower surface. The flowers are of two kinds, rarely present at the same time, the earlier ones mostly solitary, pedicelled, with bright yellow corolla, from 2 to 3 cm. in breadth, hairy calyx, about 30 stamens and a 3-carpelled pistil, producing an ovoid capsule, about 6 or 7 mm. in length; later flowers smaller, nearly sessile, apetalous, in the axils of leaves, with only 4 stamens and a pistil, the latter maturing to form a capsule about 4 mm. in length. The odor of the drug is slightly aromatic. The taste is astringent and bitter.

Constituents.—Volatile oil, tannin,bitter principle, etc.

Uses.—Bitter tonic, astringent and alterative.

FLACOURTIACEÆ (FLACOURTIA FAMILY)

A family of chiefly tropical trees and shrubs with simple, alternate leaves, staminate, pistillate and hermaphrodite flowers, frequently dioecious or polygamous, with a 1-celled ovary. The fruits are either berries, drupes or rarely capsules. The seeds are albuminous.

OLEUM CHAULMOOGRÆ (CHAULMOOGRA OIL)

Synonym.—Kalaw Tree Oil.

Botanical Origin.—*Taraktogenos Kurzii* King.

Part Used.—The fixed oil expressed from the seeds.

Habitat.—Burma.

Plant.—*Taraktogenos Kurzii* is a tree attaining the height of 40 to 50 ft. whose young branches, leaves and flower clusters are tawny-pubescent. the trunk and older branches being covered with a grayish bark. Its mature leaves are alternate, lanceolate or oblong-lanceolate or occasionally elliptic, shiny, subcoriaceous with 6 to 7 pairs of main nerves. The inflorescence is a many-flowered axillary cyme. The staminate flowers which alone have been described by King are said to be about 3 in. in diameter and possess 4 ovate sepals, 8 broadly ovate petals having ciliate edges and 24 stamens. The fruit is a fawn-colored, globular berry about the size of an orange with a minutely granular, velvety rind and containing numerous irregularly oval, brownish-yellow seeds imbedded in a fleshy pulp.

Production and Commerce.—The seeds are collected by the natives of the Chittagong hills of Burma from the ripe fruits and sent to Calcutta where they are washed, dried in the sun, shelled and subjected to hydraulic pressure for the expression of the fixed oil. The cold drawn oil is then filtered. Oil containing chaulmoogric and hydnocarpic acids is also obtained from the seeds of *Hydnocarpus Wightiana* Blume and *H. anthelmintica* Pier. (Fam. *Flacourtiaceæ*) and can be legitimately substituted for Chaulmoogra oil, if agreeing with the latter in physical and chemical characters and its source be designated. The commercial supplies come from India or indirectly through London.

Constituents.—Chaulmoogric acid ($C_{18}H_{32}O_2$), palmitic acid, hydnocarpic acid, etc.

Uses.—Chaulmoogra oil is employed as a germicide in the treatment of leprosy. It has also been used in rheumatism, psoriasis and tuberculosis; it is the source of Ethyl Chaulmoograte U.S.P.

TURNERACEÆ (DAMIANA FAMILY)

Tropical herbs, shrubs (*Turnera*) or trees. Isolated groups of sclerenchyma fibers occur in the pericycle and numerous tannin cells in the cortex. Leaves alternate, simple, petioled, exstipulate, having in several species large nectar glands along the margin and base of the leaves. Flowers perfect, regular, axillary, pentamerous with one-celled ovary. Fruit a capsule with three valves. Seeds strophiolate with albuminous embryo.

DAMIANA N. F. (DAMIANA)

Synonyms.—Turnera, Damiana Leaves; *Ger.* Turnerenthee.

Botanical Origin.—*Turnera diffusa* Willdenow ex Schultes and *Turnera aphrodisiaca* Ward.

Part Used.—The dried leaf.

Limit of Impurities.—15 per cent. of its stems and not more than 3 per cent. of other foreign matter.

Ash.—Not more than 4 per cent. acid-insoluble.

Habitat.—California, Lower California, Mexico, West Indies and S. America.

Plants.—Shrubs.

Production and Commerce.—Damiana is grown in California and Texas but most of the drug used in this country is imported from Mexico and Bolivia.

Description.—Leaves obovate to lanceolate from 10 to 30 mm. in length and from 4–10 mm. in width; short petioled; apex acute; base cuneate; margin from 2 to 10 toothed on each side; veins of the first order straight, 2 ascending and running to the sinuses of the teeth, or occasionally branched, the branches entering the teeth; upper surface pale green, smooth; lower surface with a few glandular hairs on the veins and midrib (*Turnera aphrodisiaca*) or densely tomentose over the entire surface (*T. diffusa*). Intermixed with the leaves are often found reddish-brown twigs, the young ends and buds of which are grayish pubescent (*T. aphrodisiaca*) or white floccose (*T. diffusa*). In addition to these there may also occur flower buds, yellowish flowers and ovoid capsules, the latter containing crescentic seeds, the seed coats of which are reticulate. Each seed possesses a small, thin, membranous arillus. The odor is characteristically aromatic. The taste is aromatic, bitter and resinous.

Histology.—Transverse sections made through the lamina outside of the midrib show a clearly bifacial structure. Both epidermises possess stomata, the lower also showing glandular hairs with short stalks and multicellular heads. A single row of palisade cells faces each epidermis while a narrow zone of spongy parenchyma through which vascular tissue courses is seen in the center.

Powdered Drug.—Light yellowish-green; numerous rough, thick walled non-glandular hairs, often curved near the base, up to 900μ in length and 30μ in breadth at the base; fragments of stem epidermis showing rectangular epidermal cells and a few stomata; fragments of hypodermis, the cells of which are rectangular and have lignified walls; fragments of spiral tracheæ and tracheids; few strongly lignified stone cells and sclerenchyma fibers; fragments of lignified, porous, pith parenchyma; fragments of epidermal cells and leaf parenchyma; the former with somewhat wavy vertical walls and associated with broadly elliptical stomata; numerous rosette aggregates of calcium oxalate up to 32μ in diameter; few monoclinic prisms; few simple starch grains up to about 12μ in diameter.

Constituents.—A bitter principle termed damianin, volatile oil, a hard and a soft resin, tannin, etc.

Use.—Damiana is used as an aphrodisiac but is of doubtful value as such.

Substitute.—The leaves of *Aplopappus discoideus* and *Aplopappus Venetus* (Fam. *Compositæ*).

PASSIFLORACEÆ (PASSION FLOWER FAMILY)

Herbaceous or woody vines climbing by tendrils. Leaves alternate, simple, entire, lobed or compound. Flowers perfect or imperfect, solitary; peduncles jointed at the flowers; perianth petaloid with urceolate or tubular tube and four to five or eight to ten partite and two-seriate limb, the throat usually crowned by one or more series of subulate filaments which are frequently colored; gynophore elongating, supporting the stamens and pistil. Fruit a one-celled berry(*Passiflora*), or a 3- to 5-valved, dehiscent capsule containing numerous seeds.

PASSIFLORA N.F. (PASSION FLOWER)

Synonyms.—Passion Vine, Wild Passion Flower.
Botanical Origin.—*Passiflora incarnata* Linné.
Part Used.—The dried flowering and fruiting top.

Purity Rubric.—Not more than 5 per cent. of stems over 8 mm. in diameter or other foreign matter.

Habitat.—In dry soil of the southern United States; Virginia to Florida, west to Texas and Missouri.

Plant.—A perennial herb, climbing by means of axillary tendrils; leaves alternate, palmately 3- to 5-cleft with serrate lobes; flowers large, solitary, long peduncled, whitish, with a triple purple and pink crown; fruit an ovate berry containing numerous ovoid, flattened seeds that are covered with a yellowish or brownish aril.

Production and Commerce.—The drug is gathered in summer when in flower and fruit and carefully dried. The commercial supplies come chiefly from Virginia and North Carolina.

Description.—Stems subcylindrical, glabrous or slightly pubescent above, longitudinally striate, woody and hollow, the cavity about one-half the diameter; bark thin, greenish or purplish; wood porous and showing on its inner margin a thin layer of pith. Leaves more or less broken, greenish-brown, thick; when entire, palmately 3–5 cleft; base cordate, apex acute, margin of lobes serrate; petioles up to 5 cm. in length with 2 nectar-glands near the summit. Tendrils numerous and closely coiled. Flowers solitary, axillary, peduncles as long as the petioles, usually with an involucre of 3 bracts, calyx cup-shaped of 5 sepals; corolla of 4 to 5 yellow petals inserted on the calyx; corona of the fresh flowers purple and pink; stamens 5, monadelphous; ovary unilocular, superior; fruit an ovoid, many seeded berry, about the shape and size of a pullet egg; externally green or yellow, somewhat shrivelled; seeds flat, ovate, each with a yellow or brown arillus; odor slight, taste slightly acrid.

Constituents.—Not investigated.

Uses.—Motor depressant in neuralgia; also employed in insomnia, dysmenorrhœa and diarrhœa.

CARICACEÆ (PAPAW FAMILY)

A small tropical American family of trees and shrubs containing a milky juice. Leaves in a terminal cluster, alternate, exstipulate and usually palmately lobed. Flowers pentamerous, staminate, pistillate and hermaphrodite, racemose, the pistillate and hermaphrodite with a superior 1- to spuriously 5-celled ovury containing numerous ovules. Fruit a berry. Seeds albuminous. Laticiferous tubes occur in roots, stems, leaves and fruits.

CARICA (PAPAW)

Synonyms.—Papaya, Pawpaw.

Botanical Origin.—*Carica Papaya* L.

Parts Used.—The dried latex of the unripe fruit, the green fruits and the leaves.

Habitat.—Tropical America. Naturalized in Southern Florida.

Plant.—A tree attaining the height of about 20 ft. with large, long petioled, palmately 7-lobed leaves whose lobes are in turn divided into secondary lateral lobes. The inflorescences consist of racemose cymes of yellow, staminate and pistillate flowers. The fruit is a large melon-like, edible berry up to about 15 lbs. in weight and with a salmon-pink or yellow flesh and a central cavity in which are found numerous blackish spheriodal seeds.

Production and Commerce.—The Papaw is widely cultivated in tropical America, in Hawaii and other tropical countries for its fruits and leaves which with other parts of the plant contain the proteolytic enzyme, papain

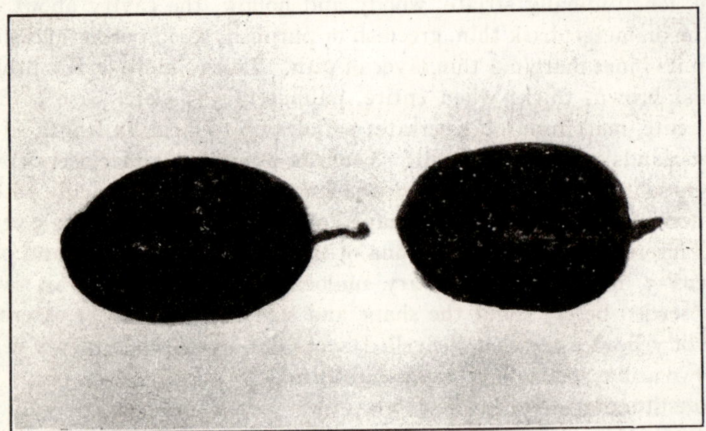

FIG. 169.—Fruits of the Paw Paw, *Carica Papaya*, × ⅛. (*Photograph by Stoneback.*)

Papain is obtained commercially by slashing the fruits and collecting the latex in porcelain-lined receptacles wherein it is permitted to evaporate until it has become granular. This constitutes the crude papain of commerce. From this the purified article (papain or papayotin) is prepared by dissolving it in water and precipitating with alcohol.

Constituents.—The latex of Papaw contains about 5 per cent. of the proteolytic enzyme, papain; a rennin-like enzyme, an amylolytic enzyme, a lipase and pectase; traces of the alkaloid carpaine, etc.

Use.—Digestant. The leaves and green fruits are eaten by the natives as vegetables.

CACTACEÆ (CACTUS FAMILY)

Herbaceous, rarely arborescent (*Cereus giganteus*), more or less succulent plants living in warm, dry (*Pereskia*), usually desert situations, rarely becoming epiphytic and correspondingly modified. Stems accordingly varying from elongate, slightly enlarged, green (*Pereskia*), to flattened and ribbed (*Selenicereus*) to flattened and shortened (*Opuntia*), to condensed (*Echinocactus*, *Echinocereus*, etc.), to greatly condensed (*Mamillaria*). Leaves alternate, stipulate or exstipulate, enlarged and more or less fleshy (*Pereskia*), becoming reduced, green and semicircular (*Opuntia*), or modified into spines, or wholly absorbed. Stems and leaves possess numerous mucilage sacs and crystals of calcium oxalate. Flowers, regular, solitary, or fascicled, in axils of leaves; sepals five; petals similar to sepals, petaloid, small to much enlarged, in color varying from yellow to white or from yellow to yellowish-pink, pink, scarlet or crimson; stamens indefinite, inserted at varying levels in the throat of a greatly expanded up-grown receptacle; pistil generally tricarpellary; ovary inferior, often deeply sunk in up-grown receptacular part; style thread-like, divided above into as many stigmas as carpels. Fruit a receptacular berry enclosing numerous small seeds. Seeds exalbuminous.

CACTUS GRANDIFLORUS N.F. (CACTUS GRANDIFLORUS)

Synonyms.—Night Blooming Cereus, Cactus, *Ger.* Königin der Nacht; *Fr.* Cierge à grandes fleurs.

Botanical Origin.—*Selenicereus grandiflorus* Brit. and Rose [*Cactus grandiflorus* Linné, *Cereus grandiflorus* Miller].

Part Used.—The fresh succulent stem of the wild growing plant.

Habitat.—Jamaica.

Plant.—A perennial creeping or climbing vine with a stout, bluish-green, ribbed stem bearing at intervals tufts of from 9 to 12 brownish, acicular spines and longer bristles together with branched roots. Its flowers are large, up to 8 or 10 inches in diameter. They open at sundown and decay the following morning.

Production and Commerce.—Both the fresh stems and the flowers are employed in the preparation of separate tinctures. The genuine article is collected only in Jamaica, the commercial supplies being shipped to this country from Kingston, Jamaica. The flowers are made into a tincture as soon as they open.

Description.—Cactus stem occurs in segments of variable length, from 1.5 to 4 cm. in diameter and with 5 to 9 angles or ribs, the latter at intervals of about 2 cm. showing tufts of from 9 to 12 acicular spines about 5 mm. in length, together with a number of bristles about 1 cm. in length; at irregular intervals along the ribs, branched roots sometimes occur; odor strong, herb-like; taste acidulous and mucilaginous.

Histology.—Transverse sections of the stem exhibit a 5 to 9 angled outline and the following internal structure: An epidermis of papillose cells, a narrow hypodermis of clear mucilage containing cells, a broad cortex of chlorenchyma tissue, a narrow circle of open collateral fibrovascular bundles separated by medullary rays and a narrow central pith. Mucilage sacs and crystal cells occur scattered through the cortex, pith and medullary rays. The crystal cells contain either solitary crystals of

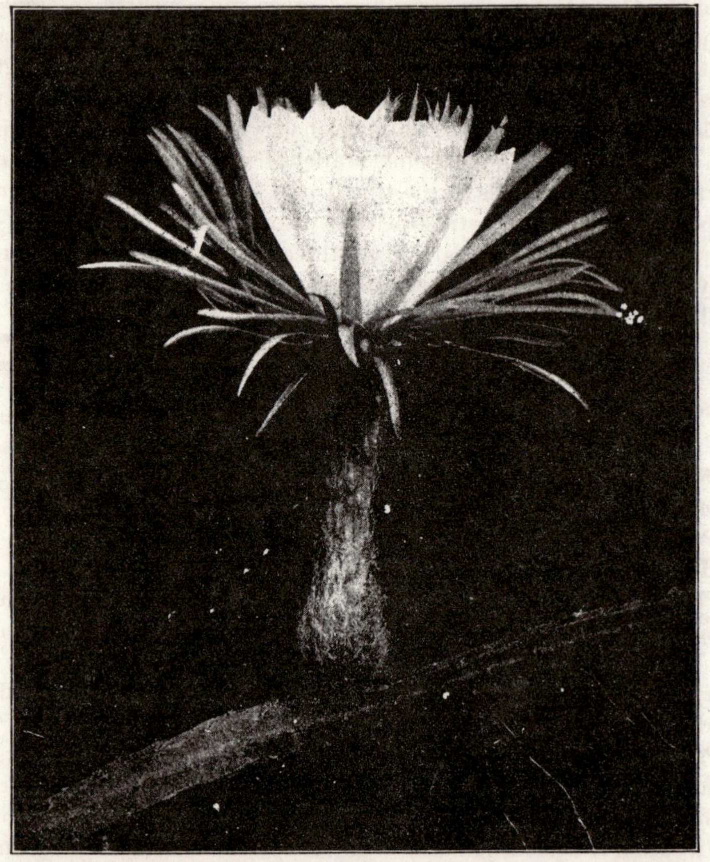

FIG. 170.—*Selenicereus grandiflorus* (L.) Britton & Rose (*Cactus grandiflorus*, Linnaeus). (*Portrait from United States National Museum through the kindness of Dr. J. N. Rose.*)

calcium oxalate up to 400μ in length or raphides of CaO. Thick walled bast fibers occur in the phloem.

Constituents.—A resinous substance, mucilage, tartaric acid, etc.

Uses.—Cactus is employed chiefly as a heart and nerve tonic.

Substitutes.—The stems of two Mexican species of *Selenicereus*, viz., *S. spinulosus* Brit. and Rose and *S. pteranthus* Brit. and Rose have long been imported and used in place of the genuine article. *Selenicereus spinulosus* may be distinguished by its usually 5-ribbed stem bearing at intervals about 8 very short dark spines which are not acicular. *S. pteranthus* possesses 4- or 6-ribbed stems, the ribs showing groups of 1 to 4 short spines which are not acicular.

THYMELÆACEÆ (MEZEREON FAMILY)

Shrubs (*Daphne Mezereum*) or low trees, usually of branching habit, the stems developing long tenacious bast fibers. Leaves alternate, rarely opposite, coriaceous, simple, varying from lanceolate to ovate, devoid of glandular hairs. The vascular bundles are bicollateral. Inflorescence a condensed raceme or spike. Flowers perfect, polygamous or diœcious, small, with calyx alone of the perianth parts developed. This is crimson-purple in *Daphne Mezereum*. Sepals usually fused to form a tube or cup-shaped perianth. Stamens usually eight in two rows of four longer and four shorter (*Daphne Mezereum*), inserted on the calyx tube. Pistil monocarpellary; ovary superior, mostly one-celled with a single pendulous ovule. Fruit a nut, drupe, or berry (*Daphne*). Calcium oxalate occurs in the form of rosette aggregates, styloids, micro-crystals or monoclinic prisms.

MEZEREUM N.F. (MEZEREUM)

Synonyms.—Mezereon, Mezereon Bark, Spurge Laurel, Wild Pepper; *Fr.* Ecorce de Mézéréon; *Ger.* Seidelbastrinde, Kellerhalsrinde.

Botanical Origin.—*Daphne Mezereum* Linné, *Daphne Laureola* Linné and *Daphne Gnidium* Linné.

Part Used.—The dried bark from the aerial stem.

Purity Rubric.—Not more than 2 per cent. of foreign organic matter.

Habitat.—Europe and Asia.

Plants.—*Daphne Mezereum* is a straggling deciduous shrub with smooth, light gray bark, the young branches being covered with dense white hairs. Its leaves are alternate, lanceolate, entire and dark green, with very short petioles. Its small purplish-pink flowers occur in clusters of 2 or 3, sessile in the axils of fallen leaves, on branches of the previous year. Its fruit is an ovoid, slightly pointed, bright red drupe.

Production and Commerce.—The bark is collected from the shrubs from November to early March, dried and made up into rolls or small bundles. It enters commerce mainly through southern France, Algeria and Thuringia.

Description.—In flexible, tough, somewhat flattened strips or quilled pieces up to 90 cm. in length, of variable breadth and up to 1 mm. in thickness; outer surface yellowish or olive-brown (*D. Mezereum*) or purplish-brown (*D. Gnidium*) or purplish-gray (*D. Laureola*), smooth, showing numerous lenticels and often brownish-black apothecia of lichens; cork readily separable from the greenish to olive brown middle bark; inner surface yellowish-white, satiny lustrous, finely striated; fracture tough, fibrous; inner bark lamellated; odor faint; taste at first slight, becoming gradually and increasingly pungent and acrid.

Histology.—Transverse sections, mounted in chloral hydrate solution exhibit the following peculiarities, when examined microscopically:

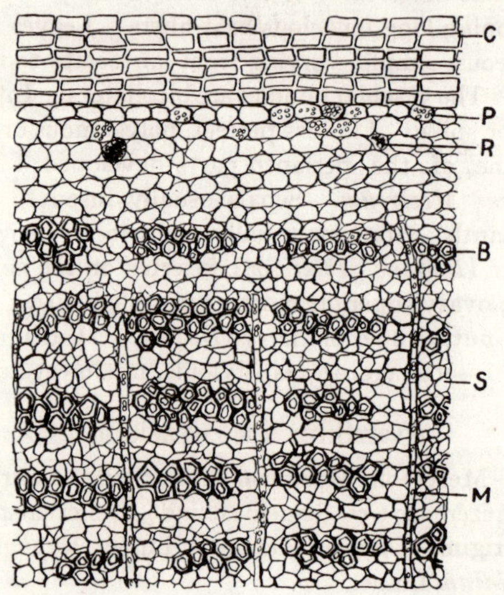

FIG. 171.—Mezereum. Transverse section of bark showing cork (*C*); collenchymatous tissue containing chloroplastids (*P*); cells containing greenish-yellow resinous substance (*R*); bast fibers (*B*); sieve tissue (*S*) and medullary-rays (*M*).

1. Cork, usually forming a broad zone of 20 to 30 layers of cells, the outer being compressed and yellowish-brown, the inner being tabular and nearly colorless.

2. Cork cambium of meristematic cells.

3. Cortex, the outer 3 to 5 rows of cells of which are collenchymatic and contain either chloroplastids or a yellowish-green resinous substance.

4. Phloem, a comparatively broad zone separated into phloem patches by means of narrow, starch-containing medullary rays, averagely 1-cell wide. Each phloem patch contains striking groups of loosely arranged, non-lignified bast fibers.

Powdered Drug.—Light grayish-brown; numerous long, non-lignified, poreless and colorless bast fibers that are often uneven or irregularly bent and considerably attenuated at their ends; fragments of yellowish-brown or colorless cork cells; fragments of starch-containing medullary rays;

fragments of cortical parenchyma containing resinous substance and chloroplasts; few nearly spheroidal starch grains up to 15μ in diameter, and 2–4 compound starch grains.

Constituents.—A greenish-brown acrid resin (mezerein) readily decomposing into mezereic acid in preparations of the bark, glucoside (daphnin), fixed oil, malic acid, sugars, starch, etc. Mezerein is the vesicant principle.

Uses.—Vesicant and counter-irritant.

GRANATACEÆ (POMEGRANATE FAMILY)

Herbs (*Cuphea*), shrubs (*Decadon*) or low trees (*Punica*) containing astringent principles. Leaves either alternate, opposite (*Punica*) or whorled, simple, usually lanceolate to ovate, entire, often glandular, viscous and containing idioblasts. Stems and leaves possess bicollateral bundles. Inflorescence a raceme, spike, or condensed cyme. Flowers perfect, usually regular, but pass more or less to irregular, sometimes very irregular as in genus *Cuphea;* sepals five to four, more or less fused below in themselves and with calyx tube; petals commonly five, often frilled or crumpled, inserted on the mouth of the calyx tube; stamens fifteen, ten, or five in alternate rows of five each, inserted hypogynously or perigynously; pistil six-, five-, four-, two-, rarely one-carpeled with as many cavities in the ovary and numerous small ovules; style elongate with pointed or knobbed stigma. Flowers of *Punica granatum* are scarlet in color. Fruit a baccate capsule (*Punica granatum*) or a capsule, dehiscing longitudinally or transversely. Seeds exalbuminous. Calcium oxalate occurs in rosette aggregates.

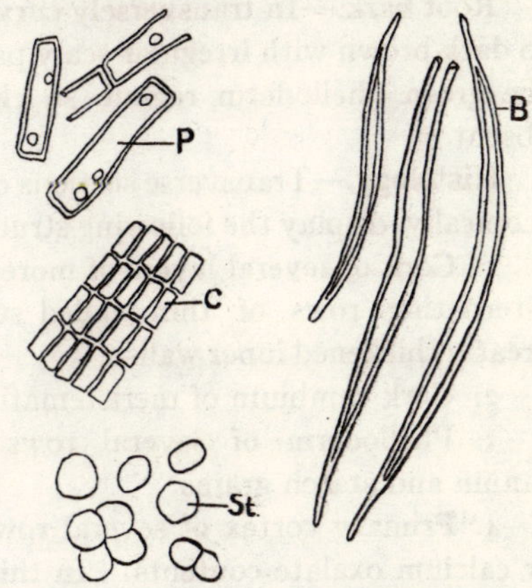

FIG. 172.—Powdered Mezereum. Parenchyma containing starch (*P*); cork tissue (*C*); starch grains (*St*); bast fibers (*B*).

GRANATUM U.S.P. (POMEGRANATE)

Synonyms.—Pomegranate Bark, Carthagenian Apple, Grenadier; *Ger.* Granatrinde; *Fr.* Ecorce de Balaustier.

Botanical Origin.—*Punica Granatum* Linné.

Part Used.—The dried bark of the stem or root.

Limit of Impurities.—2 per cent. of wood or other foreign organic matter.

Habitat.—India.

Plant.—A large shrub or small tree with oblong or obovate, shining leaves, orange-red showy flowers and large, red, many seeded, pome-like berry fruits, the seeds of which are surrounded by a succulent, red, edible flesh.

Description. Stem bark.—This occurs in transversely curved pieces or quills of variable length and up to 3.5 mm. in thickness; outer surface yellowish to grayish-brown with grayish patches of foliaceous lichens with their brownish-black apothecia, longitudinally wrinkled, also marked with small, broadly elliptical lenticels and with more or less abraded patches of cork; inner surface light yellow or yellowish-brown, finely striate; fracture short, smooth, exhibiting a greenish phelloderm; odor slight; taste astringent, somewhat bitter and nauseous.

Root bark.—In transversely curved pieces; externally brownish-yellow to dark brown with irregular scaly patches of cork; internally dark yellow, the green phelloderm region, so characteristic of the stem bark, being absent.

Histology.—Transverse sections of the *stem bark*, when examined microscopically, display the following structural characteristics.

1. Cork of several layers of more or less tabular cells and composed of alternating rows of thin walled suberized cells and lignified cells with greatly thickened inner walls.

2. Cork cambium of meristematic cells.

3. Phelloderm of several rows of cells containing chloroplastids, tannin and starch grains.

4. Primary cortex of several rows of parenchyma cells with starchy, or calcium oxalate contents. In this region there also occur large, thick walled and lamellated stone cells with branching pore canals. These are arranged singly or in small groups. Calcium oxalate crystals occur in various cells of the primary cortex both as rhombohedral crystals and rosette aggregates.

5. Phloem, a broad region of numerous narrow phloem patches separated by medullary rays most of which are one cell in width. Each phloem patch is characterized by its numerous tangential rows of cells containing rosette aggregates of calcium oxalate. Other phloem cells possess starch grains, still others contain yellowish-brown amorphous tannin masses. Bast fibers are absent.

The *root bark*, as seen in cross section, somewhat resembles the stem bark, differing mainly from the latter by the absence of primary cortex, chloroplastids, and, the presence of a broader phloem, the medullary rays of which extend nearly to the outer surface.

Powdered Drug.—Yellowish-brown to dark brown; calcium oxalate crystals numerous, in rosette aggregates, rhombohedra, or crystal fibers, the individual crystals up to 18μ in diameter; fragments of cork with lignified walls; starch grains numerous, spheroidal, ellipsoidal or irregular, simple or compound, the simple grains up to 12μ in diameter; stone cells mostly single, occasionally in small groups, the individual cells from 50 to 185μ in length and possessing thick, strikingly lamellated walls with branching pore canals; fragments of parenchyma containing yellowish-brown amorphous masses or chloroplastids. The latter are not present in ground or powdered root bark. Samples of powdered drug obtained from bark to which wood adhered show occasional slightly lignified wood fibers and porous tracheæ.

Constituents.—The liquid alkaloids, pelletierine, methylpelletierine, methylisopelletierine, isopelletierine; the solid crystalline alkaloid, pseudo-pelletierine; about 22 per cent. of tannin; starch, calcium oxalate and a yellow coloring substance. The tannin gives a bluish-black precipitate with iron solutions.

Use.—Pomegranate bark is used as a taenifuge usually in the form of a decoction.

Adulterants.—(1) Bark of *Buxus sempervirens* or Boxwood. (2) Bark of *Berberis vulgaris* or Barberry. Both of these are devoid of tannin.

MYRTACEÆ (MYRTLE FAMILY)

Rarely herbs (*Careya*) mostly shrubs or trees, some being the tallest trees known (*Eucalyptus*). Stems often tend to develop cork in flakes which separate much as in the Buttonwoods. Leaves rarely alternate nearly always opposite, entire, often glistening, subcoriaceous to coriaceous (*Eucalyptus*, *Pimenta*, etc.), frequently edge-on in position upon branches. Inflorescence cymose, at times forming scorpioid cymes, becoming condensed into small fascicles, or each cyme condensing into a solitary flower.

Flowers regular or very rarely irregular from the lop-sided development of the stamens. Symmetry rarely hexamerous, typically pentamerous, not infrequently reduced to tetramerous (*Clove*); sepals five, six or four, aposepalous, synsepalous at base, superior and inserted around the edge of an expanded, upgrown receptacular disc, varying from green and more or less expanded to short, thick, fleshy (*Clove*) or reduced to teeth (*Eucalyptus*); petals equal in number to the sepals, more or less petaloid and enlarged, rarely reduced and wanting, varying in color from green through greenish-yellow to white (*Eugenia* species) or from whitish to pink, scarlet, crimson, purple and blue, petals sometimes synpetalous and cup-like, detaching as the flower opens; stamens usually indefinite and epigynous, varying in the color of their filaments as do the petals; pistil rarely of ten to six carpels, usually of five, not infrequently as in Clove of four carpels; ovary inferior or semi-inferior, as many-celled as there are carpels and with central placentation; style elongate; stigma undivided. Fruit either a hard, woody indehiscent nut (Brazil Nut), a capsule dehiscing at apex (*Eucalyptus*) or berry (*Eugenia*). Seeds exalbuminous.

EUCALYPTUS U.S.P. (EUCALYPTUS)

Synonyms.—Blue Gum Leaves, Australian Fever Tree Leaves, Iron Bark Tree; *Fr.* Feuilles d'Eucalyptus; *Ger.* Eucalyptus Blätter.

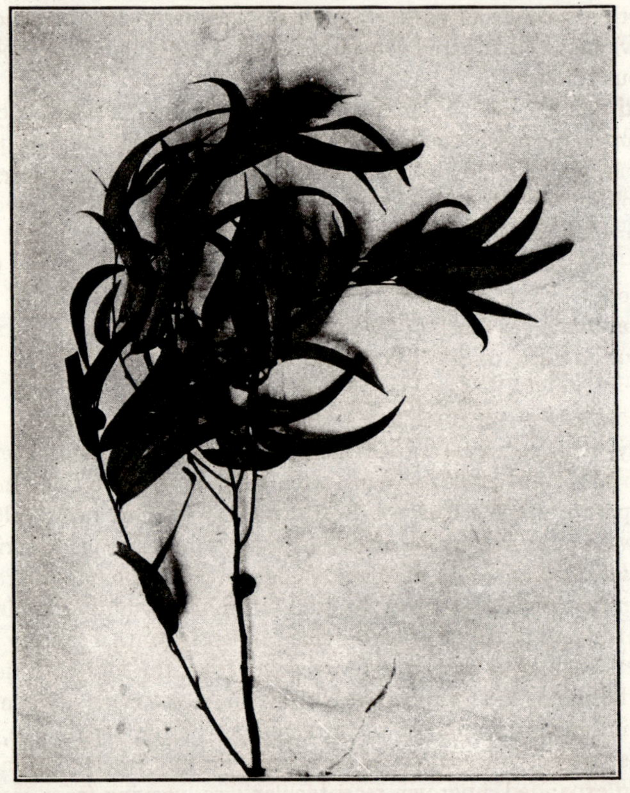

Fig. 173.—Leafy branch of *Eucalyptus globulus*, × ⅛. (*Photograph by Stoneback.*)

Botanical Origin.—*Eucalyptus globulus* Labillardière.

Part Used.—The dried scythe-shaped leaf.

Limit of Impurities.—3 per cent. of stems, fruits or other foreign organic matter.

Habitat.—Australia and Tasmania. Cultivated in California and Southern Europe.

Plant.—A very tall tree with ash-gray bark, opposite leaves on younger branches and alternate leaves on older ones, and white flowers, the calyx tube of each of which is covered by a conical lid called the operculum, and composed of the limb of the calyx and united petals. The fruit is a woody truncated capsule.

Production and Commerce.—The Eucalyptus trees are grown in Australia, Tasmania, Southern Europe and California and are amongst the tallest trees known. The leaves are gathered from older parts of the trees, dried and baled. The commercial supplies are mainly shipped to the U. S. A. from Brussels, Antwerp and Marseilles.

Description.—Petiole twisted; lamina lanceolately scythe-shaped, bifacial, from 8 to 30 cm. in length and from 2 to 7 cm. in breadth; coriaceous; apex, when present, acute or acuminate; base unequal, obtuse or somewhat rounded; margin uneven, revolute; ventral and dorsal surfaces grayish-green to pale yellowish-green, more or less glaucous, glabrous glandular-punctate, with numerous small rounded brown dots of cork; venation pinnate-reticulate, the veins of the first order running to within a short distance from the margin where they anastomose with each other and form a vein nearly parallel with the margin; odor aromatic; taste aromatic, bitter and cooling.

Histology.—1. Upper and lower epidermis composed of clear, polygonal epidermal cells with thick cutinized outer walls. Both epidermises possess sunken stomata.

2. Mesophyll (chlorenchyma) differentiated into palisade and spongy parenchyma regions, there being two palisade regions of 3 to usually 4 rows of cells each, one facing each epidermis. In each of these regions occur large, sub-globular, internal glands, lined with secretory epithelium and containing yellow oil of Eucalyptus. The spongy parenchyma region is a narrow zone of more or less loosely arranged cells between the 2 palisade zones. Some of its cells contain rosette aggregates while others possess monclinic prisms of calcium oxalate. Fibrovascular tissue courses through the spongy parenchyma. In the midrib and petiole a more or less interrupted arc of slightly lignified pericyclic fibers occurs just outside these bundles.

Powdered Drug.—Light green; fragments of chlorenchyma with embedded, broken, yellow, internal glands numerous; calcium oxalate in rosette aggregates or monoclinic prisms up to 25μ in diameter; fragments of epidermis with polygonal cells having very thick cuticle and sunken, almost invisible, stomata; fragments of selerenchyma fibers and thick walled stone cells; fragments of cork; tracheids.

Constituents.—Up to 6 per cent. of volatile oil (U.S.P.) of which 60 per cent. or more is eucalyptol (U.S.P.), the balance consisting of d-pinene and other terpenes; resins, a bitter principle, tannin, eucalyptic acid, calcium oxalate.

Uses.—Stomachic, carminative, expectorant, rubefacient, antiseptic and antiperiodic.

Adulterants.—(1) Leaves from young branches of *E. globulus* that are ovate-oblong, dorsoventral and opposite. These show stomata only on the dorsal surface and palisade parenchyma only beneath the ventral epidermis. (2) Leaves of allied species, some of which are less leathery in texture and not as fragrant in odor.

EUCALYPTI GUMMI N.F. (EUCALYPTUS GUM)

Synonyms.—Red Gum, Australian Kino, Eucalyptus Kino, Creek Gum.

Botanical Origin.—*Eucalyptus rostrata* Schlechtendal and other species of *Eucalyptus*.

Plants.—*Eucalyptus rostrata* or Red Gum is a forest tree attaining a height of 200 feet with gray bark and reddish twigs. It possesses lanceolate, acuminate leaves, axillary umbels of small flowers, each with a hemispheric calyx tube and lid, the latter beaked, and small, nearly globular, caspular fruits. Other Australian trees yielding smaller amounts of this drug include *E. amygdalina*, *E. marginata*, *E. falcifolia*, *E. Leucoxylon*, *E. Gunnii*, *E. piperita*, *E. macrorycha*, and *E. stellulata*.

Part Used.—The dried gummy exudate.

Habitat.—Australia.

Production and Commerce.—A red juice is secreted in cavities of the wood or between the bark and wood, of these trees. It is obtained by making an incision into the trunk and inserting a trough-shaped piece of tin, by means of which the liquid, as it exudes is conveyed into buckets. The juice is then boiled or allowed to evaporate spontaneously until it attains the consistency of a solid mass. This becomes friable, breaking up into fragments. The commercial supplies are shipped from Melbourne and Victoria, Australia to England, thence some reaches this country.

Description.—When first collected the juice has a syrupy consistency and a sour odor. After drying it occurs in friable masses of a blackish color or in grains; small fragments are ruby-red, have a dusty appearance, and lack the brittleness of those of Malabar Kino; odor indistinct; taste astringent, imparting a red color to the saliva. From 80 to 90 per cent. of the drug is soluble in cold water.

Constituents.—46 to 47 per cent. of kino-tannic acid; kinoin, kino red catechin and pyrocatechin.

Use.—Astringent in pharyngitis and laryngitis, in form of troches.

PIMENTA N.F. (PIMENTA)

Synonyms.—Allspice, Clove Pepper; *Fr.* Toute épice; *Ger.* Nelkenpfeffer, Allerlei-Gewürz.

Botanical Origin.—*Pimenta officinalis* Lindley.

Part Used.—The dried, nearly ripe fruit.

Purity Rubric.—Not more than 3 per cent. of stems or other foreign organic matter, not more than 0.4 per cent. of acid-insoluble ash, and not over 25 per cent. of crude fiber.

Ash.—Not more than 6 per cent. of total ash and not more than 0.4 per cent. of acid-insoluble ash (Circ. 136, U.S. Dept. Agric.).

Habitat.—West Indies, Mexico, Central America and Northern South America.

Plant.—An evergreen tree growing to the height of about 12 m. Its leaves are entire, ovate-oblong, pellucid-punctate on dorsal surface. Its

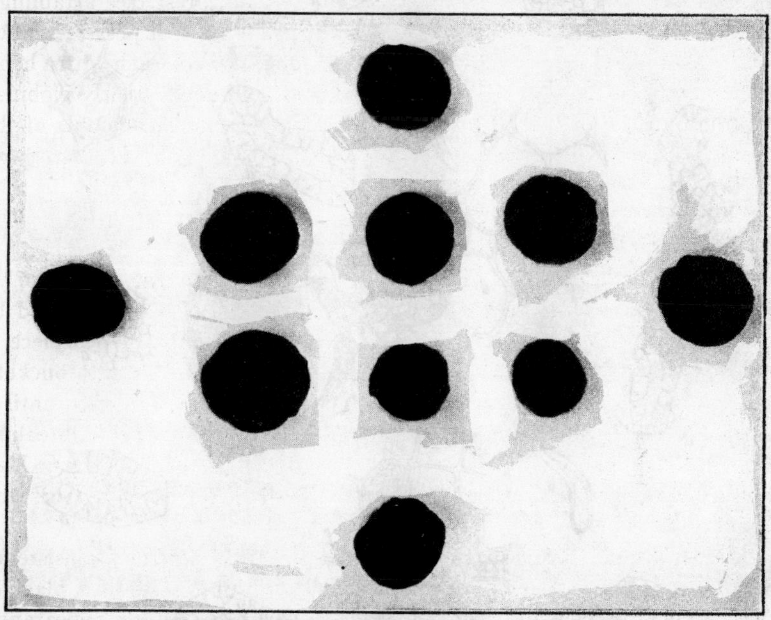

FIG. 174.—Allspice, × 1⅓. (*Photograph by Stoneback.*)

flowers are small, white and borne in racemose cymes. Its fruit is a berry crowned with a persistent calyx and style.

Production and Commerce.—The fruits are gathered when full grown but green, by breaking off the inflorescence axes and drying the twigs and berries in ovens or rarely in the sun. The dried fruits are readily separated. The commercial supplies are imported largely from Jamaica.

Description.—A mixture of entire berries and broken stems. Berry inferior, sub-globular to globular, dark brown to dark reddish-brown, the surface being rough and granular; summit with calyx ring, within which is a depression containing the remains of the style; base with short stalk or stem scar; internally exhibiting 2 or 3 chambers, separated by thin dissepiments, each chamber containing a single plano-convex to angular reddish-brown seed; odor aromatic; taste sweet and pungent.

Powdered Drug.—Reddish-brown or dark brown. Numerous stone cells of variable shape with porous, strongly lignified walls and frequently

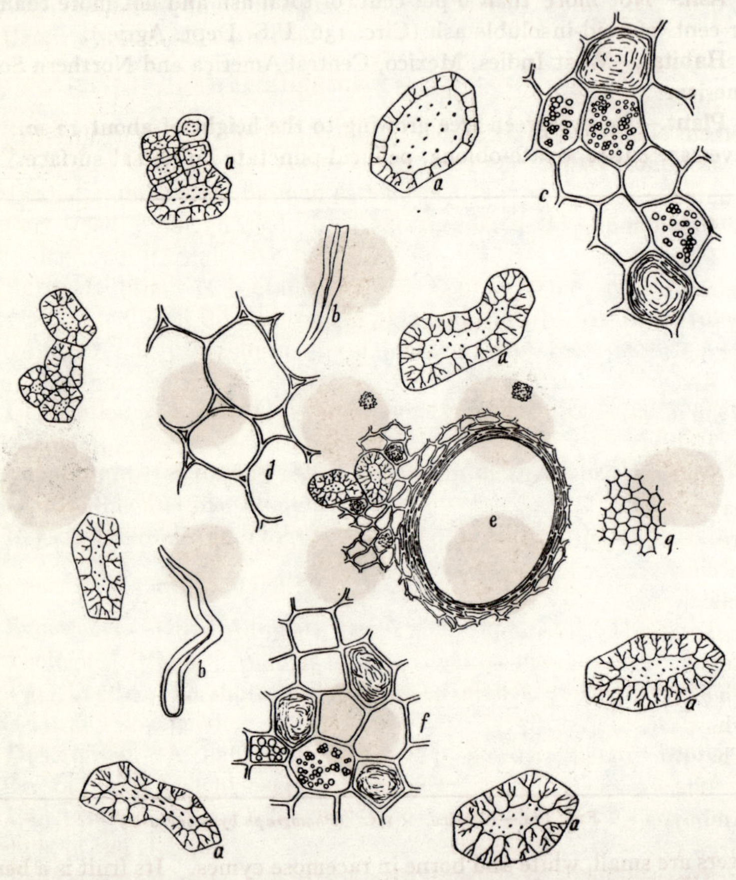

FIG. 175.—Powdered Pimenta. (*a*) Stone cells; (*b*) trichomes; (*c*) parenchyma with starch and resin; (*d*) parenchyma; (*e*) gland, stone cells and crystal bearing cells; (*f*) endosperm cells with starch and resin; (*g*) epidermal cells. (*Schneider*.)

containing a brownish amorphous substance; numerous simple or 2–3 compound starch grains, the individual grains spherical, plano-convex or polygonal with a central hilum and averagely up to 25μ in diameter; fragments of irregular shape containing internal glands with a yellowish-brown oil content; rosette crystals of calcium oxalate; few stem fragments showing somewhat curved, narrow lumened non-glandular hairs, long, narrow sclerenchyma fibers and tracheids.

Constituents.—Volatile oil (3 to 4 per cent.) containing eugenol (U.S.P.) an acrid fixed oil, tannin, resin, etc.

Adulterants of Powder.—Ground olive pits, cocoanut shells, cocoa sheels, allspice stems, etc.

Uses.—Aromatic and condiment.

CARYOPHYLLUS U.S.P. (CLOVE)

Synonyms.—Cloves; *Fr.* Girofle, Clous aromatiques; *Ger.* Gewürznelken, Nägelein.

Botanical Origin.—*Caryophyllus aromaticus* L. [*Eugenia aromatica* (L.) Kuntze].

Part Used.—The dried flower-buds.

Purity Rubric.—Not more than 5 per cent. of its stems and not more than 1 per cent. of other foreign organic matter. It yields not less than 15 per cent. of volatile ether-soluble extractive, not more than 10 per cent. of crude fiber and not more than 0.75 per cent. of acid-insoluble ash.

Ash.—Not more than 7 per cent. total ash nor more than 0.5 per cent. of ash insoluble in hydrochloric acid (Circ. 136, U.S. Dept. Agric.).

Habitat.—Molucca Islands.

Plant.—An evergreen tree attaining a height of 30 or 40 feet. The leaves are entire, smooth, coriaceous and glandular punctate. The flowers are tetramerous, rose-colored and arranged in axillary and terminal racemes of cymes. The fruit is an ovoid berry which, when nearly ripe, is collected and sold as "Mother of Cloves."

Production and Commerce.—The clove trees are cultivated in Java, Ceylon, Zanzibar, Pemba and Madagascar. The flower buds are gathered when pink and unexpanded (generally in August or September) by natives, who either pick them off the branches or beat them off with bamboo canes. They are then either dried in the sun or artificially and garbled.

The commercial supplies come mainly from Zanzibar, Madagascar, Amboyna and Penang. The finest cloves come from Penang. They are large, plump and reddish-brown.

Description.—From 10 to 17.5 mm. in length, of a dark brown, reddish-brown or brownish-black color, consisting of a stem-like, solid, inferior ovary, obscurely four-angled or somewhat compressed, terminated by four calyx teeth, and surmounted by a nearly globular head, consisting of four petals, which enclose numerous curved stamens and one style; odor strongly aromatic; taste pungent and aromatic, followed by slight numbness.

When Clove is pressed strongly between the thumb nail and finger the volatile oil becomes visible.

Stems either separate or attached to the flower-buds; sub-cylindrical or four-angled, attaining a length of 25 mm. and a diameter of 4 mm., either simple, branching or distinctly jointed, and less aromatic than the flower-buds.

Powdered Drug.—Dark brown to reddish-brown, consisting mainly of cellular fragments showing the large oil reservoirs, spiral tracheæ and a few somewhat thick-walled, slightly-lignified, spindle-shaped bast-

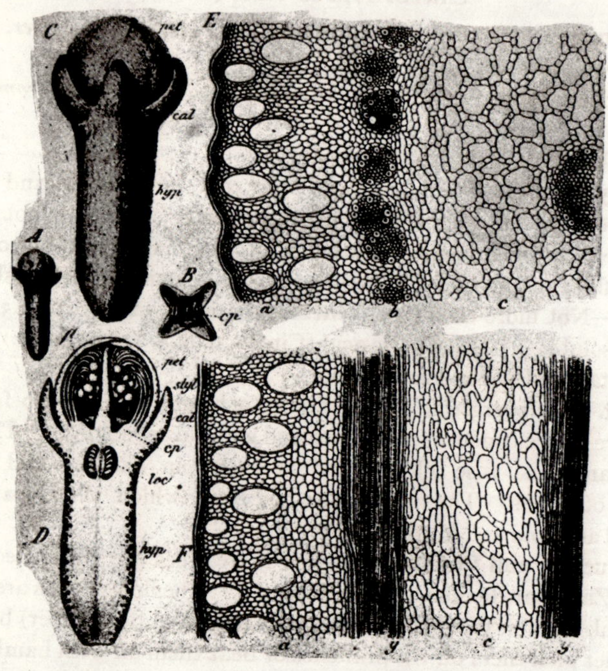

FIG. 176.—*Clove.* *A*, Whole clove (nat. size). *B*, The same viewed from above without corolla, stamens or style. *C*, A clove (enlarged). *D*, The same viewed in longitudinal section. *E*, Representative portion of a transverse section cut through the receptacle of clove, × 50. *F*, Representative portion of a longitudinal section of clove cut through receptacle, × 50. *cal*, calyx; *pet*, corolla; *cp*, carpels; *hyp*, receptacle; *st*, stamens; *styl*, style; *loc*, locule of ovary; *a*, parenchyma of receptacle containing oil glands (*t*); *b* and *y*, fibrovascular bundles containing sclerenchyma fibers; *c*, pith. (*After Berg.*)

fibers; calcium oxalate in rosette aggregates, up to 15μ in diameter; pollen grains numerous, triangular, with rounded angles and up to 20μ in diameter.

Constituents.—Volatile oil (15 to 20 per cent.) containing eugenol and caryophyllene; eugenin, vanillin, gallotannic acid, etc. The volatile oil is official in the U.S.P. as *Oleum Caryophylli*. It contains from 50 to 85 per cent. of *eugenol* which is also official.

Uses.—Cloves are used as an aromatic and condiment as well as in the manufacture of clove oil and vanillin.

Adulterants.—(1) Clove stems, identified chiefly by the presence of yellow, thick-walled stone cells, cork elements and numerous scalariform and reticulate tracheæ.

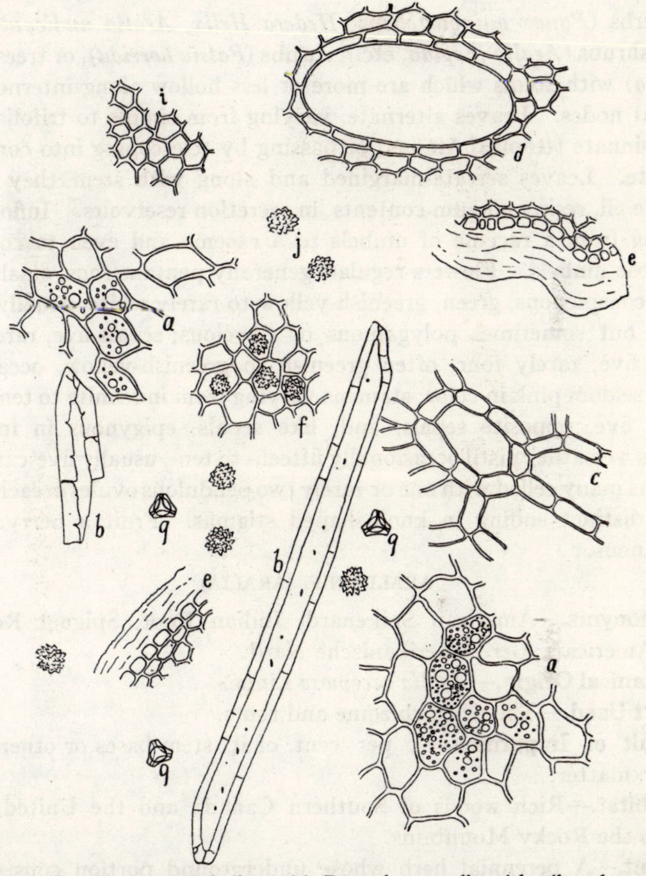

FIG. 177.—Powdered Caryophyllus. (*a*) Parenchyma cells with oil and granules; (*b*) bast cells; (*c*) inner spongy parenchyma; (*d*) oil gland; (*e*) epidermal tissue, lateral view; (*f*) crystal bearing parenchyma; (*g*) pollen grains; (*i*) epidermal cells, vertical view; (*j*) rosette aggregate crystals of calcium oxalate. (*Schneider.*)

(2) Cocoanut shells, distinguished by having many stone cells of slenderly elongated shape and brownish-yellow walls with dark brown contents that become reddish-brown when mounts are examined in potassium hydroxide solution. Used only in ground form to adulterate powdered cloves as well as other ground spices.

3. Olive pits, identified in powdered cloves by their stone cells which in water mounts are of a variety of shapes and have colorless walls and contents.

4. Cereal flours, identified by their characteristic starches, hairs, etc.

ARALIACEÆ (GINSENG FAMILY)

Herbs (*Panax quinquefolium*, *Hedera Helix*, *Aralia nudicaulis*, etc.), undershrubs (*Aralia hispida*, etc.), shrubs (*Fatsia horrida*), or trees (*Aralia spinosa*) with stems which are more or less hollow along internodes and solid at nodes. Leaves alternate, varying from simple to trifoliate or to multipinnate (tropical Aralias) or passing by telescoping into compound-palmate. Leaves serrate-margined and along with stem they develop volatile oil, resin and gum contents, in secretion reservoirs. Inflorescence varying from a raceme of umbels to a raceme and even to condensed racemose umbels. Flowers regular, generally pentamerous, small, generally inconspicuous, green, greenish-yellow to rarely white, usually hermaphrodite but sometimes polygamous or diœcious; sepals five, rarely four; petals five, rarely four, often greenish to greenish-yellow, occasionally white, seldom pink in color; stamens varying from indefinite to ten to commonly five, opposite sepals, and, like sepals, epigynous in insertion; anthers versatile; pistil occasionally fifteen- to ten-, usually five-carpellate, ovary as many celled with one or rarely two pendulous ovules in each cavity; styles distinct ending in knob-shaped stigmas. Fruit a berry. Seeds albuminous.

ARALIA N.F. (ARALIA)

Synonyms.—American Spikenard, Indian Root, Spignet Root, *Fr.* Nard Americain; *Ger.* Amerikanische Nard.

Botanical Origin.—*Aralia racemosa* Linné.

Part Used.—The dried rhizome and roots.

Limit of Impurities.—5 per cent. of its stem bases or other foreign organic matter.

Habitat.—Rich woods of Southern Canada and the United States, west to the Rocky Mountains.

Plant.—A perennial herb whose underground portion consists of a fleshly, oblique, aromatic rhizome bearing numerous roots. Its aerial portion consists of widely branched, unarmed stems arising to the height of 1 to 1.8 m. bearing ternately to quinately compound leaves, each with broadly ovate, membranous leaflets having acuminate apices, cordate bases and doubly serrate margins, and hairy on the veins beneath. The inflorescences consist of panicles of umbels bearing small, greenish-yellow flowers. Each flower is composed of a tubular calyx adnate to the ovary and with a 5 toothed limb, a corolla of 5 greenish-yellow petals, 5 stamens inserted on the epigynous disk and a central pistil composed of an inferior 5-celled ovary and 5 styles which are connate below. The fruit is a subglobular, dark purple to reddish-brown berry.

Production and Commerce.—The rhizomes and roots are gathered in autumn, frequently sliced lengthwise to facilitate drying and carefully dried. The commercial supplies come chiefly from the states of North Carolina, Virginia, Indiana, Illinois, Missouri and Washington.

Description.—Rhizome oblique, annulate between stem scars, usually cut longitudinally, up to 5 cm. in thickness; externally pale brown; nodes closely arranged, each with a prominent, depressed stem scar about 3 cm. broad; fracture fibrous; internally whitish; roots numerous of variable length, from 5 to 25 mm. in thickness, usually cut lengthwise and furrowed, sometimes with transverse ridges and cork patches; externally light brown or purplish-brown, whitish and spongy internally; fracture of bark short, of wood short and fibrous; odor aromatic; taste mucilaginous, pungent and slightly acrid.

Histology.—Sections of the root exhibit a well developed cork; one or more hypodermal layers with lignified cells up to 100μ in length and with porous wall, a broad cortex of cortical parenchyma cells, some containing spherical or angular, simple or 2-several compound starch grains, the individual grains up to 20μ in diameter, other possessing rosette aggregates of calcium oxalate up to 70μ in diameter, several rows of secretion reservoirs, containing oil and resin, course through the cortex; a cambium; a broad distinctly radiate wood showing tracheæ with reticulate or scalariform thickenings and simple or bordered pores.

Constituents.—Volatile oil, resin, starch, pectin, sugar, etc.

Uses.—Stimulant, diaphoretic and alterative. A constituent of syrup of white pine compound.

Substitute.—The rhizome of Wild or Virginian Sarsaparilla, *Aralia nudicaulis L.* This is grayish-brown, deeply longitudinally wrinkled, seldom cut longitudinally, shows alternate undeveloped buds, few roots, possesses a short fracture, the fractured surface whitish and showing a spongy and starchy pith. The taste is aromatic, bitter and pungent.

UMBELLIFERÆ (PARSLEY FAMILY)

Herbs, rarely shrubs, often of rapid growth, and with upright, fistular (hollow at internodes, solid at nodes), often grooved and ridged stems. Leaves alternate, compound and usually much divided, exstipulate, but with expanded sheathing and flattened leaf base (pericladium), that ensheathes the stem. Inflorescence a simple or often compound umbel surrounded by an involucre of bracts or of bracteoles. Flowers small, pentamerous, with inferior ovary and superior floral parts. Sepals minute, tooth-like, inserted above inferior ovary, or absorbed. Petals small, usually yellow to white, rarely pink to purple, distinct, each with inflexed tip. Stamens five, epigynous, inserted below a nectariferous, epigynous disc, incurved in bud. Carpels two, fused into bicarpellate pistil. Ovary two-celled, with one pendulous ovule in each cell, ovarian wall traversed by oleoresin canals called vittæ; styles two, distinct above the nectar disc or stylopod. Fruit a dry, splitting fruit or cremocarp, that splits lengthwise into two mericarps which hang for a time by a forked carpophore. Seeds single in each mericarp, albuminous.

ANISUM N.F. (ANISE)

Synonyms.—Aniseed, Sweet Cumin; *Fr.* Anis; *Ger.* Anissame.

Botanical Origin.—*Pimpinella Anisum* Linné.

Part Used.—The dried ripe fruit.

Purity Rubric.—Not more than 3 per cent. of other fruits, seeds or foreign organic matter. It yields not more than 1.5 per cent. of acid-insoluble ash.

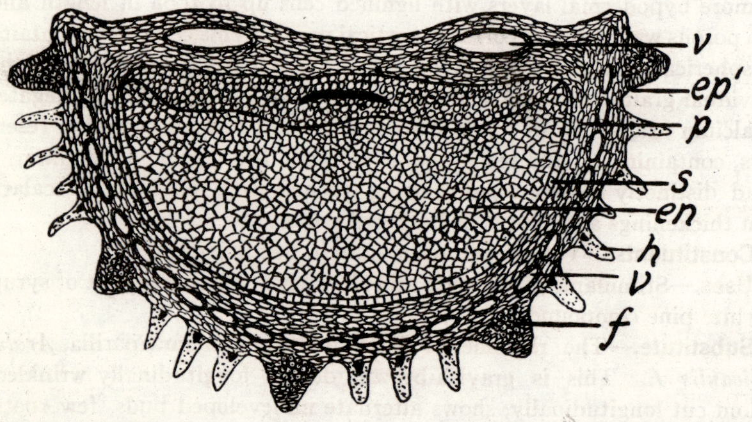

FIG. 178.—Anisum. Transverse section of mericarp. Epicarp (*ep*); parenchyma of mesocarp (*p*); vittæ (*v*); spermoderm (*s*); hair (*h*); fibrovascular tissue in one of the primary ribs (*f*); endosperm (*en*). The two larger vittæ are on the commissural side; the smaller vittæ are on the dorsal side. The layer of cells directly outside of the spermoderm is the endocarp.

Ash.—Not more than 9 per cent. of total ash nor more than 1.5 per cent. of ash insoluble in hydrochloric acid (Circ. No. 136, U.S. Dept. Agric.).

Habitat.—Asia Minor, Greece and Egypt.

Plant.—An annual herb with an erect, cylindrical, striated, smooth stem arising to the height of about .3 m. Its leaves are alternate below, opposite above, the lower long petioled, ovate to orbicular, dentate, the upper with short dilated petioles, pinnatifid or ternately pinnate with long, entire or cut, cuneate segments. The inflorescences are long stalked, 8- to 14-rayed, compound umbels. The flowers are small, white in color, each on a long hairy pedicel. The fruit is a mouse-shaped cremocarp of a small stylopod and 2 minutely pubescent mericarps which do not readily separate from the carpophore.

Production and Commerce.—Anise has been cultivated in Asia Minor and southern Europe for many centuries. It has also been cultivated in many sections of this country as a garden plant, notably in the state of Rhode Island. It is propagated from seeds (fruits) which are sown in early spring directly in the field. The soil should be moderately rich, well drained loam. When the seedlings are 2 or 3 inches high they are thinned so as to be about 8 inches apart in a row. Ample space should be allotted between the rows for cultivation. The drug should be collected as soon as the summits of the fruits assume a grayish-green color. In harvesting, the plants are pulled up by hand or mowed down and stacked in tall heaps for about 4 or 5 days until the fruits have ripened. The fruits are then separated by thrashing and carefully cleaned.

The five leading commercial varieties of Anise before the world war were as follows: Spanish, Italian, Russian, Levant and French. The Spanish or Alicante Anise, obtained from plants cultivated in Spain has been the variety in greatest demand in this country. At present the commercial supply is obtained chiefly from Spain, France and Russia. Russian anise comes through London.

Description.—Cremocarp broadly ovoid or pyriform, laterally compressed, from 3 to 7 mm. in length and from 2 to 3 mm. in breadth; mericarps usually cohering and attached to a slender pedicel from 2 to 12 mm. in length; summit with a ring-like stylopodium (disk) and two projecting, diverging styles; externally grayish-yellow (Italian, Spanish, French and Levant anise) or grayish-brown (Russian anise), slightly pubescent; each mericarp with 5 light brown filiform ridges and a carpophore, a transverse section exhibiting a pericarp containing from 15 to 45 vittæ and a somewhat reniform seed; odor aromatic; taste aromatic, resembling Illicium.

Histology.—Transverse sections of the cremocarp show the following microscopical peculiarities:

Two mericarps, each, 5 ribbed, of reniform outline and with a carpophore separating their concave commissural surfaces. Examination of one of the mericarps reveals the following:

1. Epicarp, consisting of a layer of outer yellowish brown epidermal cells having numerous papillæ and short, unicellular, non-glandular hairs with thick papillose walls.

2. Mesocarp of several layers of tangentially elongated parenchyma cells in which region are to be noted 15 to 45 vittæ. Two of these, larger than the rest, are on the commissural side, the remainder on the dorsal. In each of the primary rib parts of this region will be noted a small fibrovascular bundle surrounded by sclerenchyma fibers.

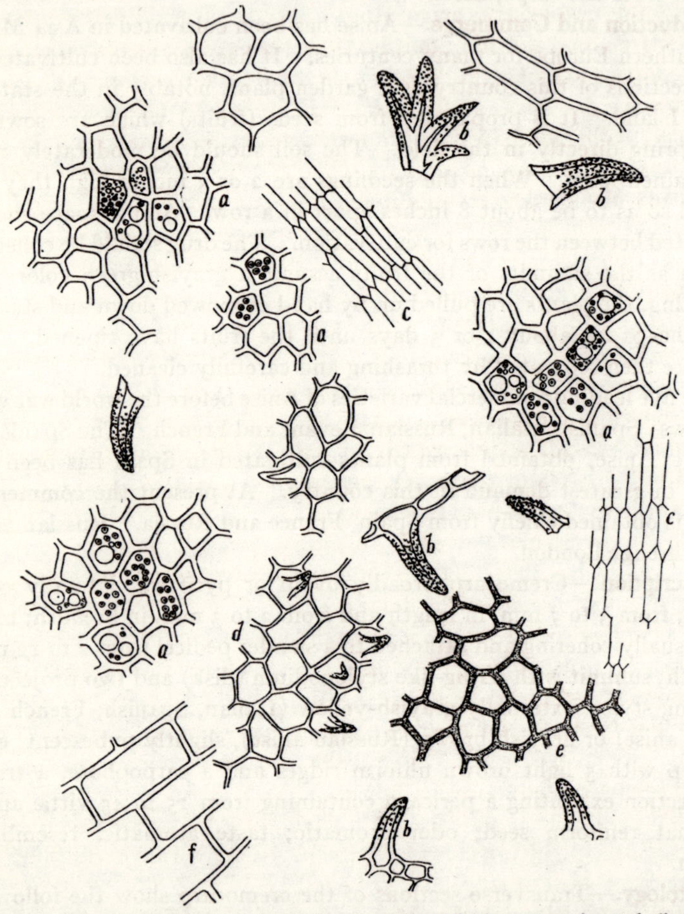

FIG. 179.—Powdered Anisum. (*a*) Endosperm cells with aleurone grains and oil globules; (*b*) trichomes; (*c*) thin-walled parenchyma of testa; (*d*) epidermal cells of pericarp with trichomes; (*e*) reddish-brown cells of pericarp; (*f*) parenchyma, longitudinal view. (*Schneider.*)

3. Endocarp, consisting of a layer of tangentially elongated cells closely adherent to the seed coat, except on the commissural side, where a large cavity exists, due to shrinkage of the seed coat.

4. Spermoderm or seed coat, comprising a layer of tangentially elongated cells with yellowish-brown walls.

5. Endosperm of numerous thick-walled polyhedral cells containing globules of fixed oil and aleurone grains, each of the latter containing a small rosette aggregate of calcium oxalate.

Sections cut through the upper portion of the mericarp show embryo in center of endosperm.

Powdered Drug.—Yellowish-brown; numerous fragments of the pericarp showing parenchyma, imbedded in some of which will be noted the yellowish vittæ or walls of vittæ; fragments of yellowish-brown epicarp cells, some showing short papillose outgrowths, others unicellular non-glandular hairs up to 170μ long and with thick, yellowish, lamellated walls; fragments of carpophore, showing sclerenchyma fibers; fragments of fibrovascular tissue; numerous fragments of the endosperm, consisting of polygonal, thick-walled cells containing aleurone grains, in each of which will be noted a tiny rosette aggregate of calcium oxalate.

Constituents.—Up to 3 per cent. of volatile oil containing anethol; fixed oil, calcium oxalate, etc.

Uses.—Stimulant, carminative and flavoring agent; a source of Oil of Anise U.S.P.

Adulterants.—Foreign seeds, and fruits, pebbles, exhausted fruits, and Conium. The latter is poisonous and may readily be detected by triturating a portion of a suspected sample with an alkaline solution, when an odor resembling mouse urine develops.

FŒNICULUM N.F. (FENNEL)

Synonyms.—Fennel Seed, Fennel Fruit; *Ger.* Fenchelsamen; *Fr.* Fenouil.

Botanical Origin.—Cultivated varieties of *Fœniculum vulgare* Miller.

Part Used.—The dried ripe fruit.

Limit of Impurities.—4 per cent. of foreign organic matter.

Ash.—Not more than 9 per cent. of total ash, nor more than 2 per cent. of ash insoluble in hydrochloric acid (S.R.A. No. 23).

Habitat.—Southern Europe and Asia Minor.

Plants.—Perennial aromatic herbs attaining a height of about 1 m. with green, glaucous, furrowed, branched stems bearing alternate, twice pinnate leaves with narrow pinnæ, small yellow flowers in compound umbels and oblong cremocarps.

Production and Commerce.—Fennel is cultivated on a large scale in Saxony, Germany, in Spain, Italy, Russia, France, Roumania, India and Japan and to a lesser extent as a garden herb in this country. It thrives best in well drained garden soil which has been limed. It is propagated from fruits sown directly in the field after preparation of the ground or by sowing in seed beds first and later transferring seedlings to the field. The seedlings should stand about 15 inches apart in rows with ample space left between these for cultivation. The fruits are collected similarly to those of anise and packed in bags for shipment.

German Fennel is shipped largely through Hamburg, Roumanian Fennel through Hamburg and Trieste, Italian Fennel through Naples and Siaeca, French Fennel from Marseilles, Levant from Trieste, and Indian Fennel through Bombay and London. There is quite a difference between these fennels. The German large is preferred. It is green in color. The French, Italian, Levant and Indian fennels are yellow. The Roumanian is a small green fruit which is not highly prized.

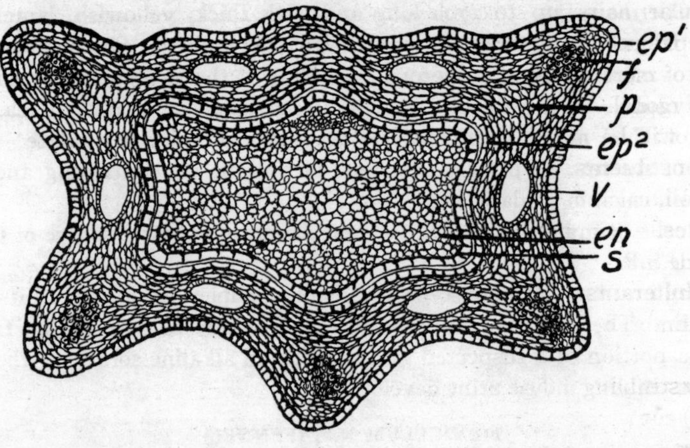

FIG. 180.—Fœniculum. Transverse section of mericarp. Epicarp (ep^1); parenchyma of mesocarp (*p*); fibrovascular bundle in primary rib (*f*); vitta (*v*); endocarp (ep^2); spermoderm (*s*); endosperm (*en*).

Description.—Mericarps usually separate, each being broadly elliptical, more or less curved from 4 to 15 mm. in length and from 1 to 5 mm. in breadth, some having a slender pedicel; dorsal surface convex, yellowish-green to grayish-brown, with 3 prominent, longitudinal primary ribs and at the summit a short, conical stylopodium; commissural surface grooved with alternate light and dark areas; odor and taste characteristically aromatic.

Histology.—Transverse sections of the mericarp, when examined with a hand lens, show a pentagonal outline, four of the edges being nearly equal and slightly concave, the other or commissural surface being considerably longer and somewhat undulate. The ribs are larger and wing-like. When examined under a compound microscope the following microscopical details are noted:

1. Epicarp, consisting of a layer of clear, tangentially elongated epidermal cells.

2. Mesocarp of several layers of thin-walled porous or reticulate parenchyma cells; in the commissural region of this zone are usually 2, occasionally 4 large elliptical vittæ with brown walls; in the dorsal region between each 2 primary ribs will be observed similar vittæ, there being 6 to 8 in the entire mesocarp; in the center of each of the rib portions of the mesocarp occurs a nearly circular fibrovascular bundle with a few tracheæ and numerous strongly lignified sclerenchyma fibers.

3. Endocarp, a narrow layer of cells, transversely elongated, except over the regions of bundles.

4. Spermoderm or seed coat, consisting of a layer of somewhat broadened epidermal cells attached to the endocarp, beneath which are several layers of more or less collapsed cells which are best defined in the region of the raphe. The raphe will be found as a somewhat crescent-shaped band of thick-walled cells just outside the center of the commissural region of the seed coat.

5. Endosperm, a large somewhat reniform zone of thick-walled polygonal cells containing aleurone grains and fixed oil globules. Each aleurone grain generally contains a rosette aggregate of calcium oxalate about 2μ in diameter and one to two globoids.

6. Embryo, embedded in the endosperm of the upper region of the seed.

Constituents.—Up to 6.5 per cent. of volatile oil (*Oleum Fœniculi* U.S.P.) containing anethol and fenchone, fixed oil, calcium ocalate, etc.

Uses.—Stimulant, carminative, galactagogue and condiment; source of volatile oil of fennel.

Adulterants.—(1) Fruits of other *Umbelliferæ*, notably *F. piperitum* (from Italy) which has a bitter taste; (2) Fruits of grasses, cereals, etc. (3) Undeveloped fennel fruits; (4) Moldy fennel fruits; (5) Dirt.

CARUM U.S.P. (CARAWAY)

Synonyms.—Carawayseed, Caraway Seed; *Ger.* Kümmelsamen; *Fr.* Carui.

Botanical Origin.—*Carum Carvi* Linné.

Part Used.—The dried fruit.

Purity Rubric.—Not more than 3 per cent. of other fruits, seeds or foreign organic matter. It yields not more than 1.5 per cent. of acid-insoluble ash.

Ash.—Not more than 8 per cent. of total ash, nor more than 1.5 per cent. of ash insoluble in hydrochloric acid (Circ. No. 136, U.S. Dept. of Agric.).

Habitat.—Asia and Europe. Naturalized in United States and Canada.

Plant.—A biennial herb sending up the first season a cluster of bi-to tri-pinnate root leaves. During the second year there arises a slender stem bearing alternate, pinnate to bipinnate leaves, the terminal segments of which are quite narrow and pointed. These cauline leaves have large sheathing brown petioles. The inflorescence is a long-stalked compound umbel bearing small white flowers with small calyx teeth, the petals ovate and notched, the stylopod conical. The fruits are oblong, laterally compressed, dark brown cremocarps.

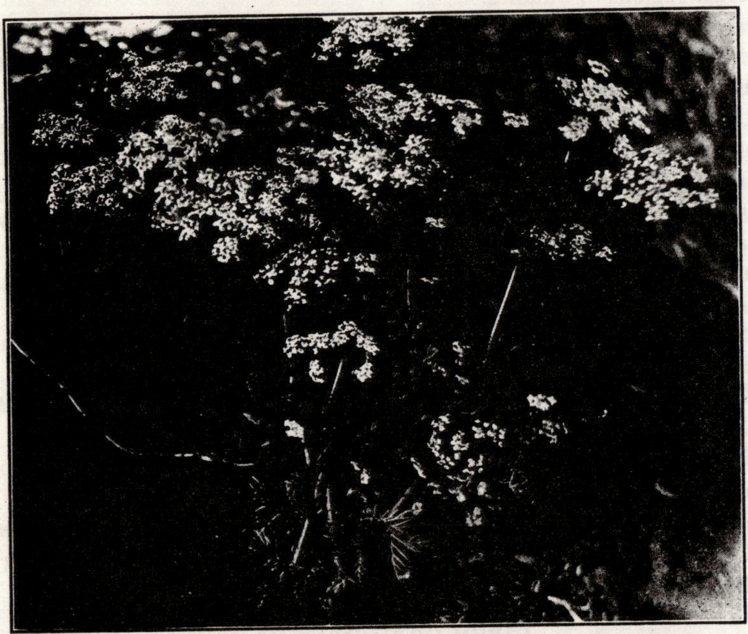

FIG. 181.—Caraway plant (*Carum Carvi*). (*Photograph by Hogstad.*)

Production and Commerce.—Caraway has long been cultivated in Germany, Holland, Morocco, Spain, Norway, Russia, England and to a lesser extent in the northern part of the United States. The plant thrives well in clay soil containing some humus. The seeds are sown in spring in drills about 18 inches apart. Shallow cultivation is essential to keep down weeds. The plants are mowed down when the oldest fruits are ripe, dried in the field or in the barn loft until they have lost most of their moisture, after which the fruits are thrashed out, cleaned and stored in bags. Most of the commercial supply used by this country comes from Amsterdam and Rotterdam, Holland in burlap bags. Occasional lots of African seed are imported through Marseilles and London. This usually comes in "bearded" form, having the pedicels attached. The drug should be stored in tightly closed containers.

Description.—Mericarps usually separated, crescent shaped, 3 to 7 mm. in length 1.5 to 2 mm. in diameter, externally dark brown with 5 yellowish filiform ribs; in cross section nearly equilaterally pentagonal, the commissural surface with 2 vittæ, the dorsal surface with a vitta between each two primary ribs; oily endosperm large, embedded in the upper end of which is a small embryo; odor and taste characteristically aromatic.

Histology.—Transverse sections, cut through the center of the mericarp, show the following structures;

1. Epicarp consisting of an outer layer of slightly tangentially elongated cells with thick outer wals.

2. Mesocarp, a zone of several rows of more or less collapsed, tangentially elongated parenchyma cells. In each of the rib portions of this zone will be noted a fibrovascular bundle surrounded by a layer of thick walled sclerenchyma fibers. On the commissural side will be noted 2 large vittæ, and, at the middle portion, 2 large transverse hollow spaces formed by the separation of the tissues of the seed coat on one side and the pericarp on the other. On the dorsal side there are 4 large vittæ, one between each 2 primary ribs. Each vitta is elliptical, brown, and lined by small epithelial secretory cells.

3. Endocarp, composed of a layer of broad, tangentially elongated cells closely adherent to the seed coat.

4. Spermoderm, a layer of somewhat collapsed brownish cells.

5. Endosperm, a large zone of thick-walled, polygonal, reserve parenchyma cells containing droplets of fixed oil and aleurone grains, the latter not infrequently containing a small rosette aggregate of calcium oxalate.

Powdered Drug.—Yellowish-brown to brown; numerous polygonal endosperm cells containing aleurone grains, each aleurone grain usually containing a rosette aggregate about 1μ in diameter; fragments of light yellow vittæ together with yellowish-brown endocarp and spermoderm cells; fragments with yellow or yellowish-brown walls of vittæ; fragments containing slightly lignified sclerenchyma fibers, having oblique walls, sometimes associated with a few tracheæ.

Constituents.—Volatile oil (5–7 per cent.), fixed oil, tannin. The volatile oil contains carvol and carven.

Uses.—Stimulant, carminative and condiment; source of oil of caraway U.S.P.

Adulterants.—(1) Ergotized Caraway, detected by bluish-black sclerotia; (2) Mogador Caraway from Morocco; (3) Cumin which is the fruit of *Cuminum Cyminium*, indigenous to northeast Africa. This fruit may readily be distinguished from Caraway by its mericarps which are usually coherent, forming an oblong cremocarp, which is rough hairy along the ribs, and by its peculiar odor.

APII FRUCTUS N.F. (CELERY FRUIT)

Synonyms.—Celery Seed; *Ger.* Epich; *Fr.* Ache celeri.

Botanical Origin.—*Apium graveolens* Linné.

Part Used.—The dried ripe fruit.

Purity Rubric.—Not more than 5 per cent. of unsound or foreign fruits or other foreign organic matter. It yields not more than 3 per cent. of acid-insoluble ash.

Ash.—Not more than 10 per cent. of total ash, nor more than 2 per cent. of ash insoluble in hydrochloric acid (S.R.A. No. 22).

Habitat.—Southern Europe.

Plant.—A biennial (sometimes annual) herb widely cultivated in this country and abroad for its leaves, root and fruit. The mature leaves are averagely 6 to 15 in. long and possess 3 pairs and a terminal leaflet, all coarsely serrate and ternately lobed or divided. The inflorescence is a compound umbel of small white flowers. The fruit is a minute, brown, roundish-ovate cremocarp.

Commercial.—Celery fruit is shipped to the United States in bags chiefly from Marseilles. Smaller lots are imported from London and Nimes.

Description.—Mericarps usually separated, ovoid, slightly curved, from 1 to 2 mm. in length, and about half as broad and thick, deep brown; inner surface flat, the outer convex, smooth, except for very slender light colored ribs, two of which are marginal, three dorsal; oil tubes (vittæ) in the mesocarp, 2 on the commissural and generally 1 to 3 between each 2 primary ribs on the dorsal side; odor agreeably aromatic; taste aromatic, warm and pungent.

Histology.—Transverse sections cut through the middle region of a mericarp show it to be nearly equilaterally pentagonal with somewhat convex surfaces and to exhibit the following internal structures:

1. Epicarp, a layer of tangentially-elongated epidermal cells with a thick cuticle, a few of the cells being papillose.

2. Mesocarp composed of a matrix of polygonal-shaped parenchyma cells imbedded in which are 2 vittæ on the commissural side and generally 1 to several vittæ between each 2 primary ribs on the dorsal side. In this region, also, will be noted a fibrovascular bundle in each primary rib that is surrounded by thick walled, lignified sclerenchyma fibers.

3. Endocarp, composed of a layer of tangentially elongated cells with brown walls.

4. Spermoderm, of collapsed brown cells.

5. Endosperm, of polygonal, thick-walled, reserve parenchyma cells containing globules of fixed oil and aleurone grains, the latter containing rosette aggregates of calcium oxalate varying from 2 to 8μ in diameter.

Constituents.—Up to 3 per cent. of a colorless volatile oil containing d-limone which is found, as in other umbelliferous fruits, in the vittæ; fixed oil, etc.

Uses.—Stimulant and condiment.

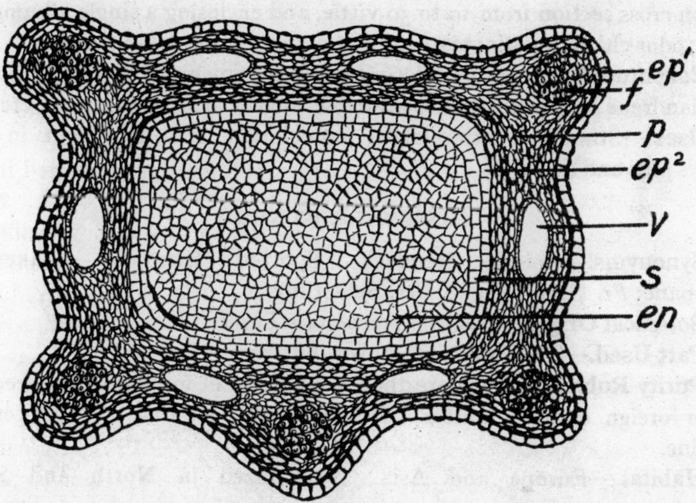

FIG. 182.—Celery fruit (Apii Fructus). Transverse section of mericarp. Epicarp (ep^1); parenchyma of mesocarp (p) in which are imbedded the vittæ (v); fibrovascular bundle in primary rib (f); spermoderm (s); endosperm (en); endocarp (ep^2)

ANGELICÆ FRUCTUS N.F. (ANGELICA FRUIT)

Synonym.—Angelica Seed, *Ger.* Angelicasamen; *Fr.* Semence d' angélique.

Botanical Origin.—*Angelica Archangelica* Linné and other species of *Angelica*.

Part Used.—The dried ripe fruit.

Limit of Impurities.—3 per cent. of foreign fruits, seeds or other foreign matter.

Habitat.—Northern Europe and Siberia.

Plant.—Angelica Archangelica is an herb with smooth, purple-green, hollow stems, twice pinnate leaves and greenish-white flowers.

Commercial.—Angelica fruit is imported in bags from Belgium, France and England.

Description.—Cremocarps oval, externally greenish-yellow or pale yellowish-brown, from 4 to 10 mm. in length, 3 to 6 mm. in breadth and from 1 to 2.5 mm. in thickness, the summit bearing five minute calyx teeth and the remains of a style; the two mericarps joined by their broad commissural faces or separate; each mericarp nearly flat upon the commissural surface, which bears a central longitudinal groove and has sharp, slightly upturned margins, convex upon the dorsal surface which shows 3 strong ribs, separated from one another by narrow grooves and from the margin by broad grooves; pericarp soft, rather tough and corky showing on cross section from 10 to 30 vittæ, and enclosing a single albuminous seed; odor characteristic; taste aromatic, sweetish and pungent.

Constituents.—Volatile oil containing a terpene with a pepper odor, phellandrene and cymol; bitter principle, angelic acid, resin, sugar, etc.

Uses.—Stimulant, stimulating expectorant and ingredient in Warburg's pills and tinctures.

CONIUM N.F. (CONIUM)

Synonyms.—Poison Hemlock, Spotted Hemlock, Snakeweed, Cowbane; *Fr.* Grand Ciguë; *Ger.* Schierling.

Botanical Origin.—*Conium maculatum* Linné.

Part Used.—The dried full grown, but unripe fruit.

Purity Rubric.—Not more than 2 per cent. of foreign fruits, seeds, or other foreign organic matter. It yields not less than 0.5 per cent. of coniine.

Habitat.—Europe and Asia. Naturalized in North and South America.

Plant.—A large, branching, poisonous, biennial herb found growing in waste places. Its stems are spotted and attain a height of from .6 to 2 m. Its leaves are large and decompound with lanceolate pinnatifid leaflets which are dark green above and glossy beneath. The flowers are white and appear in mid summer in long peduncled compound umbels. The poisonous juice of this plant was employed by the ancient Greeks as a potion which was given at the Athenian prison to criminals and philosophers as capital punishment. Socrates, Phœcion and other literary celebrities were put to death by this means.

Production and Commerce.—In North America, Poison Hemlock occurs wild, in waste places, from Canada to Indiana, California, Utah and Mexico. The fruits are collected from wild plants of the second year's growth while green, but full grown, screened, and dried with little exposure to light. They should be carefully stored in air tight, light proof containers. After having been kept for two years, Conium is unfit for use. The commercial supply of this drug is largely obtained from Europe.

Description.—Cremocarp ovoid, greenish-gray, the 2 mericarps of most of the fruits separated, each about 3 mm. in length, and about 1.5 mm. in diameter, ovoid, somewhat curved, the inner flattened side marked by a deep longitudinal groove, the outer convex side with 5, pale yellow, somewhat crenate ribs; pericarp without oil tubes (vittæ); odor slight, but when triturated with potassium hydroxide solution, strong, disagreeable, and mouse-urine like; taste characteristic, disagreeable, afterwards acrid.

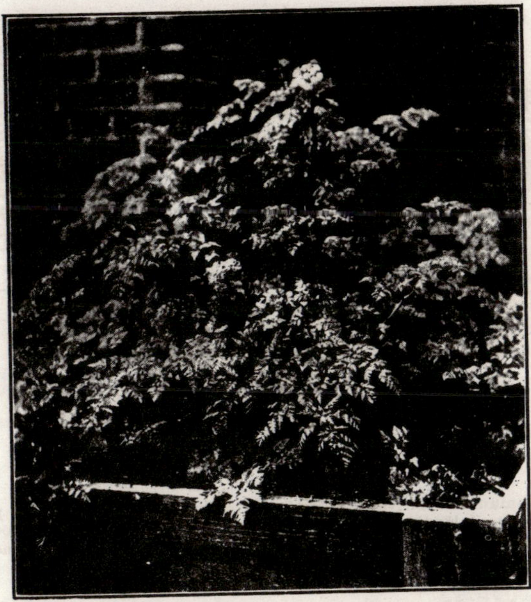

FIG. 183.—Poison hemlock (*Conium maculatum*) growing on roof garden of the Philadelphia College of Pharmacy and Science.

Histology.—Transverse sections of the mericarp exhibit a pentangular outline, the angles projecting and forming the ribs, four of the sides being almost equal in length, the fifth or commissural side being about twice as long as one of the dorsal sides and usually concave near the middle; a distinct fibro-vascular bundle at each angle composed of thick-walled fibers about 0.013 mm. in diameter and a few tracheæ; epidermis consisting of one layer of cells which are sometimes slightly centrifugally developed, hairs are absent; pericarp thin, without vittæ, enclosing a single seed and extending inwardly on the commissural side for about one-third the diameter of the section; the inner epidermis of the pericarp composed of two layers of cells with yellowish-brown walls, the outer layer with cells from 0.06 mm. to 0.14 mm. in tangential length and with thickened radial and inner walls, the inner layer with thin-walled cells from 0.03 to 0.06 mm. in tangential length and about 0.03 mm. in radial diameter; the seed coat composed of small, thick-walled cells about 0.015 mm. in radial diameter; often obliterated; a large endosperm or central portion being somewhat pentangular-rounded in outline, with a deep channel on the commissural side and composed of polygonal parenchyma cells; the latter contain globules of fixed oil and aleurone grains with rosette aggregates of calcium oxalate, the latter up to 8μ in diameter.

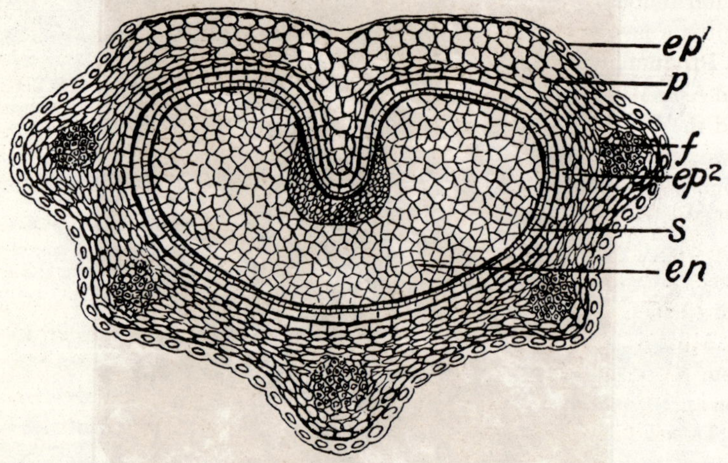

FIG. 184.—Conium. Transverse section of mericarp. Epicarp (ep^1); parenchyma of mesocarp (*p*); fibrovascular tissue in a primary rib (*f*); endocarp (ep^2); spermoderm (*s*); endosperm (*en*); between the spermoderm and the endocarp is a clear layer of more or less tangentially elongated cells containing coniine. Vittæ are absent in this drug.

Constituents.—Up to 3 per cent. of the poisonous liquid alkaloid, coniine; conydrine, pseudoconydrine, coniciene, fixed oil, calcium oxalate, etc.

Uses.—Conium is employed as a motor depressant in tetanus, convulsions, delirium tremens, spasmodic chorea, etc.

CORIANDRUM N.F. (CORIANDER)

Synonyms.—Coriander Seed, Coliander; *Ger.* Koriandersamen; *Fr.* Coriandre.

Botanical Origin.—*Coriandrum sativum* Linné.

Part Used.—The dried ripe fruit.

Purity Rubric.—Not more than 5 per cent. of other fruits, seeds, or other foreign organic matter. It yields not more than 1.5 per cent. of acid insoluble ash, nor less than 0.5 per cent. of volatile ether-soluble extractive.

Ash.—Not more than 7 per cent. of total ash, nor more than 1.5 per cent. of ash insoluble in hydrochloric acid (S.R.A. No. 22).

Habitat.—Mediterranean and Caucasian regions. Naturalized in the United States.

Plant.—An annual fetid smelling herb with erect, slender, smooth stem, branched in the upper part. The lower leaves long-petioled, pinnate with nearly sessile, ovate to sub-orbicular, deeply lobed leaflets, crenate-dentate on margin; upper leaves nearly sessile, bi- or tri-pinnate with ultimate segments strap shaped or linear. The inflorescences are compound umbels of white or pink flowers. No involucre is present. The fruit is a nearly spherical cremocarp.

Production and Commerce.—Coriander grows wild in southern Europe and Asia Minor and is cultivated there as well as in India, northern Africa, and the United States. The plants are propagated from seeds which are sown thickly in fertile garden soil, in the spring. The rows should be from 1½ to 3 feet apart for cultivation purposes. When sufficiently strong, the plants are thinned to stand about 5 inches apart in the row. The plants are mowed down when most of the fruits are ripe, partially cured in the field and dried under cover. The fruits are then thrashed out and cleaned.

Most of the drug used in the United States is now imported in bags from Morocco, Marseilles, Germany, Bombay, Madras, Casablanca, London and Amsterdam. The German seed is the most highly esteemed.

Description.—Mericarps usually coherent; cremocarp nearly globular, from 3 to 5 mm. in diameter; externally light brown or rose colored; summit with 5 calyx teeth and a short stylopodium, each mericarp with 5 prominent, straight, longitudinal primary ribs and 4 undulate secondary ribs; mericarps easily separated, deeply concave on the commissural or inner surface and showing in transverse section 2 vittæ on the inner surface of each.

Histology.—Transverse sections of each of the component mericarps show the following microscopical peculiarities.

1. Epicarp consisting of a layer of small, thick-walled epidermal cells.

2. Mesocarp of several rows of thin-walled, somewhat collapsed parenchyma, separated from a broad continuous zone of thick-walled sclerenchyma fibers; two or three rows of large thin-walled parenchyma containing prominent intercellular-air-spaces. Imbedded in this zone on the commissural side are two large elliptical vittæ.

3. Endocarp, of a layer of large tabular cells with thick, yellowish inner walls, adherent to the seed coat except on the commissural side, where a large elliptical cavity occurs.

4 Spermoderm or seed coat of tangentially elongated brownish cells.

5. Endosperm, of reniform outline and consisting of polygonal thick-walled cells containing numerous large aleurone grains and globules of fixed oil. Each aleurone grain contains a rosette aggregate or prism of calcium oxalate from 3 to 10μ in diameter.

6. Embryo, enveloped by endosperm in the upper end of the seed.

Constituents.—Up to 1 per cent. of volatile oil containing coriandrol; fixed oil, calcium oxalate, and tannin.

Uses.—Aromatic stimulant, corrective of purgative preparations and source of oil of coriander U.S.P.

PETROSELINUM (PARSLEY FRUIT)

Synonyms.—Parsley Seed, Common or Garden Parsley.

Botanical Origin.—*Petroselinum sativum* Hoffman.

Part Used.—The dried ripe fruit.

Habitat.—Mediterranean Region.

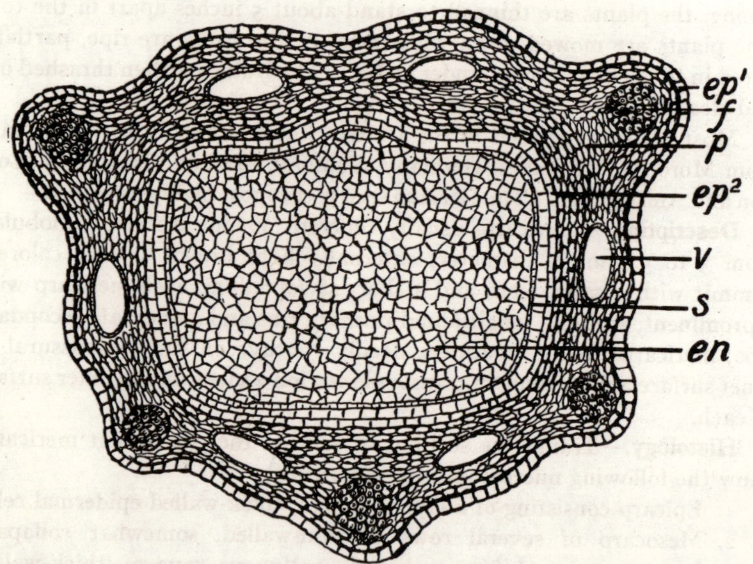

FIG. 185.—Petroselinum (parsley fruit). Transverse section of mericarp. Epicarp (ep^1); parenchyma of mesocarp (p); endocarp or inner epidermis of pericarp (ep^2); vittæ (v); spermoderm (s); endosperm (en); fibrovascular bundle in primary rib (f).

Plant.—An aromatic biennial herb with ternately pinnate, decompound leaves, the leaflets being small, ovate, 3 cleft and toothed. The flowers are yellow and borne on compound umbels showing many parted involucels.

Production and Commerce.—Parsley has been cultivated on a large scale in United States and Europe for its fruit, leaves and root which are

DISTINCTIONS BETWEEN IMPORTANT UMBELLIFEROUS FRUITS

	Anisum	Carum	Conium	Coriandrum	Fœniculum	Petroselinum
Synonym	Anise seed	Caraway seed	Poison hemlock	Coriander seed	Fennel seed	Parsley seed
Botanical origin	Pimpinella Anisum	Carum carvi	Conium maculatum	Coriandrum sativum	Foeniculum vulgare	Petroselinum sativum
Habitat	Asia Minor, Egypt, and Greece	Europe, Asia	Europe	Mediterranean Basin	Europe and Asia	So. Europe and Asia Minor
Plant	Annual herb	Biennial herb	Biennial herb	Annual herb	Perennial herb	Biennial herb
Occurrence	Entire cremocarps with few mericarps; pedicel adhering	Mericarps usually separated	Mericarps usually separated	Entire cremocarps generally	Mericarps usually separated	Mericarps usually separated
Vittæ in mesocarp of each mericarp	2 on commissural side; 15-45 on dorsal side	2 vittæ on commissural side; a vitta between each of primary ribs on dorsal side	None present	2 vittæ on commissural side; none on dorsal side	2 occasionally 4 vittæ on commissural side; one vitta between each of primary ribs on dorsal side	2 vittæ on commissural side; one vitta between each of the primary ribs on dorsal side
Hairs	Numerous unicellular; non-glandular hairs present	Absent	Absent	Absent	Absent	Absent
Constituents	Volatile oil containing anethol	Volatile oil containing carvol	The liquid alkaloid, coniine; conydrine	Volatile oil containing coriandrol	Volatile oil containing anethol, fenchone	Volatile oil containing apiol, and a terpene; resin, etc.
Adulterants	Conium	Cumin Ergotized Caraway		Bombay or Indian Coriander	Roman fennel, wheat, etc.	

employed for culinary purposes as well as in medicine. The plants thrive best in a rich moist soil with a certain amount of shade. The plants are propagated from seeds (fruits) which are sown in early spring in cold frames. The seedlirgs, when 2 or 3 inches tall are transferred to the garden or field, where they are planted about 6 inches apart in rows about a foot apart.

The fruits are gatherd the second year when ripe and carefully dried. The leaves may be gathered when full grown from both first and second year plants. The root is dug up at the end of the second growing season in October, the thicker roots cut longitudinally to facilitate drying and all well washed and carefully dried by artificial heat. The Hamburg or turnip-rooted variety is preferred for the root.

Description.—Cremocarp ovate; mericarps usually separated, crescent shaped, from 2 to 3 mm. in length and about 1 mm. in diameter; externally grayish to grayish-brown showing 5 yellowish primary ribs alternating with roughened furrows; nearly hemispherical in transverse section, there being 2 vittæ in the commissural and 1 to 2 vittæ between each of the primary ribs in the dorsal region of the fruit wall; endosperm large, oily, enclosing a small embryo near summit of seed; odor and taste characteristically aromatic, the odor being most pronounced when the fruit is bruised.

Constituents.—Up to 3 per cent. of volatile oil consisting of apiol (parsley camphor) and a terpene; resin, fixed oil mucilage, etc.

Use.—Emmenagogue in amenorrhœa and dysmenorrhœa.

ANGELICÆ RADIX N.F. (ANGELICA ROOT)

Synonyms.—Archangel Root, Holy Ghost Root. *Ger.* Angelikawurzel, Erzengelwurzel; *Fr.* Racine d'angélique, Racine du St. Esprit.

Botanical Origin.—*Angelica Archangelia* Linné and other species of *Angelica.*

Part Used.—The dried rhizome and roots.

Purity Rubric.—Not more than 5 per cent. of its stem bases or other foreign organic matter. It yields not more than 4 per cent. of acid-insoluble ash.

Habitat and Plants.—See Angelicæ Fructus.

Production and Commerce.—The plants are cultivated in northern Europe. The rhizomes and roots are dug up in autumn, cleaned, the thicker rhizomes cut into longitudinal slices and carefully dried. The commercial supplies reach this country through London and Hamburg.

Description.—Rhizomes vertical, short and thick 5 to 10 cm. long, sometimes split, upper portion frequently crowned with leaf and stem bases; roots, fleshy, up to 20 cm. long and from 5 to 7 mm. thick at the base and gradually tapering to about 1 mm., frequently twisted and braided together and attached to rhizome; externally dark gray brown to reddish and purplish brown, deeply furrowed; fracture short and smooth; internally light and yellow with a spongy bark showing radial rows of brownish oleoresin reservoirs, a broad radiate and porous wood, and a pith in the rhizome; odor aromatic; taste sweetish, pungent, aromatic and bitter.

Constituents.—Up to 1 per cent. of volatile oil containing a terpene with a pepper-like odor, phellandrene and cymol; resin, a bitter principle, angelic acid, valeric acid, tannin, starch, etc.

Uses.—Aromatic bitter and carminative.

SUMBUL N.F. (SUMBUL)

Synonyms.—Musk Root; *Fr.* Racine de sumbul; *Ger.* Moschuswurzel, Bisamwurzel.

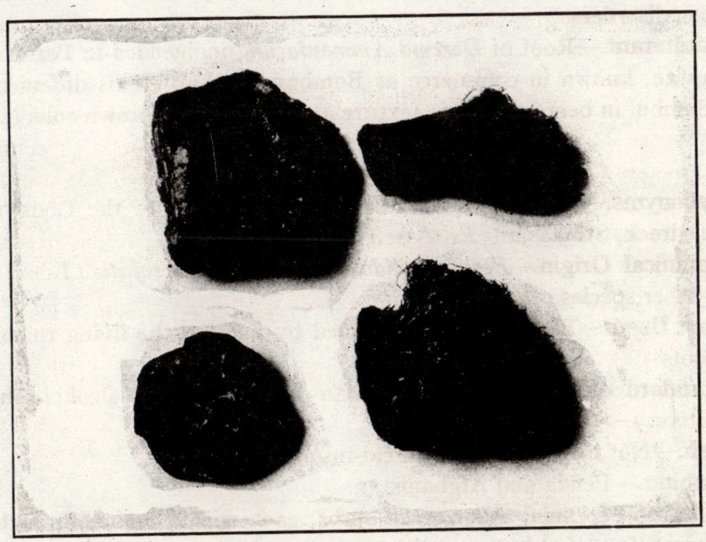

FIG. 186.—Sumbul, × ½. (*Photograph by W. J. Stoneback.*)

Botanical Origin.—*Ferula Sumbul* (Kauffmann) Hooker filius or other closely related species of *Ferula* possessing a characteristic musk-like odor.

Part Used.—The dried rhizome and roots.

Purity Rubric.—Not more than 2 per cent. of foreign organic matter.

Habitat.—Asia.

Commercial.—The commercial supplies are obtained from Turkey.

Description.—It occurs as short, more or less cylindrical segments of the rhizome and roots up to 10 cm. long and 7 cm. wide; extremely light in weight; externally brown, the rhizome distinctly annulate, cork readily separable; crown of rhizome branched, with fibrous remnants of stem bases, occasional circular scars or leaf bases; fracture short, irregular, fibrous and spongy sometimes strong and tough; internally, dark brown, wood yellowish-white, porous and spongy, showing a very irregular arrangement of the bundles; odor aromatic, musk-like; taste bitter and pungent.

Powdered Drug.—Gray brown; numerous isolated reticulate tracheæ up to 100μ in width; fragments of yellowish-brown polygonal cork cells; numerous fragments of sieve tissue; few fragments of parenchyma with spherical starch grains from 3 to 12μ in diameter; fragments of reticulate and pitted tracheæ; irregular masses of brownish resin.

Constituents.—Volatile oil with a mint taste up to 1 per cent., an alcohol-soluble resin, an ether-soluble resin, bitter principle, fixed oil, umbelliferone, valeric, angelic and methyl-crotonic acids.

Uses.—Musk root is used as a calmative in hysteria and some other nervous disorders.

Adulterant.—Root of *Dorema Ammoniacum*, indigenous to Persia and Turkestan, known in commerce as Bombay Sumbul. This differs from true Sumbul in being of denser texture and of a reddish-brown color.

ASAFŒTIDA U.S.P. (ASAFETIDA)

Synonyms.—Gum Asafetida, Devil's Dung, Food of the Gods; *Ger.* Teufelsdreck, Stinkasant; *Fr.* Assefétide.

Botanical Origin.—*Ferula fœtida* Regel, *Ferula Asafœtida* Linné and some other species of *Ferula*.

Part Used.—The gum-resin obtained by incising the living rhizomes and roots.

Standard of Assay.—Not less than 50 per cent. of alcohol-soluble extractive.

Ash.—Not over 15 per cent. acid-insoluble.

Habitat.—Persia and Afghanistan.

Plants.—Perennial monœcious herbs, each with a conical, branching root, erect, furrowed but smooth, green, succulent stem attaining a height of about 3 m., and ternately compound leaves. The inflorescences are compound umbels of yellow flowers. The fruit is a cremocarp.

Collection and Commerce.—In spring of the year, the stems of the Asafoetida yielding plants are cut down and a slice cut off the crown of each root, when a milky juice exudes. The exposed surface is then covered with a dome-shaped structure made of twigs and earth to protect the exudate from the heat of the sun. About a month later the collectors return and find a thick, reddish, gummy exudate which they scrape off and place in leather bags. Collection is repeated at intervals of 10 days until exudation ceases. The product obtained from numerous plants is mixed and allowed to harden in the sun. Most of the drug is collected in Eastern Persia and Afghanistan. It is sent to the main trade centers, Herat and Kandahar, from whence it is shipped to dealers in various European and Asiatic countries. The present supply of the drug to this country comes from London.

Description.—This drug generally occurs as irregular hard or soft masses or as tears, occasionally as an almost semi-liquid mass, usually admixed with vegetable fragments; when in mass form, the tears imbedded in a brownish matrix. Tears ovoid, the freshly fractured surface being milky-white, changing gradually on exposure to air to pinkish, reddish-purple or reddish-brown; upon moistening with water the tears become milky-white; odor garlic-like and persistent; taste bitter, garlic-like and acrid. When triturated with water, it forms a milky-white emulsion, which becomes yellowish on the addition of alkaline solutions. An alcoholic solution of the drug acquires a cherry-red color upon the addition of solution of phloroglucin and hydrochloric acid.

Powdered Drug.—This is prepared by drying the crude article over freshly burnt lime or by currents of warm air (air at about 30°C.) until it ceases to loose weight and then comminuting it at low temperatures. The U.S.P. permits the use of diluents of starch or magnesium carbonate in order to maintain it in powdered form.

Adulterants.—(1) Galbanum, a gum resin obtained from *Ferula galbaniflua* a perennial herb growing in Persia and Afghanistan. It may be detected in Asafoetida by making an alcoholic solution of the suspected sample adding hydrochloric acid to it until a faint turbidity results, when the development of a bluish-green color that fades on standing would indicate its presence.

2. Rosin. If this be present, a petroleum benzin solution of the sample will give a bluish-green color on shaking it with a freshly made (1–20) solution of copper acetate.

3. Ammoniac, a gum resin obtained from *Dorema Ammoniacum*, a perennial herb, indigenous to Persia and Turkestan. The presence of Ammoniac is indicated when an aqueous emulsion of the suspected sample is colored red upon the addition of sodium hypobromite test solution.

4. Vegetable Tissues. 5. Gums. 6. Cereal flours. 7. Gypsum. 8. Pebbles. 9. Sand. 10. Marble.

Constituents.—About 60 per cent. of a reddish-brown resin; from 3 to 6 per cent. of a volatile oil containing hexenyl sulphide and disulphide, cadinene and pinene; vanillin, ferulaic acid, formic, malic, acetic and valeric acids, etc.

CORNACEÆ (DOGWOOD FAMILY)

Herbs (*Cornus canadensis*, etc.), shrubs (*Cornus sanguinea*, etc.) or trees (*Cornus florida*, *Nyssa sylvatica*, etc.). Leaves simple, alternate (Sour Gum), or opposite (Dogwoods). Inflorescence an umbel or head, the whole being surrounded by an enlarged and more or less petaloid involucre. Flowers regular, rarely pentamerous, more frequently tetramerous; sepals usually four, small, tooth-like or absorbed; petals usually four, small, greenish to yellowish to white (*Cornus florida*), rarely pink or crimson; stamens four or five, alternate to the petals and inserted with the sepals epigynously around and between the nectar disc, pistil syncarpous, bicarpellate, rarely tricarpellate; ovary as many celled with one pendulous ovule in each cavity; style usually simple, ending in rounded or slightly bilobed stigma. Fruit a one- to two-seeded drupe. Seeds albuminous.

CORNUS N.F. (CORNUS)

Synonyms.—Dogwood Bark, Flowering Dogwood; *Fr.*, Ecorce de Cornouiller à grandes fleurs; *Ger.* Grossbluthige Kornelrinde.

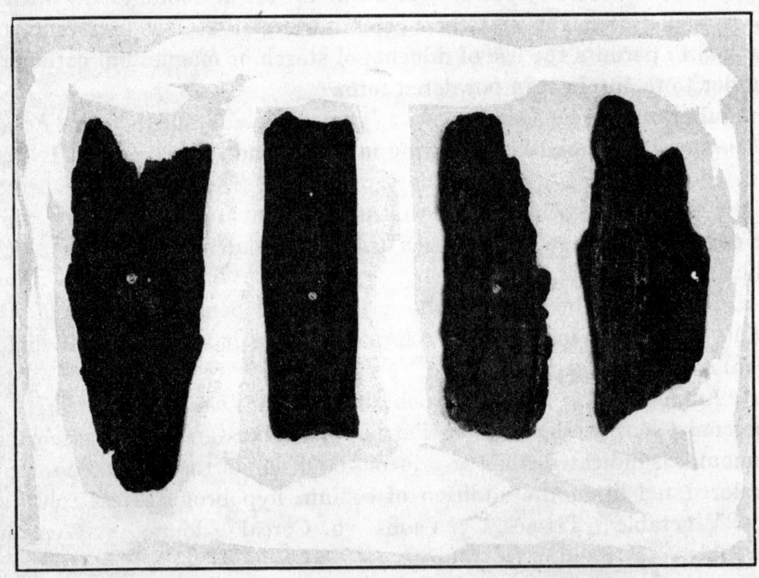

FIG. 187.—Dogwood bark (*Cornus florida*) ×½. The 2 pieces on the left show outer surface. The 2 on the right, inner surface. (*Photograph by Stoneback.*)

Botanical Origin.—*Cornus florida* Linné.

Part Used.—The dried bark of the root.

Purity Rubric.—Not more than 5 per cent. of adhering wood or more than 2 per cent. of other foreign organic matter.

Habitat.—In woods of eastern and central United States.

Plant.—A small tree with alligator-like bark, a low, broad crown bearing opposite branches, red or occasionally greenish twigs, small lateral buds covered with bases of leaf stalks, and spherical flower buds. Its leaves are opposite, simple, ovate, acute, at apex, cuneate at base, entire to undulate along margin, dark green above, pale green beneath, with prominent pinnate veins. Its flowers appear in April, in the Philadelphia neighborhood, on glomerules. Each glomerule consists of a dense cluster of small perfect, greenish florets imbedded on a compound receptacle that is surrounded by a white, corolla-like involucre of 4 obcordate bracts. The fruit is a scarlet ovoid drupe with a grooved putamen, appearing about October.

Commercial.—The commercial supplies come from Virginia and Illinois.

Description.—In irregular chip-like pieces or parts of quills of varying length and from 1 to 4 mm. in thickness; outer surface dingy-brown, somewhat fissured and thin scaly or reddish, where cork has been abraded, inner surface pink-brown to red-purple, short striated; fracture short; fractured surface whitish with yellow striæ, except in inner bark region which is light purple; odor indistinct; taste bitter and astringent.

Constituents.—A bitter principle termed cornin, resin, fixed oil, tannin and gallic acid.

Uses.—Tonic, astringent and antiperiodic.

SUB-CLASS B.—SYNPETALÆ

Those dicotyledonous plants in which the flowers possess both calyx and corolla, the latter with petals more or less joined along their margins.

ERICACEÆ (HEATH FAMILY)

Sub-herbaceous (*Chimaphila*), suffruitcose (*Erica*), fruticose (*Azalea*, *Rhododendron*, *Kalmia*, etc.), rarely sub-arborescent (*Arbutus unedo* or Strawberry Tree) plants. Roots fibrous, often saprophytically associated, rarely tuberous or more or less enlarged. Stem upright, ascending or creeping, more or less woody, rarely through saprophytic connection becoming soft, annual and pale above ground (*Monotropa uniflora*). Leaves alternate, simple, entire, exstipulate, rarely soft, delicate, herbaceous (*Azaleas*), usually leathery to wiry and evergreen. more rarely (*Pterospora*, *Monotropa*, etc.) becoming greenish-blue, bluish-yellow, yellowish-white to white and correspondingly saprophytic. Inflorescence typically a raceme (*Pyrola*, *Andromeda*, *Gaylussacia*, *Vaccinium*, *Erica*, *Artostaphylos Uva Ursi*, etc.) but raceme condensed into a racemose umbel (*Azalea*, *etc.*) or further reduced to a few flowers or, in the degraded saprophytic condition, to one flower (*Monotropa uniflora*). Flowers regular, passing to irregular (*Rhododendron*), pentamerous or tetramerous; sepals five to four, rarely fewer, apo- to synsepalous, usually green, sometimes brightly petaloid; petals five, more rarely four, slightly to deeply synpetalous, cup-shaped (*Kalmia*) to urceolate (*Arctostaphylos*, *Andromeda*, etc.), yellow to white or through yellow pink to scarlet to crimson to crimson-purple; stamens ten to eight in two circles of five to four each, becoming by absorption of inner circle four only, hypogynous, epipetalous or epigynous; anthers two-celled, dehiscing by apical pores (*Arctostaphylos*) or apical slits; pollen sometimes agglutinated into long viscous threads; pistil five- to four-, rarely six- to eight carpeled, superior, rarely semi-inferior to inferior (*Vacciniœ*); ovary as many celled as there are carpels; style elongated, filiform, usually five- to four lobed. Fruit a capsule (*Trailing Arbutus*), berry (*Vaccinium*) or false drupe (*Gaultheria*). Seeds small, anatropous. Arbutin, ericolin and ursone as well as tannin and gallic acid occur in a number of plants of this family.

CHIMAPHILA N.F. (CHIMAPHILA)

Synonyms.—Pipsissewa, Prince's Pine, Bitter Wintergreen, Ground Holly; *Fr.* Herbe de Pyrole ombellée; *Ger.* Doldenblüthiges Harnkraut.

Botanical Origin.—*Chimaphila umbellata* (Linné) Barton.

Part Used.—The dried leaves.

Limit of Impurities.—5 per cent. of its stems or other foreign organic matter.

Habitat.—Northern America, Europe and Asia, in dry woods.

Plant.—A low perennial herb with long extended subterranean shoots sending up aerial stems which bear whorled and scattered cuneate-lanceolate, sharply serrate, coriaceous, shiny leaves and a terminal 2–8 flowered raceme of pinkish flowers, the anthers of which are violet colored. The fruit is a capsule.

Commercial.—The commercial supplies come largely from Virginia, North Carolina and Michigan.

Description.—This drug occurs as entire and broken leaves usually admixed with a few stems. Leaves, oblanceolate, 2.5 to 7 cm. in length and from 8 to 20 mm. in breadth, the distal portion coarsely and sharply serrate, acute or somewhat obtuse, the proximal wedge-shaped and nearly entire; coriaceous, smooth, shiny, and uniformly dark green on the ventral surface, paler beneath, the veins prominent; odor slight; taste astringent and bitter.

Powdered Drug.—Brownish-green. Fragments of epidermis composed of cells with clear, unevenly thickened, porous and wavy vertical walls, those from the lower epidermis showing broadly elliptical stomata; fragments of mesophyll, some of the cells of which contain chloroplastids, others tannin; fragments of parenchyma containing a reddish-brown amorphous substance; fragments of the epidermis of the stems, the cells of which contain a purplish pigment that is colored yellowish-red with acids and green with alkalies; calcium oxalate in rosette aggregates up to 65μ in diameter; starch grains few, simple, spheroidal, up to 16μ in diameter or 2 to 4-compound; fragments of sclerenchyma fibers; tracheæ of stems with spiral or annular thickenings.

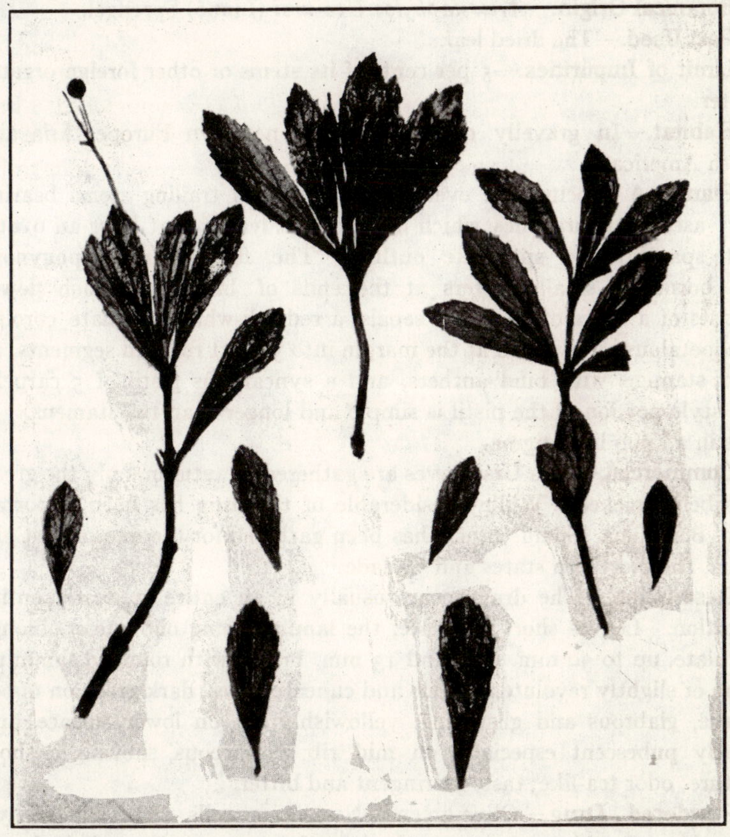

FIG. 188.—Pipsissewa (*Chimaphila umbellata*). Leaves and leafy stems.

Constituents.—The glucosides, ericolin and arbutin; a neutral principle, chimaphilin; tannin, gallic acid, etc. Arbutin is resolved by hydrolysis into dextrose and hydroquinone.

Uses.—Chimaphila is used as a diuretic, astringent and mild disinfectant to urinary tract; in cystitis, gonorrhœa, etc.

Allied Plant.—*Chimaphila maculata* or Spotted Wintergreen is a perennial herb growing in North America frequently in localities where Pipsissewa abounds. Its leaves are lanceolate or ovate-lanceolate, obtuse at the base, toothed, the upper surface spotted with white.

UVA URSI U.S.P. (UVA URSI)

Synonyms.—Red Bearberry, Bearberry, Mountain Box, Rockberry; *Ger.* Bärentraubenblätter, *Fr.* Rasin d'ours.

Botanical Origin.—*Arctostaphylos Uva-ursi* (Linné) Sprengel.

Part Used.—The dried leaf.

Limit of Impurities.—5 per cent. of its stems or other foreign organic matter.

Habitat.—In gravelly or sandy soil of northern Europe, Asia and North America.

Plant.—A procumbent evergreen shrub with trailing stems bearing short ascending branches which in turn bear leaves that have an ovate, ovate-spatulate to spatulate outline. The flowers are hypogynous and borne in small clusters at the ends of branches. Each flower consists of a calyx of 5 reddish sepals, a reddish-white urceolate corolla, gamopetalous but divided at the margin into 5 short reflexed segments, 10 short stamens with bifid anthers, and a syncarpous pistil of 5 carpels. The style portion of the pistil is simple and longer than the stamens. It ends in a knob like stigma.

Commercial.—Uva Ursi leaves are gathered in autumn, only the green ones being picked. While considerable of the drug has been imported from Barcelona, Spain, much has been gathered for the market in California, the Northern states and Canada.

Description.—The drug occurs usually in an entire or nearly entire condition. Leaves short petiolate, the laminæ being obovate or oblong-spatulate, up to 30 mm. long and 13 mm. broad, with rounded summits, entire or slightly revolute margins and cuneate bases, dark green on upper surface, glabrous and glistening, yellowish-green on lower surface and slightly pubescent especially on mid rib, coriaceous, showing a short fracture; odor tea-like; taste astringent and bitter.

Powdered Drug.—Olive-green. Numerous cells of the mesophyll with chloroplastids and frequently irregular masses of a carbohydrate; fragments of fibrovascular bundles showing spiral tracheæ and narrow lignified sclerenchyma fibers associated with which are crystal fibers containing monoclinic prisms of $Ca\bar{O}$; fragments of epidermis with polygonal cells and broadly elliptical stomata surrounded by 5 to 8 neighboring cells; numerous fragments of cells having a yellowish-brown content colored a bluish-black with ferric chloride T.S. If a small quantity of the powder be placed in a watch crystal and covered with microscopic slides and the powder gently heated, a crystalline sublimate of hydroquinone is formed consisting of long rods and feather like aggregates.

Constituents.—The glucosides, arbutin and ericolin, ursone, tannic acid, gallic acid, calcium oxalate, etc.

Uses.—Diuretic and mild disinfectant to urinary tract.

SAPOTACEÆ (STAR APPLE FAMILY)

Tropical shrubs or trees (*Palaquium*) characterized by the presence of rows of laticiferous sacs in the pith and cortex of the stems and adjoining the veins of the leaves. Leaves alternate, exstipulate, evergreen and coriaceous. Flowers perfect, large and axillary. Fruit a berry (*Palaquium*) rarely a capsule (*Ponteria*).

GUTTA PERCHA (GUTTA PERCHA)

Synonyms.—Gummi Plasticum, Gutta Pertscha, Gutta Taban.

Botanical Origin.—Trees of the genera *Palaquium* and *Payena*.

Part Used.—The purified, coagulated, milky exudate.

Habitat.—Malay Archipelago.

Plants.—Stately trees with reddish-gray bark, alternate, exstipulate, evergreen, coriaceous, obovate-lanceolate leaves, yellow or white flowers and ovoid berries. The leaves are smooth and bright green on the upper surface, yellowish-brown and silky on the lower surface.

Production and Commerce.—A number of species of *Palaquium* yield this drug, but the best article is obtained from *Palaquium gutta*, *Palaquium oblongifolia* and *Payena Leerii* growing on the islands of the Malay Archipelago, the Phillippine Islands, and Sumatra. The grayish-white latex is formed in laticiferous sacs arranged in rows in the cortex, phloem and pith as well as in the leaves. It is usually obtained, during the wet season, by felling the trees, chopping off the branches and removing the bark in circular strips, forming channels about an inch wide and about a foot apart along the trunk. The latex exudes and fills these channels from which it is removed and boiled in open vessels over wood fires. It is then kneaded, some impurities such as wood removed, and made into blocks or cakes. Some gutta percha is also obtained by making V-shaped incisions in the living tree. It is sent from British. American and Dutch possessions to Singapore, thence to London, from whence we receive our supply. Most of the commercial article is at present produced in Sumatra. The crude article is purified by washing chopped or sliced pieces in hot water, passing through a wire strainer to remove dirt and kneading by machinery to remove water. (Alkaline solutions or light petroleum are occasionally used to remove resin from the crude article.) It is then passed, while still hot and plastic, through rolling machines and comes out as sheets of varying degrees of thickness. The value of the drug is directly proportionate to the amount of the hydrocarbon, gutta, it contains.

Description.—Gutta Percha occurs in pliable and elastic masses, sticks or sheets of variable size and shape. It is tough, yellowish-white, usually with reddish streaks. It is insoluble in water and partly soluble in carbon disulphide, chloroform, petroleum benzin, or oil of turpentine, there being left not more than 10 per cent. of undissolved residue. It is slowly dissolved by sulphuric and nitric acids. It should be preserved under water, for when exposed to air and sunlight it absorbs oxygen and becomes hard and brittle.

Constituents.—Up to 85 per cent. of gutta ($C_{10}H_{16}$) which is soluble in ether, chloroform, petroleum ether and in volatile and fixed oils; from 13 to 20 per cent. of two oxygenated resins, viz., alban ($C_{10}H_{16}O$) (soluble in hot alcohol) and fluavil ($C_{20}H_{32}O$) (soluble in cold alcohol); guttan, etc.

Uses.—Gutta percha is used in the manufacture of insulating material, surgical instruments, splints, supports, etc. It is sometimes dissolved in chloroform or carbon disulphide and applied as a protective covering to a wounded surface.

CHICLE

Synonyms.—Gum Chicle, Mexican Chicle, Sapodilla Gum, Gum Zapotl.

Botanical Origin.—*Achras Sapota* Linné.

Part Used.—The dried latex.

Habitat.—Mexico and Central America.

Plant.—A tall evergreen tree which is cultivated in Tropical America and on the Florida Keys for its edible fruit known as the "Sapodilla."

Production and Commerce.—The bark of *Achras Sapota* contains a milky latex known as chicle, which is obtained by tapping the trunk of the tree and scraping the thickened exudate from the bark. This product is known as "*crude chicle*" or "loaf chicle," and is exported from Mexico.

Description.—*Crude chicle* occurs in irregular, pinkish to cherry-red or reddish-brown pieces with a considerable amount of adherent bark and usually with admixtures of stones, twigs and numerous insect remains. The extraneous matter varies from 25 to 40 per cent. with different varieties of Mexican Chicle which are designated as "dark," "medium" and "light" chicle. Dark chicle is cherry-red in color, medium chicle, reddish-brown and light chicle, flesh colored.

Purified chicle occurs as an amorphous, pale pink colored powder, insoluble in water and ordinary solvents and when heated, forming a tenacious sticky mass which, upon cooling, possesses a pink color. Upon ageing, it undergoes partial oxidation, becomes yellowish-brown to brown and very brittle. The purified article is prepared by first breaking the crude chicle into small pieces, placing them in a revolving screen drum and washing in a bath of strong alkali solution to remove extraneous matters. The drum and contents are then lifted out and placed in a bath of sodium acid phosphate to neutralize the alkalinity. The material is next washed with water until free from soluble salts and subsequently dried and powdered.

Constituents.—Similar to Gutta Percha but with less gutta and more resin.

Use.—Chicle is employed in the manufacture of medicated chewing gums.

Allied Product.—**Balata** is a dried latex obtained from *Mimusops Balata* Miq. (*Mimusops globosa* Gærtner) a tree indigenous to the West Indies and South America. It possesses the general properties of gutta percha and chicle and is employed in the manufacture of the bubble-balloon chewing gums. The crude article which is solid and somewhat crumbly is frequently adulterated with sticks, stones and other foreign matter. It is imported into this country from Mexico, Central America and Africa.

STYRACEÆ (BENZOIN FAMILY)

Shrubs or low trees mostly indigenous to tropical America, many of which yield balsamic resins. Leaves alternate to opposite, entire, often acuminate. Flowers hermaphrodite, regular, rarely sub-irregular, either in condensed fascicles or solitary in the axils of the leaves; sepals and petals typically five each; corolla often white, rarely pinkish or yellowish; stamens many to four to two, perigynous or sub-hypogynous; pistil bicarpellary or four to five carpellate. Fruit either fleshy or dry, often winged and rarely as many-celled as there are carpels.

BENZOINUM U.S.P. (BENZOIN)

Synonyms.—Gum Benjamin, Benzoin Laurel, Benjamin Tree; *Ger.* Benzoe; *Fr.* Benzoin.

Botanical Origin.—*Styrax Benzoin* Dryander and some other species of *Styrax*.

Part Used.—A balsamic resin.

Purity Rubric.—Sumatra Benzoin yields not less than 75 per cent. of alcohol-soluble extractive and not more than 1 per cent. of acid-insoluble ash. Siam Benzoin contains not more than 1 per cent. of foreign organic matter, yields not less than 90 per cent. of alcohol-soluble extractive, and not more than 0.5 per cent. of acid-insoluble ash.

Habitat.—East Indies.

Plants.—Trees of medium height, having gray bark, oblong-ovate, acuminate, hairy leaves and axillary pink or white flowers which are borne on branched peduncles.

Production and Commerce.—The species of *Styrax* yielding Benzoin grow on hills and in plantations of Borneo, Java, Sumatra and Siam. The uninjured bark of these plants has been found by Lüdy to contain tannin, traces of wax, phloroglucin and sugar but no balsamic resin. The same investigator has shown that neither a secretion nor secretion cells occur in the uninjured bark but instead large quantities of tannin and further that the formation of balsam first takes place in those parts of the injured bark containing the tannin. Since the balsam contains a large amount of alcohol reacting like tannin, viz., resinotannol, it seems probable that the drug is at least in part produced from the tannin in the bark under morbid influence. The balsamic resin is collected during the summer and autumn from both wild and cultivated trees of 5 to 6 years or more growth by making incisions through the bark of the trunk with an axe. The balsamic resin slowly exudes as a white liquid. When dry and hard it is scraped and picked off, placed in appropriate receptacles and assorted according to sizes, cleanness, etc. The trees yield the resin for about 12 years. The first three year's product is more fragrant and contains more white tears. This is known to the natives as "head benzoin." The next 7 to 9 year's yield is somewhat brown and termed "belly benzoin." The trees are subsequently felled and the trunk split. The product that is scraped off is of poor quality, of a dark-brown color, admixed with wood, bark, dirt and known as "foot benzoin." There are two officially recognized commercial varieties, namely, Siam and Sumatra Benzoin. Siam Benzoin, yielded by indefinitely determined species of *Styrax*, occurs in pebble-like tears of variable size, sometimes agglutinated with a reddish-brown substance. It is produced in the province of Luang Prabang of Siam where it is packed in cases for shipment. The largest amounts are imported into the U.S.A. from Paris and Tonkin. Smaller lots have been received from Bangkok, Geneva and London.

Sumatra Benzoin yielded by *Styrax Benzoin*, occurs as irregular, reddish-brown, reddish-gray or grayish-brown masses. It is produced in Sumatra and Java mainly, wrapped in matting and conveyed to Padang, Penang and Singapore, where it is packed in chests weighing about 100 lbs. and sent into commerce. Most of it is imported from Sumatra, Padang and Penang, although occasional lots come to us from London and Amsterdam.

Description. Siam Benzoin.—It occurs as compressed, yellowish-brown to rusty-brown, pebble-like tears of variable size, separate or slightly agglutinated with a reddish-brown resin; fracture milky-white;

hard and brittle at ordinary temperatures but softened by heat and becoming plastic on chewing; odor balsamic, vanilla-like; taste aromatic and slightly acrid. The alcoholic solution becomes milky upon the addition of water. Upon boiling an acidulated solution of Siam benzoin with potassium permanganate, no odor of benzaldehyde should be evident (absence of cinnamic acid). Upon the addition of an ethereal solution of Siam benzoin to a small quantity of sulphuric acid in a porcelain dish, the solution should be colored purplish-red.

Sumatra Benzoin.—It occurs in the form of irregular, marbled masses of variable size, made up of tears imbedded in a reddish-brown, reddish-gray or grayish-brown resinous substance; tears externally yellowish or rusty-brown, milky-white on fresh fracture; hard and brittle at ordinary temperatures, but softened upon heating and becoming gritty on chewing; odor aromatic and upon digesting with boiling water exhibiting an odor of storax or cinnamic acid; taste aromatic and slightly acrid. The alcoholic solution becomes milky upon the addition of water. Upon boiling an acidulated solution with potassium permanganate, benzaldehyde is produced (presence of cinnamic acid).

Upon the addition of an ethereal solution of Sumatra benzoin to a small quantity of sulphuric acid in a porcelain dish, the solution should be colored brownish-red.

Constituents.—**Siam Benzoin** contains lubanol benzoate, siaresinol benzoate, *d*-siaresinolic acid, vanillin, benzoic acid both free and combined, about 3 per cent. of cinnamic acid, etc. **Sumatra Benzoin** contains two alcohols, one known as benzoresinol combined with cinnamic acid, about 10.3 per cent. of free cinnamic acid, about 6.5 per cent. of free benzoic acid, phenylpropyl ester of cinnamic acid, benzaldehyde, cinnamic cinnamate, etc.

Uses.—Siam Benzoin is used chiefly in the manufacture of toilet preparations and as a fixative in the manufacture of perfumes. Sumatra Benzoin is employed internally as a stimulating expectorant and externally as a stimulant and antiseptic. Benzoin is also employed by the confectionery trade in the preparation of vanilla creams, etc. and by the leather trade as an ingredient of leather dressings.

OLEACEÆ (OLIVE FAMILY)

Oleaceæ or Olive Family.—Shrubs (***Forsythia***, ***Chionanthus***, ***Syringa***, etc.) or trees (***Fraxinus***, ***Olea***, etc.) with stems possessing close white wood, and slightly swollen or enlarged nodes. Leaves opposite, decussate, simple, rarely pinnately compound (Ash). Stems and leaves with bicollateral bundles. Inflorescence dichesial or scorpioid cymes but tending constantly toward condensation and so, in the Lilac, the inflorescence becomes a clustered raceme of cymes (thyrsus). Flowers regular, pentamerous or tetramerous; sepals small, green, rarely petaloid, synsepalous; petals synpetalous, elongated into a narrow tube, expanding above into a stellate limb; stamens very rarely five, rarely four to three, nearly always two, epipetalous and high set on corolla tube; pistil bicarpellate, rarely of three to four carpels; ovary two-celled with two to one pendulous ovules in each cavity. Fruit either a capsule (Lilac), drupe (Olive), berry (Privet) or a winged indehiscent akene (Ash). Seeds with moderate to scanty albumen becoming occasionally albuminous.

MANNA U.S.P. (MANNA)

Synonyms.—Manna Ash; *Fr.* Manne; *Ger.* Manna.

Botanical Origin.—*Fraxinus Ornus* Linné.

Part Used.—The dried saccharine exudation.

Purity Rubric.—Not less than 75 per cent. of anhydrous alcohol-soluble extractive, when extracted with boiling 90 per cent. alcohol, by volume.

Habitat.—Southern Europe.

Plant.—A small tree bearing imparipinnate leaves, each with 7 ovate, acuminate, serrate leaflets, and panicles of small white flowers. The fruit is a winged akene (samara).

Production and Commerce.—The manna ash is cultivated for the drug chiefly in Italy and Sicily. When the trees are about 8 years of age transverse incisions are made in the bark of one side of the stem, daily, beginning from the ground upward at succeeding higher levels. The manna exudes as a clear liquid which, after hardening, is collected either from the side of the trunk or in special receptacles.

Five Italian provinces supply most of the world's consumption of manna which occurs in 6 commercial varieties, as follows:

Manna, flake, Capaci, 62.15 per cent. mannite
Manna, flake, Geraci, 62 per cent. mannite
Manna, flake, Frassino, 47 per cent. mannite
Manna, sorts, Capaci, 37–55 per cent. mannite
Manna, sorts, Geraci 37 per cent. mannite
Manna, sorts, Castelbuono, 28–30 per cent. mannite

The present supply to the United States comes from Palermo, Italy, packed in cases.

Description.—In irregular, more or less elongated, flattened, 3-sided pieces, externally yellowish-white or cream colored; friable, somewhat waxy; internally nearly white, porous and crystalline from 10 to 25 cm. in length (*large flake manna*) or in shorter yellowish-white to yellowish-gray pieces (*small flake manna*), or in irregular yellowish-brown masses consisting of agglutinated tears and vegetable fragments (*manna in sorts*); odor slight; taste sweet, slightly bitter and faintly acrid.

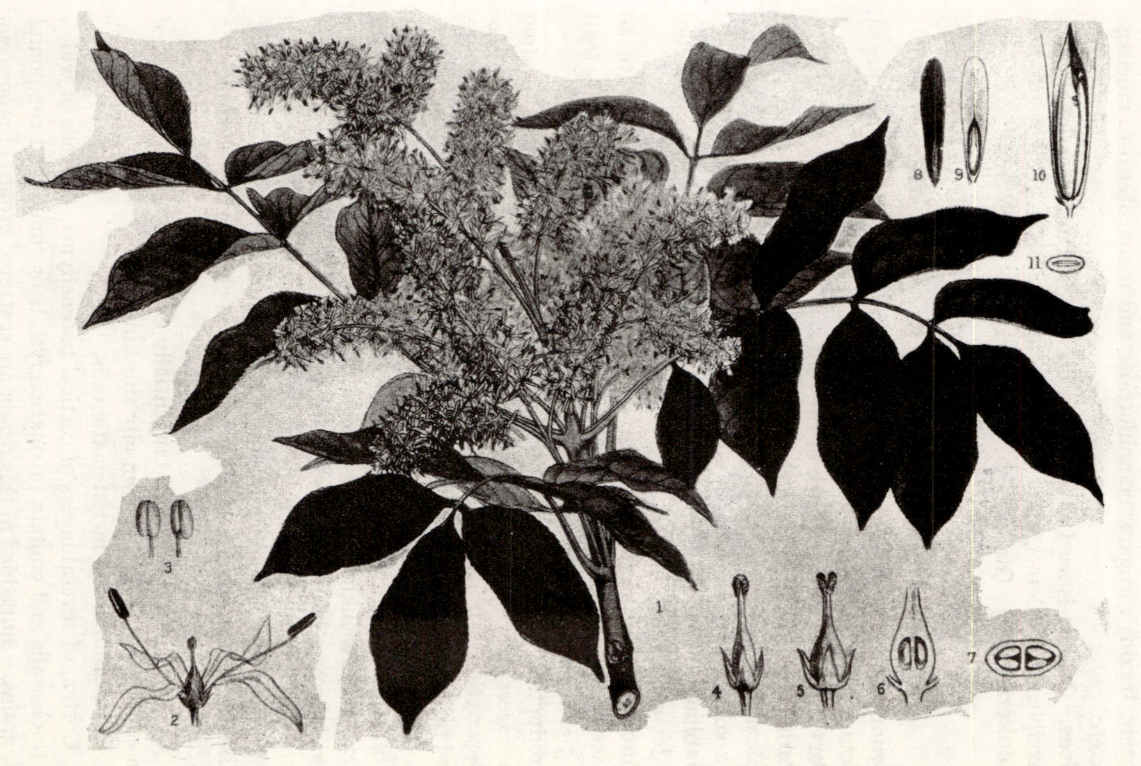

FIG. 189.—The Manna Ash, (*Fraxinus Ornus*). I. Flowering branch. 2. Expanded flower. 3. Unopened anthers. 4, 5. The calyx and pistil. 6. Vertical- and 7. Transverse section of same. 8. Fruit (a single samara). 9. Vertical section of same and seed. 10. Fruit with a part of the pericarp removed, showing the ripe seed. 11. Transverse section of seed. (*After Bentley and Trimen.*)

Constituents.—Up to 60 per cent. of mannitol (mannite); a bitter glucoside, fraxin; 2 sugars, manninotriose and manneotetrose, mucilage, resin, etc.

Uses.—Manna is used as a laxative for children and occasionally as a pill excipient for calomel, etc.

Adulterants.—1. Glucose. 2. Bread crumbs. 3. Sucrose.

CHIONANTHUS N.F. (CHIONANTHUS)

Synonyms.—Fringe Tree Bark, Flowering Ash, Old Man's Beard.

Botanical Origin.—*Chionanthus virginica* Linné.

Part Used.—The dried bark of the root.

Purity Rubric.—Not more than 5 per cent. of wood and other foreign organic matter. It yields to 70 per cent. alcohol not less than 25 per cent. of non-volatile extractive.

Habitat.—Southern United States as far north as Pennsylvania and New Jersey.

Plant.—A low deciduous tree with opposite, petiolate, ovate to obovate-lanceolate leaves and drooping panicles of white flowers, each with 5 or 6 linear petals. The fruit is an ovoid, purple drupe.

Production and Commerce.—The bark is collected in autumn from roots of trees growing in Virginia and North Carolina and carefully dried.

Description.—It occurs as irregularly broken, flat, or as more or less quilled pieces of variable length and from 2 to 10 mm. in thickness; heavy, some pieces of the whole drug sinking when thrown into water; outer surface rough, usually reddish-brown, occasionally grayish-brown, with few transverse wrinkles, whitish cork patches, and root scars; inner surface yellowish brown, longitudinally striate and undulate; fracture short, hard and coarsely granular, due to projecting groups of stone cells; fractured surface yellowish-white; odor aromatic; taste bitter.

Histology.—Transverse sections mounted in chloral show the following characteristics:

1. Cork of several layers of tangentially elongated cells, a number of which contain a yellowish-brown oily substance.

2. Cork cambium of meristematic cells.

3. Cortex, of several layers of cortical parenchyma, the cells of which have thick walls and contain prismatic crystals or simple and compound starch grains. Imbedded in this region are scattered groups of stone cells and a few bundles of sclerenchyma fibers.

4. Phloem, a broad zone of sieve tubes, companion cells and phloem parenchyma. Imbedded in this region are a few groups of sclerenchyma fibers. The medullary-rays are 1 to 3 cells wide.

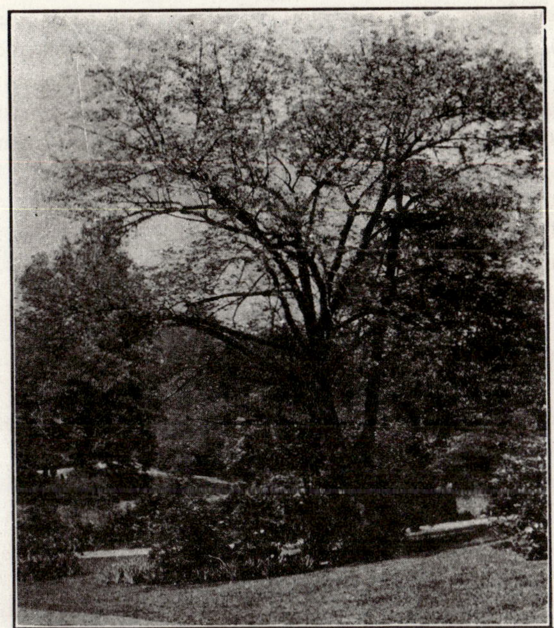

FIG. 190.—White ash (*Fraxinus americana*).

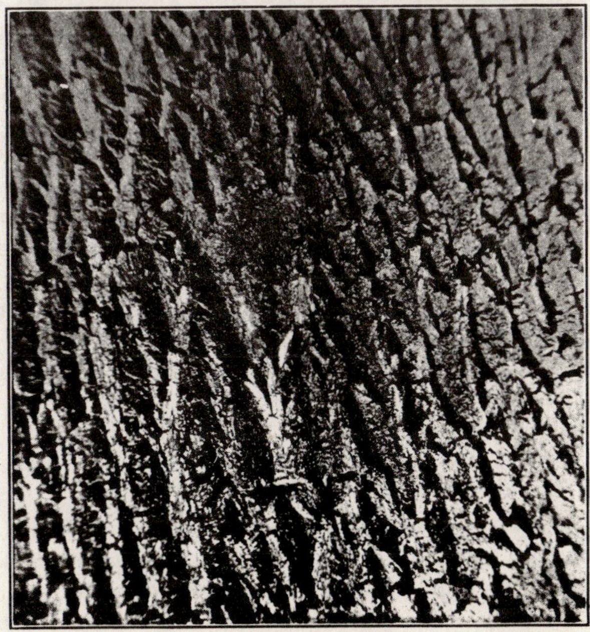

FIG. 191. White ash bark before removal of cork.

Powdered Drug.—Light-brown; numerous porous stone cells with thick, lignified walls; numerous brownish, resin masses; fragments of light brown cork tissue; fragments of parenchyma, many of the cells filled with small prismatic crystals, some with starch; starch grains spheroidal, simple or 2- to 4-compound, the individual grains up to 20μ in diameter; a few fibers with lignified porous walls and truncated ends.

Constituents.—A bitter glucoside, chionanthin, etc.

Uses.—Bitter tonic, diuretic and aperient.

Adulterant.—(1) Stem bark of *Chionanthus virginica.*

FRAXINUS (WHITE ASH BARK)

Synonyms.—White Ash, Cane Ash, American Ash; *Ger.* Esche; *Fr.* Frené.

Botanical Origin.—*Fraxinus americana* Linné and probably other species of *Fraxinus.*

Part Used.—The dried bark, deprived of cork.

Habitat.—Eastern and central North America, in rich woodland.

Plant.—A dioecious shade and timber tree which, when grown in the open, develops a pyramidal or ovoid crown with long lateral branches. Its leaves are imparipinnate with 5 to 11 oblong-lanceolate, ovate or obovate petioulated leaflets, acuminate at apex, rounded or cuneate at base, entire or crenate-serrate along margin. The flowers are dioecious; calyx campanulate, 4 lobed; petals none; stamens 2 or 3; stigma 2-cleft. The fruit is a single samara, winged only from near the apex.

Production.—The White Ash is grown mainly as a timber and ornamental tree. The bark of its trunk and root are removed, by those associated with the lumber industry. After removing the cork, it is then carefully dried.

Description.—In flat pieces of variable length and breadth, from 3 to 7 mm. in thickness; outer surface grayish-brown with warty ridges, where cork is present, otherwise yellowish-brown; inner surface pale brown to yellowish, longitudinally striate; fracture uneven and coarsely fibrous; odor slightly aromatic; taste bitter and weakly acrid.

Constituents.—Fraxin (glucoside), fraxetin (bitter substance), tannin, volatile oil, mannite, gum, etc.

Uses.—Diuretic and emmenagogue, but of doubtful value.

LOGANIACEÆ (NUX VOMICA FAMILY)

Herbs (*Spigelia*, etc.), woody vines (*Gelsemium*, etc.) or trees (*Strychnos Nux Vomica*, etc.) with a bitter juice usually containing alkaloids. Stem, rarely herbaceous, usually woody, often long-climbing and rope-like (*Gelsemium*), usually with a bicollateral bundle system. Leaves opposite, stipulate or exstipulate. Inflorescence racemose or cymose (*Spigelia*), scorpioid cyme (*Strychnos*), sometimes condensed into solitary, axillary flowers. Flowers perfect, usually regular; calyx gamosepalous; corolla gamopetalous, hypogynous, rotate, campanulate or infundibuliform; stamens inserted on the corolla tube or throat and with thread-like filaments; ovary superior, two-celled; style elongate with bifid stigma; ovules numerous. Fruit usually a capsule, septicidally dehiscent (*Gelsemium sempervirens*), or loculicidally dehiscent (*Spigelia marilandica*), sometimes a berry (*Strychnos Nux Vomica*) or drupe. Seeds numerous or solitary, sometimes winged.

GELSEMIUM N.F. (GELSEMIUM)

Synonyms.—Yellow Jasmine, Yellow Jessamine, Trumpet Flower; *Ger.* Giftjasmin; *Fr.* Jasmine sauvage.

Botanical Origin.—*Gelsemium sempervirens* (Linné) Persoon.

Part Used.—The dried rhizome and roots.

Purity Rubric.—Not more than 2 per cent. of foreign organic matter.

Habitat.—Eastern United States from Virginia to Florida and Texas.

Plant.—A perennial woody twiner with purplish stem and opposite, short petioled, ovate-lanceolate to lanceolate entire leaves, axillary clusters of yellow funnel-form or trumpet-shaped flowers and 2-celled, flat, capsular fruits containing several winged seeds in each cell.

Production and Commerce.—The rhizomes and roots are dug up in autumn, washed and dried. The commercial supplies of Gelsemium are collected in Virginia, North and South Carolina, Tennessee and Georgia.

Description.—The drug occurs as segments of the cylindrical rhizome with attached wiry roots. Rhizome horizontal, the segments from 3 to 30 cm. in length and from 3 to 35 mm. in diameter; externally light-yellowish-brown or purplish, frequently spirally twisted, longitudinally wrinkled, with purplish-brown longitudinal lines and transverse fissures; upper surface with few stem scars, the under lateral portions with several roots and root scars; fracture tough, splintery; internally exhibiting a narrow purplish-brown bark, a broad, pale yellow, finely radiated wood and a minute disintegrated pith; odor indistinct; taste strongly bitter.

Roots up to 20 cm. in length and from 2 to 19 mm. thick, light brown, nearly smooth and wiry; fracture one-half transverse, the other oblique or splintery.

Histology.—Transverse sections of the rhizome show the following microscopical peculiarities.

1. Cork, of several layers of yellowish-brown more or less lignified cells.
2. Cork cambium of meristematic cells.

3. Cortex of numerous layers of parenchyma cells containing spherical starch grains. In the outer part of this region occur scattered groups of sclerenchyma elements.

4. Outer Phloem, a narrow zone of phloem patches, containing sieve tubes and phloem cells, separated from each other by phloem portions of medullary-rays which show a marked contrast to the xylem portions of

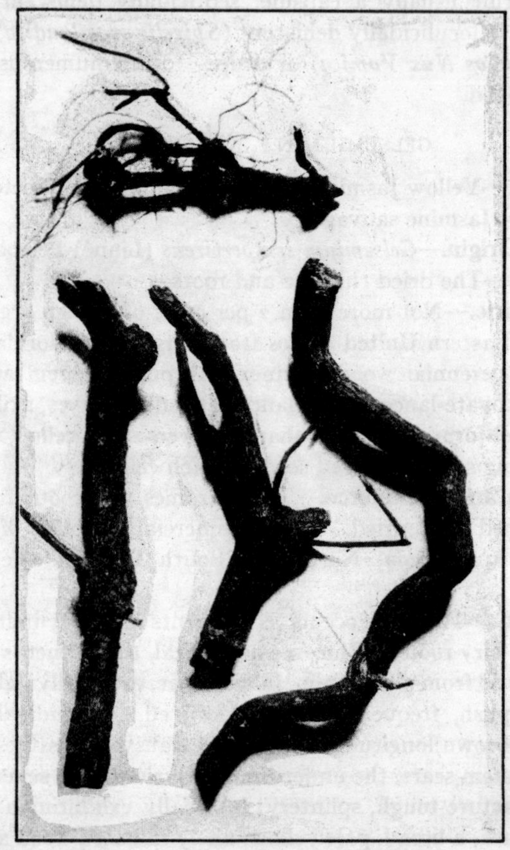

FIG. 192.—Gelsemium. Note the slender wiry roots emanating from the rhizomes. Characteristic fissures appear in the lower portion of the rhizome to the right. × 5/8.

medullary-rays in being non-lignified. In various cells of the medullary rays of the phloem occur long monoclinic prisms of calcium oxalate.

5. Cambium, of small meristematic cells.

6. Xylem, a broad radiate zone composed of wedge-shaped xylem patches consisting of large, broad, porous tracheæ and small, narrow porous tracheids. Each xylem patch is separated from its neighbor by a mulit-

celleate xylem medullary ray, the cells of which contain starch and have lignified walls.

7. Cambium, of meristematic cells.

8. Internal Phloem, consisting usually of 4 masses of sieve tubes and phloem parenchyma.

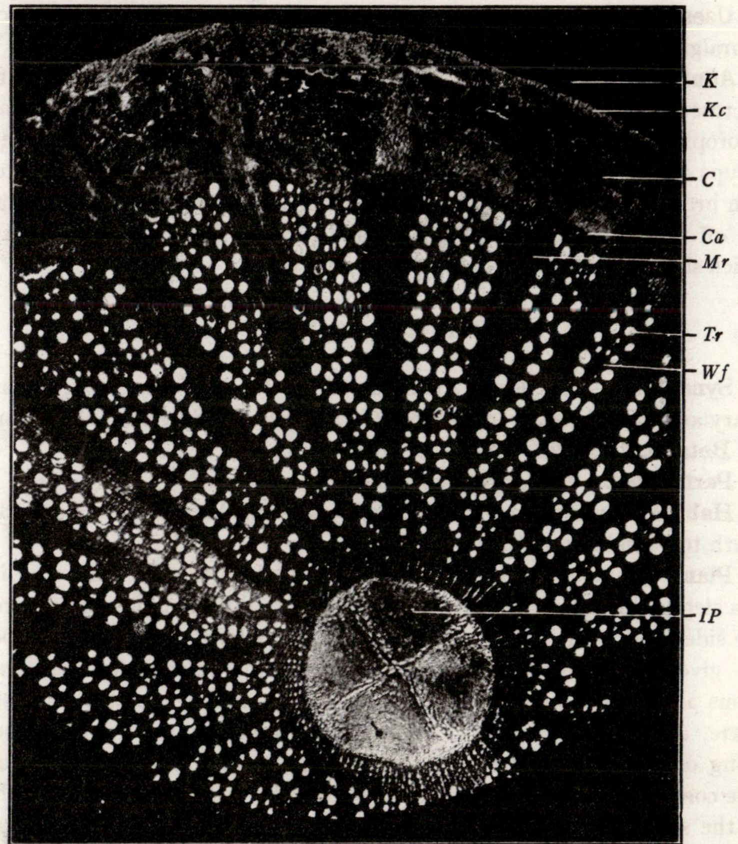

FIG. 193.—Transverse section through representative part of *Gelsemium* rhizome showing cork (*K*); cork cambium (*Kc*); cortex (*C*); cambium (*Ca*); xylem portion of medullary ray (*Mr*); trachea (*Tr*) and wood fibers (*Wf*) of xylem; intraxylary phloem (*IP*). Phloem, between *Ca* and *C*.

9. Pith, a very small central zone of more or less disintegrated non-indurated cells; in very old rhizomes completely absent.

Powdered Drug.—Dark yellow; numerous tracheæ with bordered pores and tracheids with lignified walls; a few spiral tracheæ; numerous spheroidal starch grains up to 12μ in diameter; occasional groups of stone cells and narrow sclernchyma fibers with lignified walls; monoclinic prisms of calcium oxalate from 15 to 30μ in length; fragments of more or less lignified cork; fragments of lignified xylem medullary-rays the cells of which contain starch.

Constituents.—The crystalline alkaloid, gelsemine, the amorphous alkaloids gelseminine and gelsemoidine; emodin monomethyl ether, gelseminic acid, fixed oil, resins, gallic acid, etc.

Uses.—Motor depressant. Employed in the treatment of facial neuralgia, migraine, asthma, spasmodic dysmenorrhœa, etc.

Adulterants.—(1) Aerial stems of *Gelsemium sempervirens*. These differ microscopically from the rhizome in showing collenchyma containing chloroplasts in the outer cortex and in having an interrupted circle of groups of sclerenchyma fibers in the pericycle. They are frequently reddish brown to dark brown externally and show greenish bark, upon scraping off the cork. (2) The rhizome and roots of *Jasminum fructicans* L. which shows bast fibers outside of each seive mass.

SPIGELIA (SPIGELIA)

Synonyms.—Pink Root, American Worm Root, Worm Grass, Indian-, Maryland-, Carolina-, or India Pink; *Ger.* Spigelie, *Fr.* Spigélie du Maryland.

Botanical Origin.—*Spigelia Marilandica* L.

Parts Used.—The dried rhizome and roots.

Habitat.—In rich woods from New Jersey and Maryland to Kentucky, south to Florida and Texas.

Plant.—A perennial herb, the underground portion of which consists of a slender branched, knotty, horizontal, or slightly oblique rhizome from the sides and lower surface of which numerous long slender fibrous roots are given off. From the upper surface of the rhizome several aerial stems arise that attain a height of .3 to .6 m. and bear opposite, sessile, ovate, acute, entire leaves. The tubular-funnel-shaped flowers appear along one side of the terminal portion of the stem from May to July. The corolla of each flower is scarlet-red outside, yellow within and 5-lobed at the summit. The fruit is a 2 chambered, loculicidally dehiscent capsule containing yellowish seeds.

Production and Commerce.—Pink root was formerly collected in large amounts in North Carolina and Tennessee but is becoming very scarce in these states at present. Most of the commercial article is now gathered in Mississippi.

Description.—Rhizome more or less branched, entire or in pieces 1.5 to 7 cm. in length and from 2 to 5 mm. in diameter; externally dark brown finely annulate, the upper surface knotty from stem bases, the latter attaining a length of 6 cm. and a diameter of 3 mm. and possessing nodes with opposite leaf scars; the lower and lateral portions of the rhizome bearing many long, coarse, finely branched, brittle roots; fracture short, brittle and uneven, the inner surface showing nearly equal zones of white bark, yellow wood and dark pith. Roots up to 10 cm. long, few if any of which show terminal portions with bark removed from the wood.

Histology of Rhizome.—1. Epidermis of dark brown epidermal cells with thickened outer walls. 2. Cortex of from 10 to 15 layers of isodiametric cells containing spheroidal to somewhat polygonal starch-grains up to 6μ in diameter. 3. Phloem, of sieve tubes and phloem parenchyma, this zone up to 150μ broad. 4. Cambium. 5. Xylem, a compact zone

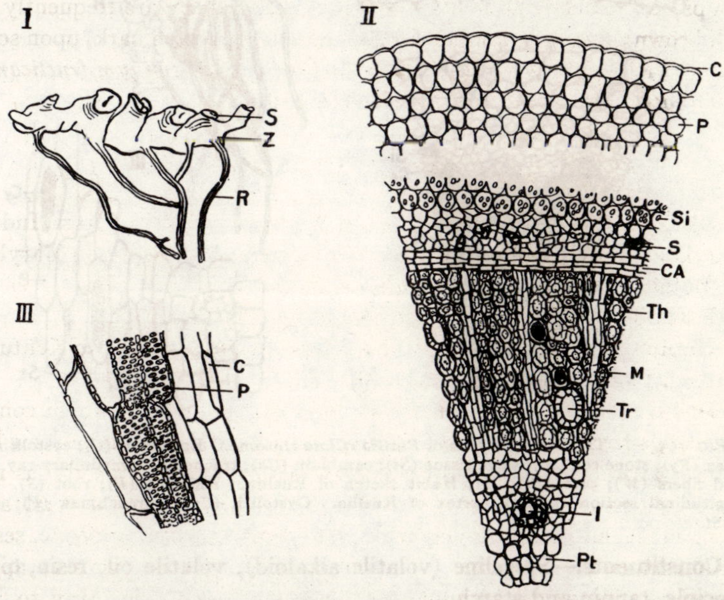

FIG. 194.—*I*, Habit sketch of Spigelia. Stem scar (*S*); rhizome (*Z*); root (*R*). *II*, Transverse section of a rhizome of Spigelia. Cuticle of yellowish-brown color, covering epidermis (*C*); cortical parenchyma (*P*); starch parenchyma (*Si*); sieve tissue (*S*); cambium (*CA*); trachea (*Tr*); tracheids (*Th*); internal phlœm (*I*); medullary-ray (*M*); pith (*Pt*). *III*, Longitudinal view of porous tracheæ (*P*) and parenchyma (*C*).

of radially arranged, lignified tracheids and tracheæ with bordered pores, a few with spiral thickenings. 6. Intraxylary phloem, a narrow zone containing groups of sieve tubes surrounded by phloem parenchyma. 7. Pith, of thin-walled parenchyma, many of the cells containing small starch grains.

Histology of Root.—Transverse sections of the root show a hairy epidermis, a broad cortex of somewhat rounded parenchyma cells containing numerous small starch grains, an endodermis and pericambium and a central stele of 6 to 8 xylem and phloem patches forming a radial fibrovascular bundle.

Powdered Drug.—Grayish-brown. Fragments of lignified tracheæ and tracheids having bordered pores. Starch grains simple, spheroidal or more or less polygonal, 2 to 6μ in diameter. Fragments of reddish-brown epidermal cells and starch parenchyma.

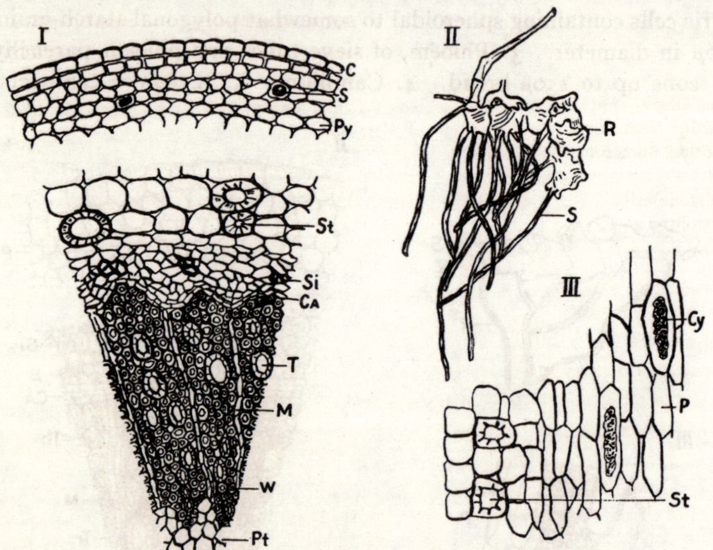

FIG. 195.—*I.* Transverse section of *Ruellia ciliosa* rhizome. Epidermis (*C*); cystolith (*S*); cortex (*Py*); stone cell (*St*); sieve tissue (*Si*); cambium (*Ca*); trachea (*T*); medullary-ray (*M*); wood fibers (*W*); pith (*Pt*). *II*, Habit sketch of Ruellia. Rhizome (*R*); root (*S*). *III*, Longitudinal section through cortex of Ruellia. Cystolith (*Cy*); parenchyma (*P*); stone cell *St*.

Constituents.—Spigeline (volatile alkaloid), volatile oil, resin, bitter principle, tannin and starch.

Use.—Pink root is used as an anthelmintic; often in combination with senna.

Substitutes and Adulterants.—The most common substitute and adulterant has been the rhizome and roots of *Ruellia ciliosa* Pursh. (Fam. *Acanthaceæ*), commonly known as East Tennessee Pink Root, a perennial herb, somewhat resembling Spigelia and often found growing in vicinities where the latter abounds. The rhizome and roots of *Phlox ovata* L. (*Phlox Carolina*) (Fam. *Polemoniaceæ*), the Carolina Pink of So. U. S., have been occasionally admixed with the drug. The important differences between Spigelia, Ruellia and Phlox underground portions may be tabulated as follows:

Spigelia	Ruellia	Phlox
Rhizome: Horizontal or slightly oblique.	*Rhizome:* Oblique	*Rhizome:* Vertical
Rootlets arising from sides and lower surface.	Rootlets arising from sides and lower surface.	Rootlets arising laterally from nodes (2 to 4 from each node).
Cystoliths absent in cortex and pith.	Cystoliths present in cortex and pith.	No cystoliths.
Intraxylary phloem present.	Intraxylary phloem present.	Intraxylary phloem absent.
Stone cells generally absent.	Stone cells in cortex much elongated and lignified.	Stone cells short or elongated, less thickened than those of Ruellia.
Root: Bark not readily detached from wood.	*Root:* Bark readily detached.	*Root:* Bark readily removable.
Rootlets numerous.	Rootlets numerous.	Rootlets few and thicker than those of Spigelia and Ruellia
No stone cells.	Stone cells numerous.	No stone cells.
Cystoliths absent.	Cystoliths present.	No cystoliths.

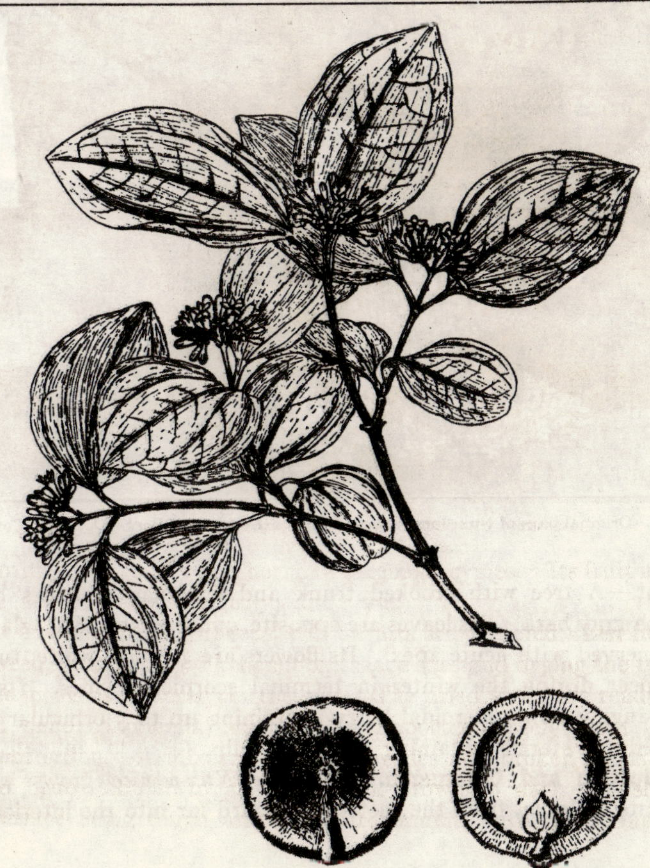

FIG. 196.—*Strychnos Nux-vomica*—Flowering branch and seeds. (*Sayre.*)

NUX VOMICA U.S.P. (NUX VOMICA)

Synonyms.—Dog Button, Quaker Button, Poison Nut; *Ger.* Brechnuss; *Fr.* Noix-vomique.

Botanical Origin.—*Strychnos Nux-vomica* Linné.

Part Used.—The dried ripe seed.

Standard of Assay.—Not less than 2.5 per cent. of the alkaloids of Nux Vomica.

Habitat.—India.

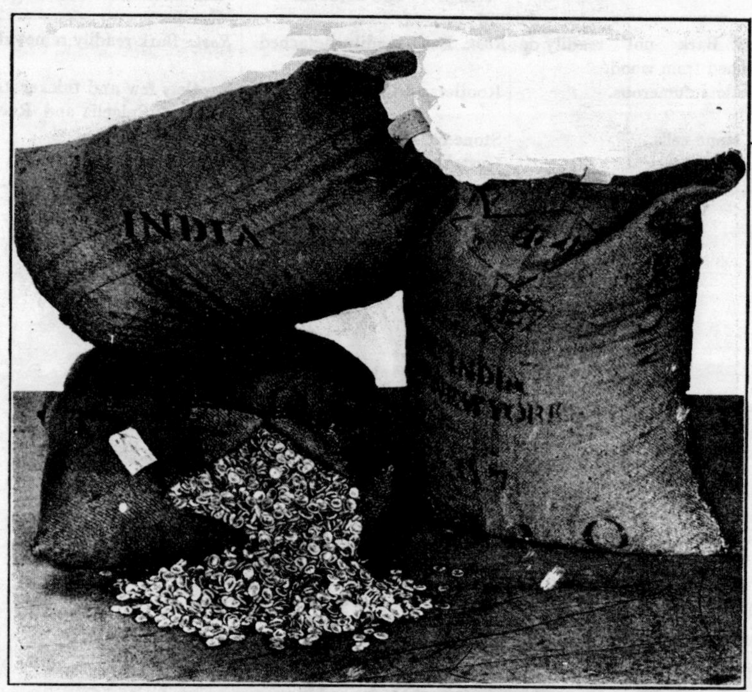

FIG. 197.—Original bags of Nux Vomica from India. (*Courtesy of Parke, Davis and Company.*)

Plant.—A tree with crooked trunk and irregular branches having yellowish-gray bark. Its leaves are opposite, ovate, exstipulate, glabrous, 3- to 5-nerved with acute apex. Its flowers are greenish-white, tubular, and appear during the winter in terminal scorpioid cymes. Its fruit is an orange-yellow spheroidal berry containing up to 5 orbicular seeds, imbedded in a starch-containing, glutinous pulp.

Production and Commerce.—*Strychnos Nux-vomica* grows wild in the forests of India, from the eastern seaboard far into the interior, and also in the forests of Ceylon, Burmah, Siam, Cochin China and northern Australia. Two-thirds of the world's supply of Nux vomica is furnished by the Madras Presidency of India. The drug is gathered and prepared in the hills of Travancore and Cochin, along the Malabar coast and in the Ganjam, Godavery and Nellore districts on the Coromandel coast. The forest tribes gather the fruits when dead ripe and wash off the pulp or

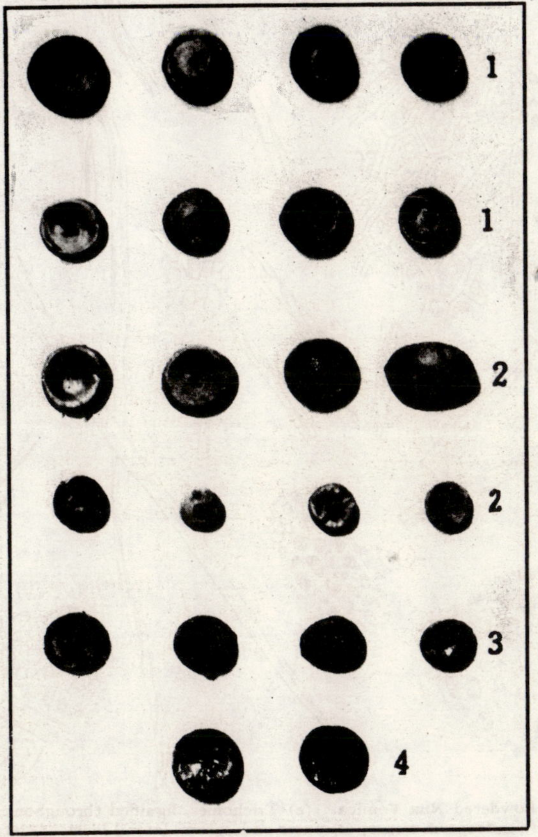

FIG. 198.—Commercial varieties of Nux Vomica. (1) Ceylon; (2) Cochin; (3) Madras; (4) Tellicherry. × ½.

permit it to rot off and then spread the seeds on mats in the sun to dry. The seeds are then sold to small middlemen from whence they pass through the hands of larger middlemen to the large exporters at Madras, Cochin and Coconada. The exporters wash and sort the seeds, separating the broken ones and the "floaters" (underweight seeds). They are then packed in burlap bags, each containing 162 or 182 poudds of seed and exported chiefly to the United States and Great Britain. The cullings and broken seeds are imported for alkaloid manufacture. The commercial supplies are imported into the United States from Madras, Cochin, Coconada, Calcutta, Bombay and London. The important commercial varieties are the Madras, Cochin, Tellicherry and Ceylon.

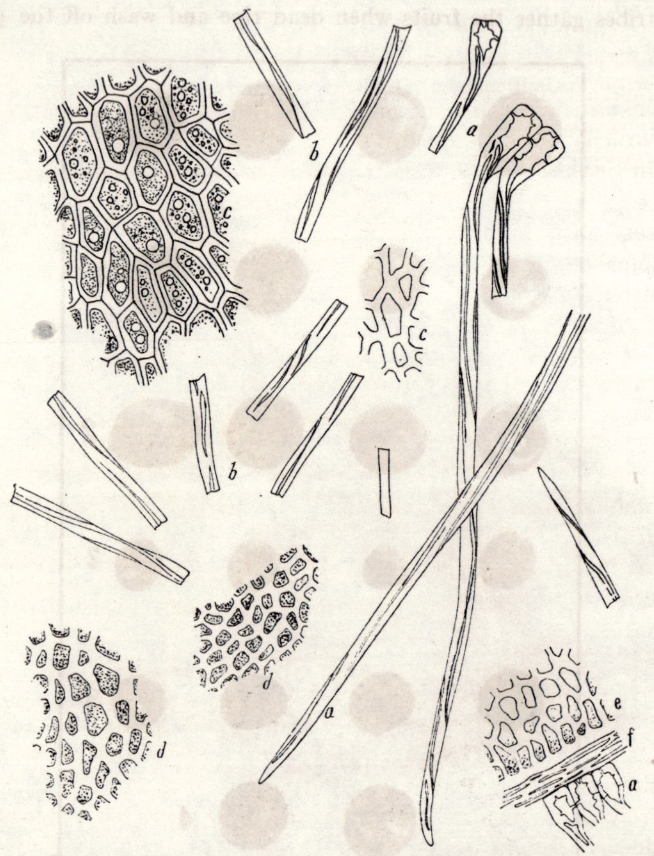

FIG. 199.—Powdered Nux Vomica. (*a*) Trichomes, lignified throughout; (*b*) trichomatic fragments; (*c, d*) endosperm tissue; (*e*) outer endosperm, lateral view; (*f*) hypodermal tissue. (*Schneider*.)

Description.—Orbicular, nearly flat, occasionally irregularly bent, from 10 to 30 mm. in diameter and from 3 to 5 mm. in thickness, very hard when dry; externally silver-yellow, grayish or greenish-gray, covered with appressed hairs giving it a silky luster, hilum indicated by a circular scar at the center of one of the flattened sides and connected with the micropyle at the edge by a ridge; internally showing a thin, hairy seed-coat and a large grayish-white endosperm at one end of which is embedded a small embryo with two broadly ovate, 5- to 7-nerved cotyledons; inodorous; taste intensely and persistently bitter.

Powdered Drug.—Light gray; consisting chiefly of thick-walled endosperm cells containing globules of a fixed oil and a few small aleurone grains, and fragments of strongly lignified, non-glandular hairs, the walls of the latter possessing large, circular, or long, slit-like pores. In the tissues of the adhering pulp occur a few small, nearly spherical starch grains.

Constituents.—From 1.84 to 5.3 per cent. of the alkaloids strychnine and brucine; a glucoside termed loganin, igasuric acid, protein, fixed oil, etc.

Uses.—Nux Vomica is employed as a spinal stimulant (excito-motor), and bitter tonic.

IGNATIA N.F. (IGNATIA)

Synonyms.—Saint Ignatius Bean, Ignatia Amara; *Fr.* Feve de Saint-Ignace; *Ger.* Ignazbohne, Bittere Fiebernuss.

Botanical Origin.—*Strychnos Ignatii* Bergius.

Part Used.—The dried ripe seed.

Purity Rubric.—Nor less than 2 per cent. of Ignatia alkaloids and not more than 1 per cent. of foreign organic matter.

Habitat.—Philippine Islands.

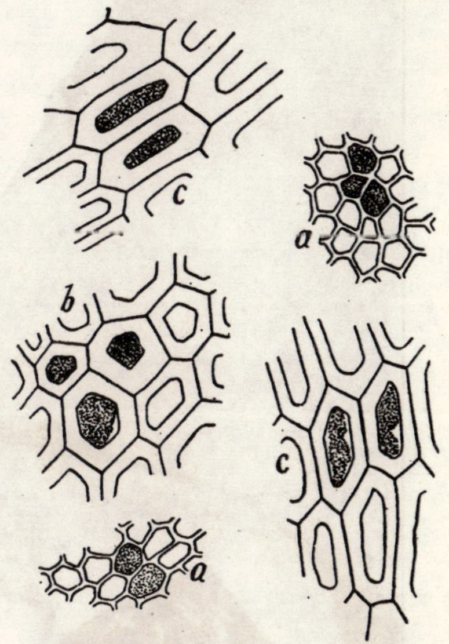

FIG. 200.—Powdered Ignatia. (*a*) Epidermal cells, vertical view; (*b*) endosperm; (*c*) endosperm. (*Schneider.*)

Plant.—A tall climbing shrub with opposite, exstipulate, ovate, glabrous leaves and white tubular flowers. The fruit is a large pyriform berry containing up to 24 pebble-like seeds imbedded in a bitter pulp.

Commerce.—The commercial supplies of this seed are obtained from the Philippine Islands.

Description.—Heavy, hard, angularly ovate with obtuse angles, from 20 to 30 mm. in length and about 15 mm. in breadth and thickness; externally grayish or reddish-black, nearly smooth with few or no hairs; fracture granular and translucent in small fragments; a small irregular cavity in the center. Nearly inodorous and intensely bitter.

Powdered Drug.—Grayish-brown; exhibiting thin cells of the epidermis and the subjacent layer of the seed coat, polygonal cells with thickened, pitted walls; hairs characteristic, spreading and thickened at the base and having linear markings; endosperm tissue, the outer cells small, con-

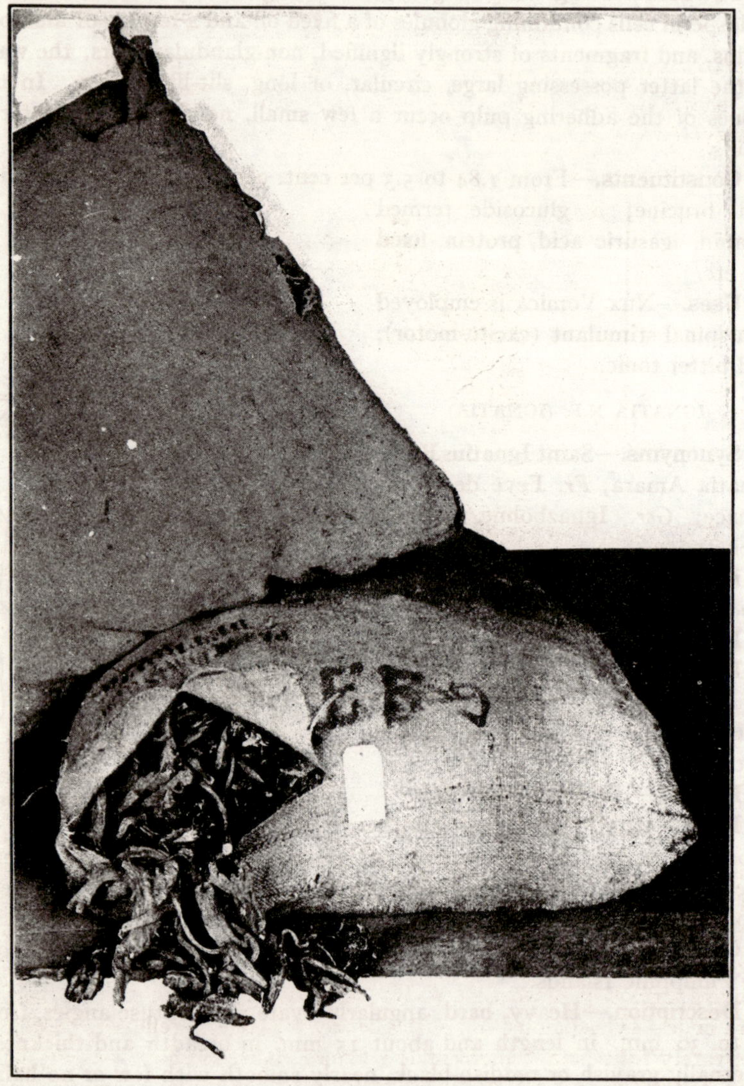

FIG. 201.—Original bags of Gentian root as imported into this country. (*After a photograph by Parke, Davis and Co.*)

tents granular, the inner larger, with thickened walls; lumen irregular in size and shape.

Constituents.—From 2.5 to 3 per cent. of the alkaloids strychnine and brucine; igasuric acid, loganin, fixed oil, proteids, etc.

Uses.—Spinal stimulant and bitter tonic.

GENTIANACEÆ (GENTIAN FAMILY)

Herbs, often low-growing and containing bitter principles. Roots and short stems sometimes more or less thickened (*Gentiana lutea*). Interxylary and intraxylary phloem occurs in some of the genera. Pith

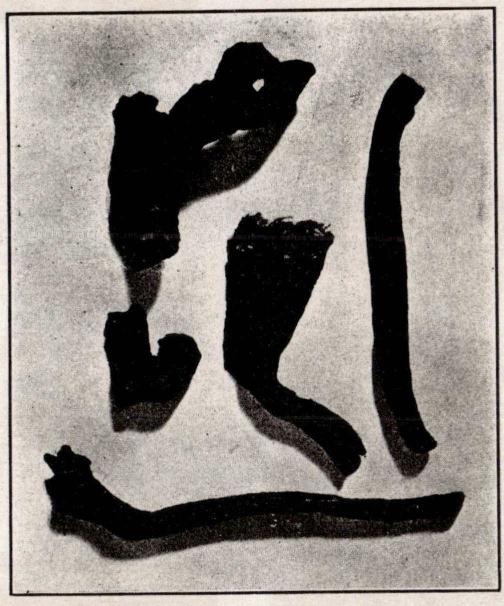

FIG. 202.—Gentian. Portions of rhizomes and roots which constitute the crude drug. Note that the rhizome is annulated while the root is deeply longitudinally wrinkled and twisted. Broken rhizome is shown in upper left hand corner. × ½.

bundles have been observed in *Gentiana*. The medullary rays are narrow and in some roots entirely absent. Leaves opposite, decussate, entire, exstipulate. Inflorescence cymose (*Gentiana lutea*) or condensing to a single, solitary, terminal flower (*Gentiana verna*, *G. acaulis*, etc.) Flowers regular, perfect, pentamerous or tetramerous, sepals five to four, green, more or less synsepalous, not infrequently everted or reflexed, corolla of five, rarely four petals, more or less synpetalous, in shape passing from open-stellate, as in *Gentiana lutea*, through many stages of connation to long-tubed as in *Gentiana acaulis;* stamens five, epipetalous; pistil bicarpellate; ovary one-celled or incompletely two-celled; style more or less elongated with bilobed to divided stigma. Fruit a capsule. Seeds albuminous.

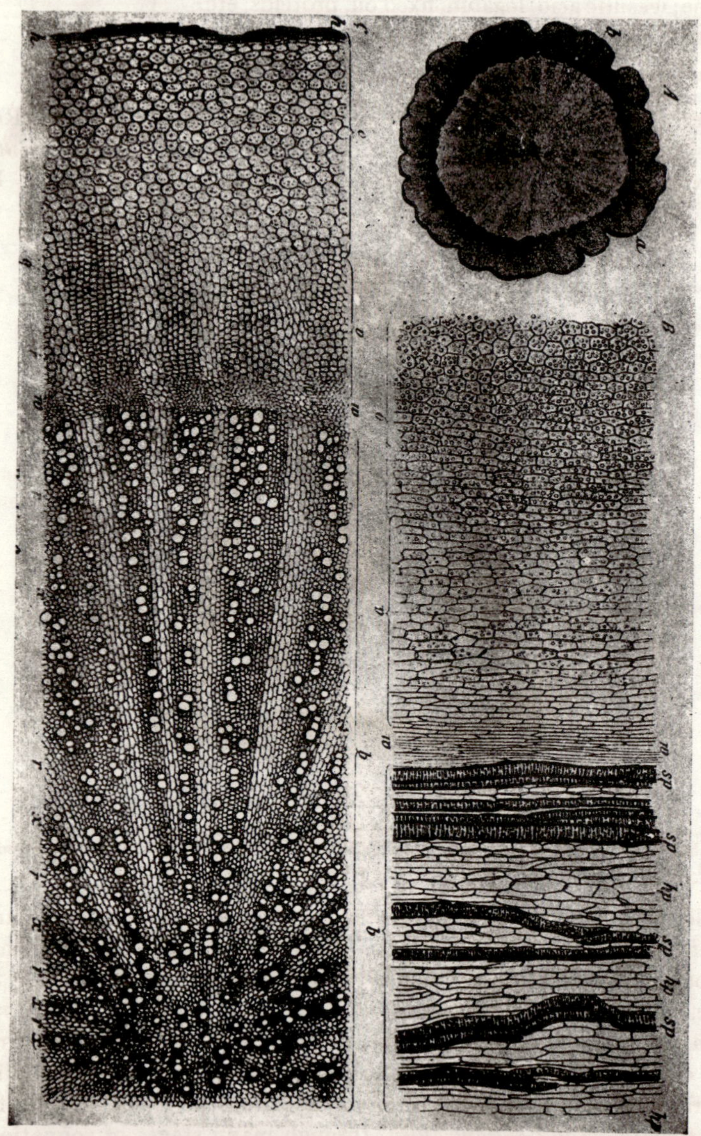

FIG. 203.—*Gentiana lutea.* *A*, Transverse section of root, × 2. *B*, Longitudinal-radial section of root from the center of cortex to within part of the xylem, × 100. *C*, Transverse section of root from cork to center of xylem, × 65. *a*, bark; *b*, xylem; *hp*, wood parenchyma; *o*, cortex; *v*, phloem, *r*, medullary rays; *sp*, tracheæ; *w*, cambium; *x*, xylem patches. (*After Berg.*)

GENTIANA U.S.P. (GENTIAN)

Synonyms.—Bitter Root, Yellow Gentian Root, Felwort; *Ger.* Bitterwurzel, Enzianwurzel; *Fr.* Racine de Gentiane jaune.

Botanical Origin.—*Gentiana lutea* Linné.

Part Used.—The dried rhizome and roots.

Purity Rubric.—Not less than 30 per cent. of water soluble extractive.

Habitat.—Mountainous regions of central and southern Europe.

Plant.—A perennial herb growing to the height of about 1 m. with thick, hollow stem bearing large, opposite, 5 to 7 nerved, ovate leaves and axillary cymes of orange-yellow open-stellate flowers. The fruit is an ovate capsule containing winged seeds.

Production and Commerce.—The rhizomes and roots are dug up in autumn, the thick fleshy parts occasionally longitudinally sliced and the slender rhizomes and roots cut into segments of variable length. The drug is then slowly dried, during which it develops its characteristic odor, internal color and taste. During the drying process the internal color changes from white to yellowish-brown and much of the gentiopicrin disappears, being hydrolyzed by an enzyme into gentiogenin and dextrose.

It is packed in burlap bales and bags for shipment. Most of our commercial supplies are imported from Marseilles, Bordeaux, Paris, Antwerp, Brussels, Hamburg, Trieste and Budapest. The chief cause of inferiority is moldiness.

Description.—In subcylindrical, often branched segments, rarely as entire roots or rhizomes of variable length and up to 38 mm. in diameter; externally light brown, the rhizome vertical and annulate from leaf bases, the roots deeply longitudinally wrinkled and sometimes twisted; fracture short and brittle when dry but tough and flexible when damp; internally yellowish-brown exhibiting a bark up to 2 mm. in thickness and yellowish-brown, a dark brown cambium, a somewhat radiate wood and, in the rhizome, a brownish-yellow pith; odor characteristically aromatic; taste at first sweet, then persistently bitter.

Histology.—Transverse sections of the root show a narrow zone of about 4 to 6 layers of thin-walled cork cells, a cork cambium, a broad zone of cortex with thick walled parenchyma cells, practically devoid of starch, but containing oily globules, a narrow zone of phloem composed of collapsed phloem parenchyma and sieve tubes, a distinct cambium and a broad xylem, the latter composed largely of brown, thin-walled wood parenchyma, scattered through which are tracheæ which are isolated or in small groups. The medullary rays are indistinct.

Powdered Drug.—Dull yellowish-brown. Fragments of reticulate, scalariform and porous tacheæ, fragments of brownish cork tissue, adhering to which are frequently thick-walled cells, numerous collapsed, large parenchyma cells; starch grains few or absent. Stone cells and sclerenchyma fibers are absent.

Constituents.—The bitter crystalline glucoside, gentiopicrin, some of which disappears during the curing of the drug; the glucosides gentiamarin (amorphous) and gentianin (crystalline); gentisin, gentianose, glucose, etc.

Use.—Simple bitter.

Adulterants.—(1) The rhizomes and roots of other European species of the genus *Gentiana*, particularly *G. purpurea*, *G. punctata* and *G. pannonica*. (2) The root of *Frasera caroiinensis* (American Columbo) which has a yellowish color, lacks sieve tubes in xylem, but contains gentiopicrin. (3) The ground drug has been adulterated with ground almond shells.

CENTAURIUM N.F. (CENTAURY)

Synonyms.—Bitter Herb, Herba Centaurii Minoris, Lesser Centaury Tops; *Ger.* Tausendgüldenkraut, *Fr.* Petite centaurée.

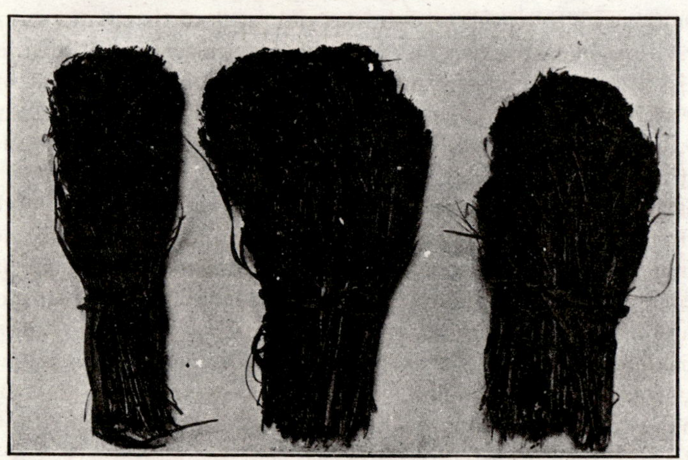

FIG. 204.—Centaurium in original bundles, × ¼. (*Photograph by Stoneback.*)

Botanical Origin.—*Erythræa Centaurium* (Linné) Persoon.

Part Used.—The dried flowering herb.

Purity Rubric.—Not more than 3 per cent. of foreign organic matter.

Habitat.—Europe.

Plant.—An annual herb growing to the height of 5dm., much branched, with opposite, entire, ovate, obovate and lanceolate leaves, terminal compound cymes of rose-colored flowers and capsular fruits.

Production and Commerce.—The entire plant or the aerial portion thereof is collected in the summer after some of the fruits have been partially ripened. The plants are dried in the sun, after which they are tied in bundles. While the plant has been introduced into this country and Canada, practically all of the drug on the American market is imported from Halle and Hamburg, Germany and Trieste.

Description.—Stems glabrous, slender, some 4-angled, others cylindrical and with brown ridges or wings, variable in color, sparsely leafy, having a fibrous fracture and hollow pith; leaves opposite, entire, sessile, mostly 3-nerved, the basal leaves obovate, 2 to 5 cm. in length with obtuse apex and narrowed base, those higher up ovate to linear-lanceolate with acute apex, 2 to 3.5 cm. in length; flowers rose-colored and arranged in terminal compound cymes; calyx tubular, deeply 5-parted, the tube being short and angled; corolla salver-form, the tube being nearly twice the length of the calyx, the lobes of the limb oblong or oval; stamens 5, yellow, perigynous, their anthers twisted when old; pistil bicarpellary with slender style; fruit an ovoid, two-valved capsule containing numerous small seeds; odor characteristic; taste very bitter.

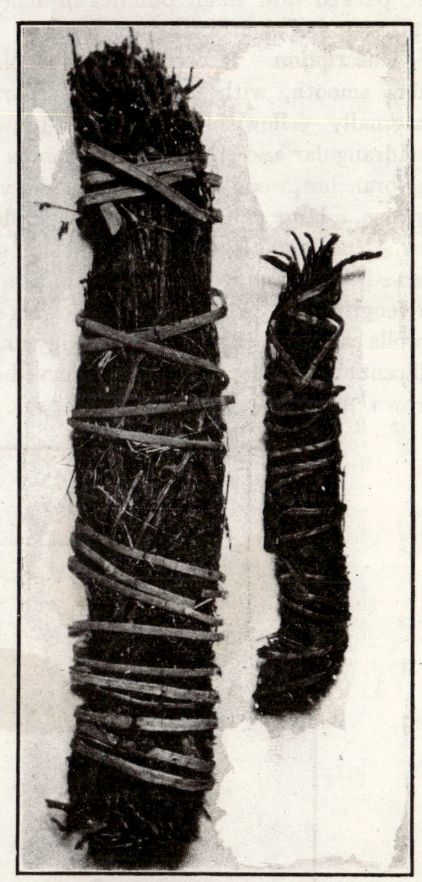

FIG. 205.—Chirata, tied in bundles with bamboo—the condition in which it is imported.

Constituents.—Erytaurin (glucoside), bitter principle, volatile oil, resin, mucilage, etc.

Use.—Simple bitter.

CHIRATA N.F. (CHIRATA)

Synonyms.—Chiretta, Bitter Stick, Chirayta; *Fr.* Chirette; *Ger.* Chiretta, Ostindischer Enzian.

Botanical Origin.—*Swertia Chirayita* (Roxburgh) Lyons.

Part Used.—The dried plant.

Purity Rubric.—Not more than 3 per cent. of foreign organic matter.

Habitat.—Mountainous regions of Northern India.

Plant.—An annual, smooth herb attaining a height of 1 m.

Production and Commerce.— The plants are gathered in the fruiting condition, carefully dried and tied in bundles with bamboo strips. These are packed into small bundles or bales and imported into the United States from Calcutta.

Description.—It occurs as entire plants or as broken pieces thereof; stem smooth, with thin readily separable bark, about 1 m. in length, externally yellowish- or purplish-brown, cylindrical in basal region, quadrangular and slightly winged above, with numerous opposite, ascending branches; wood of stem porous and yellow, enclosing, in the internodal regions, a large yellowish, easily separable pith; root simple, conical with few, slender rootlets; leaves opposite, sessile, entire, ovate-lanceolate, 5-nerved, with rounded base, acuminate apex and entire margin, up to 9 cm. in length and 3 cm. in width; flowers numerous in panicles; calyx and corolla each 4-lobed; stamens 4, perigynous; ovary unilocular with 2 parietal placentæ; style slender with 2 recurved stigmas; fruit an ovoid, yellowish-brown, unilocular, many seeded capsule; odor indistinct; taste very bitter.

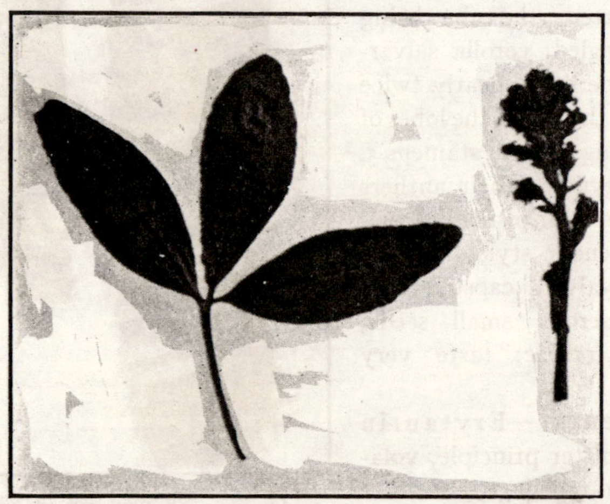

FIG. 206.—*Menyanthes trifoliata.* Leaf and inflorescence. × ⅔1.

Powdered Drug.—Yellowish-brown. Numerous fragments of stem tissues, the sclerenchyma fibers long, lignified and with oblique pits, the tracheæ with spiral or porous markings, the parenchyma of pith large celled, more or less lignified and pitted; fragments of leaf epidermis with cells having straight vertical walls, the lower epidermis alone possessing stomata, which are surrounded by 4 to 5 neighboring cells; pollen grains foot-ball shaped, about 35μ in diameter; resin and tannin cells with yellowish or brown contents.

Constituents.—Chiratin (a bitter glucoside), chiratogenin, ophelic acid, resin, and tannin.

Use.—Simple bitter.

Adulterants.—Entire plants of *Swertia augustifolia* and *Swertia pulchella* both of which are less bitter and possess little or no pith in their square stems.

MENYANTHES (MENYANTHES)

Synonyms.—Buckbean, Bogbean, Marsh Trefoil, Water Shamrock; *Ger.* Bitterklee, Wasserklee; *Fr.* Ményanthe.

Botanical Origin.—*Menyanthes trifoliata* Linné.

Part Used.—The dried leaves.

Habitat.—In shallow water and bogs of Europe and Asia. Naturalized in Canada and Northern United States.

Plant.—A perennial herb with a thick, horizontal rhizome from which arises long petioled, trifoliate leaves, each with 3 obovate leaflets, as well as a long naked scape bearing a raceme of white or slightly reddish flowers. Each flower consists of a 5-cleft calyx, an infundibuliform, 5-cleft corolla, bearded on its upper surface, 5 stamens, a bicarpellary pistil with slender style and 2-lobed stigma. The fruit is a many seeded unilocular capsule.

Production and Commerce.—The leaves are collected from late April to June and dried.

Description.—Leaves usually broken, when entire, trifoliate with broad, flattened and striated petioles up to 16 cm. in length, the base of which when present is sheathed with broad membranous stipules; leaflets sessile or nearly so, each 5 to 8 cm. long, obovate in outline with obtuse or acute apex, entire or coarsely undulate margin and cuneate base, ash-green; odor indistinct; taste strongly bitter.

Constituents.—The glucoside, meliatin; fatty acids, etc.

Use.—Simple bitter.

APOCYNACEÆ (DOG BANE FAMILY)

Herbs, rarely shrubs, not infrequently clambering or climbing in habit (Climbing Dogbane). Stem and branches show bicollateral bundles. Stem, leaves and flowers have latex tubes which ramify through the cortex and mesophyll tissues. Leaves alternate, opposite or verticillate, simple, entire, deciduous or evergreen. Inflorescence cymose. Flowers regular, pentamerous, rarely tetramerous; sepals five, gamosepalous, green, rarely subpetaloid to petaloid; petals five, slightly to deeply gamopetalous, in shape varying from open tubular, stellate, to elongate tubular to elongate funnel-shaped, in color varying from greenish-yellow to white or from yellow to yellow-red to crimson to crimson-purple to nearly purple-blue;

stamens five, epipetalous; pistil usually bicarpellate; ovary two-celled with central placentation; style more or less elongate with a terminal brush of hairs, knobbed or multifid; stigma circular band or circular spur beneath terminal style swelling. Fruit two follicles (*Apocynum*, etc.), a berry,

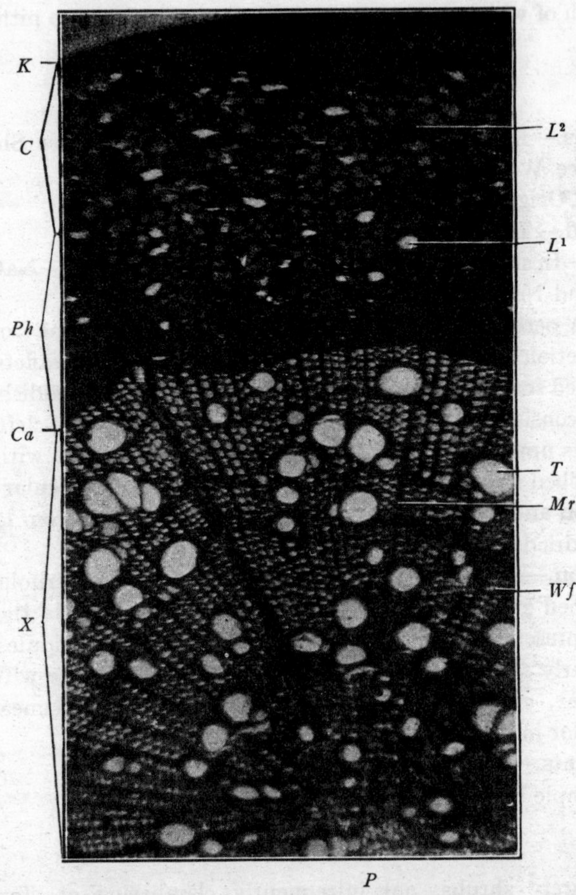

FIG. 207.—Transverse section of *Apocynum cannabinum* rhizome. Cork (*K*); cortex (*C*); phloem (*Ph*); empty latex cell (L^1); latex cell containing latex (L^2); cambium (*Ca*); xylem (*X*); medullary-ray (*Mr*); trachea (*T*); wood fibers (*Wf*); pith (*P*).

drupe, or capsule. Seeds flattened, frequently with a tuft of silky hairs at one end, albuminous.

APOCYNUM N.F. (APOCYNUM)

Synonyms.—Canadian Hemp, Wild Cotton, Rheumatism Weed; *Ger.* Canadische Hanfwurzel; *Fr.* Chanvre du Canada.

Botanical Origin.—*Apocynum cannabinum* Linné.

Part Used.—The dried rhizome and roots.

Limit of Impurities.—5 per cent. of its stems or other foreign organic matter.

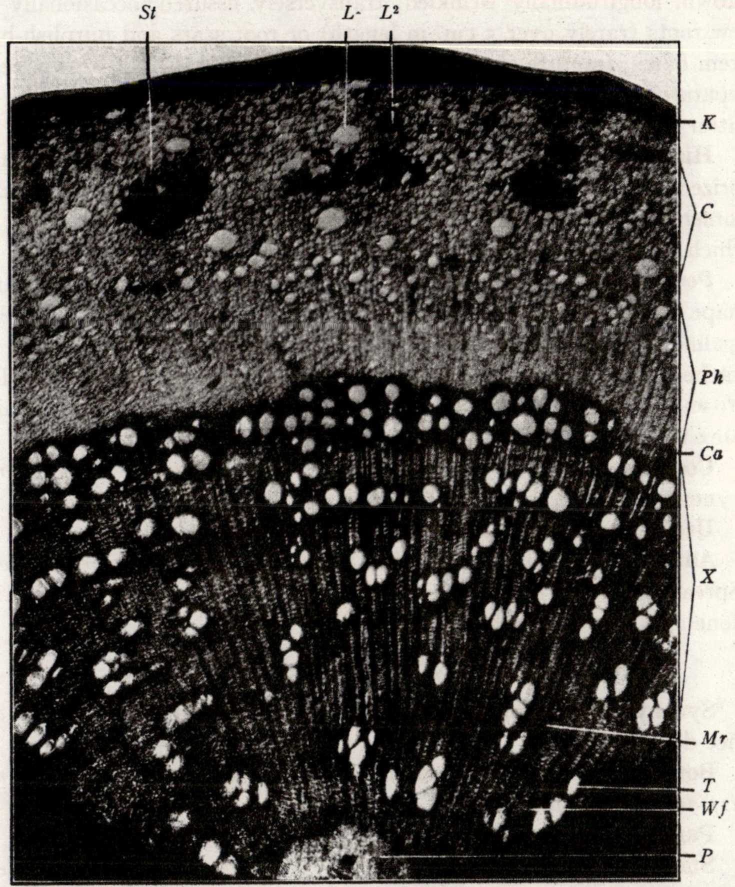

FIG. 208.—Transverse section of *Apocynum androsæmifolium* rhizome. Cork (*K*); cortex (*C*); phloem (*Ph*); group of stone cells (*St*); empty latex cell (*L*[1]); latex cell containing latex (*L*[2]); cambium (*Ca*); xylem (*X*); medullary-ray (*Mr*); trachea (*T*); wood fibers (*Wf*); pith (*P*).

Habitat.—United States and Canada.

Plant.—A smooth perennial herb with nearly erect branches, attaining a height of about 2 m. The leaves are ovate-oblong to lanceolate, pale green, short petioled on the main stem and nearly sessile on the branches. The flowers are small, greenish-white, bell-shaped and arranged in dense cymes. The fruit consists of paired slender follicles.

Description.—The drug occurs as cylindrical, sometimes branched segments of the rhizome and roots up to 10 cm. in length and up to 1.5 cm. in diameter; rhizome horizontal, externally light brown or grayish brown, longitudinally wrinkled, transversely fissured, occasionally with few roots (rarely over 5 cm. in length) or root scars and purplish-brown stem bases; fracture short; internally bark thin and light brown, readily separating from the yellowish and porous wood; odor indistinct; taste bitter and acrid.

Histology.—Transverse sections of both rhizome and root are characterized by exhibiting a porous, radiate wood and a cortex containing numerous scattered latex cells. The rhizome in addition contains pith which also contains latex cells.

Powdered Drug.—Light brown; numerous starch grains of varying shape up to 20μ in diameter, sometimes altered, swollen and with a central hyaline cleft; numerous fragments of lignified wood fibers associated with tracheæ with bordered pores and spiral thickenings; fragments of reddish-brown suberous tissue; fragments of latex and parenchyma containing latex tubes.

Constituents.—The glucosides apocynin, apocynein, apocynamarin (cynotoxin); resin, volatile oil, starch, etc.

Uses.—Cardiac stimulant, and diuretic in dropsy.

Adulterant.—The rhizomes and roots of *Apocynum androsæmifolium* (Spreading Dogbane). These may be readily detected by containing stone cells in cortex and pith (rhizome).

STROPHANTHUS U.S.P. (STROPHANTHUS)

Synonyms.—Strophanthus Seeds; *Ger.* Strophanthussamen; *Fr.* Semence de Strophanthe.

Botanical Origin.—*Strophanthus Kombé* Oliver and *Strophanthus hispidus* De Candolle.

Part Used.—The dried, ripe seed deprived of the awns.

Standard of Assay.—The official tincture, properly diluted and injected into the ventral lymph sac of a frog has a minimum systolic dose (the minimum dose producing in one hour a stoppage of the ventricle of the heart in systole) not greater than 0.00006 cc. of tincture, equivalent to 0.0000005 Gm. of ouabain, for each gramme of body weight of frog.

Habitat.—Africa.

Plants.—Perennial woody climbers, whose scandent stems arise to the summits of tall trees and dangle downward in festoons. The inflorescence is a terminal cyme of cream-colored, purplish-spotted flowers, the corolla of which possesses long tailed and twisted lobes. The fruit is a thick skinned, lance-ovate follicle, occurring in pairs. Each follicle contains numerous closely packed lance-ovoid, hairy seeds with their long awns.

Production and Commerce.—*Strophanthus Kombé* is native to forests of Eastern Africa and yields that commercial variety of seed known as "Green Strophanthus." *Strophanthus hispidus* is native to forests of West Africa and yields the seeds known in commerce as "Brown Strophanthus." The fruits are gathered when ripe, in June and July, by the natives who peel off the epicarp and mesocarp and dry the seeds in the endocarp. The seeds are later deprived of their long awns, generally before being exported to this country. Green Strophanthus seeds are considered the best, since they generally contain the greater percentage of strophanthin. Most of our commercial supply of the drug is imported in bags from East African ports through Hamburg.

Description.—Usually as entire seeds, lance-ovoid to oblong lanceolate, somewhat compressed, with obtuse base and acute to narrowly acuminate apex; from 7 to 22 mm. in length, 4 to 6 mm. in breadth and up to 3 mm. in thickness; externally yellowish-green when recent, light fawn brown with a greenish tinge when kept for a year or more, silky lustrous from a dense covering of appressed hairs (*S. Kombé*); or light to dark-brown, sparingly hairy (*S. hispidus*), bearing on one side a distinct raphe running from the center to the summit; fracture short and soft; the broken surface whitish and oily; odor heavy when the seeds are crushed and moistened; taste strongly bitter.

Histology.—Sections of Green Strophanthus seeds show the following structures, passing from periphery toward the center;

1. *Spermoderm*, consisting of outer epidermis and several layers of more or less collapsed thin-walled cells. Growing out of the epidermis are numerous thin-walled, unicellular, non-glandular hairs which are lignified at their bases. If sections are cut through the raphe, fibrovascular elements are visible.

2. *Endosperm* of from 9 to about 30 rows of somewhat polygonal cells with slightly thickened walls, and containing strophanthin, aleurone grains and globules of fixed oil. When sections are transferred from water to 50 per cent. sulphuric acid, the strophanthin gradually dissolves, imparting a bright green color to the cells containing it. This color gradually changes to blue, violet and red.

3. Two large wavy-convex *cotyledons* in the center, each showing a prominent epidermis enclosing numerous reserve parenchyma cells, each of which contains aleurone grains, oil and occasionally strophanthin. Fibrovascular tissue extends through each cotyledon.

Powdered Drug.—Grayish-brown to brown. Numerous fragments of thin-walled, slightly lignified hairs in *S. Kombé*, fewer in powder of *S. hispidus*, numerous fragments of thin-walled parenchyma of endosperm and cotyledons containing small aleurone grains and fixed oil, some strophanthin; spiral tracheæ; no calcium oxalate.

Constituents.—Up to 3 per cent of the bitter glucoside, strophanthin; (U.S.P.), fixed oil, kombic acid, etc.

Uses.—Cardiac stimulant (of digitalis group) and diuretic.

Adulterants.—(1) *Strophanthus Courmontii* seeds, which are averagely shorter, and contain prismatic crystals of calcium oxalate in the seed coat. (2) Seeds of *Strophanthus Nicholsonii* which are averagely thicker, wooly with long white shaggy hairs. (3) Seeds of *Strophanthus gratus* which are somewhat spindle-shaped, compressed, brown and almost devoid of hairs. These contain the crystalline glucoside, ouabain. (4) Seeds of *Kickxia Africana* which are acuminate at both ends, devoid of hairs, and reddish-brown in color. Sections of these adulterants take on a reddish coloration when mounted in sulphuric acid.

ASPIDOSPERMA (ASPIDOSPERMA)

Synonyms.—Quebracho, White Quebracho, Quebracho Bark; *Fr.* and *Ger.* Quebracho.

Botanical Origin.—*Aspidosperma Quebracho-blanco* Schlectendal.

Part Used.—The dried bark.

Limit of Impurities.—2 per cent. of wood or other foreign matter.

Habitat.—Argentine Republic.

Plant.—A stately ornamental tree with a huge trunk and large crown, found growing in Argentine Republic and adjacent countries.

Production and Commerce.—Most of the commercial supply comes from Argentina. That country also ships large quantities of extract of the bark of *Loxopterygium Lorentzii* (Fam. *Anacardiaceæ*), commonly known as "*Quebracho Colorado*," which is employed in the tanning industry.

Description.—The drug occurs in broken, irregular, flat, chip-like or partially quilled pieces up to 18 cm. in length, 7 cm. in breadth and 3.5 cm. in thickness; cork layer from 3 to 25 mm. in thickness, grayish- or reddish-brown, deeply furrowed, frequently netted with shallow transverse and longitudinal fissures; outer surface, when deprived of cork, light brown or reddish-brown; inner surface pale yellowish- or reddish-brown, finely striated longitudinally, often with adhering wood; fracture short-fibrous with projecting bast fibers; odor indistinct; taste bitter and aromatic.

Histology.—Sections of the bark exhibit the following structural characteristics.

1. Cork, a very broad zone of reddish-brown cells of polygonal outline with somewhat lignified walls.

2. Cork cambium of meristematic cells.

3. Cortex consisting of a matrix of starch- and tannin-containing parenchyma cells, amongst which are scattered large groups of stone cells and sclerenchyma fibers.

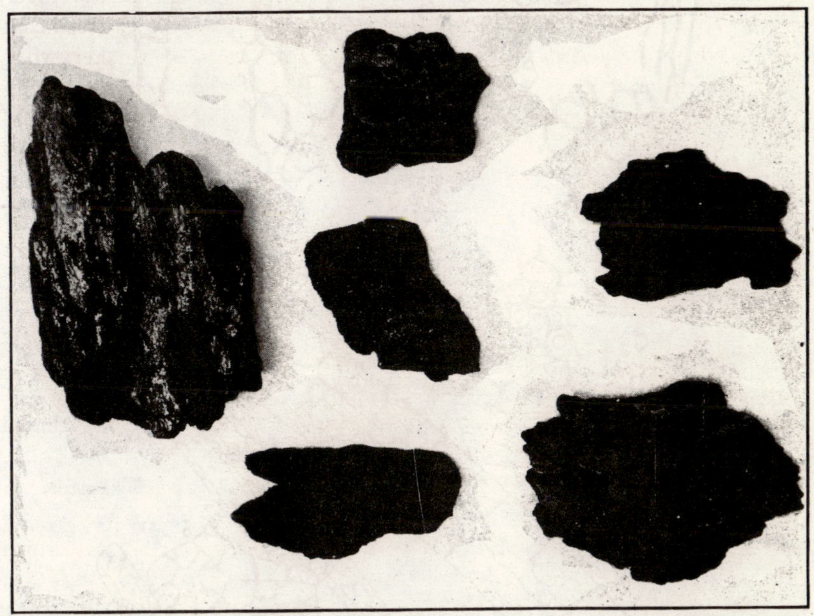

Fig. 209.—Aspidosperma, × 1⅓₀. The 4 pieces to left show outer surface while the 2 pieces to the right show the inner surface of this bark. (*Photo by Stoneback.*)

4. Phloem, a broad zone of sieve tubes, phloem cells and companion cells separated into irregular shaped phloem patches by starch containing medullary rays, the latter being 1 to 5 cells broad. Imbedded in the phloem patches are large groups of stone cells with included bast fibers. The sclerenchyma fiber groups of both cortex and phloem are more or less surrounded by crystal fibers the cells of which contain monoclinic prisms.

The starch grains found in cortex, phloem and medullary rays, when examined in scrapings of the bark mounted in water, are found to be simple or 2- to 4-compound, the separate grains of spheroidal, plano-convex or irregular outline and up to 25μ in diameter.

Constituents.—The alkaloids aspidospermine, quebrachine, aspidospermatine, aspidosamine, quebrachamine, and hypoquebrachine; tannin, a sugar, etc.

Uses.—Aspidosperma is used as a respiratory stimulant in emphysema, chronic bronchitis and pneumonia.

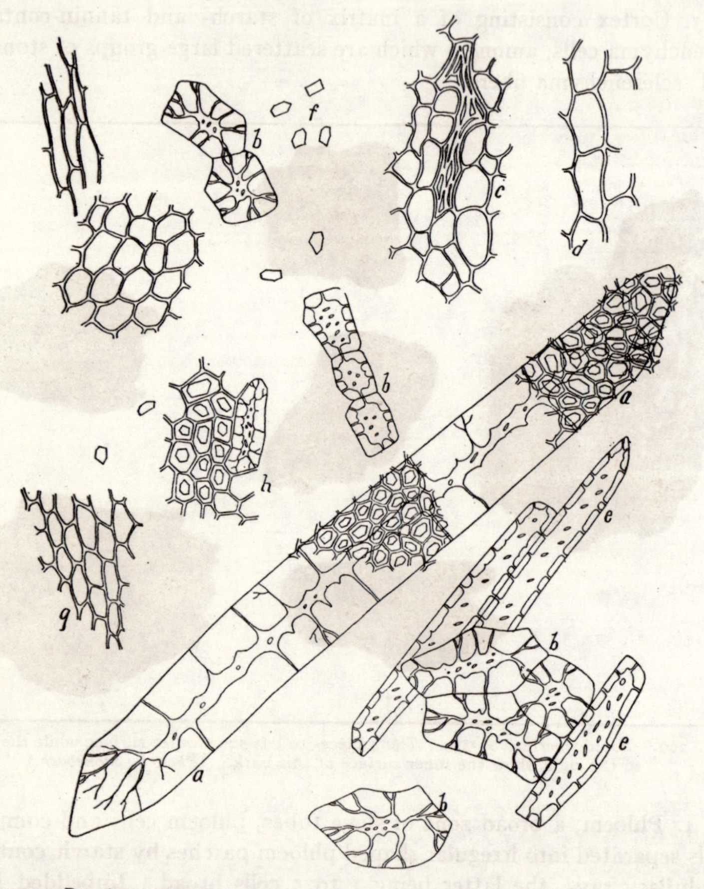

FIG. 210.—Powdered Aspidosperma. (*a*) Very large bast fiber, all lined with crystal bearing cells; (*b*) stone cells; (*c*) parenchyma with phloem group; (*d*) parenchyma; (*e*) sclerenchymatous tracheids; (*f*) prismatic crystals; (*g*) small celled parenchyma; (*h*) crystal bearing parenchyma and stone cell. (*Schneider.*)

ASCLEPIADACEÆ (MILKWEED FAMILY)

Herbs or shrubs containing a milky juice, many species yielding rubber. Leaves entire, more or less fleshy, sometimes verticillate. Inflorescence usually a dichesial or scorpioid cyme. Flowers regular, pentamerous; sepals wooly, small, synsepalous; petals five, rarely four, synpetalous, elongated into awls; the corolla varying in shape from stellate to campanulate and in color from pale green to yellow, to greenish-brown, chocolate, or from white to yellow, to scarlet, to crimson, to purple, to blue; stamens five, epipetalous, fused in relation, forming a cylindrical swollen mass around the central pistil; filaments flattened and furnished with a crown having various appendages; anthers two-celled, each cell containing a pollen mass (pollinium), adhering to the glandular prominences of the stigma; pistil bicarpellate, superior. Fruit typically two dry follicles (*Asclepias*), rarely becoming succulent or bladdery. Seeds numerous, compressed, imbricate, with a comose appendage

ASCLEPIAS N.F. (ASCLEPIAS)

Synonyms.—Pleurisy Root, Orange Milk Weed Root, Butterfly Weed Root. *Ger.* Knollige Schwalbenwurzel; *Fr.* Racine d'asclépiade tubéreuse.

Botanical Origin.—*Asclepias tuberosa* Linné.

Part Used.—The dried root.

Limit of Impurities.—5 per cent. of foreign organic matter.

Habitat.—United States.

Plant.—A perennial herb with erect, hirsute stem frequently branched near the summit. Leaves alternate, sessile or short petiolate, lanceolate or oblong-lanceolate with acute or obtuse apex and rounded or cordate base. Inflorescences terminal cymes of many flowered umbels, the peduncles of which are shorter than the leaves. Calyx small and 5 parted; corolla deeply 5 parted, the segments greenish orange; corona of 5 erect, oblong, orange hoods, each bearing a filiform horn; stamens with filaments united to form a tube and winged anthers; stigma flat, 5 lobed. The fruit consists of finely hairy, acuminate follicles, each containing numerous seeds.

Description.—It occurs as entire fusiform roots up to 25 cm. in length and up to 5 cm. in diameter or as transverse segments or longitudinal slices of variable length; externally orange brown or grayish-brown, longitudinally furrowed, annulate in upper region, the crown with short hollow stem bases and circular or elliptical scars; fracture of thicker parts, tough and uneven, of thinner parts short; inner surface whitish and showing many cavities; odor indistinct; taste starchy, bitter and acrid.

Histology.—Transverse sections of the root show the following microscopic structures, passing from periphery toward the center.

1. *Cork,* of tangentially elongated, slightly lignified cells.
2. *Phellogen,* of meristematic cells.
3. *Secondary Cortex,* a broad cone of parenchyma cells, some of which contain starch grains, others rosette aggregates of calcium oxalate. In the

outer region of this zone occurs a closed band of stone cells, each of which has thick, lignified walls and branching pores.

4. *Phloem,* of narrow phloem patches separated by phloem portions of medullary rays.

5. *Cambium,* of more or less collapsed meristematic cells.

6. *Xylem,* a broad zone of xylem patches composed mostly of starch- and crystal-containing wood parenchyma and wood fibers, scattered amongst which are a few broad porous and scalariform tracheæ. Separating the xylem patches from each other are broad medullary rays, the cells of which are thin-walled and contain starch.

Scrapings of the fractured surface of the drug, when mounted in water, show that the starch grains are simple or 2- to many-compound, the individual grains being spheroidal, polyhedral or plano-convex, with a central hilum and up to 15μ in diameter. The calcium oxalate crystals will be noted in the form of rosettes up to 50μ in diameter.

Constituents.—The glucoside, asclepiadin; resins, volatile oil, tannin, fixed oil, gum, calcium oxalate, etc.

Uses.—Pleurisy root is used as a diaphoretic, diuretic and alterative.

Adulterants.—Rhizomes and roots of other species of *Asclepias* which differ from the official drug by possessing latex cells and contents.

CONDURANGO N.F. (CONDURANGO)

Synonym.—Condurango Bark, Eagle-vine Bark, Condor-vine Bark; *Ger.* Kondurangorinde; *Fr.* Ecorce de condurango.

Botanical Origin.—*Marsdenia Condurango* (Triana) Nichols.

Part Used.—The dried bark.

Purity Rubric.—Not more than 2 per cent. of wood or other foreign organic matter.

Habitat.—Ecuador.

Commercial Source.—Colon and Cristobal.

Plant.—A climbing vine growing in various parts of South America.

Description.—In quills or transversely curved pieces of variable length and from 1 to 6 mm. in thickness; outer surface grayish-brown to dark-brown, nearly smooth and with numerous lenticels, or more or less scaly and rough, the scales rough; inner surface finely longitudinally striated, grayish yellow to light brown; fracture short fibrous and granular; odor slightly aromatic; taste aromatic and bitter.

Histology.—1. Cork of several layers of suberized cells having yellowish brown contents.

2. Secondary cortex of about 10 layers of parenchyma cells, some containing simple or 2- to 4-compound starch grains, others prismatic membrane crystals.

3. Primary cortex, some of the cells of which contain the characteristic starch grains noted above, others rosette aggregates of calcium oxalate. Scattered here and there are large groups of stone cells.

4. Pericycle of tangentially-elongated parenchyma in which are arranged latex cells and groups of thick walled, lignified, bast fibers.

5. Phloem of numerous phloem masses separated by narrow medullary-rays, 1 to 2 cells wide. Each phloem patch contains sieve tubes, companion cells and phloem parenchyma as well as numerous latex cells, isolated bast fibers and occasionally groups of stone cells.

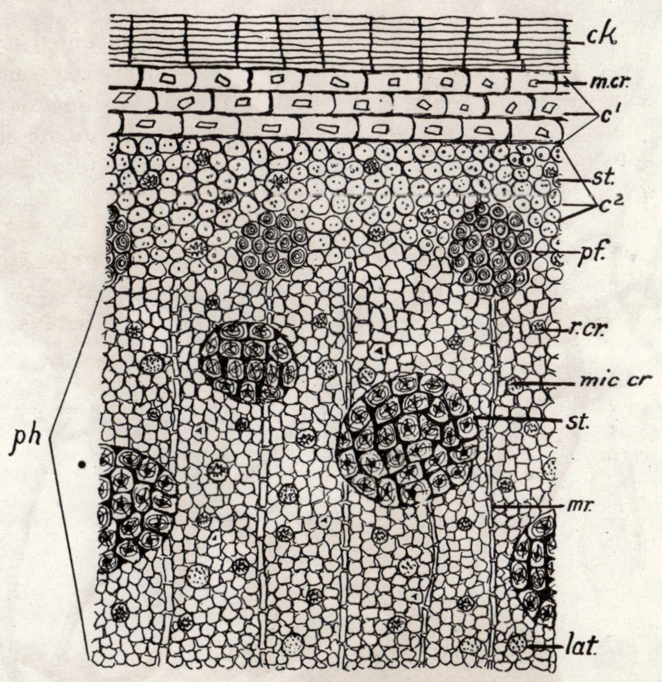

FIG. 211.—Condurango. Transverse section of drug (diagrammatic) showing cork (*ck*); secondary cortex (c^1) containing monoclinic prisms (*m.cr.*); primary cortex (c^2) containing starch (*st*); group of pericyclic fibers (*pf*); phlœm (*ph*); group of stone cells (*st*); rosette aggregate of calcium oxalate (*r. cr*); micro-crystals of calcium oxalate (*mic. cr*); latex cells (*lat*); medullary-ray (*mr*).

Powdered Drug.—Pale yellow-brown; numerous groups of stone cells; parenchyma containing rosette aggregates (up to 40μ in diameter) and prisms (up to 35μ in length) of calcium oxalate as well as starch grains; starch grains simple or 2- to 4-compound, the individual grains from 3 to 20μ in diameter; fragments of long sclerenchyma fibers; fragments of latex tubes; fragments of cork tissue.

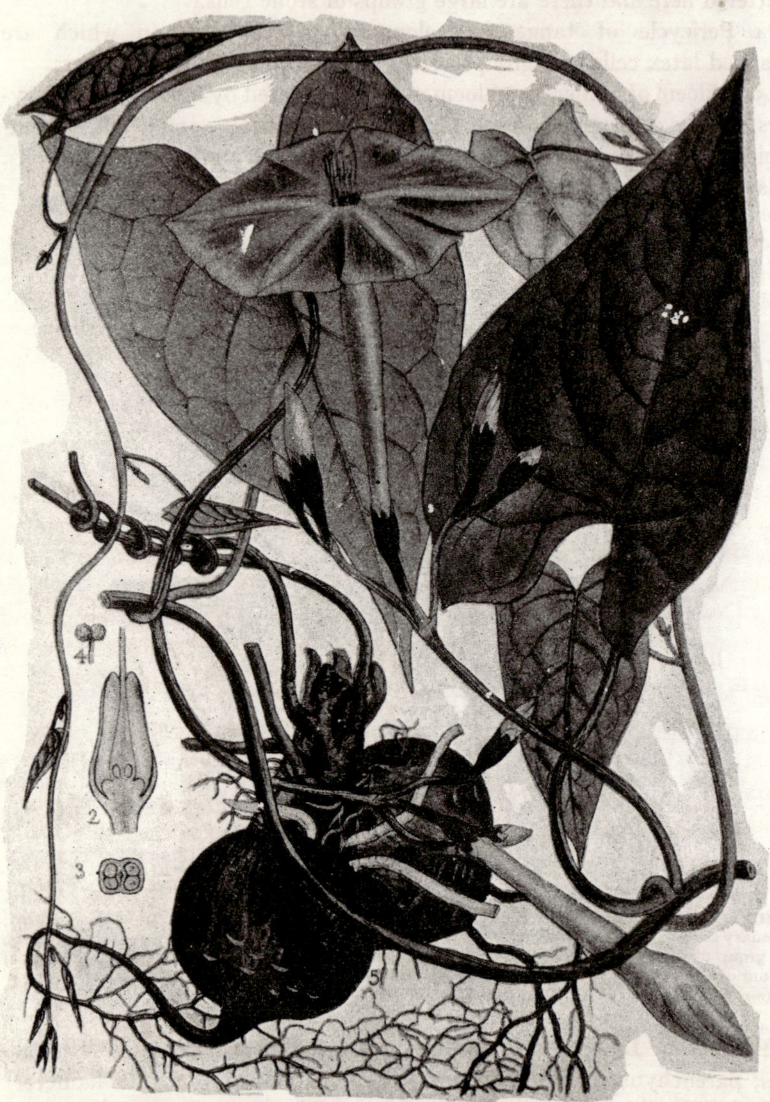

FIG. 212.—*Exogonium Jalapa.* 1. Portion of stem bearing flowers and leaves. 2. Vertical-, and 3. Transverse section of ovary. 4. Stigma. 5. Base of stem and tuberous roots. (*After Bentley and Trimen.*)

Constituents.—Condurangin, resin, fixed oil, tannin, starch, etc.
Use.—Aromatic bitter.

CONVOLVULACEÆ (MORNING GLORY FAMILY)

Frequently herbaceous, more rarely sub-woody to woody, perennial climbing plants with underground parts sometimes swollen into tuberous roots (Jalap, Sweet Potato, Wild Man of the Earth). Stems rarely short, upright or tufted, usually elongate and circumnutating in action. Vascular bundles frequently bicollateral. Leaves alternate, simple, exstipulate, varying from cordate to cordate-sagittal, to broad reniform to reniform, palmately-lobed to palmatifid to palmately-compound (*Ipomœa* shows all these transitions). Stem and leaves frequently contain a dull, viscous, watery to milky-white juice. Inflorescence a scorpioid cyme, becoming reduced in some forms to a solitary flower. Flowers pentamerous; sepals five, green, gamosepalous; corolla varying in shape from rotate to funnel-like with expanded mouth, in color from greenish-yellow to white or through yellowish-pink to scarlet, crimson, purple or blue; stamens five, often with the bases of the filaments expanded; pistil bicarpellate; ovary two celled, superior, often surrounded by a nectar girdle; style filiform with bilobed or bifid stigma. Fruit usually a capsule (*Exogonium*, etc.), dehiscing septifragally, rarely a berry. Seeds scantily albuminous to exalbuminous.

JALAPA U.S.P. (JALAP)

Synonyms.—Radix Jalapæ, Jalap Root, Vera Cruz Jalap; *Ger.* Jalapenwurzel, Jalapenknollen; *Fr.* Jalap tubéreux.

Botanical Origin.—*Exogonium Jalapa* (Nuttall et Coxe) Baillon.

Part Used.—Dried tuberous root.

Standard of Assay.—Not less than 7 per cent. of the total resins of Jalap.

Habitat.—In moist, rich woodlands of Eastern Mexico.

Plant.—A perennial twining herb whose underground portion consists of a tuberous root system. Its aerial portion consists of many slender, furrowed, purplish, twining stems which may attain a length of 5 or 6 m. These bear alternate, long petioled, exstipulate, cordate, entire leaves and 3-flowered cymes of purple, salver shaped flowers. The fruit is a septifragally dehiscent capsule.

Production and Commerce.—The plant grows wild in rich woodland soil at an elevation of from 5,000 to 8,000 feet in Eastern Mexico. It is extensively cultivated in the vicinity of Jalapa, Mexico, in the Neilgherry mountains of India, and grown to some extent in Jamaica. The roots are gathered at various seasons of the year. The best time for gathering is the fall. They are washed, placed in nets and dried over fires which gives them a smoky odor. The largest roots are longitudinally sliced before drying. The drug is placed in bags for shipment. During recent years the drug has been imported wholly from Vera Cruz and Mexico City, Mexico.

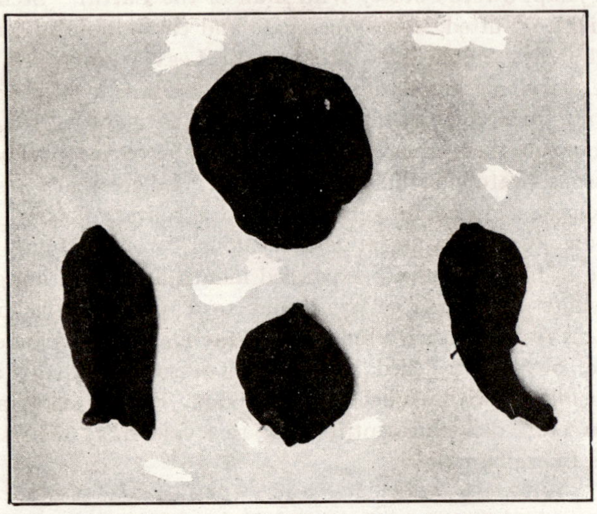

FIG. 213.—Jalap, × ⅓. (*Photograph by Stoneback.*)

Description.—The tuberous roots occur either in the entire or cut condition. The entire roots are either fusiform, globular, ovoid, or pyriform (pear-shaped), the upper end being somewhat rounded, the lower slightly tapering; from 4 to 15 cm. in height and from 1 to 10 cm. in diameter; externally dark brown, longitudinally wrinkled or furrowed and with numerous lenticels; hard, compact and resinous; when broken, internally dark brown, horny or waxy, exhibiting a distinct brown primary cambium, and mottled wood containing numerous bundles and brown resin cells; odor distinct, smoky; taste sweet and acrid.

Histology.—Transverse sections, cleared in potassium hydroxide solution, exhibit the following structural peculiarities, passing from periphery toward the center.

1. Cork, a zone of numerous layers of cork cells with brownish contents.

2. Cork cambium.

3. Cortex, a narrow zone of more or less tangentially elongated starch containing cells, scattered amongst which will be noted yellowish-brown resin cells.

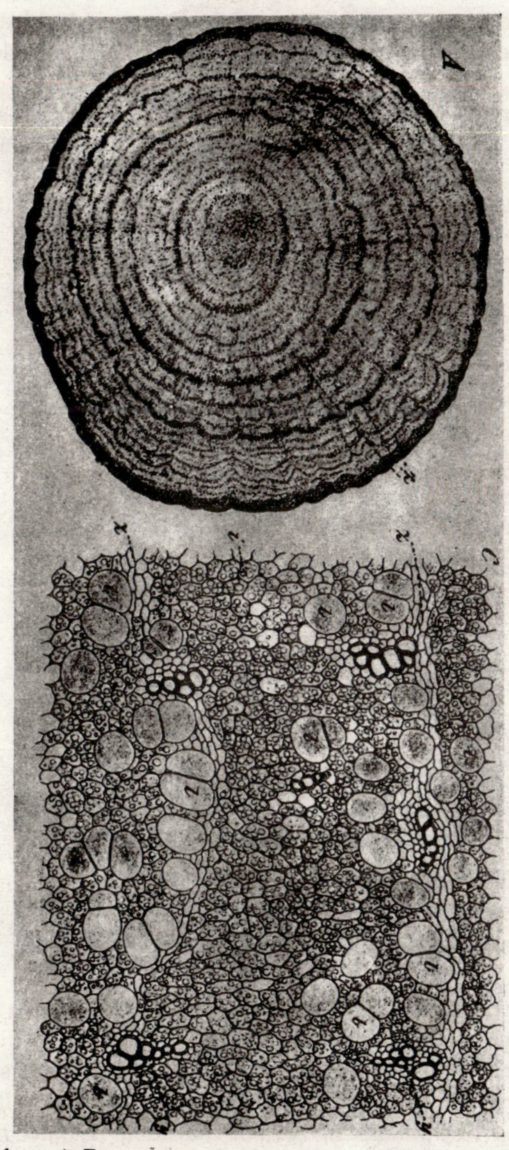

FIG. 214.—Jalap. *A*, Transverse section (nat. size). *C*, Segment of A through 2 secondary cambium zones, × 65. *z*, secondary cambia; *i*, starch parenchyma; *l*, resin cells; *y*, fibrovascular bundles. (*After Berg.*)

4. Primary cambium, on the outer surface of which will be noted small groups of sieve elements and on the inner surface interrupted groups of tracheæ.

5. A broad central zone of starch parenchyma imbedded in which are interrupted concentric zones of bicollateral bundles developed from secondary cambia and numerous resin cells with yellowish-brown contents.

Powdered Drug.—Light brown; starch grains numerous, single or 2 to 3 compound, often swollen, ellipsoidal or ovoid with concentric or

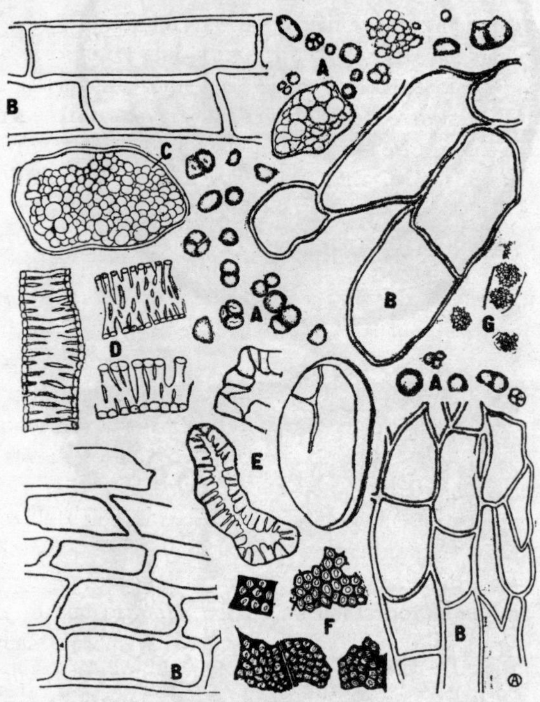

Fig. 215.—Powdered Jalap, × 183. A, Starch grains. B, Parenchyma cells. C, Paren chyma cells filled with starch. D, Tracheæ. E, Stone cells. F, Fragments, of tracheæ with bordered pores. G, Rosette aggregates of calcium oxalate. (*After Sayre.*)

excentral lamellae and radiating or crescentic clefts, from 3 to 35μ in diameter; calcium oxalate in rosette aggregates from 10 to 36μ in diameter; tracheæ short, broad with elliptical shaped bordered pores; fragments of brown resinous masses; few sclerenchyma fibers with thick walls.

Constituents.—The resins convolvulin (insoluble in ether but soluble in alkaline solutions) and jalapin (soluble in ether and alkalies); volatile oil, gum, starch, calcium oxalate and sugar.

Uses.—Hydragogue cathartic and source of Resina Jalapæ U.S.P.

Adulterants.—The root of *Piptostegia Pisonis* Mart. (Fam. *Convolvulaceæ*) known as **"Piptostegia Root"** and **"Brazilian Jalap"** has for the past 5 years appeared in the American and European markets. It occurs in transverse, circular or oval sections, varying from about 2.5 to 8 cm. in diameter and from about 0.3 to 0.6 or 0.8 cm. in thickness, its cut surface pale yellowish-brown, marked with several concentric rings and many resin dots. It somewhat resembles Poke, Mexican Scammony and Bryonia roots. Farwell (Jour. A. Ph. A., Vol. vii, No. 10, p. 854) describes its histology as follows:

"The cambium forms complete circles and together with the phloem are, in the commercial drug, noticeable as dark concentric circles shrunken a little below the level of the surrounding tissues. In the sections observed the tissues were all of secondary growth; that is, spiral or annular tracheæ usually associated with primary meristem could not be detected. The center of the root in the smaller sections is nearly solid xylem, there being four narrow strands of secondary cortex, thus making the structure of the root a tetrarch. The larger sections are very similar but may have less xylem and more cortex. The cambium of the collateral bundles soon ceases its activity and the cortex gives rise to another meristematic region beyond the phloem and this operation is continued repeatedly. producing in this unusual way its growth in thickness. The xylem forms a very small bundle of few vessels and these are rather widely separated forming an interrupted circle with wide spaces between the bundles. The medullary ray is usually one cell, sometimes two cells, in width. The vessels of the bundle are reticulated tracheæ, often 0.13 mm. in diameter with walls 0.008 mm. thick, and these constitute the greater portion of the strengthening tissue of the root; tracheids and wood fibers are frequent in the central circles but absent or only occasional in the outer ones. Rosette crystals of calcium oxalate are frequent just internal to the cork, scattered through the cortex, and form crystal fibers close to the xylem. Starch is present only in a very small amount; the grains are simple and range from 0.002 mm. to 0.024 mm. in diameter. Bast fibers are absent or at least were not detected; but most of the bast parenchyma and some of the cells of the medullary rays and secondary cortex, while retaining comparatively thin walls, are stained brown with chloro-iodide-of-zinc, indicating suberization or cutinization. The cells of the cortex are more or less polygonal and average about 0.044 mm. in diameter, the walls are thin and the air space between the cells is very small. The cork layer is about 0.123 mm. thick and is composed of a series of thin-walled, more or less tubular cells (0.008 mm. by 0.048 mm.), only the outermost series having thickened cell walls. The tracheids average about 0.44 mm. in length, 0.026 mm. wide, and have a wall about 0.003 mm. in thickness. The wood fibers oblique pores and range from 0.62–0.78 mm. in length, 0.013–0.020 mm. wide, and have a lumen varying from 1/5–3/4 the width of the fiber." This drug contains about 20 per cent. of resin which is mostly insoluble in ether.

Male or Orizaba Jalap (Mexican Scammony) consists of the tuberous roots of *Ipomoea Orizabensis* Ledenois, a plant growing in Mexico. This

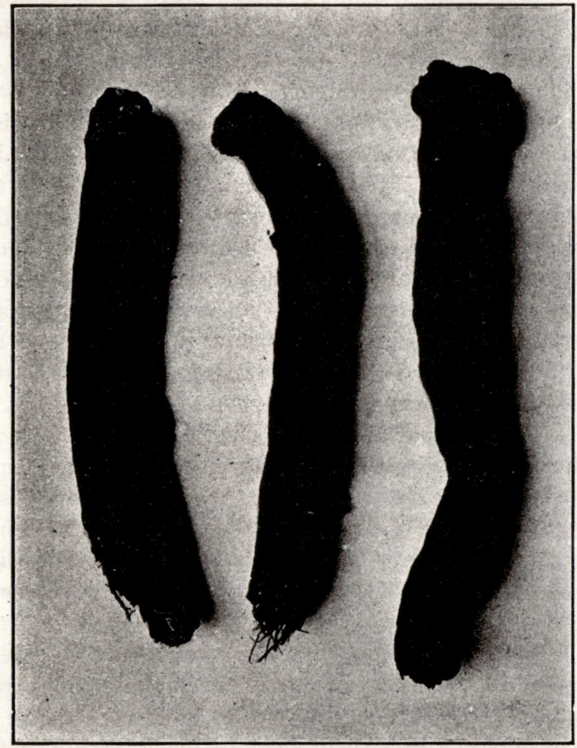

FIG. 216.—Levant Scammony, × ½. (*Photograph by W. J. Stoneback.*)

substitute for Jalap has also been used to adulterate Levant Scammony and in numerous instances has been substituted for the latter. When found as an adulterant for Jalap it occurs as entire fusiform roots or long segments of these. These are light to dark brown externally, deeply wrinkled with a tough fibrous fracture exposing a light brown inner surface which shows numerous alternating rings of fibrovascular tissue and parenchyma containing latex tubes with brownish contents. It contains averagely from 12 to 18 per cent. of resin of which about 65 per cent. is ether-soluble.

Resina Drastica from an unidentified Mexican plant probably belonging to the *Convolvulaceæ* somewhat resembles Brazilian Jalap and Orizaba Jalap. It differs from both of these by having no rosette crystals and in yielding a lemon yellow colored resin.

IPOMŒA U.S.P. (IPOMEA)

Synonyms.—Orizaba Jalap Root, Mexican Scammony Root, Male Jalap Root.

Botanical Origin.—*Ipomœa orizabensis* Ledenois.

Part Used.—The dried root.

Purity Rubric.—Not less than 15 per cent. of the total resins of Ipomœa and not more than 3 per cent. of acid-insoluble ash.

Habitat.—Mexico.

Plant.—A climbing perennial vine whose underground portion consists of a large fusiform, somewhat branching, yellowish root which when freshly gathered is milky-white internally. Its aerial portion consists of cylindrical, slightly villous stems bearing large, petiolate, cordate and acuminate leaves and reddish-purple, bell-shaped flowers. The fruit is a capsule.

Production and Commerce.—The root is gathered in the vicinity of Orizaba in the Mexican Andes, cut transversely into disks and dried in the sun. It is packed in burlap bags and exported from Mexico City to the United States.

Description.—It occurs in more or less circular transverse slices from 2 to 12 cm. in diameter and from 1 to 5.5 cm. in thickness; externally brown and deeply wrinkled; fracture tough and fibrous; the cut surface light brown and showing concentric rings of bundles from which coarse fibers protrude; odor distinct, somewhat aromatic; taste slightly sweet becoming acrid.

Histology.—Transverse sections of the macerated drug exhibit the following microscopic structures:

1. *Cork* of several rows of thin-walled, brownish, tabular cells.
2. *Cork cambium* of collapsed meristematic cells.
3. *Cortex* of numerous layers of cortical parenchyma and divisible into an outer zone of a few layers of thin-walled, colorless cells and an inner broad zone of thick-walled, more or less tangentially elongated cells. Some of these cells contain starch, others rosette aggregates or rhombohedral crystals of CaO, while still others contain a brown resinous latex.
4. *Collateral fibro-vascular bundles* arranged in concentric circles alternating with layers of parenchyma containing latex cells with brown resinous content.

5. *Medullary-rays* separating the bundles and composed of cells containing either starch, calcium oxalate or latex.

Powdered Drug.—Grayish-brown; numerous single or 2- to 4-compound starch grains, the individual grains with a central cleft hilum and up to 35µ in diameter; numerous rosette aggregates and fewer rhombohedra of $Ca\overline{O}$; numerous fragments of yellowish-brown latex cells or their contents; fragments of tracheæ having bordered pores and of strongly-lignified wood fibers.

Constituents.—From 6 to 22 per cent. of a glucosidal resin containing the glucoside and methylpentoside of jalapinolic acid and its methyl ester; also fat, β-methylæsculetin, dihydroxycinnamic acid, phytosterol, starch and calcium oxalate.

Use.—Hydragogue cathartic and source of Resina Ipomœæ U.S.P.

HYDROPHYLLACEÆ (WATER LEAF FAMILY)

Annual, herbaceous, rarely perennial woody plants whose stems, branches, leaves and sepals are often viscous and glandular hairy. Leaves alternate, exstipulate, from simple linear to pinnatipartite to pinnate, usually possessing unicellular non-glandular and glandular hairs with multicellular heads. Inflorescence rarely expanded, usually scorpioid cymes. Flowers small to large, funnel-form in *Eriodictyon californicum;* sepals five, green; petals five, regular; corolla varying from small stellate with slightly fused petals to large rotate, campanulate or tubular, in color varying from greenish-white or yellow to rarely white; often pink, purple or blue; stamens five, rarely with alternate staminodes; pistil bicarpellate. Fruit a two-celled capsule dehiscing usually septicidally.

ERIODICTYON U.S.P. (ERIODICTYON)

Synonyms.—Yerba Santa, Consumptives Weed, Gum Bush, Mountain Balm, Bear's Weed; *Fr.* Feuilles d'Eriodictyon; *Ger.* Eriodictyon.

Botanical Origin.—*Eriodictyon californicum* (Hooker and Arnott) Greene.

Part Used.—The dried leaf.

Purity Rubric.—Not more than 5 per cent. of its stems or more than 2 per cent. of other foreign organic matter.

Habitat.—In hilly and rocky regions of California and Mexico.

Plant.—An evergreen shrub with alternate oblong-lanceolate leaves, infundibuliform, violet or white colored flowers and capsular fruits.

Collection.—Yerba Santa is collected for the market in Lake county and also near Los Angeles, California.

Description.—The drug occurs as fragments of leaves mixed with stem segments and entire leaves; when entire, leaves lanceolate, short petiolate coriaceous, brittle, with acute apex, tapering base, irregular serrate or crenate-dentate margin, the upper surface yellowish-brown, coated with resin, the under surface grayish-white or grayish-green conspicuously

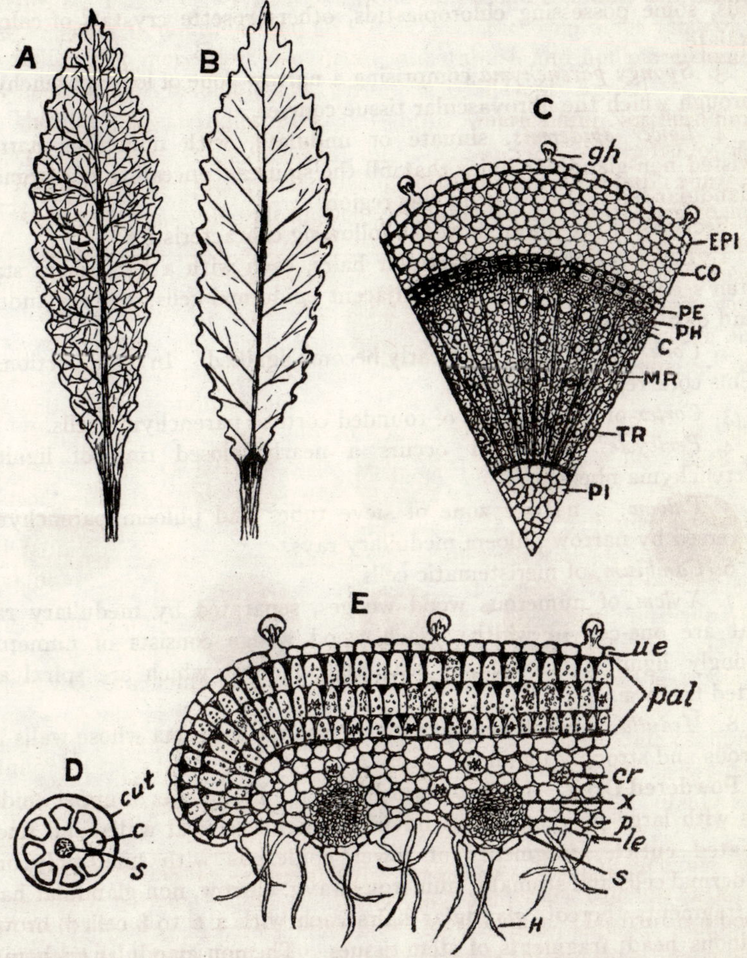

FIG. 217.—Eriodictyon. *A*, Lower surface of leaf. (*B*) Upper surface of leaf. (*C*) Transverse section of stem. Epidermis (*EPI*); glandular hair (*gh*); cortex (*CO*); pericyclic fibers (*PE*); phloem (*PH*); cambium (*C*); medullary-ray (*MR*); trachea (*TR*) of xylem; pith (*PI*). (*D*) Glandular hair in vertical view showing cuticle (*c*); stalk (*s*) and cells of head (*c*). (*E*) Transverse section through portion of leaf blade. Upper epidermis (*ue*); palisade parenchyma (*pal*); rosette crystals of calcium oxalate (*cr*); xylem (*x*) and phloem (*p*) of fibrovascular bundle; lower epidermis (*le*); stoma (*s*); unicellular curved hairs (*H*).

pinnate-reticulate; tomentose between the reticulations; odor balsamic; taste balsamic and bitter.

Histology.—Transverse sections of the **lamina** show the following structural peculiarities:

1. *Upper epidermis* of large sized, clear epidermal cells and numerous glandular hairs with short one celled stalks and 6- to 8-celled heads.

2. *Palisade parenchyma* consisting of 2 to 6 rows of narrow palisade cells, some possessing chloroplastids, others rosette crystals of calcium oxalate.

3. *Spongy parenchyma* comprising a narrow zone of loose parenchyma through which the fibrovascular tissue courses.

4. *Lower epidermis*, sinuate or undulate, with numerous narrow, twisted non-glandular hairs that fill the sinuses, concealing the stomata. Glandular hairs also occur in this region.

Sections of the **stem** show the following characteristics:

1. *Epidermis* bearing glandular hairs, each with a very short stalk, often seen wedged in between adjacent epidermal cells, and a glandular head of 6 to 8 cells.

2. *Cork*, the cells of which early become lignified. In older portions of stems cork replaces epidermis.

3. *Cortex* of several rows of rounded cortical parenchyma cells.

4. *Pericycle*, in which occurs a nearly closed ring of lignified sclerenchyma fibers.

5. *Phloem*, a narrow zone of sieve tubes and phloem parenchyma, traversed by narrow phloem medullary rays.

6. *Cambium*, of meristematic cells.

7. *Xylem* of numerous wood wedges, separated by medullary rays that are one-cell in width. Each wood wedge consists of numerous strongly lignified wood fibers scattered amongst which are spiral and pitted tracheæ.

8. *Medulla*, a broad central zone of pith parenchyma whose walls are porous and strongly lignified.

Powdered Drug.—Light brownish-green. Fragments of upper epidermis with large polygonal cells having straight vertical walls and linear striated cuticle, fragments of lower epidermis with small polygonal epidermal cells and stomata; numerous wavy, narrow, non-glandular hairs or fragments thereof; glandular hairs each with a 6 to 8 celled, brown, resinous head; fragments of stem tissues. The non-glandular trichomes, when entire, are up to 250μ in length.

Constituents.—Resin, volatile oil, eriodictyonon, tannin, gum, fixed oil, xanthoeriodictyol, sugar, etc.

Use.—Expectorant.

Adulterant.—Leaves of *Eriodictyon tomentosum* which has oval, obtuse and larger leaves of lighter color and shorter villous hairs.

VERBENACEÆ (VERVAIN FAMILY)

Herbs (*Verbena*), shrubs (*Clerodendron*), rarely trees (some *Premna spp.*, *Tectona grandis* or Teak-wood) whose stems and branches are usually quadrangular and rarely scented. Leaves generally opposite, exstipulate, simple or compound. Inflorescence a terminal panicle of spikes (*Verbena hastata*), a cyme (*Callicarpa*) or head (*Lippia lanceolata*). Flowers white, pink or blue (*Verbena hastata*) irregular, more or less 2-lipped; calyx gamosepalous, tubular; corolla gamopetalous, hypogynous, tubular, with a 4- to 5-fid limb; stamens generally 4, didynamous and inserted on the corolla tube or throat; pistil of 2 to 4 carpels, with a superior ovary, a terminal style and undivided stigma. Fruit a drupe or 2- to 4-celled berry, usually splitting into as many nutlets. Seeds exalbuminous.

VERBENA (VERBENA)

Synonyms.—Blue Vervain, Wild Hyssop; *Ger.* Eisenkraut; *Fr.* Verveine.

Botanical Origin.—*Verbena hastata* Linné.

Part Used.—The dried aerial portion.

Habitat.—In moist fields and meadows of eastern and central United States.

Plant.—A rough puberulent herb with erect, quadrangular, puberulent stem, branched above. Leaves opposite, petioled, lanceolate or oblong-lanceolate, acute or acuminate at apex, base tapering, margin serrate, some times pinnatifid, the lower leaves occasionally and hastately 3-lobed at base. Inflorescence a terminal panicle of densely flowered spikes of usually blue (occasionally white or pink) flowers.

Production and Commerce.—The plants are cut down during flowering and dried in the sun. The commercial supply is obtained from wild plants.

Description.—In broken or cut pieces; stem 4-sided, rough, pubescent; leaves opposite, petioles 12 to 25 mm. long, blades up to 12 cm. in length, lanceolate, acute or acuminate, shortly and sharply serrate, or the lower hastately 3-lobed, deep green above, paler beneath, prominently veined, inflorescence a panicle of dense interrupted spikes, each spike being cylindraceous, each flower subtended by a lanceolate acute bract; calyx tubular, 5 lobed; corolla small blue, white or pink, salverform, hairy externally, 5 lobed; fruit 4 nutlets; odor heavy on moistening; taste bitter and unpleasant.

Constituents.—A bitter principle, tannin, etc.

Uses.—Verbena is employed in the form of a hot infusion as a diaphoretic, tonic and expectorant.

TONGA N.F. (TONGA)

Botanical Origin.—*Premna arborea* (Forster filius) Farwell (Fam. *Verbenaceæ*) and *Epipremnum pinnatum* (Linné) Engler (Fam. *Araceæ*).

Parts Used.—The bark of *Premna arborea* and the root of *Epipremnum pinnatum* in equal parts.

Purity Rubric.—Not more than 5 per cent. of foreign organic matter.

Plants.—*Premna arborea* is a tree with opposite leaves, cymose flowers and drupaceous fruits.

Epipremnum pinnatum is a climbing tropical aroid with fibrous rope-like roots, spadicious flowers and berry fruits.

Habitat.—Fiji Islands.

Description.—The bark occurs in small chips or quills of varying length and up to 3 mm. in thickness; outer surface brownish and striated with irregular, sometimes pale yellow longitudinal ridges; fracture short and hard. The root occurs in cylindrical pieces about 6 cm. in length and 3 cm. in diameter; outer surface brownish with cork often partly exfoliated, upon bending the interior separates into numerous tough fibers; odor and taste slight.

Constituents.—The volatile alkaloid, tongine, volatile oil, etc.

Uses.—Tonga is used either in the form of a fluidextract or in an elixir combined with sodium salicylate, cimicifuga, colchicine and pilocarpine nitrate in the treatment of neuralgia and rheumatism.

LABIATÆ (MINT FAMILY)

Herbs producing creeping runners that spread out and root at the nodes. Stems quadrangular, rarely cylindrical in outline. Leaves opposite, decussate, mainly petiolate; leaf margin nearly always serrate, dentate or crenate. Stems and leaves further characterized by the presence of glandular hairs containing aromatic volatile oil. These hairs consist of a short one-celled stalk and a head (gland) of six or eight cells. Inflorescence a raceme or spike of verticillasters (double dichesial cymes) or, as in the Ground Ivy, a reduced verticillaster. Flowers typically pentamerous, rarely tetramerous; sepals five, synsepalous, ribbed and forming a tubular, regular or irregular bilabiate (Scullcap, etc.) calyx whose upper lip is bifid and lower trifid; corolla of five to four gamopetalous petals, hypogynous, frequently two-lipped, the upper lip bifid, the lower trifid; stamens four, didynamous, rarely one pair alone fertile and the other pair reduced, in some cases almost or quite to disappearing point (*Salvia* and *Monarda*); pistil bicarpellate, embryologically two-celled with two ovules in each cavity, becoming, at time of flowering, four-celled with one ovule in each cavity. Style embryologically terminal, but, upon opening of flower, deeply gynobasic, elongate, slender, with two stigmatic surfaces. Fruit consisting of four nutlets enclosing as many exalbuminous seeds.

THYMUS N.F. (THYME)

Synonyms.—Common Thyme; Garden Thyme, Mother of Thyme; *Fr.* Thym; *Ger.* Thymian.

Botanical Origin.—*Thymus vulgaris* Linné.

Part Used.—The dried leaves and flowering tops.

Purity Rubric.—Not more than 3 per cent. of stems over 1 mm. in diameter or other foreign organic matter, and not more than 4 per cent. of acid-insoluble ash.

Habitat.—Southern Europe.

Plant.—A low aromatic shrub, 20 to 30 cm. in height with ascending, quadrangular, grayish-brown to purplish-brown branches bearing oblong-lanceolate to ovate-lanceolate grayish-green leaves that are pubescent beneath. The flowers are pale purple in color and appear in verticillasters and terminal dense cymes. The fruit consists of 4 ovoid nutlets.

Production and Commerce.—Thyme, while native to Spain, France and Italy, has been extensively cultivated in Germany and various other countries both for seasoning and for its volatile oil. It is propagated readily from seeds sown in drills in the spring and from cuttings rooted in sand under glass and later transplanted to mellow upland soil. The crude drug is obtained by cutting off the flowering tops when in full bloom and carefully drying in the shade. The entire plants are collected for the production of volatile oil, when they are in full bloom, and distilled by steam without drying. The commercial supplies of the crude drug are largely obtained from France and arrive in burlap bags and bales.

Description.—The drug occurs as segments of the flowering tops, leaves and flowers. Stems mostly 4-angled, grayish-brown or purplish, simple or opposite-branched, pubescent, of variable length and usually 0.5 to 1 mm. in diameter, occasionally with attached opposite leaves; leaves linear, linear-lanceolate or ovate-oblong, up to 8 or 10 mm. in length and up to 2 mm. in breadth, lamina apex acute, base obtuse, tapering into a petiole from 0.5 to 2 mm. in length; upper surface grayish green, short hairy, lower surface, grayish, pubescent and glandular punctate margin revolute, flowers polyganous in axillary or terminal custers; calyx tubular-bilabiate, about 4 mm. in length, pubescent, 9 to 13 nerved, upper lip 3-toothed, lower lip with 2 hairy attenuate divisions; corolla about twice as long as the calyx, purplish, bilabiate, upper lip emarginate, lower spreading and 3-lobed; stamens 4, didynamous; ovary 4-parted; stigma bifid; nutlets spheroidal, finely tuberculate; odor aromatic; taste aromatic and warming.

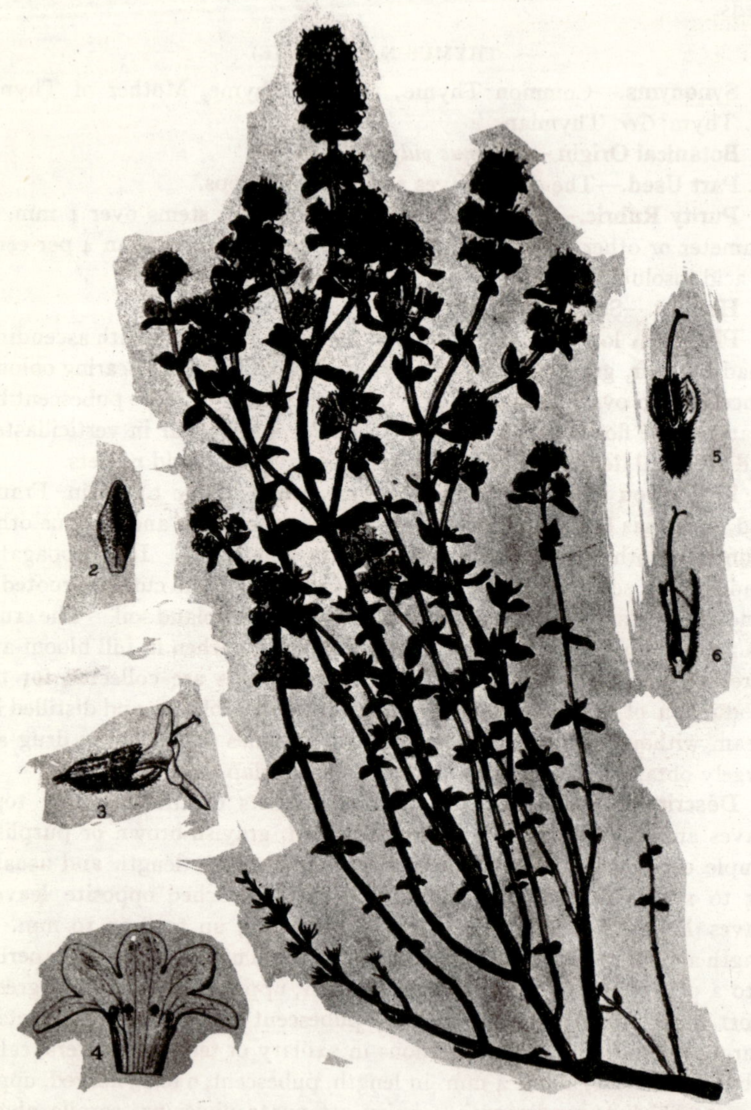

FIG. 218.—*Thymus vulgaris*. 1. Branch with numerous leaf and flower bearing twigs. 2. Leaf. 3. Pistillate flower. 4. Corolla laid open. 5. Calyx and style. 6. Section of calyx showing pistil within. (*After Bentley and Trimen.*)

Constituents.—Volatile oil (Oleum Thymi N.F.), about 2.5 per cent., containing thymol, thymene, cymene and l-pinene; tannin, etc. Thymol U.S.P. is also found in the volatile oils of Ajowan fruit (*Carum copticum*)

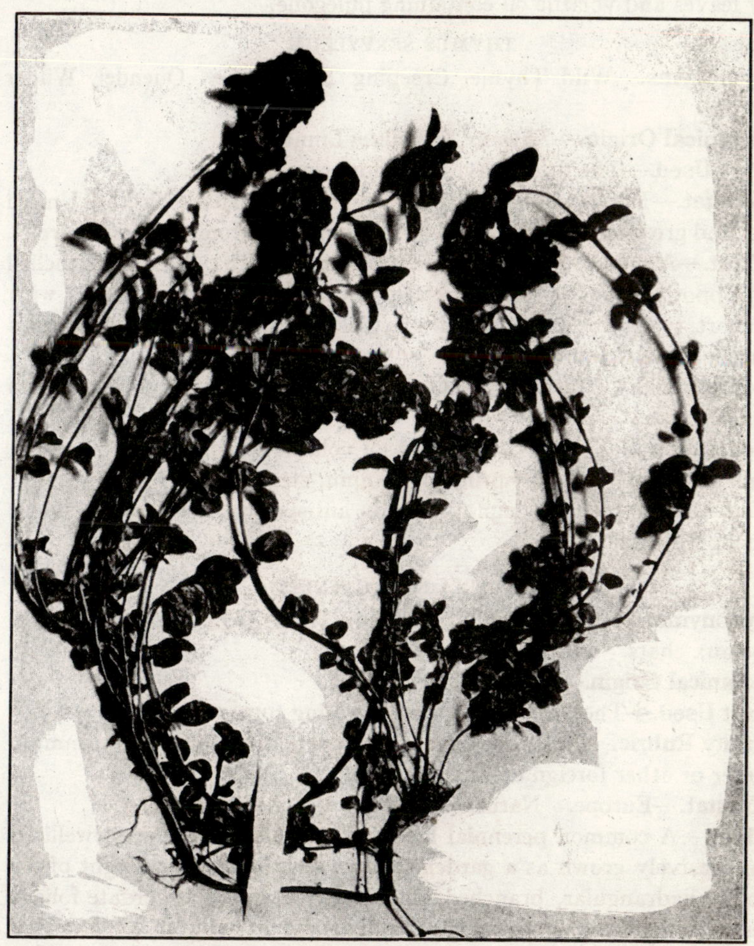

FIG. 219.—*Thymus Serpyllum* (Wild Thyme).

and various species of *Monarda* (horsemints). It is used as an antiseptic and anthelmintic (for hook worm).

Uses.—Antispasmodic and carminative.

Adulterants.—(1) The leaves and flowering tops of *Origanum creticum* or Spanish hops, indigenous to southern Europe. This substitute may be distinguished from Thyme by its yellowish to light-brown stems, palmately 5-veined, ovate leaves, ovoid or cylindrical spikes, papillated nutlets, and oil containing carvacrol ($C_{10}H_{14}O$).

(2) The leaves and flowering tops of *Origanum Dictamnus* or Cretan Dittany, indigenous to Crete has reddish-brown stems, elliptical, densely hairy leaves and volatile oil containing pulegone.

THYMUS SERPYLLUM

Synomyms.—Wild Thyme, Creeping Thyme; *Ger.* Quendel, Wilder Thymian.

Botanical Origin.—*Thymus Serpyllum* Linné.

Part Used.—The dried leaves and flowering tops.

Habitat.—Europe and Northern Asia. Naturalized in the United States and growing in fields. The drug is imported from southern Europe.

Plant.—A low, prostrate, creeping perennial with pubescent branched stem, opposite, short petioled, ovate, entire, obtuse, green leaves with very short, tooth-like hairs on their margins, and small terminal glomerules of purplish-spotted flowers.

Commercial.—The commercial supplies of the drug are obtained from central Europe.

Constituents.—About 0.5 per cent. of volatile oil containing carvacrol, thymol and cymene; bitter principle, tannin, etc.

Use.—Wild thyme is employed as an antispasmodic in the treatment of whooping-cough.

CATARIA N.F. (CATNEP)

Synonyms.—Catnip, Cat Mint, Cat's Wort; *Ger.* Katzenminze; *Fr.* Herbe aux chats.

Botanical Origin.—*Nepeta Cataria* Linné.

Part Used.—The dried leaves and flowering tops.

Purity Rubric.—Not more than 5 per cent. of its stems over 4 mm. in diameter or other foreign organic matter.

Habitat.—Europe. Naturalized in the United States.

Plant.—A common perennial herb, widely distributed near dwellings and extensively grown as a garden plant. It arises to the height of 0.8 m., has quadrangular, branched, downy stems, opposite cordate foliage leaves with deeply crenate margins, and dense, interrupted, axillary and terminal spikes or racemes of flowers that are whitish, dotted with purple.

Production and Commerce.—The plants are propagated either from seeds or by division of their roots. After they have reached a height of about 5 inches they should be thinned to stand 1 to 1½ feet apart. Plants that are grown from seed planted in the fall and properly cultivated produce a vigorous growth of herb. The leaves and flowering tops are gathered in late summer, when the plants are in full bloom, and carefully

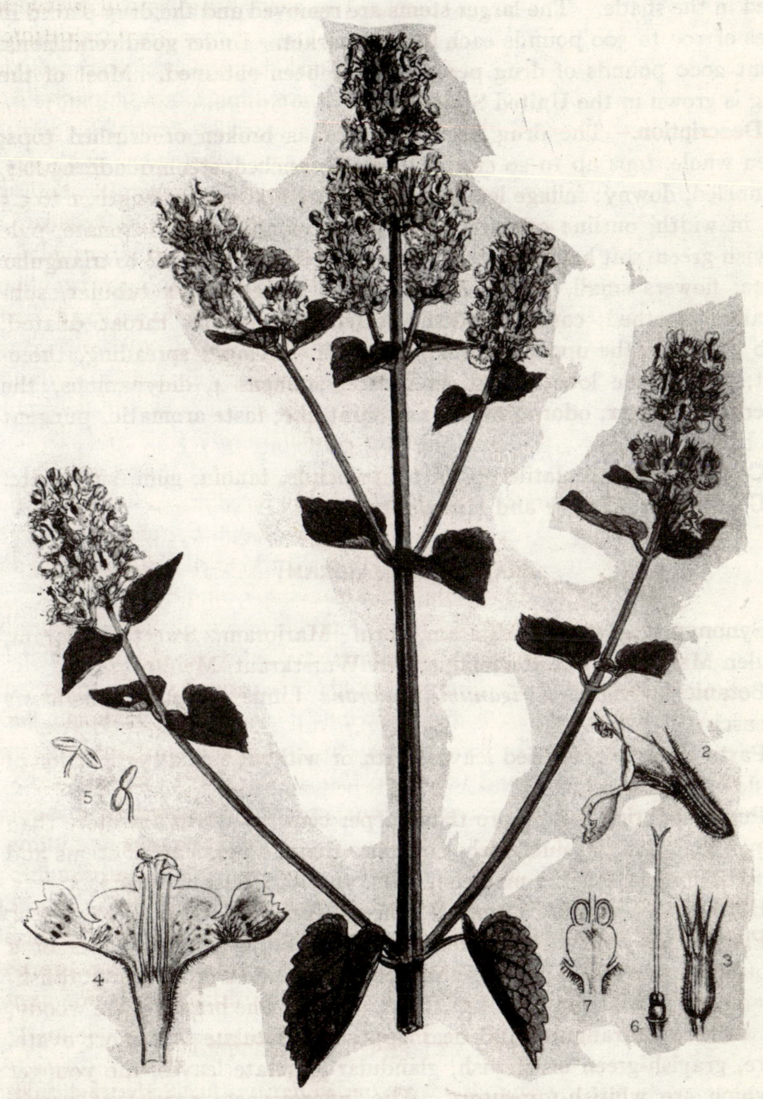

FIG. 220.—*Nepeta Cataria.* 1. Upper part of a flowering stem. 2. Flower. 3. Calyx. 4. Corolla laid open. 5. Anthers. 6. Pistil. 7. Section through gynophore. (*After Bentley and Trimen.*)

dried in the shade. The larger stems are removed and the drug placed in bales of 100 to 300 pounds each for the market. Under good conditions, about 2000 pounds of drug per acre have been obtained. Most of the drug is grown in the United States.

Description.—The drug usually occurs as broken or crushed tops; when whole, tops up to 20 cm. in length, branched; stems quadrangular, channeled, downy; foliage leaves petiolate, 2 to 15 cm. in length, 1 to 5.5 cm. in width, outline cordate, apex acute, margin deeply crenate, pale grayish-green, soft hairy above, downy beneath; bracts ovate to triangular ovate; flowers small, in dense interrupted spikes; calyx tubular, subequally 5-toothed; corolla whitish, dotted with purple, throat dilated, limb bilabiate, the upper lip erect, two-cleft, the lower spreading, three-cleft, the middle lobe largest, crenulate; stamens 4, didynamous, the lower pair shorter; odor aromatic and mint like; taste aromatic, pungent and bitter.

Constituents.—Volatile oil, bitter principle, tannin, gum, sugar, etc.

Uses.—Carminative and stimulant.

MAJORANA (MAJORAM)

Synonyms.—Sweet Marjoram, Leaf Marjoram, Sweet Majoram, Garden Marjoram; *Fr.* Marjolaine; *Ger.* Wurstkraut, Meiran.

Botanical Origin.—*Origanum Majorana* Linné (*Majorana hortensis* Moensch).

Parts Used.—The dried leaves, with or without a small proportion of the flowering tops.

Purity Rubric.—Not more than 16 per cent. total ash nor more than 4.5 per cent. acid-insoluble ash, nor more than 10 per cent. of stems and harmless foreign organic matter (F.I.D. 194, U.S. Dept. Agric.).

Habitat.—Southern Europe, Northern Africa and Asia.

Plant.—An annual herb whose underground portion consists of a fibrous root system. From this arises the aerial, much branched, purplish-brown stem attaining a height of about 30 cm. The branches are woody, thin hairy, quadrangular and bear opposite, spatulate and short ovate, entire, grayish-green or grayish, glandular-punctate leaves, the younger of which are whitish-tomentose. The inflorescences consist of nearly globular spikes of small reddish-white bilabiate flowers, and 4 rows of thin, rounded, pale green bracts.

Production and Commerce.—Sweet marjoram is widely cultivated in Europe and the United States as a seasoning herb. The leaves are gathered while the plant is in flower. Most of the drug, however, is imported in large bales from France, Tunis and Germany.

Description.—Leaves ovate, oblong, obovate or spatulate, short petiolate, averagely 4 cm. in length; apex obtuse, margin entire, upper and lower surfaces gray green and covered with glandular and non-glandular hairs; texture soft; veins forming loops; bracts similar in outline

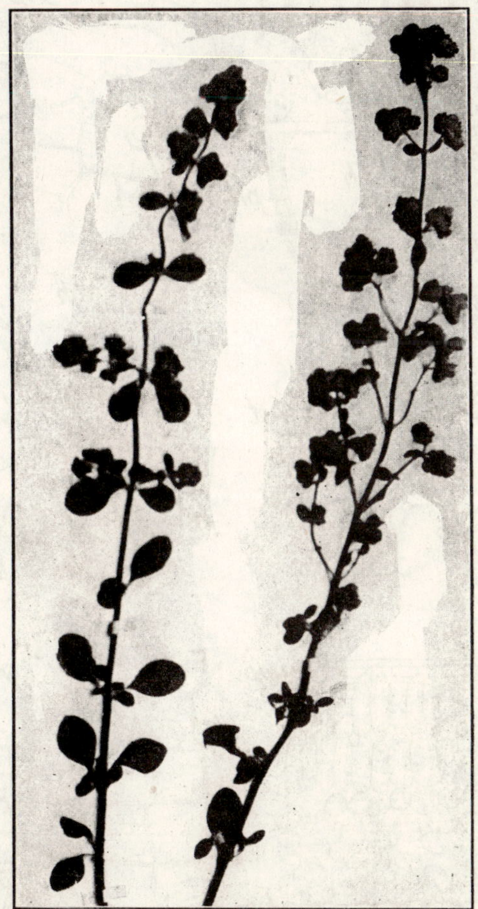

FIG. 221.—Sweet Marjoram (*Origanum Majorana*).

to foliage leaves and small as well as densely pubescent; odor aromatic characteristic; taste aromatic and slightly pungent.

Histology.—Passing from upper to lower surface the following microscopic structures are evident, when viewed in surface and cross sections.

1. Upper epidermis with thin cuticle, and epidermal cells having slightly wavy and knotty vertical walls. In surface view scars of the bases of hairs are evident, encircled by cells.

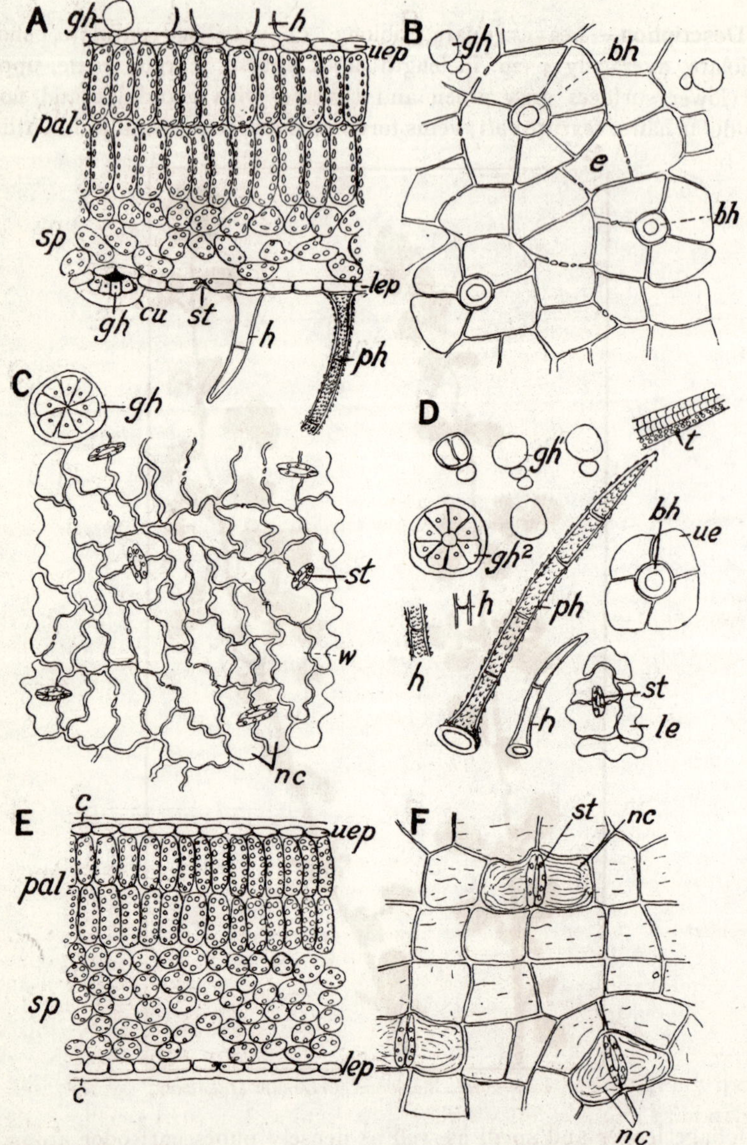

FIG. 222.—*Sweet Marjoram* (*A, B, C* and *D*) and *Coriaria* (*E* and *F*). *A,* Transverse section of sweet marjoram (*Origanum Majorana*) leaf, showing upper epidermis (*uep*); lower epidermis (*lep*); stoma (*st*); spongy parenchyma (*sp*); palisade parenchyma (*pal*); non-glandular hairs (*gh*). *B,* Vertical view of upper epidermis of leaf. Epidermal cell with porous vertical walls (*e*); glandular hair (*gh*); bases of non-glandular hairs (*bh*), characteristically surrounded by cells of epidermis. *C,* Vertical view of lower epidermis of leaf. Wavy-walled epidermal cells (*w*); neighboring cells (*nc*) perpendicular to guard cells surrounding stomata (*st*); 8-celled head of glandular hair (*gh*). *D,* Characteristic elements of powdered drug. Non-

2. Mesophyll, showing differentiation into an upper palisade region of 2 layers of columnar cells (occupying ⅔ of the entire mesophyll area) and a lower spongy parenchyma containing numerous air spaces. Through this region course the vascular bundles.

3. Lower epidermis with thin cuticle and epidermal cells exhibiting deeply sinuous, knotty, walled cells. Scattered through this region are numerous small stomata, the guard cells of which are surrounded by two neighboring cells.

DISTINCTION BETWEEN SWEET MARJORAM AND CORIARIA MYRTIFOLIA

	Sweet marjoram	Coriaria
Leaf	Soft hairy.	Thick, coriaceous with brittle fracture, no pubescence.
Venation	Veins forming indistinct loops.	3-nerved, the smaller veins indistinct.
Odor	Agreeably aromatic.	Indistinct.
Color	Grayish-green on both surfaces.	Green, paler green on lower surface.
Epidermis	Thin cuticle.	Thick cuticle.
Palisade	2 layers.	2 to 3 layers.
Upper epidermis	Cells with slightly wavy, knotty vertical walls.	Cells with rectilinear vertical walls and a wrinkled cuticle.
	Non-glandular hairs, uniseriate, 2–5 cells in length, more or less bent inward at apex, some papillose.	Hairs absent.
	Glandular hairs of 2 kinds, one with a 1- to 2-celled stalk and 1- to 2-celled glandular head, the other with no stalk and a large 8-celled head, the latter sunk in depressions of the epidermis.	
Lower epidermis	Cells with sinuous, knotty, vertical walls; stomata with 2 neighboring cells.	Cells with rectilinear vertical walls; stomata with 2 neighboring cells, more distinctly wrinkled than other epidermal cells.

Both glandular and non-glandular hairs occur on both epidermises. The glandular hairs are of two kinds, viz: one with a 1- to 2-celled stalk and a 1- to 2-celled glandular head, a second with no-stalk and an 8-celled,

glandular hairs and fragments of same (*h*); glandular hairs (*gh*); vertical view of glandular hair with 8-celled head (gh^2); upper epidermis with base of hair (*ue*); lower epidermis (*le*) with stomatal apparatus (*st*); papillose hair (*ph*), tracheæ (*t*). *E*, Transverse section of *Coriaria myrtifolia* leaf. Upper epidermis (*uep*); lower epidermis (*lep*); cuticle (*c*); palisade parenchyma (*pal*); spongy parenchyma (*sp*). *F*, Surface section of lower epidermis of *Coriaria* leaf. Note that the neighboring cells have a distinctly wrinkled cuticle and are parallel to the guard cells of the stomata. The walls of the epidermal cells are rectilinear to slightly curvilinear. (*Drawing by Miss A. Goldberg.*)

glandular, cup-shaped head sunken in a depression of the epidermis, the head portion exhibiting an up-raised cuticle. The non-glandular hairs are uniseriate, 2 to 5 cells in length, often finely warty and curved at the apex.

Constituents.—Volatile oil containing camphor and borneol, tannin, etc.

Use.—Sweet Marjoram is chiefly used as a poultry-seasoner. It has also been employed medicinally as a stimulant, carminative and emmenagogue.

Adulterants.—(1) The leaves of *Coriaria myrtifolia* or Tanner's Sumac (Fam. *Coriariaceæ*) which are frequently cut into narrow segments before being intentionally added to cheapen the article. This adulterant is dangerous on account of its poisonous constituent, *coriariamyrtin*, which acts similar to picrotoxin found in fish berries. (2) The cut leaves of *Cistus albidus* (Fam. *Cistaceæ*). (3) The powdered drug has been adulterated with Thyme and Wild Thyme.

ROSMARINUS (ROSEMARY)

Synonyms.—Garden Rosemary; *Ger.* Rosmarin; *Fr.* Romarin.

Botanical Origin.—*Rosmarinus officinalis* Linné.

Part Used.—The dried leaves.

Habitat.—Mediterranean regions.

Plant.—A bushy, low, much branched perennial shrub attaining a height of about 1 m. and bearing aromatic, evergreen, opposite, sessile, linear leaves and verticillasters of pale blue flowers.

Commercial.—The present commercial supplies of leaves come from France.

Description.—Leaves linear to linear-lanceolate from 1.5 to 3.5 cm. in length and up to 2.2.cm in breadth, coriaceous; upper surface dark green, lower surface wooly, glandular punctate and showing a prominent midrib; margin revolute; odor aromatic, characteristic; taste pungently aromatic, camphoraceous and bitter.

Constituents.—About 1 per cent. of volatile oil containing borneol; resin, bitter principle and tannin. Oleum Rosmarini U.S.P. is distilled from the fresh flowering tops.

Uses.—Stimulant, carminative and diaphoretic.

LAVANDULA (LAVENDER)

Synonyms.—Lavender Flowers, Spike Lavender, Garden Lavender; *Fr.* Lavande; *Ger.* Lavendelblüthen.

Botanical Origin.—*Lavandula spica* Linné (*Lavandula officinalis* Chaix, *Lavandula vera* DC.).

Part Used.—The carefully dried flowers.

Habitat.—Mediterranean regions.

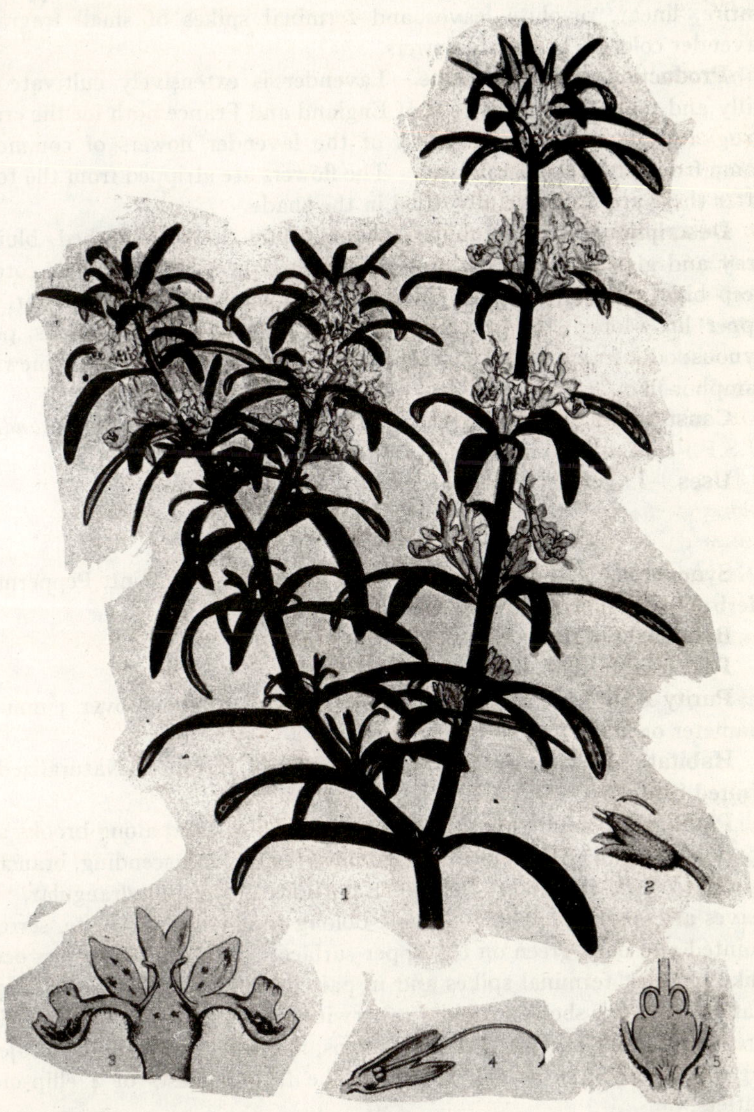

FIG. 223.—*Rosmarinus officinalis.* 1. Branch with leaves and verticillasters of flowers. 2. Calyx. 3. Corolla laid open. 4. Vertical section of calyx with pistil. 5. Section of ovary. (*After Bentley and Trimen.*)

Plant.—A crooked, much branched, low shrub with sessile, opposite, entire, linear, revolute leaves and terminal spikes of small fragrant, lavender colored, bi-labiate flowers.

Production and Commerce.—Lavender is extensively cultivated in hilly and mountainous districts of England and France both for the crude drug and its volatile oil. Most of the lavender flowers of commerce come from France and England. The flowers are stripped from the tops, after these are first carefully dried in the shade.

Description.—Calyx tubular, about 5 mm. long, 5-toothed, bluish-gray and glandular hairy, the upper tooth largest and rounded; corolla deep blue, tubular-bilabiate, about 8 mm. long, hairy and glandular, the upper lip 2-lobed, the lower lip 3-lobed; stamens 4, didynamous, perigynous; odor fragrant and characteristic; taste aromatic, bitter, somewhat camphor-like.

Constituents.—Up to 3 per cent. of volatile oil (*Oleum Lavandulæ* U.S.P.) containing l-linalyl acetate; resin, tannin, etc.

Uses.—Lavender flowers are chiefly used as a perfume.

MENTHA PIPERITA U.S.P. (PEPPERMINT)

Synonyms.—Lamb Mint, American Mint, Brandy Mint, Peppermint Herb; *Ger.* Pfefferminze; *Fr.* Mentha poivrée.

Botanical Origin.—*Mentha piperita* Linné.

Part Used.—The dried leaves and tops.

Purity Rubric.—Not more than 2 per cent. of stems over 3 mm. in diameter or other foreign organic matter.

Habitat.—In low, wet soil along brooks of Europe. Naturalized in United States.

Plant.—A perennial herb common in meadows and along brooks and spreading rapidly by runners. Its stems are erect or ascending, branched and 1 to 3 ft. in height, the upper portions always quadrangular. Its leaves are opposite, petiolate, ovate-oblong to oblong lanceolate, serrate, pointed and dark-green on the upper surface. Its purplish flowers occur alike in thick terminal spikes and in paired axillary cymes in the upper leaf axils. Each shows a tubular calyx with 5 sharp, hairy teeth, a purplish, irregular, 4-cleft corolla, 4 short stamens, a 4-celled ovary and a projecting style ending in a bifid stigma. The fruit consists of 4 ellipsoidal nutlets.

Production and Commerce.—The drug is harvested in July, August, and September, while the plants are in flower. It is cut and dried like hay. Most of the crude drug is subjected to steam distillation for its volatile oil content. The best Peppermint comes from Michigan, Northern Indiana, New York. Oregon, Indiana and Germany, where the herb is

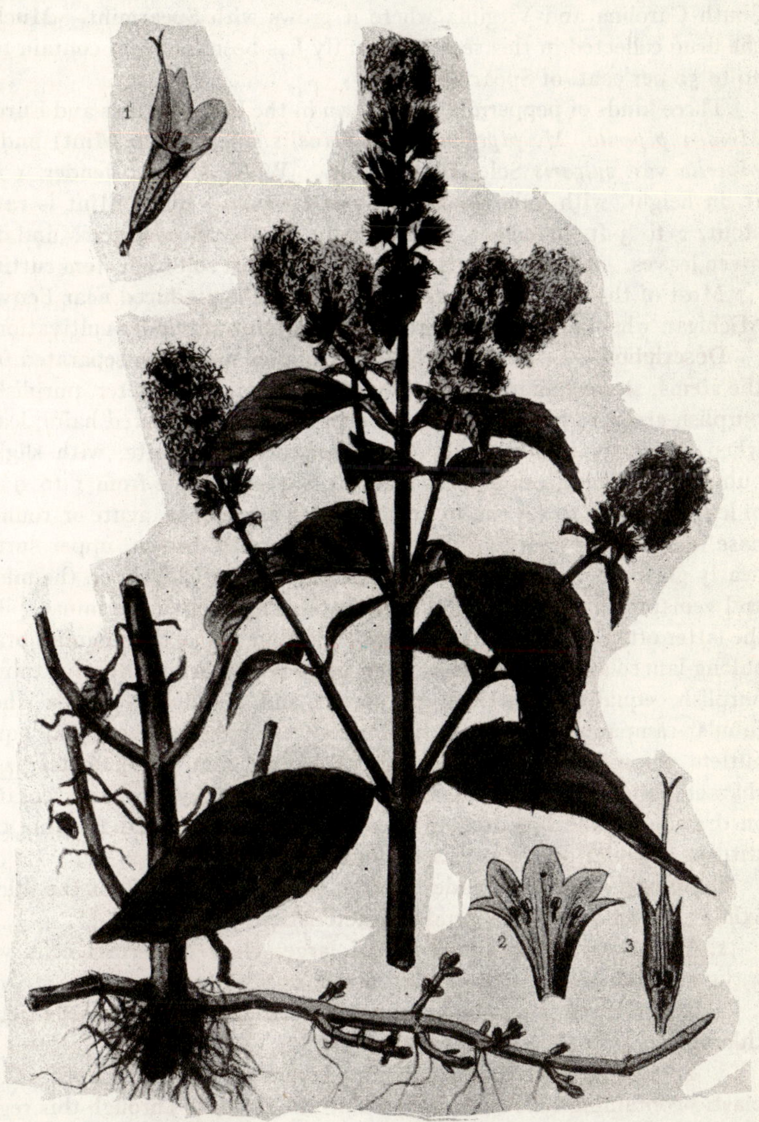

FIG. 224.—*Mentha piperita*. 1. A flower. 2. Corolla cut open. 3. Vertical section of calyx and ovary. (*After Bentley and Trimen.*)

cultivated on a large scale. Inferior Peppermint comes from North and South Carolina and Virginia where it grows with Spearmint. Much of the drug collected in this section recently has been found to contain from 30 to 50 per cent. of Spearmint.

Three kinds of peppermint are grown in the United States and Europe: *Mentha piperita*, *M. piperita* var. *officinalis* Sole (**White Mint**) and *M. piperita* var. *vulgaris* Sole (**Black Mint**). White Mint is slender, 1 to 2 ft. in height, with light green stems and leaves. Black Mint is rather stout, 2 to 3 ft. in height, with usually purple colored stems and dark green leaves. All of these may be grown in moist soil from stem cuttings.

Most of the oil of peppermint of commerce is produced near Fenville, Michigan where about 4000 acres of peppermint are under cultivation.

Description.—Leaves more or less crumpled and often separated from the stems; stems quadrangular, from 1 to 3 mm. in diameter, purplish to purplish-green to green, glabrous except for a few scattered hairs; leaves when entire ovate-oblong to oblong-lanceolate, opposite, with slightly pubescent petiole from 4 to 12 mm. in length; laminæ from 1 to 9 cm. in length and up to 2.5 cm. in breadth, with acute apex, acute or rounded base, and serrate margin, light green to purplish-brown, upper surface nearly glabrous, lower surface glandular hairy, particularly on the midrib and veins; inflorescences both verticillasters and compact terminal spikes, the latter often interrupted at the base and rounded at the summit; bracts oblong-lanceolate, acuminate at apex, up to 7 mm. in length; calyx tubular purplish, equally 5 toothed, pubescent and glandular; corolla short, tubular-campanulate, light purple, 4-cleft; stamens 4, short and equal; nutlets ellipsoidal, blackish-brown, about 0.5 mm. in diameter; odor characteristically aromatic; taste aromatic followed by a cooling sensation on drawing in the breadth. This sensation is due to the menthol constituent stimulating the cold spots in the mouth.

Histology.—Sections made through the lamina outside of the midrib exhibit the following structural characteristics.

1. Upper epidermis composed of large, clear epidermal cells with wavy vertical walls and possessing few or no stomata.

2. Palisade parenchyma, comprising a layer of columnar cells rich in chloroplasts.

3. Spongy parenchyma, of about 5 layers of irregular shaped chloroplastid-containing cells and intercellular-air-spaces. Through this region the veins course.

4. Lower epidermis, of small epidermal cells with wavy vertical walls and numerous elliptical stomata. This epidermis in the region of veins and midrib exhibits as outgrowths non-glandular and glandular hairs. The non-glandular hairs are uniseriate, papillose, 1- to 8-celled. The

glandular hairs have a 1- to 2-celled stalk and a 1- to 8-celled glandular head. These hairs contain the oil of peppermint. In the drug obtained from cultivated plants, the terminal cell of the non-glandular hair often becomes glandular.

Powdered Drug.—Green. Fragments of epidermis with thin, wavy, vertical walled cells and stomata; fragments of mesophyll containing chloroplasts; non-glandular hairs, with thin papillose walls, 1- to 8-cells in length; glandular hairs with a 1- to 2-celled stalk and a 1- to 8-celled, often balloon-shaped head; fragments of collenchyma and epidermis of stem; fragments of flowers, the pollen grains of which are spheroidal and smooth; fragments of vascular tissue, the tracheæ being slightly lignified and with spiral, simple pore or bordered pore markings, the sclerenchyma fibers, thin walled and non-lignified; fragments of stem parenchyma.

Constituents.—About 1 per cent. of volatile oil containing up to 60 per cent. of menthol (U.S.P.); resin, tannin, acetic acid, etc. Oil of Peppermint U.S.P. represents the volatile oil which is distilled from the fresh overground parts of the plant.

Uses.—Carminative and flavoring agent.

Adulterants.—(1) Spearmint. (2) Leaves of varieties of *Mentha piperita*.

MENTHA VIRIDIS U.S.P. (SPEARMINT)

Synonyms.—Mint, Common Garden Mint, Lady's or Mackerel Mint; *Ger.* Grüne Münze, Römische Münze; *Fr.* Menthe vert, Baume vert.

Botanical Origin.—*Mentha spicata* Linné (*Mentha viridis* Linné).

Part Used.—The dried leaves and tops.

Purity Rubric.—Not more than 2 per cent. of stems over 3 mm. in diameter or other foreign organic matter.

Habitat.—Europe, in wet places. Naturalized in United States.

Plant.—A perennial herb of a lighter shade of green than Peppermint and found in similar localities. Its leaves are opposite, ovate lanceolate, unequally serrate and nearly sessile. Its purplish flowers are borne in slender, interrupted, terminal spikes.

Production and Commerce.—The leaves and flowering tops are cut down during the late summer while the plant is in full bloom. They are dried similar to Peppermint. The plant is extensively cultivated in Michigan, Virginia, North and South Carolina both for its volatile oil and for sale as the crude drug Because of its prevalence in regions where Peppermint abounds, the drug is often admixed with this herb. Like Peppermint, that coming from the southern states, recently, has contained the more admixture and so has been of rather inferior quality.

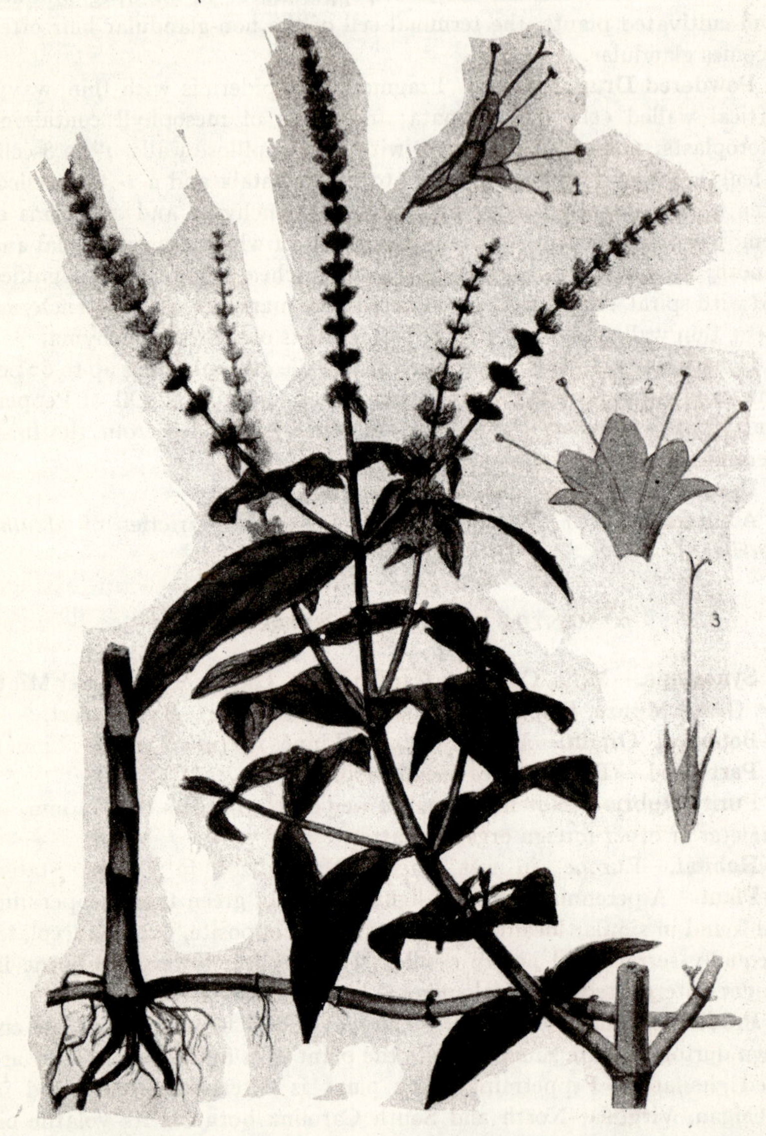

FIG. 225.—*Mentha viridis*. 1. A flower. 2. Corolla cut open. 3. Vertical section through calyx and ovary. (*After Bentley and Trimen.*)

Description.—Leaves more or less crumpled and mixed with numerous segments of brownish and purple stems; stems quadrangular, often with opposite branches, usually from 1 to 3 mm. in width, nearly glabrous; leaves when entire, ovate-lanceolate, unequally serrate, nearly sessile or with a petiole less than 5 mm. in length, bright-green, glandular hairy on lower surface; inflorescences both verticillasters in upper axils and terminal densely crowded, lanceolate spikes; bracts linear-lanceolate, subulate from 7 to 10 mm. in length, subtending the flower clusters; calyx tubular, 5-toothed, glandular-hairy and pubescent near the teeth; corolla 4-lobed white or light brown; stamens 4, extending beyond the corolla tube; taste characteristically aromatic but not followed by a cooling sensation on drawing in the breath.

Constituents.—From 0.2 to 0.5 per cent. of volatile oil of which about 55 per cent. is carvone; resin, tannin, etc. Oil of Spearmint U.S.P. represents the volatile oil distilled from the fresh, over-ground parts of the flowering plant.

Uses.—Carminative and flavoring agent.

Adulterants.—(1) Peppermint. (2) Other species of *Mentha.*

SCUTELLARIA N.F. (SCUTELLARIA)

Synonyms.—Scullcap, Quaker Bonnet, Madweed, Hoodwort, Mad Dog Scullcap; Helmet Flower; *Ger.* Schildkraut, Helmkraut; *Fr.* Scutellaire.

Botanical Origin.—*Scutellaria lateriflora* Linné.

Part Used.—The dried overground portion.

Ash.—Not more than 12 per cent.

Habitat.—In wet woods of United States and Canada.

Plant.—A perennial, smooth herb with erect, freely branched stem attaining a length of 80 cm. The leaves are opposite, lance-ovate or ovate-oblong, prominently petiolate, the lamina with acute apex, rounded or sub-cordate base and coarsely serrate margin. The inflorescences are axillary and terminal racemes, occasionally 1-sided racemes of blue, or rarely white or pink, bilabiate flowers. The fruit consists of 4 brown nutlets, enclosed by a persistent calyx having the shape of a Quaker's bonnet. The plant is gathered for medicinal purposes from July to September when in flower and dried.

Description.—Scutellaria occurs either in the whole, crushed, chopped or pressed condition. When entire, stem quadrangular, 50–80 cm. in length and averagely 1 to 4 mm. thick, varying in color from base upward from purplish-brown to brown to yellowish-green, longitudinally furrowed with distinct nodes and nearly glabrous, except on inflorescence axes; fracture short. Leaves opposite, from 2 to 7 cm. in length, long petiolate, ovate-lanceolate or ovate-oblong; apex acute or acuminate; base acute or obtuse; margin coarsely serrate; venation pinnate-reticulate, the veins of the first order anastomosing near the margin; upper surface dark green, nearly glabrous; lower surface pale green with few appressed non-glandular hairs and many glandular hairs. Flowers in axillary and terminal 1-sided

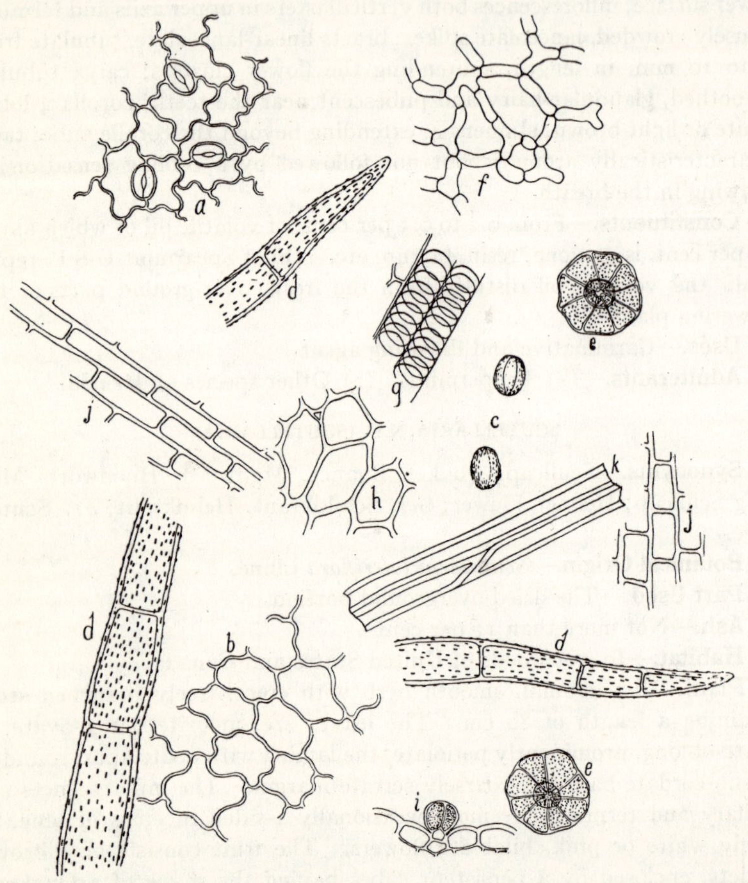

FIG. 226.—Scutellaria. (*a*) Lower epidermis; (*b*) upper epidermis; (*c*) pollen grains; (*d*) trichomes; (*e*) glands, top view; (*f*) spongy tissue of leaves; (*g*) spiral ducts; (*h*) parenchyma; (*i*) small gland and epidermal cells, profile view; (*j*) parenchyma. (*Schneider.*)

racemes; calyx light green, hairy, campanulate-bilabiate and toothed; corolla blue, rarely pink or white, tubular-bilabiate; stamens 4, hairy, the anthers of the 2 lower stamens 1-celled, those of the 2 upper ones 2-celled and cordate; ovary deeply four-lobed; style 2-cleft. Fruit composed of 4 ellipsoidal, tuberculate, brown nutlets about 1 mm. in length, enclosed within a persistent helmet shaped calyx. Subterranean portion consisting of a stoloniferous shoot giving rise to numerous fibrous and branched, slender roots. The odor is characteristic. Taste slightly bitter and somewhat aromatic.

Histology.—Transverse sections of the internodal portion of the stem are quadrangular in outline and exhibit the following structures, passing from periphery toward the center.

1. Epidermis of small epidermal cells with cutinized and striated outer walls.

2. Hypodermis of 2 to 4 layers of collenchymatous cells.

3. Cortex, a narrow zone of rather loosely arranged cortical parenchyma cells.

4. Pericycle, containing an interrupted band of thick-walled pericyclic fibers.

5. Phloem, a narrow zone of sieve tubes and phloem parenchyma becoming broadest in the regions of the angles.

6. Cambium, of more or less collapsed meristematic cells.

7. Xylem, mainly limited to regions of angles, and composed in these regions of radially arranged xylem patches composed of thick-walled, narrow wood fibers and rows of tracheæ with bordered pore or scalariform markings. The medullary-rays separating the xylem patches are 1 cell in width. Little interfacicular wood is developed.

8. Pith, a broad zone of parenchyma, usually hollow in center. Sections of the leaves show these to be distinctly dorsoventral in character and showing the following diagnostic microscopical characteristics:

A few recurved non-glandular hairs from 1–3 cells in length, with a sharp pointed distal cell occur on the upper epidermis. The cells of this epidermis are wavy-walled in surface view and devoid of stomata. The mesophyll or leaf parenchyma is differentiated into an upper layer of palisade cells and a loosely arranged spongy parenchyma region between the palisade zone and the lower epidermis. Calcium oxalate is absent. The lower epidermis consists of wavy-walled epidermal cells and numerous elliptical stomata. Growing out of this epidermis are to be observed numerous glandular trichomes having a 1- to 2-celled stalk and a 6- to 8-celled glandular head.

The pollen grains are nearly spheroidal and smooth.

Constituents.—A bitter amorphous, microscopically varnish-like glucoside, known as scutellarin; tannin, volatile oil, resin, etc.

Uses.—Bitter tonic and antispasmodic.

Adulterants.—(1) The dried overground portion of *Scutellaria cordifolia* Muehl. (*Scutellaria versicolor* Nutt.), commonly known as Heart-Shaped or Southern Scullcap, has been the chief constituent in several samples examined by the writer which were labelled "Southern Scullcap." The plant is found in the mountainous districts of Virginia, southward and southwestward. It may be distinguished from *S. lateriflora* by its stems showing abundant non-glandular and glandular hairs, by its leaves being cordate at the base (excepting upper ones) and having crenate-dentate margins, and by the non-glandular hairs on its stems and leaves being from 2 to 6 cells in length.

(2) The dried overground portion of *Scutellaria canescens* Nutt., commonly known as Western Scullcap, has almost entirely replaced the official article within recent years. This plant grows along streams from Ontario south to Northern Alabama and west to Kansas and Arkansas. It is best distinguished from *S. lateriflora*, by its glandular hairs consisting of a 2- to 6-celled stalk and a large 6- to 8-celled glandular head. Other diagnostic characters are as follows: (1) Non-glandular hairs 3 to 7 cells in length. (2) larger blue flowers than in *S. lateriflora* and usually more plentiful. (3) Interfascicular wood pronounced. (4) Leaves and stems abundantly hairy.

(3) The dried overground portion of *Scutellaria galericulata* L.

MARRUBIUM

Synonyms.—Horehound, Hoarhound, White Hoarhound, Marvel; *Ger.* Andorn, Apfelkraut; *Fr.* Marrube blanc.

Botanical Origin.—*Marrubium vulgare* Linné.

Part Used.—The dried leaves and flowering tops.

Habitat.—Europe and Central Asia.

Plant.—A perennial herb which is cultivated in various parts of the United States and which grows wild in numerous sections of North America. The underground portion consists of a short rhizome bearing numerous slender rootlets. The aërial stem is erect, quadrangular, .3 to .8 m. high, 3 to 5 mm. in diameter, branched, the branches ascending. Its white-wooly aspect is very striking. The leaves are opposite, petiolate, exstipulate, varying from ovate to broadly ovate to nearly orbicular in outline, 1.5 to 6 cm. in length, 9 to 25 mm. in breadth; apex obtuse; base narrowed or rounded or sub-cordate; margin coarsely crenate; upper surface downy-whitish, lower surface woolly; venation pinnate-reticulate. The infloresence is a verticillaster with flowers arranged in dense axillary whorls, each having a tubular, sparsely pubescent calyx 6 to 7 mm. long, with 10 subulate, recurved, bristle-like teeth, a whitish bilabiate corolla, four parallel stamens ascending under the upper lid of the corolla, and a bi-carpellary pistil with a four-celled ovary. The fruit consists of four nutlets. The odor is aromatic upon crushing; the taste aromatic and bitter.

Production and Commerce.—Horehound is cultivated in many parts of the United States and Europe. The leaves and flowering tops are best gathered when the plant is in flower and carefully dried. The bulk of the commercial article is imported from Europe and arrives in tight bales. Recent supplies were shipped from Marseilles, Hamburg, Budapest, Nimes and Rotterdam.

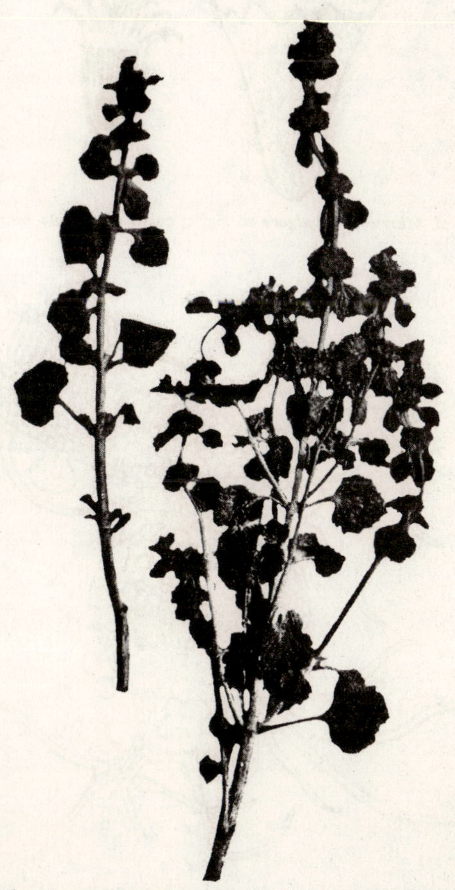

FIG. 227.—Aerial portion (to right) and branch (to left) of *Marrubium vulgare* L. × ⅓.

Histology.—The leaf shows the typical dorsoventral lamina common to the genus *Marrubium*. Transverse and surface sections show an upper epidermis, devoid of stomata, composed of tabular cells with somewhat undulate outer walls, a layer of vertically elongated palisade cells, several layers of spongy parenchyma cells traversed by collateral bundles, and a lower epidermis similar to that of the upper, but possessing stomata. Non-glandular and glandular trichomes are present as outgrowths on both upper and lower epidermis. They are, however, more numerous on the lower epidermis. The non-glandular trichomes are either simple or

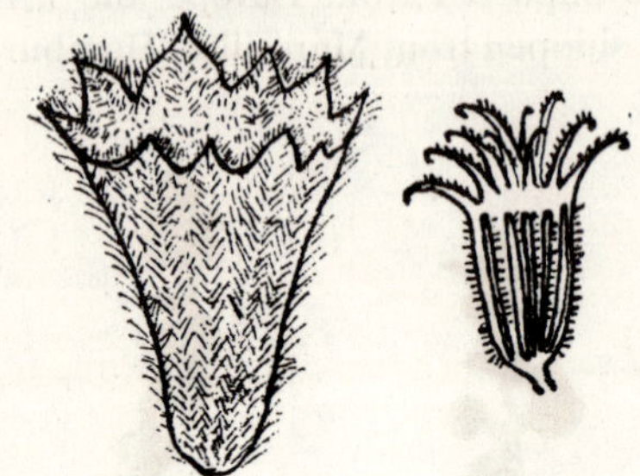

FIG. 228.—Calyx of *Marrubium vulgare* to right; calyx of *Ballota hirsuta* to left. × 4.

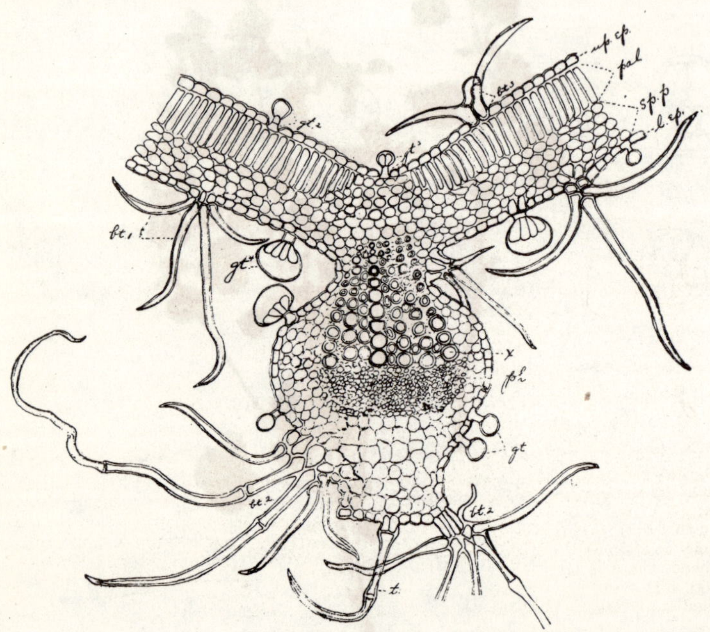

FIG. 229.—Cross-section through one of the stronger veins and portion of the lamina of *Marrubium vulgare*. (*up. ep.*) upper epidermis; (*l, ep.*) lower epidermis; (*pal*) palisade parenchyma; (*sp.p.*) spongy parenchyma; (*x*) xylem; (*ph*) phloem; (*t*) long-pointed non-glandular trichome; (bt^1, bt^2) branched trichomes, more or less stalked; (bt^3) sessile branched trichome; (gt, gt^2, gt^3 gt^4) several types of glandular trichomes. × 120.

branched, the latter type predominating. The simple trichomes are, for most part, unicellular and almost invariably slightly curved. There occur, however, a scattering of much elongated, characteristically curved and twisted (in dried material) unicellular hairs which type predominate on the stem, giving this part its white-wooly aspect (Fig. 230j). In addition to these, uniseriate 2-celled hairs with long pointed and bent distal cell have been met with occasionally.

The branched trichomes are of two kinds, viz.: (1) those that project directly out of slightly elongated epidermal cells and which are two to three branched and (2) those which consist of a more or less elongated central multicellular stalk with radiating branches (Fig. 229bt[2]). As many as fifteen branches have been observed on this type. Of these, those emanating from the base of the stalk are unicellular, and more frequently curved than straight, while those issuing from points higher up are either unicellular or two- or three-celled, the distal cell of these last being characteristically long, pointed and curved. The central stalk of the branched trichome does not usually attain the great length of the similar part of the branched trichome of *Ballota hirsuta*.

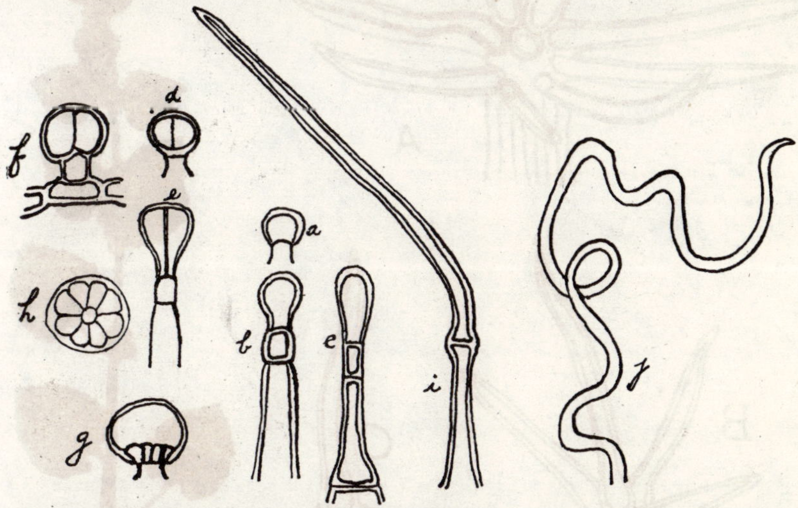

FIG. 230.—Various types of hairs found on *Marrubium vulgare*. (*a*, *b*, *c*, *d* *e*, *f*, *g*, *h*) Glandular hairs, and (*i*) non-glandular two-celled hair, all found on the foliage leaves and calyxes; (*j*) curled unicellular-non-glandular hair, a type abundantly found on the stem that gives to this part its white-woolly appearance; (*a*, *d*, *f*) glandular hairs with a one-celled stalk and a one- to two-celled head; (*b*, *c*, *e*) glandular hairs with two-celled uniseriate stalk and 1–2-celled head, the distal cell of the stalk being considerably shortened and forming the "neck cell;" (*g*) side view, and (*h*) view from above of large balloon-shaped glandular hair with one-celled stalk and 8-celled head. (All highly magnified.)

The glandular trichomes have either a one- to two-celled short or long stalk and a one-, two- or eight-celled balloon-shaped glandular head. The large number of the last mentioned (balloon) type which possess unicellular short stalks is very striking (Figs. 229 and 230).

Sections made through the calyx show in modified degree the peculiar microscopic structure of the foliage leaf. The lamina is thinner and more trichomes of the glandular variety are evident.

Constituents.—A bitter principle called marrubin, volatile oil, tannin resin, etc.

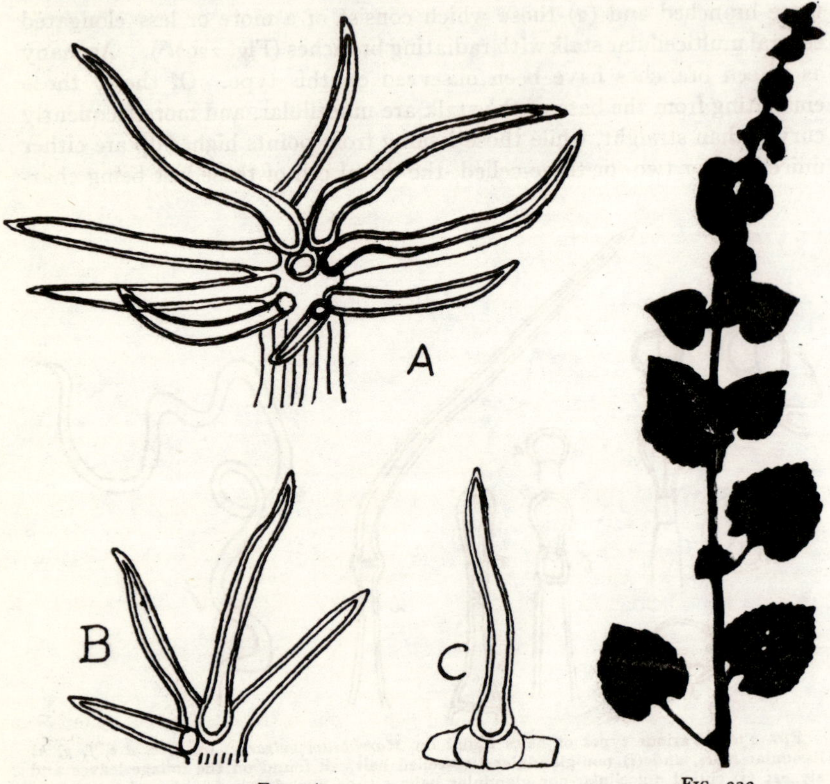

FIG. 231. FIG. 232.

FIG. 231.—Non-glandular hairs from calyx of *Marrubium vulgare*. *A*, Many branched hair with somewhat elongated stalk; (*B*) branched hair with short stalk and few branches; (*C*) unicellular, non-glandular hair (highly magnified).

FIG. 232.—*Ballota hirsuta* Benth. Aerial foliage and floral stem. Note the dense axillary clusters of flowers. × ⅓.

Uses.—Bitter tonic and expectorant.

Adulterants.—Horehound has been adulterated with the leaves and flowering tops of *Ballota hirsuta*, *Ballota nigra* and *Marrubium peregrinum* (Black Horehound). The most recent adulterant has been *Ballota hirsuta*.

The leaves and flowering tops of *Ballota hirsuta* Benth., a perennial hirsute herb indigenous to Mediterranean countries, (Fig. 232) shows the following macroscopic peculiarities: Stem quadrangular, pubescent but not white-woolly like *Marrubium*. Leaves, opposite, petiolate, ovate to orbicular, coarsely hairy on upper surface, coarsely whitish-woolly on under surface, apex obtuse, base sub-cordate, margin crenate, venation pinnate-reticulate. Inflorescence a verticillaster, the hermaphrodite flowers appearing in dense axillary clusters and usually fewer in number than in the verticillasters of *Marrubium*. Each flower consists of a bilabiate

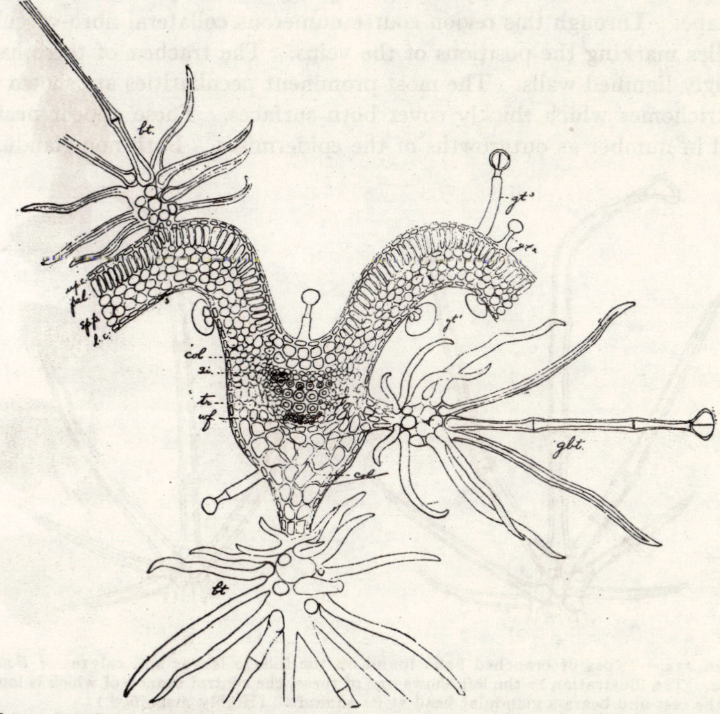

FIG. 233.—Cross-section of foliage leaf of *Ballota hirsuta* made through a stronger nerve and portion of the lamina. (*up. e*) Upper epidermis; (*l. e.*) lower epidermis; (*pal.*) palisade parenchyma; (*sp. p.*) spongy parenchyma; (*s*) stoma; (*col.*) collenchyma; (*si.*) sieve tissue; (*tr.*) trachea; (*wf.*) wood fibers; (*bt.*) branched trichomes; (*gbt.*) branched trichome with central branch the longest and bearing a two-celled glandular head; gt^1, gt^2, gt^3, glandular trichomes. ×98.

infundibuliform calyx, up to 10 mm. long (Fig. 228) with limb showing a margin of 10 broadly acute or mucronate teeth, a distinctly bilabiate corolla, four included stamens, and a bi-carpellary pistil. The fruit consists of four nutlets.

MICROSCOPICAL CHARACTERISTICS OF *BALLOTA HIRSUTA* BENTH.

Transverse sections (Fig. 233) made through the lamina region of the foliage leaf show typical dorsoventral structure. Passing from ventral to dorsal surface the following structures present themselves for examination:

Upper epidermis, devoid of stomata and composed of tabular cells with outer walls more or less convex and showing a rather thick cuticle. Directly beneath this tissue is a layer of somewhat loosely arranged vertically elongated palisade cells, the average being shorter than those found in *Marrubium vulgare*. Beneath the palisade layer are several layers of more or less loosely arranged spongy parenchyma cells, irregular in shape. Through this region course numerous collateral fibro-vascular bundles marking the positions of the veins. The tracheæ of these have strongly lignified walls. The most prominent peculiarities are shown by the trichomes which thickly cover both surfaces. These appear nearly equal in number as outgrowths of the epidermises. Both non-glandular

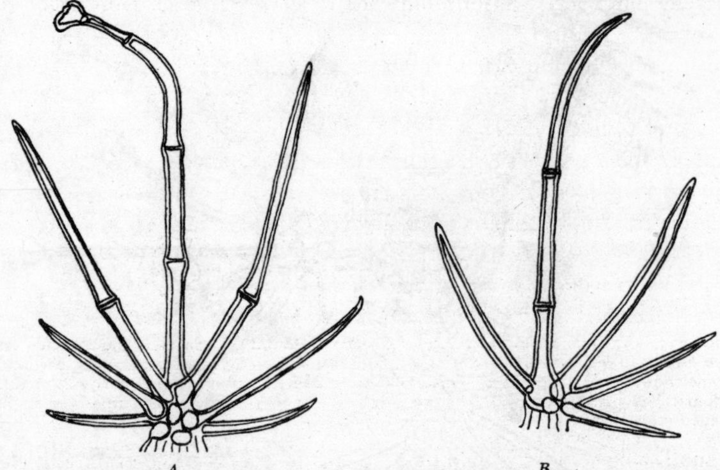

Fig. 234.—Types of branched hairs found on the foliage leaves and calyxes of *Ballota hirsuta*. The illustration to the left shows one of these, the central branch of which is longer than the rest and bears a glandular head at its summit. (Highly magnified.)

and glandular types are represented. As for *Marrubium vulgare*, so for this leaf, the non-glandular trichomes fall into three categories, viz.: unicellular, uniseriate, and branched. The unicellular variety are either short or long, straight or bent over toward the epidermis. The individual cells of the uniseriate hairs form distinct articulations. By far the most conspicuous and diagnostic elements are the branched hairs (Fig. 234). These are easily distinguished from those of *Marrubium vulgare* by their generally longer basal stalks, thicker walls and more rigid looking branches. As many as eighteen branches have been counted emanating from the central stalk. The shortest branches arise from the basal portion, the rest becoming longer as the stalk is ascended. Most of the branches vary from one to three cells in length. The central or longest branch, however, may be uniseriate, four-celled and attain a length of 3 mm.

A form of branched trichome has been observed by the writer that stands out preëminently as constituting the most easy and practical histologic means of distinguishing *Ballota hirsuta* from *Marrubium vulgare.* This trichome resembles the other branched forms seen in *Ballota* but differs from these in respect to the central branch which has a two to four celled uniseriate stalk and a glandular head of one or two to four cells (Fig. 234, *A*).

The glandular trichomes exhibit various forms (Fig. 235) viz.: (*a*) short one-celled stalk and small unicellular head; (*b*) short unicellular stalk and large four to eight-celled balloon-shaped head; (*c*) long one-celled stalk

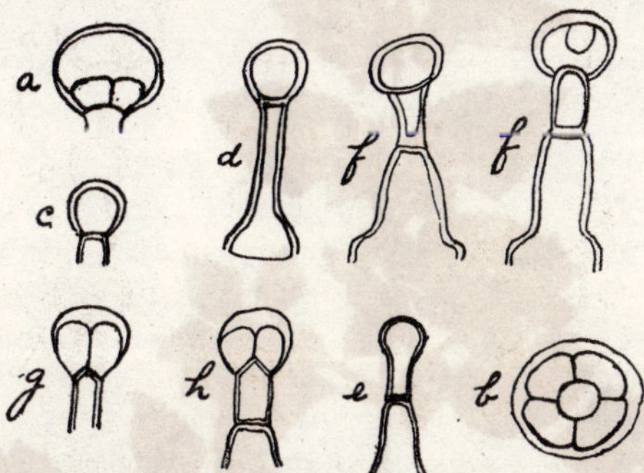

FIG. 235.—Various types of glandular trichomes found on the calyx and foliage leaf of *Ballota hirsuta.* (*a*) Lateral view, and (*b*) view from above of the balloon type of glandular trichome showing (in *a*) the short, unicellular stalk and the lateral aspect of the head, and (in *b*) a four-celled glandular head; (*c, d, e, f, g*) other types of glandular trichomes having a 1–2-celled stalk and a 1–2-celled glandular head. (All highly magnified.)

and small spheroidal unicellular head; (*d*) long one-celled stalk and elongated unicellular head; (*e*) one-celled stalk and two-celled head; (*f*) short two-celled stalk and two-celled head; (*g*) long two-celled stalk, the distal cell ("neck cell") being shorter than the proximal one and bearing a one-celled head. Many of the hairs have their basal portions lignified. These take a pinkish to reddish coloration with phloroglucin and concentrated hydrochloric acid.

The calyx of *Ballota hirsuta* shows a microscopic structure similar to that of the foliage leaf, but on a reduced scale. The tendency for more of the branched hairs to show the central branch glandular has been observed.

The chief practical diagnostic differences between *Ballota hirsuta* and *Marrubium vulgare* are as follows:

1. The calyx, which in *Ballota hirsuta* is densely hairy, distinctly bi-labiate-infundibuliform with limb margin showing 10 broadly acute or

mucronate teeth, whereas in *Marrubium vulgare* it is sparsely hairy, distinctly tubular with ten, bristle-like, recurved teeth.

2. The absence in *Marrubium vulgare* and presence in *Ballota hirsuta* of certain branched trichomes, the central branch of which bears a glandular head of one, two, or four cells.

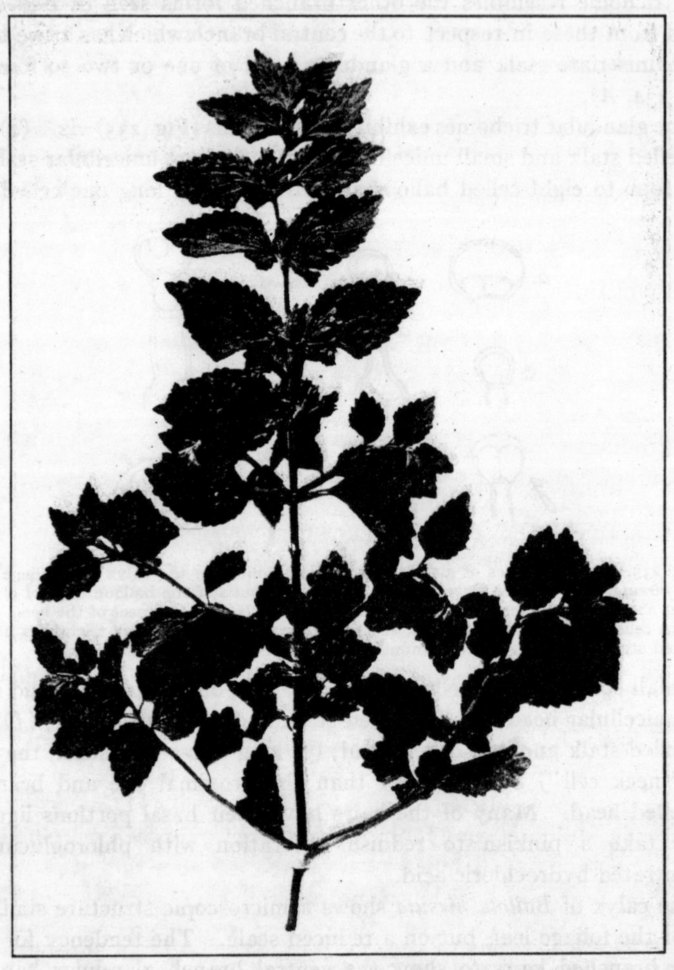

FIG. 236.—*Ballota nigra*, one of the adulterants of Marrubium.

3. The branched trichomes of *Ballota hirsuta* show on the average longer basal stalks, thicker walls and more rigid branches than those of *Marrubium vulgare*.

4. A number of trichomes of *Ballota hirsuta* are lignified at their bases, whereas in *Marrubium vulgare* no such lignification has been observed.

SALVIA (SAGE)

Synonyms.—True Sage, Garden Sage, Meadow Sage; *Fr.* Sauge; *Ger.* Salbeiblätter.

Botanical Origin.—*Salvia officinalis* Linné.

Part Used.—The dried leaf.

Purity Rubric.—It contains not less than 1 per cent. of volatile ether extract, not more than 25 per cent. of crude fiber, not more than 10 per cent. of total ash, nor more than 1 per cent. of ash insoluble in hydrochloric acid (Circ. 136, U.S. Dept. Agric.).

Habitat.—Mediterranean regions.

Plant.—A perennial low shrub or subshrub from 6 inches to 1½ feet high. From an underground fibrous root system there arises a grayish, much branched, pubescent stem with branches opposite. In early summer the upper branches bear blue, rarely pink or white, bilabiate flowers followed by blackish nutlets borne in open cups.

Production and Commerce.—The plant is cultivated in various parts of Europe and the United States from seeds, which are sown in early spring in ordinary garden soil, or from cuttings. The leaves are gathered while the plant is in flower and carefully dried in the shade and marketed. The drug is largely imported from Trieste and Prague. Greek Sage is imported from Greece, the usual shipping port being Chios. Spanish Sage is imported from Mexico. The last two sages have frequently been substituted for the true sage.

Description.—Leaves opposite, long petiolate, petiole up to 4.5 cm. in length, laminæ elliptical, ovate-oblong or oblong-lanceolate, 2 to 10 cm. in length, 1 to 2.6 cm. in breadth; apex acute or obtuse; base rounded or subcordate, uneven or lobed; margin crenulate; upper surface grayish-green (gray and densely pubescent in young leaves) with depressed midrib; lower surface grayish or pale grayish-green, densely pubescent; venation pinnate-reticulate, the reticulations being very small; midrib and veins prominent; texture velvet-like; odor strongly aromatic on crushing; taste aromatic and bitter.

Histology.—Sections of the dorsoventral lamina exhibit the following structures passing from ventral to dorsal surface.

1. *Epidermis*, undulate with thick-walled epidermal cells which are polygonal in vertical view. Numerous non-glandular and glandular hairs emanate from this epidermis, the non-glandular type predominating.

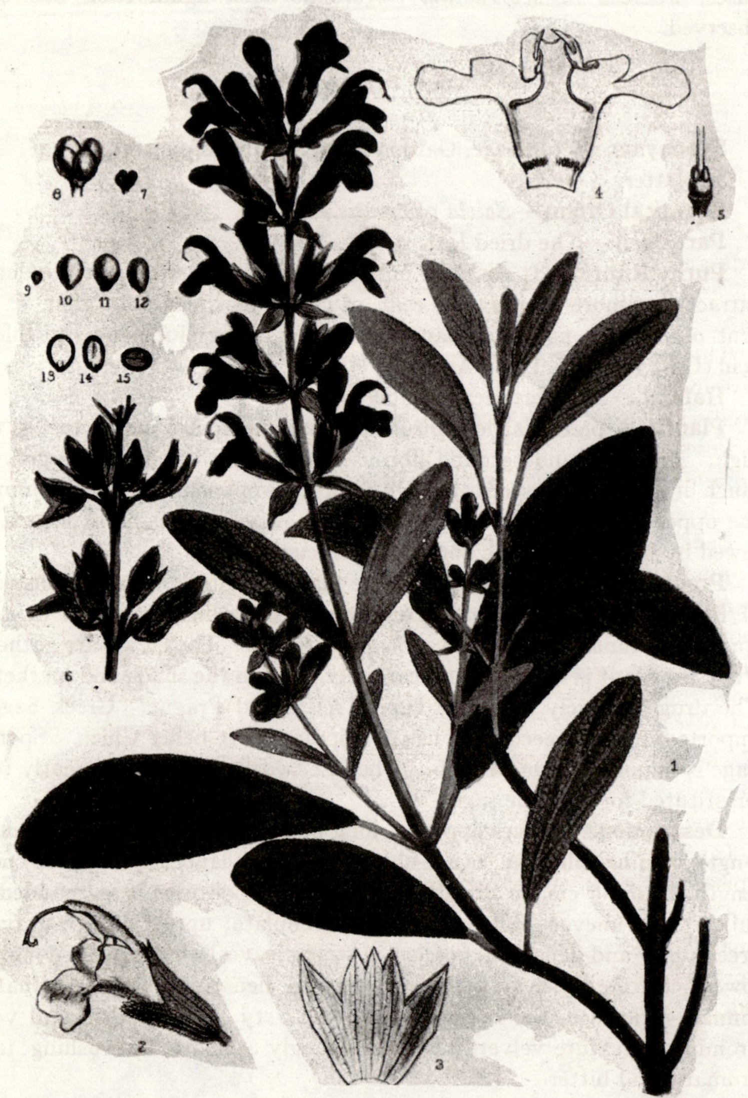

FIG. 237.—*Saliva officinalis*. 1. Portion of plant with leaves and flowers. 2. Flower. 3. Calyx laid open. 4. Corolla laid open. 5. Ovary. 6. Part of flowering stem in fruit. 7, 8. Fruits consisting of groups of 4 nutlets. 9–12. Nutlets. 13, 14. Vertical-, and 15. Transverse section of nutlet. (*After Bentley and Trimen.*)

2. *Palisade parenchyma*, consisting of 1 layer of irregularly columnar cells containing chloroplastids.

3. *Spongy parenchyma*, a zone of rounded parenchyma cells, most of which contain chloroplastids, a few resin.

4. *Lower epidermis*, undulate, consisting of wavy walled epidermal cells and numerous stomata. This epidermis is densely covered with non-glandular and glandular hairs. The non-glandular hairs found on both epidermises are uniseriate, 2- to 5-celled, the end portion being frequently reflexed. The glandular hairs include those having a 1-celled stalk and a 2-celled head, those possessing a 2- to 4-celled stalk and a 1-celled head, and still others which possess an 8-celled glandular head and no stalk.

The midrib shows abundant collenchyma above and below the vascular bundles. Some of the cells contain resin. The medullary rays are 1-cell wide.

Constituents.—Up to 2.5 per cent. of a greenish-yellow volatile oil containing borneol, a sesquiterpene, pinene, thujone and cineol; bitter principle, resin and a tannin.

Uses.—Sage is used chiefly as a condiment but is also employed as a carminative in dyspepsia and as an ingredient in hair dressings.

Adulterants.—(1) Leaves of *Salvia lavandulaefolia* Vahl, commonly known as Spanish Sage, a perennial herb indigenous to Mexico, particularly Sierra Madra, Bolanos and other towns, where it thrives 5000 to 7000 ft. above the sea level. Its leaves are oblong-lanceolate, 1 to 1½ inches long and ¼ to ½ in. broad, smaller than those of *S. officinalis* and tending to be whorled on the stems. The apex is either acute or rounded; the base subcordate or rounded; the margin nearly entire, very slightly crenulate; the surface much smoother than that of *S. officinalis.*

(2) Leaves of *Salvia tribola* Linné, commonly known as Greek Sage, a perennial herb indigenous to Mediterranean countries.

Greek Sage may readily be distinguished from Sage by the leaves usually being broader, shorter, thicker, more wooly and having a very short petiole, and a less pronounced crenulate margin and also by its odor which is characteristically aromatic.

HEDEOMA (PENNYROYAL)

Synonyms.—American Pennyroyal, Squaw Mint, Tickweed, Stinking Balm; *Ger.* Amerikanisher Poleiminze; *Fr.* Pouliot américain.

Botanical Origin.—*Hedeoma pulegioides* Persoon.

Parts Used.—The dried leaves and tops.

Habitat.—North America, in woods and along roadsides.

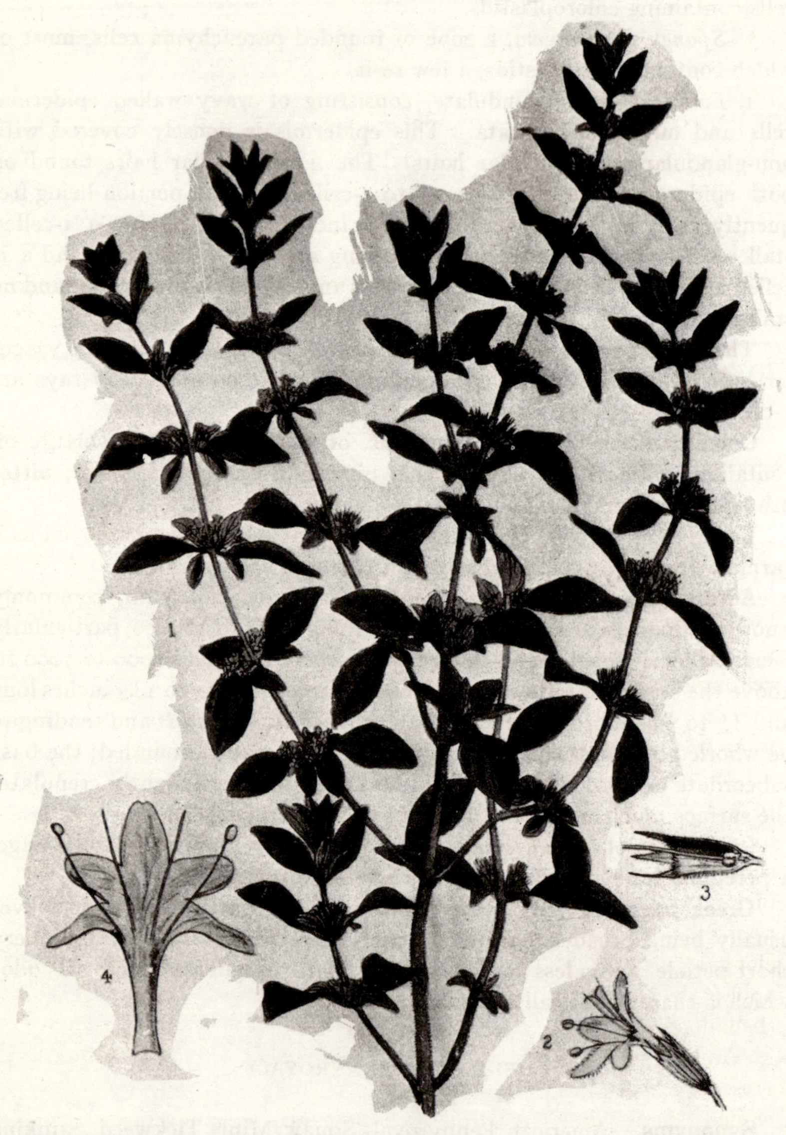

FIG. 238.—*Hedeoma pulegioides.* 1. Upper portion of plant. 2. A flower. 3. Section of calyx. 4. Corolla laid open. (*After Bentley and Trimen.*)

Plant.—An erect, much branched, annual herb from ½ to 1 ft. in height with slender, pubescent stems, opposite, ovate to oblong-ovate leaves which are slightly serrate and about 1 in. in length. The flowers are small, occurring as verticillasters in the leaf axils. Each flower consists of a tubular-bilabiate calyx, a pubescent, purple, bilabiate corolla with an emarginate, erect, flat, upper lip and a lower lip with 3 large spreading lobes, 4 didynamous, pale blue stamens, the 2 lower ones being alone fertile, and a bicarpellate pistil. The odor is characteristically mint like, the taste aromatic and pungent.

Production and Commerce.—American Pennyroyal is gathered for the market chiefly in North Carolina, Virginia and Ohio during the summer. It should be slowly dried and stored in air-tight containers.

Constituents.—Volatile oil containing pulegone ($C_{10}H_{16}O$), hedeomol ($C_{10}H_{18}O$) tannin, etc.

Uses.—Pennyroyal is used chiefly by the laity as a stimulant, carminative and emmenagogue. The oil and spirit have been employed as a mosquito repellant.

SOLANACEÆ (NIGHTSHADE FAMILY)

Stems herbaceous, rarely shrubby or arborescent, frequently with bicollateral bundles. Leaves alternate, exstipulate, entire or more or less lobed, rarely compound; often glandular-hairy. Flowers in cymes; regular or rarely irregular (Petunia, Tobacco spp.), pentamerous, perfect, synphyllous; calyx green (rarely petaloid), rotate to tubular, usually persistent and accrescent; corolla rotate (Solanum), to tubular (Atropa), to funnel-shaped (Tobacco), and so (1) open to all comers, or (2) to bees or wasps, or (3) to butterflies, moths; color, greenish-yellow, or greenish-white to white, to pink, crimson, purple, rarely blue; stamens five, epipetalous, hypogynous, along with style usually forming nectar glands. Filaments short to long, anthers dehiscing longitudinally or by apical pores; pistil bicarpellate, syncarpous, with or without nectar girdle, superior ovary, two celled with central placentation, ovules numerous, style more or less elongate with bilobed or bifid stigma. Fruit, a capsule (Tobacco, Thorn-apple) dehiscing longitudinally or transversely (Henbane); or a berry (belladonna, potato, egg-plant, tomato, red pepper). Seeds albuminous.

Among the histological features of this family are the following: The presence of intraxylary soft bast in the stems and leaves frequently accompanied by sclerenchyma fibers. The inner margin of the intraxylary phloem is often strengthened by sclerenchyma. The sclerenchyma is either in the form of a continuous ring at the margin of the pith or as isolated elements or groups of these in the medullary sheath. Isolated groups of sclerenchyma fibers occur in the pericycle. An occasional stone cell is to be found among these fibers in the genus *Brunfelsia*. The secondary phloem is commonly devoid of bast fibers. Internal secretory organs are absent. The tracheæ exhibit simple pits, bordered pores and often reticulate markings. The stomata are usually surrounded by 3 to 4 neighboring cells, but in *Brunfelsia*, *Juanulloa* and *Dyssochroma* two neighboring cells occur. Uniseriate non-glandular hairs and glandular hairs are frequent. Peltate and tufted hairs occur in the genus *Solanum*. Calcium oxalate occurs in the form of microcrystals, rosette aggregates, solitary crystals and twin prisms.

BELLADONNÆ RADIX U.S.P. (BELLADONNA ROOT)

Synonyms.—Deadly Nightshade Root, Black Cherry Root; *Ger.* Belladonna-wurzel; *Fr.* Racine de Belladonne.

Botanical Origin.—*Atropa Belladonna* Linné.

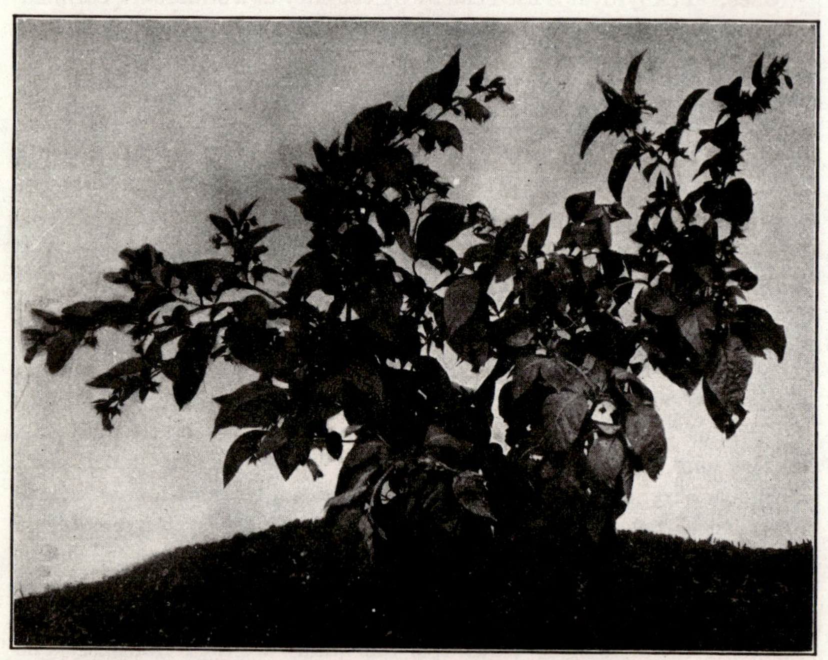

FIG. 239.—*Atropa Belladonna.* (*Photograph by Kilmer.*)

Part Used.—The dried root.

Purity Rubric.—It yields not less than 0.45 per cent. of the alkaloids of Belladonna root and contains not more than 10 per cent. of its stem bases and woody crowns, not more than 2 per cent. of other foreign organic matter. It yields not more than 4 per cent. of acid-insolule ash.

Habitat.—Central and Southern Europe and Asia Minor.

Plant.—A bushy perennial herb with dichotomously branched stems. Leaves alternate, broadly ovate to ovate, entire or nearly entire along margin, acute at summit, tapering at base, dark green. Flowers solitary or rarely in clusters of 2 or 3, axillary and drooping; calyx deeply 5-cleft; corolla dull greenish-purple or reddish-purple, campanulate, with 5 broad, spreading and recurved lobes; stamens 5, epipetalous; style exserted; stigma knob-like. Fruit a sub-glovular black berry with persistent calyx.

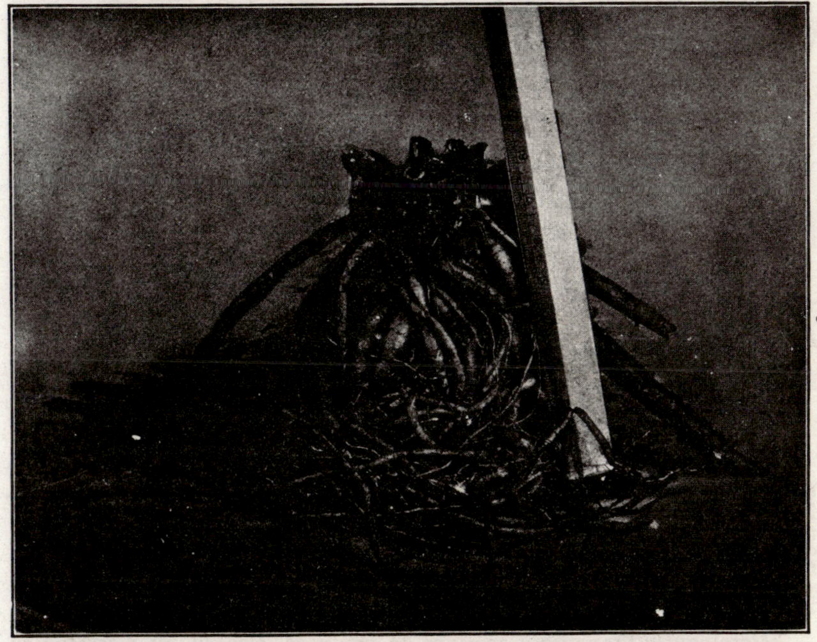

FIG. 240.—Root system of *Atropa Belladonna*. *(Photograph by Kilmer.)*

Production and Commerce.—The roots are plowed from the ground in the fall. The larger roots are split and dried. The drug is obtained largely from plants grown in this country, and Central Europe.

Description.—It occurs as cylindrical or somewhat tapering segments of roots frequently cut longitudinally, and often with a few stem bases, either attached or separate. Roots from 0.5 to 4 cm. thick, externally pale brownish-gray, longitudinally wrinkled, the cork frequently abraded and thus showing lighter patches; fracture nearly smooth, mealy, emitting a puff of dust consisting chiefly of starch grains; internally whitish with a distinct cambium zone and yellowish wood wedges; nearly inodorous, taste sweet, afterwards bitter and strongly acrid. Stem fragments light-brown or greenish-brown; finely longitudinally wrinkled, with annulations due to leaf scars and usually exhibiting a hollow pith.

Belladonna Root possesses a peculiar strongly narcotic odor on boiling.

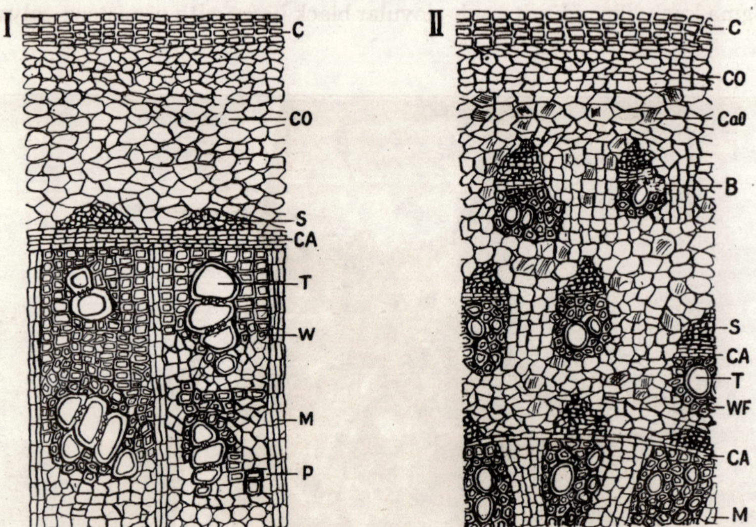

FIG. 241.—*I*, Transverse section of Belladonna root. Cork (*C*); cortex (*CO*); sieve tissue (*S*); cambium (*Ca*); tracheæ (*T*); wood fibers (*W*); medullary ray (*M*); wood parenchyma (*P*). The older the root of belladonna, the more wood fibers present. *II*, Transverse section of poke root (*Phytolacca decandra*). Cork (*C*); cortex (*CO*); raphides of calcium oxalate (*CaO*); open collateral fibrovascular bundle (*B*); phloem (*S*); cambium (*CA*); trachea (*T*) and wood fibers (*WF*) of xylem; medullary-ray (*M*).

Histology.—Transverse sections of the root, cleared by warming in chloral solution exhibit the following characteristics:

1. *Cork* composed of several rows of tangentially elongated cork cells.
2. *Phellogen* (cork cambium) of more or less collapsed meristematic cells.
3. *Secondary cortex* of cortical parenchyma cells many of which possess a grayish or black aspect, due to the presence of numerous micro-crystals. The parenchyma cells have pitted walls.
4. *Phloem*, a narrow zone of sieve tube and phloem cell masses separated by broad phloem medullary-rays. The sieve tubes and phloem cells may readily be distinguished from the cells of the cortex region by their smaller size. No bast fibers occur in this region.

5. *Cambium*, a prominent ring of somewhat collapsed meristematic cells.

6. *Xylem*, taking up the central and greater area of the section. This is seen to be composed of radially elongated xylem patches separated by broad xylem medullary rays. Each xylem patch is composed of a matrix of wood parenchyma in which are to be observed more or less radially elongated groups of tracheæ with thickened yellowish walls. Adhering to these are usually a few tracheids with thickened yellowish walls. In old woody roots, wood fibers replace considerable of the wood parenchyma. Some of the cells of the wood parenchyma and medullary rays possess a

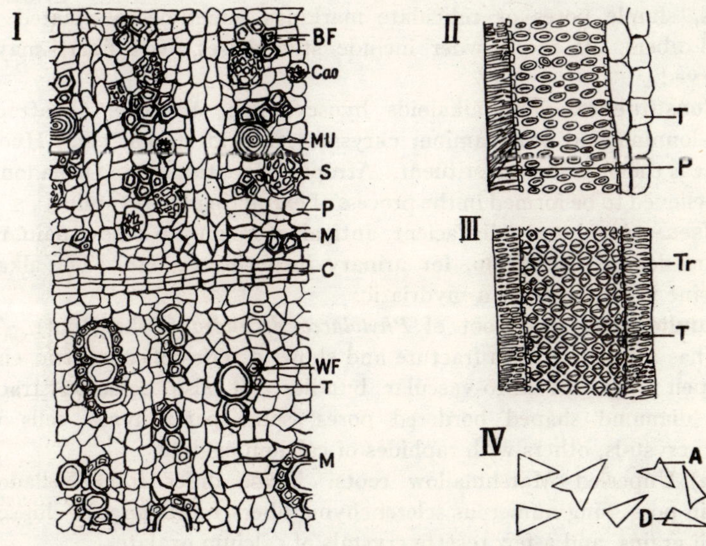

FIG. 242.—*I*, Transverse section of *Althæa* showing bast fibers (*BF*); rosette aggregates of calcium oxalate (*CaO*); mucilage sacs (*MU*); sieve tissue (*S*); phloem parenchyma (*P*); cambium (*C*); wood fibers (*WP*); tracheæ (*T*) and medullary-rays (*M*). *II*, Longitudinal section through bundle region of *Belladonna root*. Reticulate tracheid (*P*); wood parenchyma (*T*). Between *T* and *P* will be noted a broad trachea with ellipsoidal shaped bordered pores. *III*, Longitudinal section through portion of bundle of *Phytolacca root*. Trachea with diamond shaped bordered pores (*T*); reticulate trachea (*Tr*). *IV*, Micro-crystals from belladonna. (*A*) Arrow shaped; (*D*) deltoid.

grayish or blackish appearance. These contain sphenoidal micro-crystals.

Transverse sections mounted in water show that the majority of the parenchyma and medullary-ray cells are filled with starch.

Longitudinal-radial sections mounted in chloral solution show broad tracheæ with ellipsoidal bordered pores, tracheæ with simple pores, and reticulate markings, pitted tracheids, elongated and pitted wood parenchyma often associated with somewhat wavy-walled wood fibers having oblique slit-like pores. The parenchyma cells of the cortex appear somewhat axially elongated. Micro-crystals are visible in a number of praenchyma cells scattered throughout the section.

Sections of the stem bases show a circle of bi-collateral bundles, both phloem regions of each bundle exhibiting thin-walled, slightly lignified bast fibers, arranged singly and in small groups.

Powdered Drug.—Light brown; starch grains numerous, usually from 3 to 15μ, but occasionally up to 30μ in diameter, spheroidal, plano-convex, polygonal, and 2- to 6- or more compound; fragments of parenchyma, some of the cells of which contain numerous sphenoidal microcrystals the latter also occurring free in the powder and from 3 to 10μ in length; fragments of cork, fragments of tracheæ and tracheids, with bordered pores, simple pores or reticulate markings sometimes associated with wood fibers. If the powder include stem bases, bast fibers may be observed.

Constituents.—The alkaloids hyoscyamine, atropine, apoatropine, belladonnine and scopolamine; chrysatropic acid starch, etc. Hyoscyamine is the principal constituent. Atropine, apoatropine and belladonnine are believed to be formed in the process of extracting hyoscyamine.

Uses.—Anodyne, delirifacient, antigalactagogue; to relieve pain, relax spasm, decrease secretion, for urinary incontinence, etc. The alkaloid atropine is employed as a mydriatic.

Adulterants.—(1) Root of *Phytolacca decandra* (Poke Root). This root has a tough fibrous fracture and shows a series of concentric circles of open collateral fibro-vascular bundles. It also possesses tracheæ with diamond shaped bordered pores, some parenchyma cells with micro-crystals, others with raphides of calcium oxalate.

(2) Unpeeled Marshmallow roots. These differ from Belladonna root in possessing numerous sclerenchyma fibers, mucilage sacs, ellipsoidal starch grains, and a few rosette crystals of calcium oxalate.

(3) Rhizomes of *Scopolia carniolica*. These are devoid of tracheæ with bordered pores, but possess characteristic, often barrel-shaped, reticulate tracheæ.

BELLADONNÆ FOLIA U. S. P. (BELLADONNA LEAVES).

Synonyms.—Deadly Nightshade Leaves, Black Cherry Leaves, Death's Herb, *Ger.* Tollkraut, Belladonna Blätter; *Fr.* Morelle furieuse, Feuilles de Belladonne.

Botanical Origin.—*Atropa Belladonna* Linné.

Part Used.—The dried leaves and tops.

Limit of Impurities.—Not more than 3 per cent. of their stems over 10 mm. in diameter.

Standard of Assay.—Not less than 0.3 per cent. of total alkaloids of Belladonna Leaves.

Ash.—Not more than 3 per cent. acid-insoluble.

Production and Commerce.—Probably more Belladonna is grown in this country than any other drug plant. It is also extensively grown in Jugo Slavia and other Central European districts, in England and India. The plants are propagated either from seeds or roots. The seeds should be sown in a cold frame in December and the young seedlings transferred

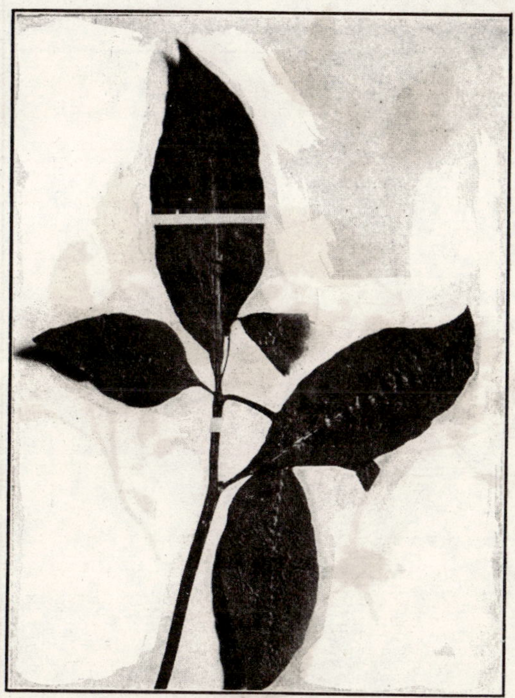

FIG. 243.—*Scopolia carniolica.* Branch, leaves and flower. An adulterant for Belladonnæ Folia.

to flats or pots in April. Potting produces a firmer root. When sufficiently strong, the seedlings should be set out 3 feet apart in each direction. The best soil is deep, well drained, moist loam, which should be well limed. Too much moisture in the soil is injurious. In propagating from roots, either whole roots may be employed or the crowns may be divided. These are planted in holes dug in the ground about 3 feet in each direction and are covered with an inch or two of soil. In localities where frost penetrates deeply into the ground, the roots should be removed in the fall and replanted in the spring. The plants should be cultivated to free the soil from too many weeds. Two crops of leaves can be gathered from first year plants. Two to four cuttings may be taken from second or third year plants. The leaves should be kept in the shade and dried with the aid of artificial heat. It is well to start with a moderate heat and gradually increase to 160° or 180° and then gradually decrease. Leaves dried artificially are generally of a richer green color and so usually demand a higher price than those dried in the sun. They are not necessarily richer in alkaloids than leaves which are sun dried and so of a more brownish-green color.

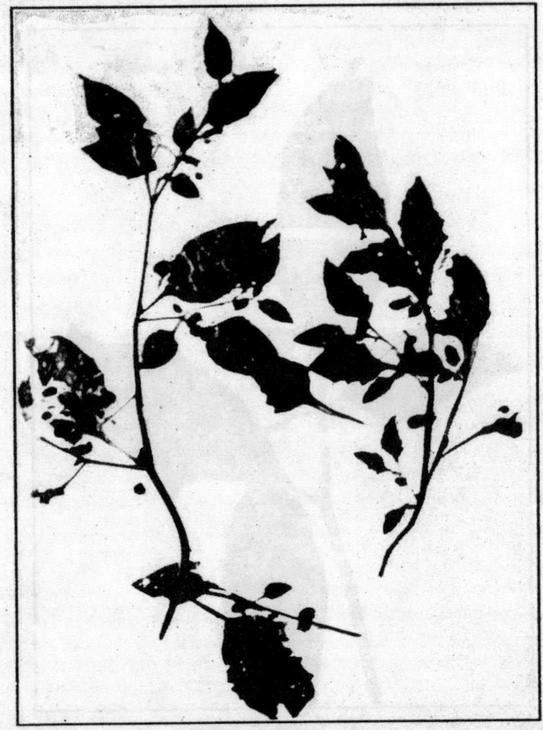

Fig. 244.—*Solanum nigrum.* The leaves and tops of this plant have been employed as an adulterant of Belladonnæ Folia.

Most of the drug used in the United States is obtained from plants cultivated in that country. On account of the great demand considerable of the drug is imported in large bales from Central Europe. The most important shipping points for the European article are Trieste, Hamburg, Rotterdam, Amsterdam, Budapest and Brussels.

Description.—Usually as matted leaves and tops with stem segments; leaves crumpled; when soaked in water and spread out, the entire leaves from 6 to 20 cm. in length 4 to 12 cm. in breadth, broadly ovate, slightly hairy, summits acute, margins entire, narrowed into the long petioles; upper surfaces brownish-green, lower surfaces grayish-green; flowers with yellowish-purple campanulate corollas; fruits globular, 2-celled berries, subtended by a 5-toothed persistent calyx and with many small seeds; odor somewhat tobacco-like especially on moistening; taste bitter and acrid. Stems of variable length and not over 10 mm. in diameter, longitudinally wrinkled, older parts smooth and usually hollow, younger parts flattened and hairy.

Histology.—Transverse and surface sections of the leaves may be prepared by placing the dried material in a moist chamber for 24 hours before the sections are cut. The epidermis may be readily separated by gently warming small fragments in solution of chloral hydrate or 1 per cent. sodium or potassium hydrate in a watch crystal for about 5 minutes, transferring to slide and exerting slight pressure on the cover slip with a rotary movement.

Both epidermises are composed of large wavy-walled epidermal cells with stomata and striated cuticle. The epidermal cells over the veins, however, have rectilinear walls, as observed in vertical view. There are a larger number of stomata on the lower than on the upper surface. Each stoma is surrounded by 3 or less often 4 neighboring cells, one of which is smaller than the rest. Non-glandular and glandular hairs occur as outgrowths from both epidermises. The former are thin-walled, uniseriate, of from 2 to 6 cells, occasionally showing terminal branching. The glandular hairs are to two kinds; one possesses a 2- to 4-celled stalk and a 1-celled head, the other a 1-celled stalk and a pluricellular head.

The mesophyll between the epidermises exhibits a layer of short palisade cells directly beneath the upper epidermis and several layers of spongy parenchyma. Most of these cells contain chloroplastids but grayish-black cells may be observed scattered here and there. These are filled with sphenoidal microcrystals (crystal sand). The midrib and veins show bicollateral bundles.

Powdered Drug.—Dark green; fragments of mesophyll containing grayish to grayish-black, to black cells scattered amongst chlorophyll parenchyma and containing microcrystals; fragments of epidermis with large, wavy-walled cells and stomata, the latter surrounded by 3 or 4 neighboring cells, one of which is smaller than the others; hairs few and generally broken the non-glandular being uniseriate and 2 to 5 cells in length, the glandular with stalks of 1 to 4 cells (usually 1–3) and 1- to many-celled heads; fragments of flowers and fruits; pollen grains few with 3 furrows; fragments of stem tissues with characteristic slightly lignified bast fibers, annular, spiral, reticulate and bordered pore tracheæ; fragments of seed coats with convolute, thickened cell walls.

Constituents.—The alkaloids, hyoscyamine (lævorotatory), atropine (optically inactive), belladonnine, scopolamine (hyoscine); chrysatropic acid, etc. Hyoscyamine is the chief constituent. The other alkaloids are thought to be formed from it in the process of extraction.

Uses.—See under Belladonna root.

Adulterants.—(1) Poke Leaves, detected by raphides in addition to microcrystals of calcium oxalate; (2) *Solanum nigrum* or Black Nightshade leaves and tops. The leaves of this plant are ovate and wavy-toothed, its corolla white and rotate. Glandular hairs were absent on the leaves examined; (3) Malva Leaves, detected by numerous stellate hairs and mucilage cells; (4) Scopolia Leaves and tops, detected by characteristic reticulate tracheæ, more lanceolate leaves, and short calyx tubes each containing a nearly spherical pyxis.

STRAMONIUM U.S.P. (STRAMONIUM)

Synonyms.—Jamestown Weed, Jimson Weed, Thorn Apple, Apple of Peru; *Ger.* Stechapfel, Dornapfel; *Fr.* Pomme-épineuse, Stramoine.

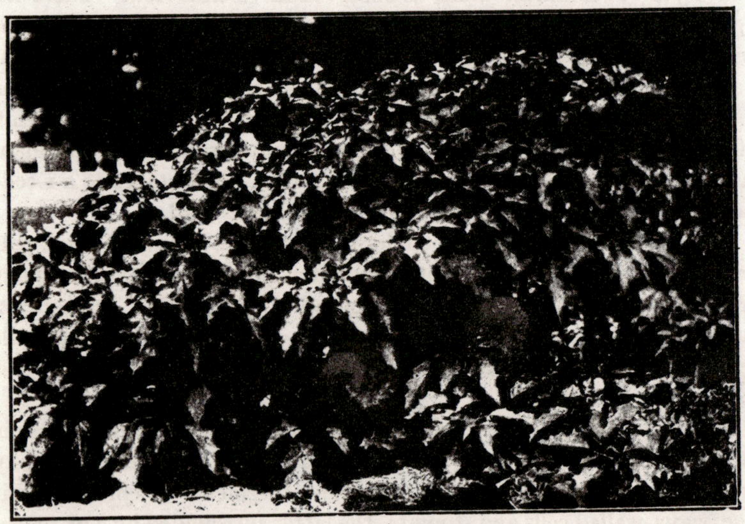

FIG. 245.—*Datura Stramonium.* Note the sinuate-dentate margins of the leaves.

Botanical Origin.—*Datura Stramonium* Linné.

Part Used.—The dried leaves and flowering tops.

Limit of Impurities.—Not more than 3 per cent. of stems over 8 mm. in diameter.

Standard Assay.—Not less than 0.25 per cent. of the alkaloids of Stramonium.

Ash.—Not more than 4 per cent. acid-insoluble.

Habitat.—Asia. Naturalized in fields, waste places and along roadsides in the United States, Canada and Europe.

Plant.—*Datura Stramonium* is an annual, rank smelling herb attaining a height of from 1 to 1.6 m. Its stem is glabrous and divides into 2 or 3 green branches, which in turn bifurcate and bear alternate inequilaterally-ovate, acuminate leaves with sinuate-dentate margins. The flowers appear in the forks of the branches on short peduncles. Each consists of a green, prismatic, 5-toothed calyx, a white funnel-shaped corolla with 5 teeth, epipetalous stamens and a bicarpellate pistil whose ovary is 4-celled below, 2-celled near the top. The fruit is a prickly, 4-valved capsule, the lower prickles of which are mostly shorter than those above. The seeds are flattened, reniform, brownish-black, with white, oily albumen surrounding an embryo which is curved parallel to the seed margin.

Datura Tatula Linné, closely resembles the former species in habit, differing mainly from it in having purplish stems, lavender colored flowers and capsules which are nearly equally prickly. This plant was recognized as an additional source of the drug in the U.S.P. ix.

Production and Commerce.—Stramonium grows abundantly as a weed on waste lots and along roadsides in the eastern and central sections of this country. It is cultivated on drug farms in several sections of the United States, Germany, France and Hungary. The plants may be propagated from seeds sown early in the spring in drills about 3 feet apart. When sufficiently strong the young plants may be transplanted to stand 2 feet apart in rows. Cultivation is necessary. The leaves are gathered while the plants are in full flower and dried in the shade at a temperature of 100° to 110°F. They are then baled for shipment. Stramonium is collected for the market in large amounts in the North Carolina section. It is also imported in large amounts from Europe. The imported article is shipped in burlap bags from Budapest, Hamburg and Leghorn.

Description.—The drug occurs as more or less matted together, wrinkled leaves and stem fragments or in the loose condition; laminæ, when entire, up to 30 cm. in length, with petioles up to 8 cm. in length; inequilaterally ovate, summits acute or acuminate, bases unequal, margins sinuate-dentate; frequently with circular perforations, which may have become filled with or surrounded by cork; upper surfaces dark green, sparsely hairy, especially upon the veins, lower surfaces light green. Stems light greenish-brown to purplish-brown, longitudinally wrinkled and furrowed, often flattened. Odor characteristically heavy and narcotic; taste disagreeable.

Histology of *Datura Stramonium* Leaves. Transverse sections cut through the lamina including the midrib and mounted in chloral solution show the following peculiarities:

1. Midrib, convex above and more greatly convex below. In the center is to be noted a concavo-convex meristele of bi-collateral bundles the phloem regions of which are devoid of bast fibers. The xylem regions of the bundles are provided with rather broad tracheæ. Directly beneath the epidermis of both upper and lower surfaces will be found several layers of collenchyma cells. Between the collenchyma and the meristele occurs parenchyma tissue, some of the cells of which are filled with

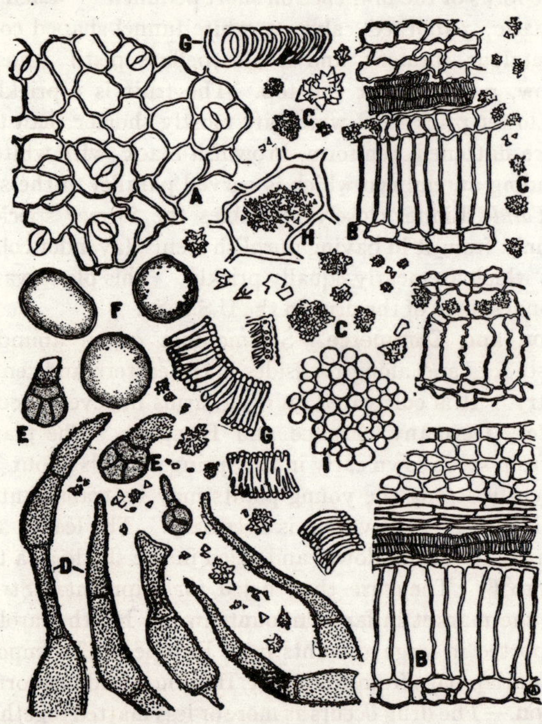

FIG. 246.—Powdered Stramonium, × 183. A, Epidermis, surface view. B, Transverse section of leaf. C, Rosette aggregates of calcium oxalate. D, Non-glandular trichomes. E, Glandular trichomes. F, Pollen grains. G, Fragments of tracheæ. H, Spongy parenchyma cell containing sphenoidal micro-crystals. I, Palisade parenchyma in surface view. (*After Sayre.*)

sphenoidal microcrystals; other although fewer cells of this region contain rosette aggregates or rod-like prisms of calcium oxalate.

2. Lamina, showing stomata on both epidermises. The mesophyll consists of a layer of elongated, narrow palisade cells with chloroplast contents and a dense spongy parenchyma. The palisade zone occupies

about one-half of the mesophyll. Directly beneath it is a layer which, while constituting the upper cells of the spongy parenchyma, is sometimes termed the crystal layer, since many of its cells possess rosette aggregates of calcium oxalate. Of the remainder of the spongy parenchyma cells, most possess chloroplastids, a few microcrystals and rod-like prisms.

Surface sections of the upper epidermis, mounted in chloral solution, exhibit mostly wavy-walled cells and elliptical stomata. The latter have 3 (or seldom 4) neighboring cells, one of which is smaller than the others. Surface sections of the lower epidermis show the cell walls to be more wavy than those of the upper epidermis. The stomata are more numerous and are surrounded by 3 or 4 neighboring cells, one of which is smaller than the rest. Both non-glandular and glandular hairs may be observed as outgrowths from both upper and lower epidermis. These are more abundant on younger than older leaves. The non-glandular hairs are uniseriate usually 2 to 3 cells in length, never more than 5 cells long. The basal cell averaged 38μ in width in 50 measured hairs. Some of the cells are more or less collapsed. The outer walls show numerous slight centrifugal projections. The glandular hairs have a 1- to 2-celled stalk and a 2- to 4-celled glandular head.

Histologic Differences Between D. Stramonium and D. Tatula Leaves

Datura Stramonium	Datura Tatula
Stomata of upper epidermis surrounded by 3, very seldom 4 neighboring cells.	Stomata of upper epidermis surrounded by 4, very seldom 3 neighboring cells.
Stomata of lower epidermis surrounded by 3 to 4 neighboring cells.	Stomata of lower epidermis surrounded by 2, 3, 4, or 5 neighboring cells.
Non-glandular hairs, uniseriate, usually 2 or 3 cells, never more than 5 cells in length.	Non-glandular hairs, uniseriate, and from 3 to 8 cells in length.

Adulterants.—(1) Leaves of *Xanthium Strumarium* Linné, which are devoid of rosette crystals and of stomata on upper surface. They possess very short, non-glandular hairs, each with a broad basal cell containing a cystolith and a pointed, terminal cell that is frequently bent over. They contain rod-shaped crystals of calcium oxalate.

(2) Leaves of *Carthamus helenoides* Desfontaines which differ from Stramonium in possessing large rectilinear epidermal cells with striated cuticle and in the absence of rosette aggregates.

(3) Leaves of *Xanthium macrocarpum* DC. (4) Leaves of *Chenopodium hybridum* Linné.

Constituents.—The alkaloid hyoscyamine, and possibly atropine and scopolamine; resin, etc.

Uses.—Stramonium is chiefly used to relax the bronchial muscle in the bronchial spasms of asthma.

HYOSCYAMUS U.S.P. (HYOSCYAMUS)

Synonyms.—Henbane, Hyoscyami folium, Black Henbane, Hog's Bean, Stinking Nightshade; *Ger.* Bilsenkrautblätter; *Fr.* Jusquiame.

Botanical Origin.—*Hyoscyamus niger* Linné.

Part Used.—The dried leaf with or without the tops.

Standard of Assay—Not less than 0.065 per cent. of the alkaloids of Hyoscyamus.

Limit of Impurities.—25 per cent. of its stems, none of which is more than 7 mm. in thickness. Not more than 12 per cent. of acid-insoluble ash.

Habitat.—Europe and Asia.

Plant.—A biennial or annual, fetid, narcotic herb growing to the height of from 0.6 to 1.4 m. Its underground portion consists of a large, brown, fleshy, branching root, somewhat resembling parsley root, for which it has been mistaken with disastrous results. Its aerial portions consists of a pubescent, branching stem bearing alternate, ovate or ovate-oblong, clasping, grayish-green leaves having a sinuate-dentate margin and acute apex. The flowers appear usually in July and August on one sided leafy spikes. Each show a green, urn-shaped, 5-toothed, hairy calyx, a 5-lobed, dull yellow, campanulate corolla, the lobes being unequal, the veins purple and reticulate, 5 stamens with purple anthers and a bicarpellary pistil with purple style. The fruit is a 2-celled pyxis, enclosed in a persistent calyx.

Production and Commerce.—Hyoscyamus grows wild in waste places of lower Canada, north central United States, Europe and Asia. It is also cultivated from seeds. Good results have been obtained by sowing the seed in small pots under glass in December and January, transplanting to 3-inch pots in March and transferring to the field in early May. The plants are set in rows about 18 inches apart. The soil should be deep loam, kept moist, well drained and limed. Like other Solanaceous plants, Hyoscyamus is susceptible to attacks of the potato beetle, which has destroyed large crops. The writer has found that occasional spraying with a dilute solution of lead arsenate is advantageous in retarding the depredations of this pest. The leaves and flowering tops should be gathered while the plants are in full flower. They should be dried in the shade. Some of the drug used in this country is procured from drug farms. Considerable, however, is imported from Europe, mainly through London.

Description.—The drug occurs as wrinkled, matted, and broken leaves intermixed with numerous stems and flowering and fruiting tops. Leaves when entire attaining a length of 26 cm., a breadth of 10 cm., ovate or ovate-oblong, inequilateral, the lower petiolate, the upper sessile, summits

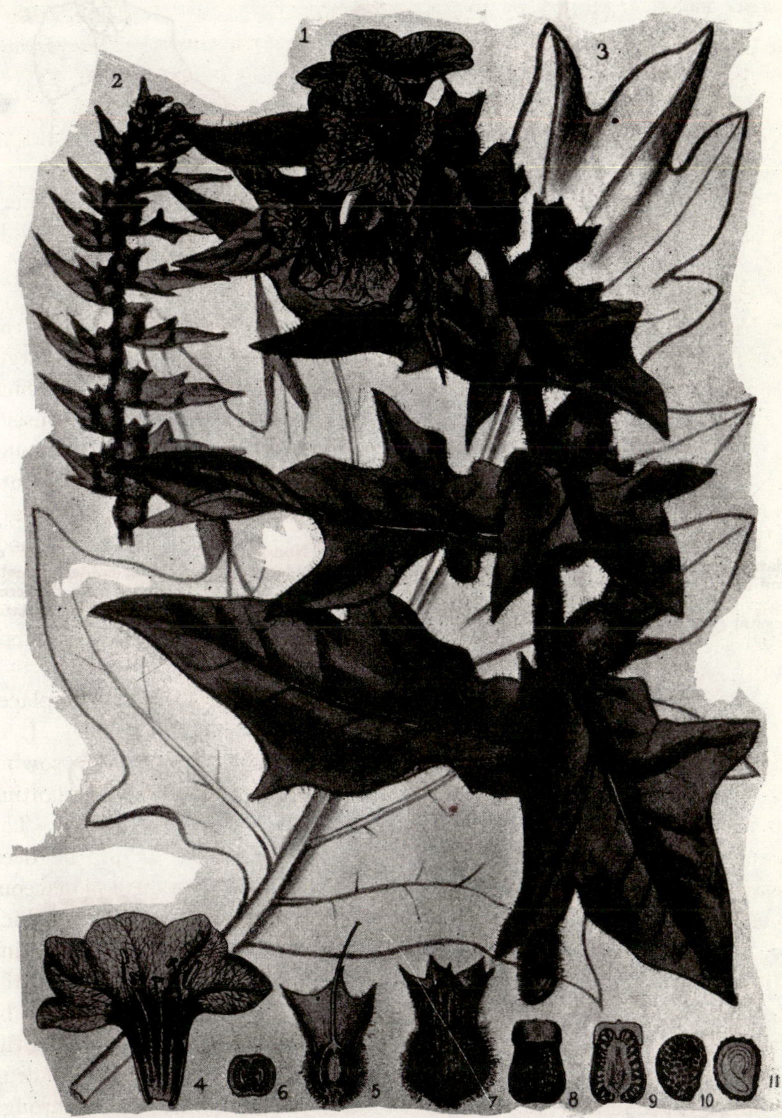

FIG. 247.—*Hyoscyamus niger*. 1. A flowering branch. 2. The same, in fruit below. 3. A radical leaf. 4. Corolla cut open. 5. Vertical section of calyx and ovary. 6. Transverse section of ovary. 7. Ripe fruiting calyx. 8. Pyxis. 9. Vertical section of pyxis. 10. Seed. (*After Bentley and Trimen.*)

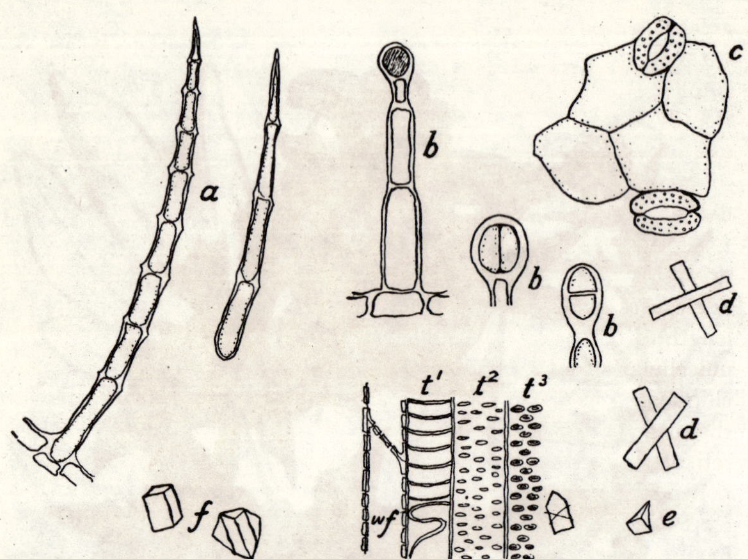

FIG. 248.—Hyoscyamus. Histological elements. Non-glandular hairs (*a*); types of glandular hairs (*b*); surface view of portion of lower epidermis (*c*), showing epidermal cells and stomata; wood fiber (*wf*); spiral trachea (t^1); porous trachea(t^2); trachea with bordered pores (t^3); twin crystals of calcium oxalate (*d*); micro-crystal (*e*); monoclinic prism and twin crystal (*f*).

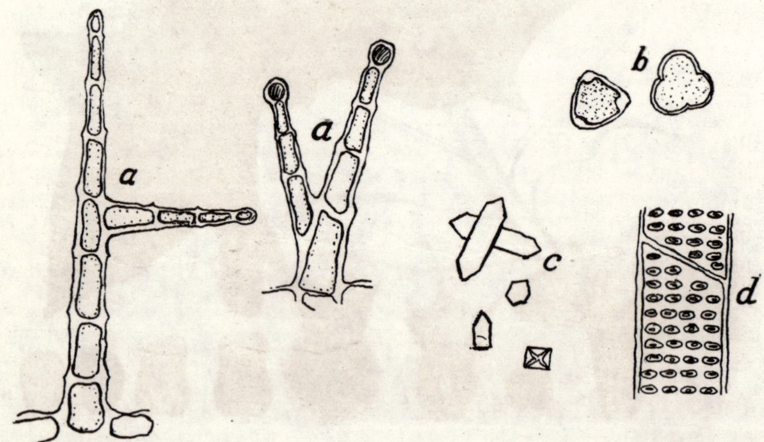

FIG. 249.—*Hyoscyamus muticus.* Diagnostic histological elements. Branched hairs (*a*); pollen grains (*b*); types of calcium oxalate crystals (*c*); portions of two adjacent tracheæ with bordered pores (*d*).

acute, margins coarsely and angularly 1- to 4-toothed or lobed, grayish-green, glandular-hairy, especially on lower surfaces; flowers nearly sessile with a 5-toothed urn-shaped, hairy calyx and a yellow campanulate corolla; fruit a 2-chambered urn-shaped pyxis, enclosed in a large urn-shaped, 5-toothed calyx; odor heavy and distinct; taste somewhat bitter and acrid. The stems are up to 20 cm. in length, from 2 to 10 cm. in diameter, compressed-cylindrical, hollow, longitudinally wrinkled and hairy.

Powdered Drug. Grayish-green; calcium oxalate in 4- to 6-sided prisms, twin crystals up to 25μ long, microcrystals, occasionally in rosette aggregates about 20μ in diameter; non-glandular hairs from 1–10 cells in length, often broken; glandular hairs with a 1- to 4-celled stalk and a unicellular or multicellular head; fragments of epidermis with broadly elliptical stomata with 3 or 4 neighboring cells, one of which is smaller than the others; fragments of tracheæ with simple or bordered pores and reticulate or spiral thickenings, often associated with sclerenchyma fibers; pollen grains nearly smooth spherical in water mounts, with a 3 radiating furrows, having a pore in the middle of each furrow, elliptical in alcohol mounts and up to about 40μ in diameter.

Constituents.—Hyoscyamine, a crystalline alkaloid, hyoscine (scopolamine), an amorphous alkaloid, hyoscypicrin, a glucoside; volatile oil, etc.

Uses.—Hyoscyamus is used to check vesical spasm in urinary incontinence and is also combined with purgatives to obviate their griping action. The alkaloids hyoscyamine and scopolamine are employed as somnifacients.

Adulterant.—The leaves and tops of *Hyoscyamus muticus* Linné from Egypt have frequently been admixed with the imported drug. This spurious article may be readily detected by peculiar branching non-glandular hairs which occur both on the leaves and stems. It has been used by some manufacturers as a source of hyoscyamine, which is present in amounts varying from 0.2 to 1.0 per cent. Samples offered to purchasers in this country have consisted chiefly of thick, broken, yellowish stems, few leaf fragments and cylindrical-shaped pyxes. (See Fig. 249.)

MANACA N.F. (MANACA)

Synonyms.—Vegetable Mercury, Manacan, Geratacaca.

Botanical Origin.—*Brunfelsia Hopeana* Benth. (*Franciscea uniflora* Pohl.).

Part Used.—The dried root.

Habitat.—Brazil and West Indies.

Plant.—A slender, twigy shrub growing along lowland streams. It possesses entire lanceolate-oblong leaves, solitary or paired violet blue flowers which later turn white and berry fruits.

Commercial Source.—Brazil.

Description.—It occurs in subcylindrical or somewhat tortuous segments of the root of variable length and up to 3 cm. in diameter; externally dark brown or reddish-brown, wrinkled and with scaly cork patches, the latter easily separating from the thin cortex which firmly adheres to the yellowish wood; fracture tough and short; odor indistinct; taste bitter.

Powdered Drug.—Pale yellow; numerous fragments of thick-walled lignified fibers associated with tracheæ having bordered pores and medullary-ray cells, the latter with lignified, porous walls; rosette aggregates of calcium oxalate; fragments of cortical parenchyma with some cells containing yellowish-brown amorphous contents, others spheroidal starch grains up to about 15μ in diameter; thick-walled stone cells.

Constituents.—The alkaloid, manacine; manaceine, a fluorescent substance, resin, starch and calcium oxalate.

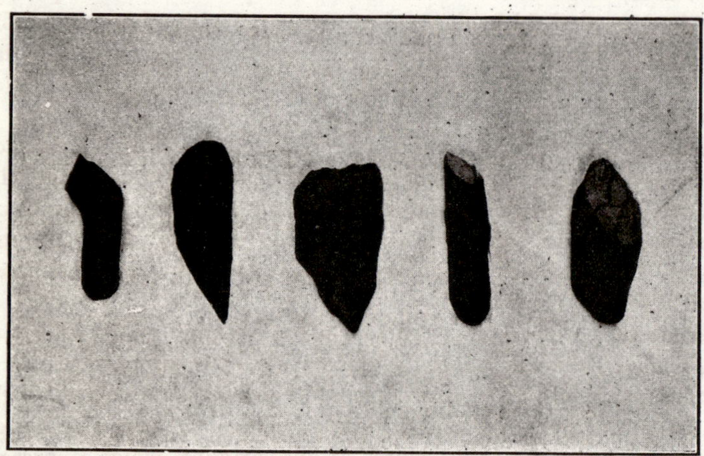

Fig. 250.—Manaca, × 28/56. (*Photograph by Stoneback.*)

Uses.—Manaca is used in the treatment of rheumatism and syphilis.

Allied Drug.—Under the aboriginal name of Miré, the rhizome, root, aerial stem and leaf of *Brunfelsia hydrangæformis* (Fam. *Solanaceæ*) are used by the natives of Bolivia as a muscular paralyzant and remedy for cutaneous parasites. For structural details of drug see Jour. A. Ph. A. vol. xiv, p. 195, 1925.

SOLANUM N.F. (SOLANUM)

Synonym.—Horse Nettle Berries.

Botanical Origin.—*Solanum carolinense* Linné.

Part Used.—The air-dried ripe fruit.

Purity Rubric.—Not more than 5 per cent. of immature fruit and not more than 2 per cent. of foreign organic matter.

Habitat.—Eastern United States in fields and waste places.

Plant.—A rough, pubescent, perennial herb with prickly stem, alternate ovate to oblong, sinuate-dentate or sinuate, pinnately-divided leaves and racemes of violet, rarely white colored flowers. The fruit is a yellowish, globular, 2-celled berry.

Production and Commerce.—Horse Nettle grows wild in dry fields from southern Canada to Illinois and south to the Gulf of Mexico. The fruits are collected when ripe during the summer and dried in the sun. The commercial supply is obtained almost entirely from plants growing wild in this country.

Description.—Berries globose, somewhat shriveled and wrinkled, from 0.8 to 2 cm. in diameter, orange-yellow, glabrous, fleshy, 2-celled, many-seeded, calyx and pedicel usually persistent; calyx pubescent, 5-lobed, the lobes enclosing half or more of the berry, seeds flat, yellow, orbicular: odor pepper-like; taste bitter and acrid.

Constituents.—Solanine (alkaloid), fat, volatile oil, resin, etc.

Use.—Horse Nettle Berries are employed in the treatment of epilepsy.

CAPSICUM U.S.P. (CAPSICUM)

Synonyms.—Cayenne Pepper, Red Pepper, African Chillies, Spanish-, Mombassa-, Mexican- or Sierra Leone Pepper; *Fr.* Capsique; *Ger.* Schlotenpfeffer.

Botanical Origin.—*Capsicum frutescens* Linné.

Part Used.—The dried ripe fruit.

Limit of Impurities.—3 per cent. of its stems, calyxes and one per cent. of other foreign organic matter.

Standard of Assay.—Not less than 12 per cent. of non-volatile extractive, soluble in ether.

Ash.—Not more than 1.25 per cent. acid-insoluble.

Habitat.—Tropical America.

Plant.—An annual herb.

Production and Commerce.—The plants are cultivated in United States, Mexico, India, Japan, and British East Africa but only the African grown fruit is officially recognized by the U.S.P. The fruits are collected when fully mature, deprived of their calyxes and carefully dried. Most of the drug used in this country is imported from Zanzibar, Mombassa, Nyasal and Sierra Leone.

Description.—Oblong-conical from 8 to 25 mm. in length and from 4 to 8 mm. in diameter; pericarp thin leathery, brownish-red or orange, shining, membranous and translucent; 2- or 3-locular with thin dissepiments and containing 6 to 20 flat, reniform, yellowish seeds each of which contains a curved embryo; seeds attached to central placenta or frequently separated from it; odor characteristic, sternutatory; taste intensely pungent, that of the dissepiments more pungent than the pericarp. The calyx, when present, is light greenish-brown, inferior, 5-toothed and generally attached to a long peduncle.

Histology.—Transverse sections of the **pericarp** of African Cayenne, mounted in chloral hydrate solution, show the following characteristics:

1. *Epicarp*, an outer layer of tangentially elongated epidermal cells, whose outer walls and greater portion of the radial walls are cutinized.

2. *Mesocarp*, composed of several layers of parenchyma cells, many containing yellowish-red oil globules and chromoplastids, others micro-crystals of calcium oxalate. Coursing through this region are a few bicollateral bundles with spiral and pitted tracheæ. The innermost layer of cells of the mesophyll consists of very large cells (giant cells).

3. *Endocarp*, comprising a single row of cells, some of which are sclerenchymatous, others parenchymatous. The former occur directly beneath the lumina of the giant cells and have thick, lignified, porous walls.

Surface sections of the **epicarp** exhibit rows of rectangular, parallel, mostly 4-sided, straight-walled epidermal cells, having a striated cuticle.

Surface sections of the **endocarp** exhibit elliptical shaped groups of stone cells separated by narrow zones of parenchyma cells. The stone cells are more or less elongated, moderately thickened, porous and slightly lignified and have wavy vertical walls.

Transverse sections of the **dissepiment** show a central zone of tangentially-elongated, more or less collapsed cells, some of which contain micro-crystals. Fibrovascular tissue courses through this region. Flanking this zone on either side is an epidermis of radially elongated cells containing capsaicin, a pungent principle. The outer walls of the epidermal cells are cutinized. Here and there, where the cuticle has has been puckered up, it is possible to see oily droplets of capsaicin.

Transverse sections of the **seeds** exhibit the following peculiarities:

1. *Spermoderm*, (*a*) Outer epidermis shows large, more or less radially elongated, stone cells with irregularly thickened radial and inner walls. The radial walls of each of these show a thickening of lignin which gradually increases toward the inner wall. The inner wall is extremely thickened in the angles, less so in the center. (*b*) A narrow zone of collapsed parenchyma. (*c*) Inner epidermis of a row of tangentially-elongated epidermal cells.

2. *Endosperm*, a broad zone of reserve parenchyma, composed of more or less thick-walled, polygonal cells containing aleurone grains.

3. *Embryo*, appearing in this kind of section as more or less circular areas of cells lined with epidermis and embedded in the endosperm. The cotyledons may be distinguished from the hypocotyl by appearing as 2 plano-convex masses with plane faces opposite, in the same circular area.

Surface sections of the *outer epidermis* of the seed coat mounted in chloral show strongly lignified, yellowish stone cells with sinuous and porous, vertical walls. Longitudinal sections cut parallel to the flat surfaces show that the embryo is curved.

Sections (both surface and transverse) of the **calyx** show stomata only on the lower epidermis. Each of these is surrounded by 3 or 4 neighboring cells, one of which is smaller than the others. Numerous glandular hairs occur on the upper epidermis. These possess 1- to 3-celled stalks and pluricellular heads. The head of each of these contains a yellow secretion. The mesophyll is composed of leaf parenchyma, some of the cells of which are filled with microcrystals.

Sections of the **peduncle** exhibit a pericyclic region containing sclerenchyma fibers.

Powdered Drug.—Yellowish-brown or brownish-red. Mounts made with chloral hydrate solution exhibit fragments of epicarp with parallel rows of rectangular cells; fragments of endocarp composed of yellow, moderately thickened, wavy-walled stone cells and parenchyma cells; fragments of seed coat with numerous yellow, sinuate, thick walled, porous stone cells, fragments of endosperm and embryo, most of the cells of which possess aleurone grains; numerous globules of yellowish-red oil; a few spiral and pitted tracheæ; cells containing microcrystals; occasionally tissues of the calyx and peduncle and a few more or less spheroidal starch grains from unripe fruits.

Constituents.—The pungent principle, capsaicin (capsacutin); a volatile alkaloid, resin, fixed oil, etc.

Uses.—Stimulant, condiment, counterirritant and stomachic.

Adulterants.—The powdered drug has been adulterated with the ground fruits of various varieties of *Capsicum annuum* known as Paprikas. These may be detected by the arrangement and shape of the epicarp cells as examined in surface view. The arrangement is irregular and the shape polygonal.

DULCAMARA N.F. (BITTERSWEET)

Synonyms.—Woody Nightshade, Wolf Grape, *Ger.* Bittersüssstengel; *Fr.* Tiges de douce-amere.

Botanical Origin.—*Solanum Dulcamara* Linné.

Part Used.—The dried stem.

Purity Rubric.—Not more than 2 per cent. of foreign organic matter.

Habitat.—Europe.

Plant.—A perennial twining undershrub which has become naturalized in North America from Kansas and Minnesota eastward. Its leaves are alternate, hastate above or with 2 auriculate lobes or leaflets at the base, ovate with cordate base below. Its inflorescences consist of axillary cymes of small lavender or blue colored flowers which bloom from May to September. Its fruit is a red berry.

Production and Commerce.—The woody stems of plants mostly growing wild in moist woodlands are collected in spring or autumn, cut into short cylindrical segments and dried. The greater portion of the drug used in this country is collected from plants growing in this country, the remainder being imported from Europe.

Description.—In short cylindrical, obliquely or transversely cut sections, from 3 to 10 mm. in length and 4 to 7 mm. in diameter; outer surface longitudinally striate, more or less warty and occasionally with leaf scars; cut surface exhibiting a thin brownish to greenish-brown bark, a broad greenish-brown or greenish-yellow wood, usually showing one or two concentric rings and a central hollow pith area; odor slight, indistinct; taste bitter, later sweet.

Powdered Drug.—Light yellowish brown; tracheæ up to 112μ in diameter and with bordered pores and spiral markings; lignified wood fibers with few pores; non-lignified bast fibers with walls up to 20μ in thickness; fragments of cork cells; few, simple, unicellular hairs up to 800μ in length, and with the lumina distinct in the lower portions only; few starch grains, spheroidal, up to 12μ in diameter; sphenoidal micro-crystals of calcium oxalate numerous, up to 7μ in length.

Constituents.—The glucoside, dulcamarin; the alkaloid, solanine; resin, gum, etc.

Uses.—Alterative and resolvent in scaly skin eruptions.

Adulterants.—Stems of *Humulus lupulus*, *Celastrus scandens* and *Lonicera Periclymenum*.

SCROPHULARIACEÆ (FIGWORT FAMILY)

Herbs (*Linaria*, *Verbascum*, *Gerardia*, *Digitalis*, etc.), shrubs (shrubby *Veronicas*, etc.), rarely trees (*Paulownia imperialis*). Stem, branches and leaves usually green and independently vegetating, but in *Pedicularis*, *Gerardia*, *Euphrasia*, *Buchnera*, *Rhinanthus*, etc., the stem, leaves, and branches are condensed from the development of a parasitic root habit. Stems cylindrical to frequently quadrangular, especially when leaves are opposite. Leaves alternate to opposite and decussate, simple, exstipulate, often hairy, but becoming by drought or parasiticism reduced to scales or almost absorbed. Inflorescence a raceme of cymes (*Paulownia*) or a simple raceme (*Foxglove*, *Linaria*, etc.) or spike (*Verbascum*

Thapsus) or, if leaves are opposite, often a whorl of axillary flowers or solitary axillary flowers. Flowers rarely regular, mostly irregular; calyx of five sepals condensed in *Veronica* to four, through absorption of one sepal by fusion of two sepals; corolla of five to four petals, deeply synpetalous, varying from rotate (*Verbascum Blattaria*, etc.) to irregular tubular to elongate, irregular bilabiate to funnel-shaped. In color, corolla varies from greenish to greenish-yellow or white (*Scrophularia*) to pure white or from red to purple to blue (*Veronica*). Stamens five, fertile, equal in length in a few *Verbascum* species or unequal in other *Verbascum* species to stamens four with a long sterile staminode (*Pentstemon*) to four didynamous stamens with a short petaloid staminode (*Scrophularia*) to four didynamous stamens with a minute often nectariferous staminode (*Linaria*), to frequently four didynamous stamens only, the two lateral or two anterior stamens stronger and longer (*Antirrhinum*) to two perfect stamens and two minute staminodes (*Calceolaria*) to two stamens alone developed (*Veronica*). Pistil bicarpellate; ovary two-celled with central placentation; style terminal with bilobed stigma; ovules numerous, small. Fruit a two-celled and usually many-seeded capsule. Seeds richly albuminous, anatropous or amphitropous.

DIGITALIS U.S.P. (DIGITALIS)

Synonyms.—Foxglove, Folk's- Fairy's- or Ladies' Glove, Dead Men's Bells, Purple Foxglove; *Ger.* Fingerhutblätter; *Fr.* Doigtier, Feuilles de digitale pourprée.

Botanical Origin.—*Digitalis purpurea* Linné.

Part Used.—The dried leaf.

Limit of Impurities.—2 per cent. of stems, flowers, browned leaves or other foreign organic matter.

Standard of Assay.—If made into the official tincture, properly diluted and injected into the ventral lymph sac of a frog, it has a minimum systolic dose not greater than 0.006 cc. of tincture, or the equivalent in tincture of 0.00,000,05 Gm. of ouabain, for each gramme of body weight of frog.

Ash.—Not more than 5 per cent. acid insoluble.

Habitat.—Europe, in meadows and pastures.

Plant.—A biennial pubescent herb whose first year's aerial growth consists of a rosette of ovate-oblong leaves. During the second year a hoary stem shoots up which arises to the height of 1 to 1.5 m., bearing alternate ovate-lanceolate to ovate-oblong, pubescent leaves and terminal racemes of purple, rarely white, tubular-campanulate flowers that are spotted within. The corolla is 4 to 5 cm. in length. The stamens are 4, didynamous. The fruit is a 2-celled pyramidal capsule.

Production and Commerce.—*Digitalis purpurea* is extensively cultivated in United States both as a garden ornamental and as a drug plant. It grows wild in many localities of this country as an escape from cultivation, notably in New York, Oregon and Washington. Considerable of the drug used here is obtained from plants cultivated on drug farms of United States and from plants growing wild in Oregon and Washington. Large amounts of this drug are also imported, the foreign article coming at present from Germany and England. It is usually shipped in bales but some of the fine English product comes in bottles.

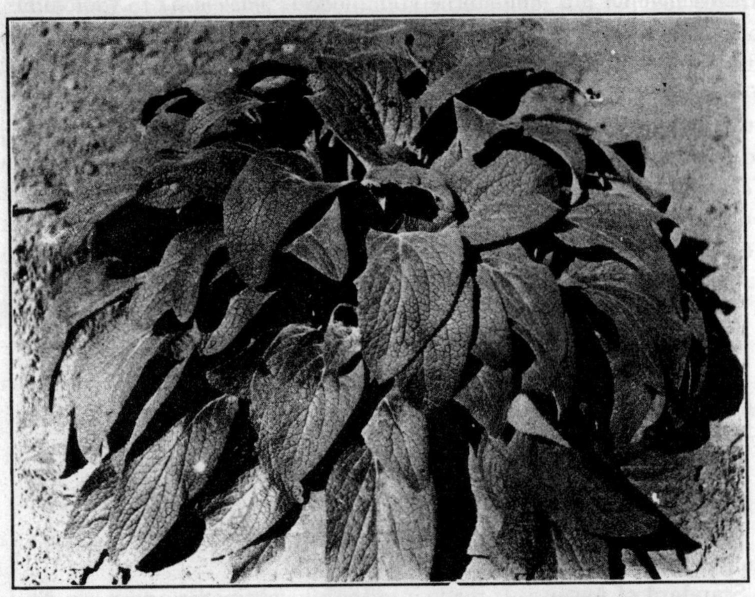

FIG. 251.—*Digitalis purpurea.* First year's growth. (*Photograph by Hogstad.*)

The plants are propagated from seeds which are mixed with sand and sown in February or March in seed pans or flats in the stove house or in cold frames. Upon the disappearance of frost, the plants should be transferred to the field where they should be planted about 1 to 1½ feet apart, in rows conveniently distanced for cultivation. The soil employed is of the ordinary garden kind but must be well drained and kept as free of weeds as possible, in order to insure a good growth of plants. The leaves are gathered from plants of the first and second year's growth. The best time to collect leaves from the second year's growth is in June, before the expansion of the flowers. These leaves are averagely richer in glucosides than leaves collected often after the flowers have opened. They are carefully dried in the shade or in ovens. They should be preserved in tightly closed containers protected from light.

Hamilton[1] has shown that the fresh leaves have greater toxicity than the dried leaves and that no more highly toxic products than those present in the crude drug are developed during the drying process.

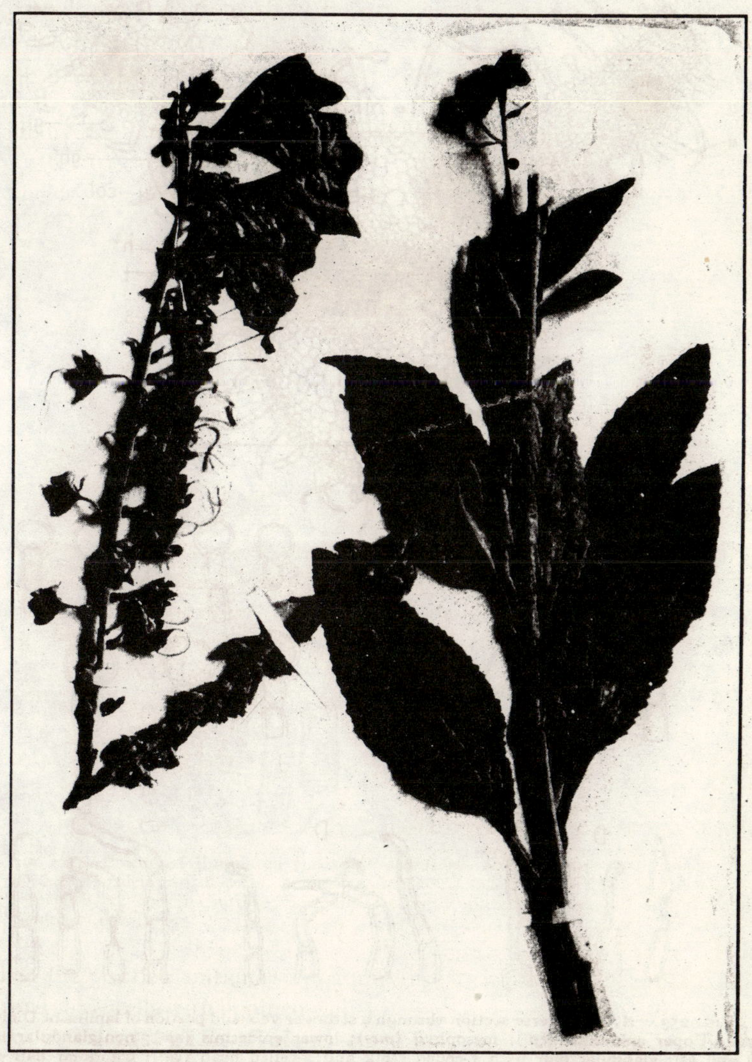

FIG. 252.—*Digitalis purpurea.* Aerial portion of second year's growth.

Description.—Leaves usually more or less crumpled and broken, when entire attaining a length of 30 cm. and a breadth of 15 cm.; laminæ, ovate, ovate-lanceolate, or ovate-oblong, abruptly contracted at bases into

[1] American Jour. Pharm., Vol. 91, p. 177, 1919.

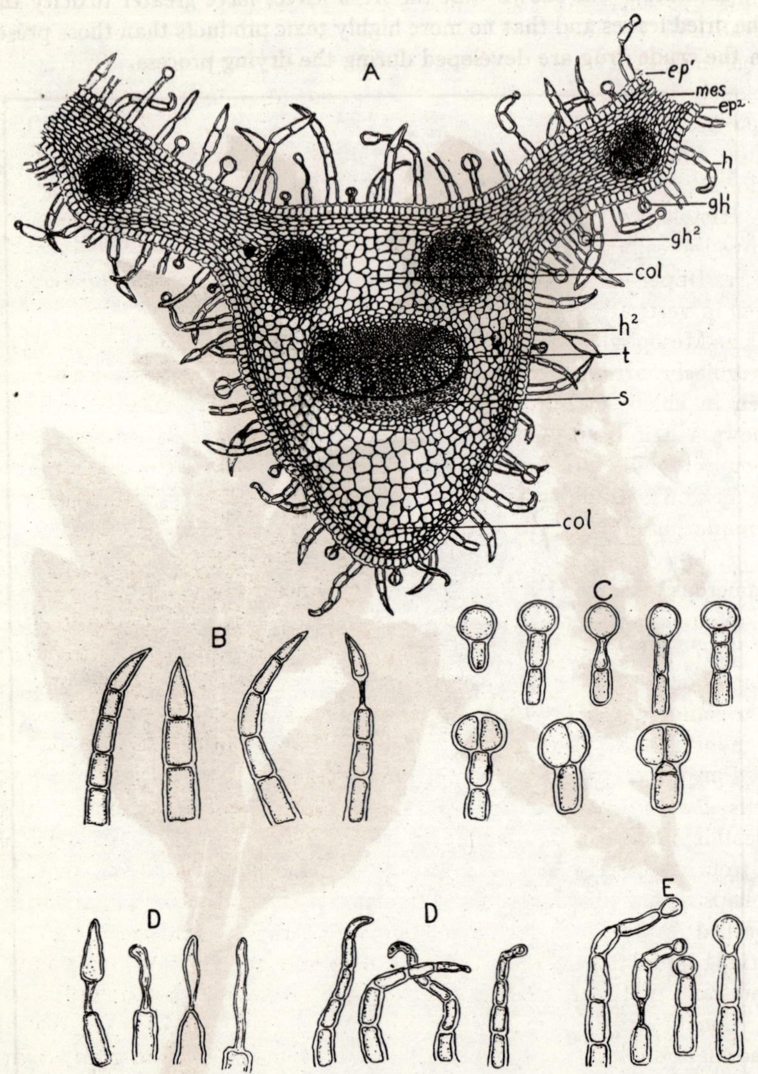

FIG. 253.—*A*, Transverse section through a stronger vein and portion of lamina of Digitalis leaf. Upper epidermis (ep^1); mesophyll (*mes*); lower epidermis (ep^2); non-glandular hairs (*h* and h^2); glandular hair with 1-celled stalk and 2-celled head (gh^1); glandular hair with 1-celled stalk and 1-celled head (gh^2); collenchyma (*col*); tracheæ (*t*) and sieve tissue (*s*) of bundles. *B* and *D*, Various types of uniseriate non-glandular hairs of digitalis. *C*, Types of glandular hairs of digitalis. *E*, Glandular hairs found on leaves of cultivated digitalis plants.

winged petioles, the latter from 5 to 10 cm. in length and up to 3 cm. in breadth or, in the smaller upper leaves, nearly absent; margin irregularly crenate or dentate; apex obtuse; upper surface dark green, wrinkled and sparsely hairy; lower surface dull, pale green and soft pubescent; venation pinnate-reticulate, the midrib and principal veins broad and flat, often purplish, the lower veins continued into the wing of the petiole; odor characteristic; taste bitter.

Histology.—Transverse and surface sections of the lamina of Foxglove leaves present the following tissues for examination:

1. Upper epidermis of slightly wavy-walled, clear epidermal cells, as seen in vertical view.

2. Mesophyll of a layer of short palisade cells and several layers irregularly arranged more or less rounded spongy parenchyma cells rich in chloroplastids. In the midrib and stronger veins, this region shows a half circle of fibrovascular bundles, the xylem portion of each group of which is fan shaped, and consists of rows of tracheæ separated by narrow medullary rays. In these parts, also, collenchymatous differentiation of the mesophyll is observed beneath each epidermis.

3. Lower epidermis of prominent wavy-walled epidermal cells and numerous stomata.

Non-glandular and glandular hairs are evident as outgrowths of cells of both epidermises. The non-glandular hairs are uniseriate, frequently curved or crooked, 2- to 8-celled, one or more of the cells being collapsed. The glandular hairs exhibit a one to two celled stalk and a one to two celled glandular head. Water stomata are present on the marginal teeth.

Powdered Drug.—Dark green; numerous fragments of mesophyll, the cells of which are devoid of calcium oxalate but contain abundant chloroplastids; numerous fragments of uniseriate, non-glandular hairs consisting of from 2- to 8-cells (usually 2- to 5-cells), some of the cells being frequently collapsed; few small glandular hairs, with a 1- to 2-celled stalk and a 1- to 2-celled glandular head; numerous fragments of epidermis with cells having undulate vertical walls and often showing stomata; fragments of veins and petioles exhibiting fibrovascular elements; no stone cells.

Constituents.—The glucosides, digitalein (gitalin), digitoxin, digitalin and digitophyllin; the saponins, digitonin, digitsaponin and gitin; volatile oil containing digitalosmin; tannin, an irritant resin termed digitalic acid, a yellow coloring substance termed digitoflavone or luteolin, an oxydase, etc. The most powerful constituent is digitoxin.

Several "digitalins" occur in commerce which vary in their composition. Nativelle's digitalin is chiefly digitoxin. Homolle's digitalin represents a mixture of digitoxin and digitalin. German digitalin (crystalline) represents digitonin. German digitalin (amorphous) is a mixture said to consist mainly of digitalein. Schmiedeberg's digitalin otherwise known as *Digitalinum Verum*, Kilani or True digitalin is pure amorphous digitalin having the chemical formula of $(C_5H_8O_2)_7$. Baljet[1] determined the localization of the glucosides in the leaves of several species of Digitalis including *D. purpurea* by means of sodium picrate reagent (a mixture of 1 drop of a 1 per cent. picric acid solution with 1 drop of a 10 per cent. solution of sodium hydroxide). He found that when sections were mounted in this reagent, the cells containing the glucosides were colored orange within one or two minutes. These glucosides were thus located in the non-glandular hairs, epidermal cells, endodermis, surrounding the vascular bundles and occasionally in the subepidermal collenchyma.

Uses.—Digitalis is extensively used as a cardiac stimulant and tonic and as a diuretic.

Adulterants.—(1) Mullein leaves (*Verbascum* species) readily distinguished from Digitalis by the presence of numerous candelabra-shaped, branching hairs.

(2) Leaves of *Inula Conyza* (Fam. *Compositæ*), the non-glandular hairs of which are thicker walled, 3- to 4-celled, the basal cell being broad. The margins are entire or dentate, the teeth with horny points.

(3) Leaves of *Salvia Sclarea* (Fam. *Labiatæ*) which have cordate bases, long petioles and glandular hairs with 8-celled heads.

(4) Leaves of *Symphytum officinale* (Fam. *Boraginaceæ*) which are ovate-lanceolate and possess stiff scattered hairs.

LEPTANDRA N.F. (LEPTANDRA)

Synonyms.—Culver's Root, Culver's Physic, Tall Speedwell or Veronica; *Fr.* Racine de Véronique; *Ger.* Leptandrawurzel.

Botanical Origin.—*Veronica virginica* Linné. (*Leptandra virginica* Nutt.)

Part Used.—The dried rhizome and roots.

Purity Rubric.—Not more than 5 per cent. of its stem bases or other foreign organic matter and not more than 6 per cent. of acid-insoluble ash.

Habitat.—In low grounds of Canada and United States as far south as Alabama and west to Minnesota and Nebraska.

Plant.—A perennial herb with erect, quadrangular stem attaining a height of 1 to 2 m. The leaves are whorled in 4's or 7's, lanceolate and serrulate. The flowers are small, pinkish to nearly white and arranged in spikes which are panicled. The fruit is an oblong-ovate capsule, opening by 4 apical teeth.

Production and Commerce.—The rhizomes and roots should be collected from plants of the second years growth. Most of the drug is gathered in the Southern Appalachian district.

[1] Schweiz. Apoth. Zeitung, 56; p. 247, 1918.

Description.—Rhizome horizontal, somewhat flattened and branched, up to 25 cm. in length and from 4 to 14 mm. in diameter, generally broken into segments 30 mm. or more in length; externally grayish-brown to purplish-brown, annulate with leaf scars, upper surface showing hollow stem bases, buds and stem scars; lower surface beset with wrinkled, fragile, rigid roots or remnants of these; fracture of rhizome, tough and uneven; internally bark and pith brown, wood yellowish, fracture of roots short; odor indistinct; taste bitter and acrid.

Histology.—Transverse sections of the older portion of the rhizome show the following characteristics, passing from periphery toward the center:

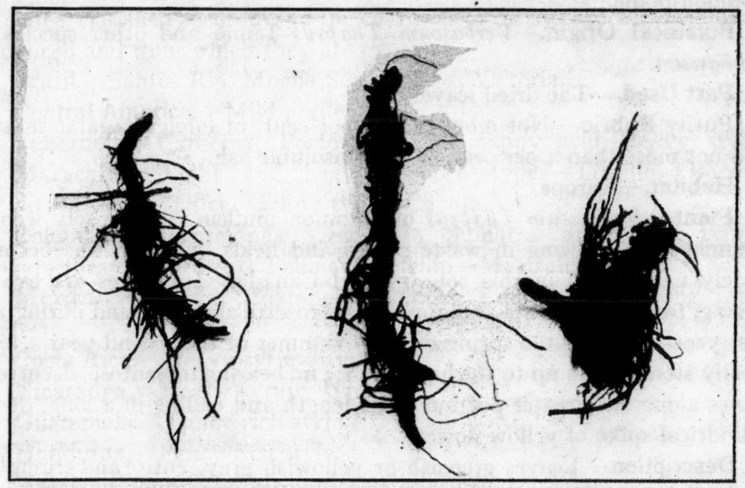

FIG. 254.—Leptandra, × 23/85. (*Photograph by Stoneback.*)

1. Cork.
2. Cork cambium.
3. Cortex containing starch and resin. The starch grains are spheroidal or polygonal and up to 8μ in diameter.
4. Pericycle, containing a closed ring of sclerenchyma.
5. Fibrovascular bundles of the open collateral type, arranged in a circle and separated from one another by medullary rays 1 cell in width. In each of these the phloem is composed of sieve tubes, companion cells and phloem parenchyma but no bast fibers; the xylem consists of numerous thick-walled, lignified wood fibers, scattered amongst which are spiral and pitted tracheæ. The protoxylem is separated from the secondary xylem by a zone of wood parenchyma.

6. Pith, composed of parenchyma cells some containing starch, others resin. Transverse sections of the rootlets of primary growth show diarch to pentarch radial fibrovascular bundles. The endodermis of these shows thickenings on the radial walls.

Constituents.—Resin, tannin, a bitter amorphous substance, volatile oil, verosterol, sugar, 3:4-dimethoxycinnamic acid, etc. Leptandrin is an impure resin obtained by precipitating a strong alcoholic tincture of the drug with water.

Use.—Cholagogue cathartic.

VERBASCI FOLIA N.F. (MULLEIN LEAVES)

Synonyms.—Common Mullein, Velvet Dock; *Ger.* Wollkraut; *Fr.* Bouillon-blanc.

Botanical Origin.—*Verbascum Thapsus* Linné and other species of *Verbascum.*

Part Used.—The dried leaves.

Purity Rubric.—Not more than 2 per cent. of foreign organic matter and not more than 4 per cent. of acid-insoluble ash.

Habitat.—Europe.

Plant.—*Verbascum Thapsus* or common mullein is a densely woolly biennial herb growing in waste places and fields, where it has become widely naturalized in this country and Canada. Its leaves are ovate-oblong, tomentose, acute and appear as a rosette above ground during the first year. During the spring or early summer of the second year a long woolly stem shoots up to the height of 1.3 m. bearing tomentose, decurrent leaves along the greater portion of its length and ending in a long, dense cylindrical spike of yellow flowers.

Description.—Leaves greenish or yellowish gray, entire and crumpled or broken, sessile, oblong, oblong-lanceolate with entire margin and densely tomentose surfaces, the latter due to long, branching, multicellular, non-glandular, candelabra-shaped hairs; odor indistinct; taste mucilaginous and slightly bitter.

Powdered Drug.—Dark green. The most diagnostic structure is the slightly-lignified, candelabra-shaped, non-glandular hair. This consists of a jointed central axis with whorls of 2 to 8 lateral cells arising at the joints or summit. Glandular hairs with a 1-celled stalk and 1-celled head are also present.

Constituents.—Mucilage, a trace of volatile oil, resin, tannin, wax, etc.

Uses.—Demulcent and emollient.

VERBASCI FLORES N.F. (MULLEIN FLOWERS)

Synonyms.—Mullen Flowers, Flores Verbasci; *Ger.* Wollkrautblumen, Königskerzenblumen; *Fr.* Fleurs de bouillon-blanc.

Botanical Origin.—*Verbascum phlomoides* Linné or *Verbascum thapsiforme* Schraeder.

Parts Used.—The dried corollas with adhering stamens.

Purity Rubric.—Not more than 2 per cent. of foreign organic matter. Flowers which have turned brown should not be used.

Habitat.—Europe and Asia.

Plants.—*Verbascum phlomoides* is a biennial herb producing a rosette of woolly oblong-lanceolate, crenulate leaves with winged petioles the first year. The second year it sends up a stout tomentose stem which arises to the height of 4 to 6 feet and bears ovate-lanceolate, crenate or entire, clasping, tomentose leaves with winged petioles. Inflorescence an elongated, terminal, spicate raceme of yellow or cream colored flowers. The calyx segments are triangular-lanceolate. Naturalized in New England and Middle Atlantic States.

Verbascum thapsiforme somewhat resembles the preceeding species but is more densely tomentose hairy, its stem leaves are narrowly decurrent from leaf to leaf, its yellow flowers are arranged in a dense spike, and the calyx segments are lanceolate.

Description.—Corolla of 5 gamopetalous, light-yellow petals forming a short tube below and expanding above into a saucer-shaped, obscurely 2-lipped limb, the outer surface woolly and grayish, the inner surface finely veined and sparsely hairy. Stamens 5, with woolly filaments, inserted on the base of the corolla, two being longer than other three; odor characteristic; taste mucilaginous.

Constituents.—Volatile oil, fixed oil, resin, mucilage, tannin, sugar, etc.

Use.—Chiefly as an ingredient of Breast Tea N.F.

RUBIACEÆ (MADDER FAMILY)

Herbs (*Galium*, *Mitchella*, etc.), shrubs (*Cephalanthus*, etc.), or trees (*Cinchona* species) with fibrous roots, sometimes, as in *Cephaëlis Ipecacuanha*, annularly enlarged. Roots, stems and to a less extent leaves rich in varied alkaloids, some of medicinal value. Leaves opposite, entire, stipulate and interpetiolate. Inflorescence a raceme of dichesial cymes occasionally condensing to scorpioids. Flowers perfect, often dimorphic, pentamerous or tetramerous; sepals five (*Cinchona*, etc.) but four in *Galium*, small, green, subtended with other flowers by one or two or more enlarged petaloid bracts; petals five (*Cinchona*, etc.) to four in *Galium*, stellate, varying from shallow-rotate to elongate-tubular or funnel-shaped with stellate limbs; stamens five to four, epipetalous; pistil nearly always bicarpellate, rarely of five to four carpels; ovary inferior, two-celled with central placentation; styles either distinct with knob-shaped stigmas or style elongate, filiform, ending in bilobed stigmas. Fruit varied, a capsule in *Cinchona*, a berry in *Coffee*, a drupe, or frequently, as in *Galium*, dry and splitting into nutlets; seeds albuminous, each with a curved embryo.

CINCHONA U.S.P. (CINCHONA)

Synonyms.—Peruvian Bark, Jesuits' Bark; *Fr.* Quinquina; *Ger.* China, Chinarinde, Peruvianische Rinde.

Yellow Cinchona = Yellow Bark, Yellow Peruvian Bark, Cartagena Bark, Calisaya Bark, Ledger Bark.

Red Cinchona = Red Bark, Red Peruvian Bark, St. Ann's Bark.

Botanical Origin.—*Cinchona succirubra* or its hybrids (Red Cinchona) or *Cinchona Ledgeriana* Moens, *Cinchona Calisaya* Weddell, and hydrids of these with other species of *Cinchona* (Yellow Cinchona or Calisaya Bark).

Part Used.—The dried bark.

Standard of Assay.—Not less than 5 per cent. of the alkaloids of Cinchona.

Habitat.—South America on the eastern slope of the Andes and western Cordilleras chain from 10° north latitude to 20° south latitude and from 3000 to about 9500 feet above the sea level.

Plants.—Evergreen trees attaining a height of 24 m. and having a trunk diameter of up to .6 m. at the base. The leaves are entire, opposite, coriaceous, elliptical or elliptical-lanceolate, petiolate and show lateral interpetiolar stipules. The flowers are pentamerous, tubular, and cymose. The fruits are septicidally dehiscent capsules, opening from the base upward and containing winged seeds.

Production and Commerce.—The Cinchona trees flourish in their wild state within forests of the Andes mountains of South America extending through Peru, Bolivia, Ecuador, New Granada, Venezuela and Colombia. They are also cultivated on a large scale in the Dutch and Anglo-Dutch plantations of Java and in the British government plantations of India. The methods of collecting the bark vary in these several districts. In South America the usual practice employed is to fell the tree during the rainy season, strip the bark from it and dry it either in the open or over a fire in huts. The bark which is stripped from the trunk is usually deprived of its cork and pressed under weights during drying constituting the "*flat bark*" or "*quina tabla;*" that stripped from the branches curls during the drying process and is known as "*quina canuto*" or "*quilled bark.*" In Java and India the methods now employed are uprooting and coppicing. Uprooting of the tree takes place when it has reached the age of about 12 years and the bark is stripped from both the root and the stem. In coppicing, the trunk is cut through above the ground, the bark stripped from

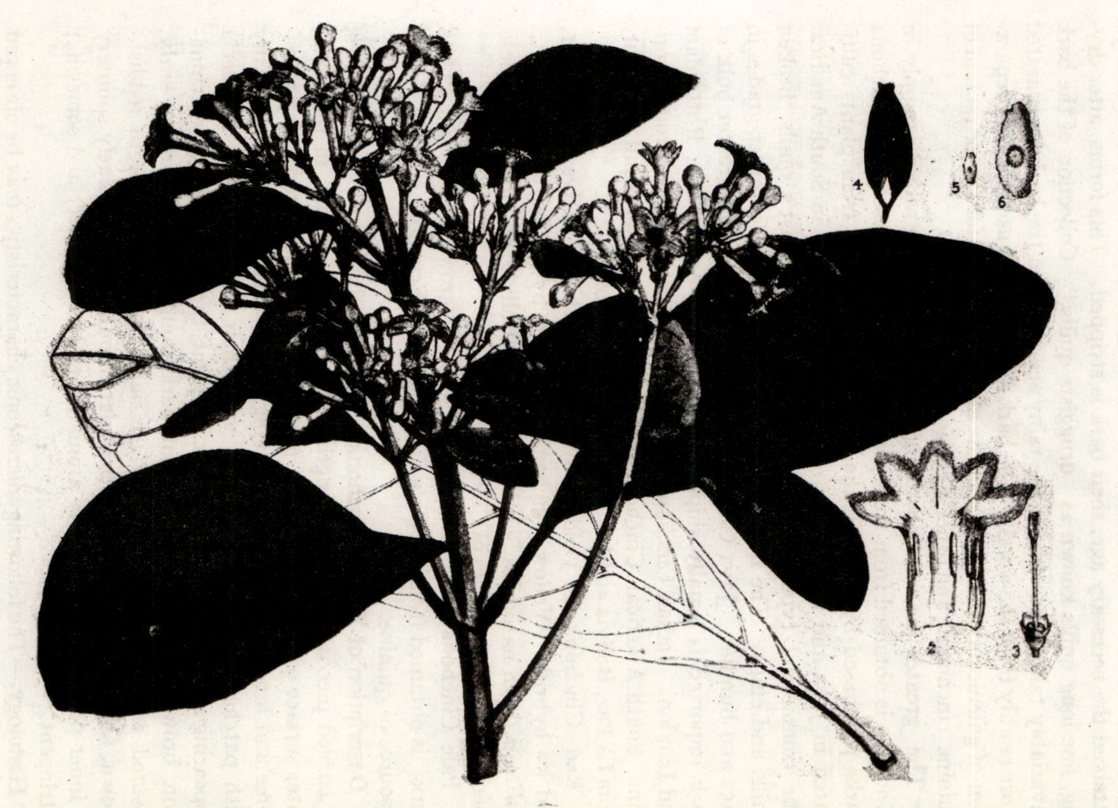

FIG. 255.—*Cinchona Calisaya.* 1. Branch with leaves and flowers. 2. Corolla laid open. 3. Calyx and pistil. 4. Fruit. 5, 6. Seeds. 7. Mature leaf. (*After Bentley and Trimen.*)

the felled portion, and the trunk left to coppice or form adventitious shoots, one or two of which are alone permitted to grow. After the shoots have attained the necessary age, their bark is stripped. This forms, after drying, fine long quills known as "druggists quills." Collection of the bark invariably takes place during the rainy season when the bark is separated more readily from the wood. The bark of the stem is used for the preparation of galenicals while that from the root is employed for the extraction of quinine, cinchonine and other alkaloids.

The greater portion (about 90 per cent.) of the world's supply of Cinchona is obtained from trees grown in Java. At present the Cinchona barks purchased by firms in the United States come from plants cultivated in Java and India and from trees growing wild in South America. The commercial types of bark imported are druggist's quills, broken quills and chips. The quills usually arrive in cases, the other grades in bags and bundles. Java Cinchona which constitutes the greater bulk of bark imported is usually shipped here through Amsterdam, Rotterdam and London. Indian Cinchona comes direct from India or through London. South American Cinchona comes direct from Guayaquil, Ecuador, from La Paz, Bolivia and from Cartagena, Colombia.

Red Cinchona is yielded by *C. succirubra*, a native of Ecuador, and its hybrids. Yellow Cinchona is yielded by *C. Ledgeriana*, and *C. Calisaya*, both natives of Southern Peru and Bolivia, and hybrids of these species with other species of Cinchona.

Pale Cinchona, also called "pale bark," "crown bark" and "Loxa bark" is obtained from *C. officinalis*, a native of Ecuador and Peru. It is a source of quinine.

Description of Yellow Cinchona.—In quills, flat pieces, broken pieces, or curved pieces of variable length and from 3 to 10 mm. in thickness; outer surface of stem bark rough, gray, with numerous intersecting transverse and longitudinal fissures, having nearly vertical sides, and usually with patches of foliaceous lichens with their brownish-black apothecia appearing as small spots; when cork is absent, the color externally is cinnamon brown; outer surface of root bark, rough, reddish brown, scaly, fissured and wrinkled; inner surface light cinnamon-brown to reddish-brown, finely striated; fracture granular in outer portion, finely splintery in inner portion; odor slightly aromatic; taste very bitter and somewhat astringent.

Histology.—The following microscopic characteristics may be observed in two of the Yellow Cinchona barks:

Cinchona Calisaya var. Micrantha	Cinchona Calisaya var. lancifolia.
Secretory latex sacs in cortex.	No secretory latex sacs in cortex.
Stone cells absent.	Stone cells in cortex.
Phloem patches cone shaped.	Phloem patches elongated and narrow.
Medullary-rays broad and wedge shaped.	Medullary-rays narrow and elongate.
Bast fibers comparatively small and less numerous.	Bast fibers comparatively large and more numerous.

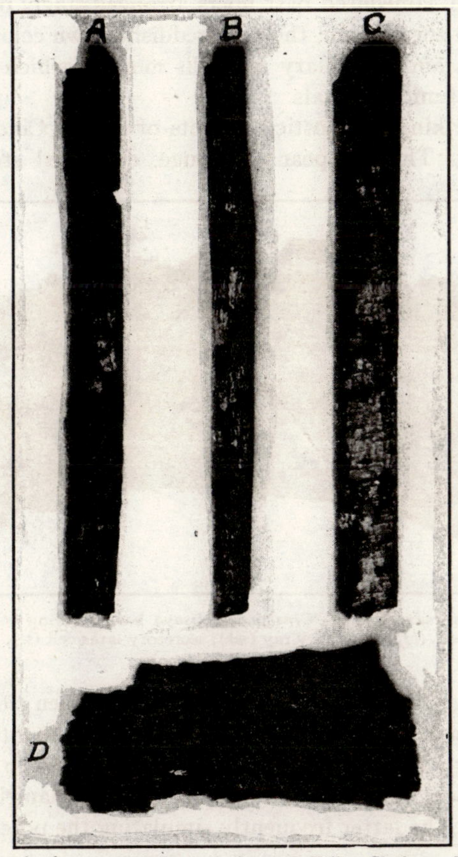

FIG. 256.—Cinchona barks. A and B, Red Cinchona; C, Yellow Cinchona; D, Tambla bark, × ⅓.

Description of Red Cinchona.—In quills or flat pieces of variable length; bark from 2 to 4 mm. in thickness, or in small broken fragments or in transversely curved pieces from 3 to 7 mm. in thickness; externally brown, brownish-gray, or reddish-brown, more or less rough from reddish, warty protuberances, and with transverse fissures which are rarely numerous or much intersected, and having their sides sloping, and with occasional patches of foliaceous lichens; inner surface reddish brown, distinctly striate; fracture short and granular in the outer bark, shortly and rather coarsely splintery in the inner bark; odor slight; taste very bitter and astringent.

Histology.—The chief diagnostic microscopical features of pure Red Cinchona bark are: The presence of an interrupted row of large, ovate secretory latex cells at the junction of the cortex with the phloem, the presence of large, lamellated bast fibers arranged singly or in radial rows or groups within the phloem, the deep reddish-brown color of the walls of the parenchyma and medullary ray cells most of which contain starch, some, sphenoidal microcrystals.

The most striking diagnostic elements of all the Cinchona barks are the bast fibers. These appear like huge, elongated stone cells, when

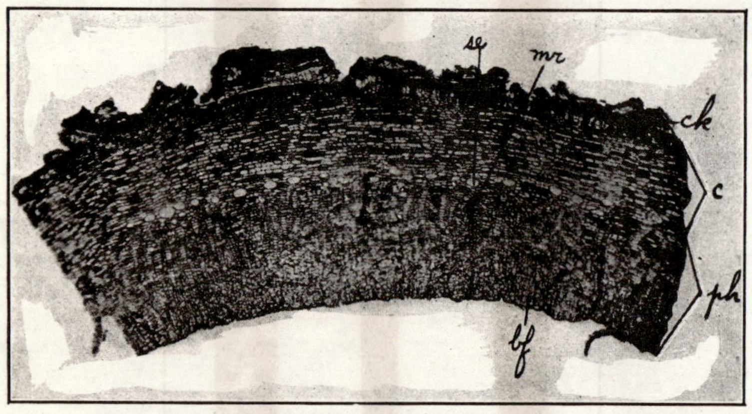

FIG. 257.—Transverse section of *Cinchona Calisaya* bark showing cork (*ck*); cortex (*c*), phloem (*ph*); bast fibers (*bf*); medullary ray (*mr*); secretory latex cell (*se*). Photomicrograph × 15.

examined in longitudinal sections which have first been cleared with weak alcoholic solution of ammonia, in order to remove pigments from adjacent cells. They vary in length from 300 to 1350μ and in diameter from 30 to 135μ, possess yellowish, strongly lignified and lamellated walls and prominent pores, the latter frequently simulating the pore canals of stone cells.

The cells of the cortex and medullary rays for the most part contain starch grains. Scattered here and there grayish-black cells will be noted. These contain sphenoidal microcrystals. Numerous cells contain brown to reddish-brown amorphous masses.

Scrapings of the bark mounted in water show the starch grains to be simple or 2- to 5-compound. The individual grains are spheroidal or plano-convex and from 3 to 15μ in diameter.

Sections mounted in solution of gold chloride show the alkaloids occur mainly in the cells of the cortex.

Powdered Cinchona.—Brown to reddish brown; bast fibers spindle-shaped, yellowish, from 300 to 1350μ in length and with thick, lamellated, strongly lignified, porous walls; starch grains simple or 2- to 5-compound, the individual grains spheroidal or plano-convex, from 3 to 20μ in diameter; numerous minute sphenoidal microcrystals; cells containing brown to reddish-brown amorphous masses.

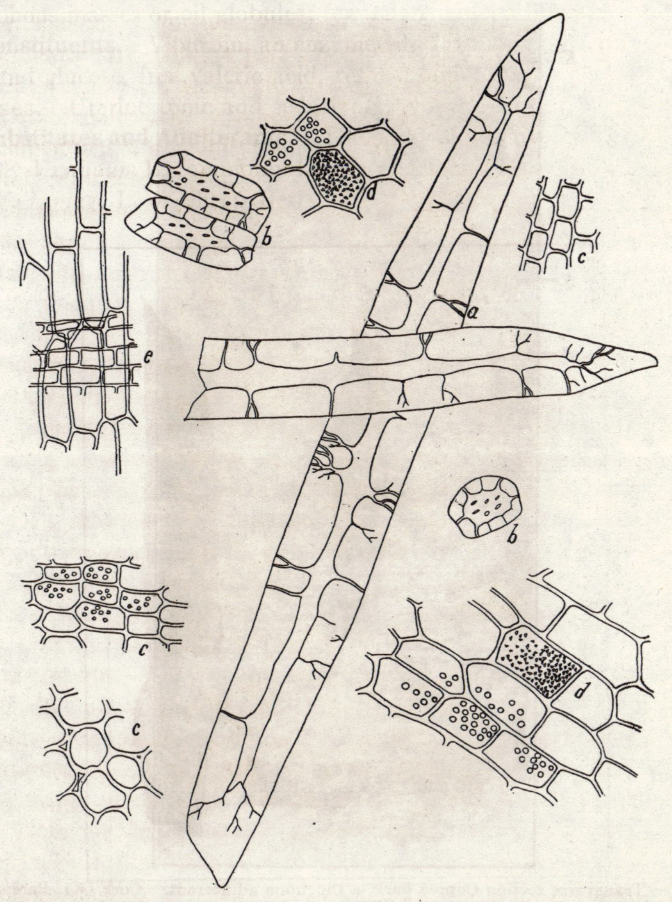

FIG. 258.—Powdered Cinchona. Red. (*a*) Large bast fibers; (*b*) sclerenchyma cells; (*c*) bark parenchyma; (*d*) cells with crystal sand; (*e*) medullary ray, (*After Schneider*.)

Constituents.—A number of alkaloids, the most important being quinine, quinidine, cinchonine and cinchonidine; cinchotannic acid, cinchona red, etc.

Uses.—Cinchona is used as a simple bitter, tonic, antimalarial and antipyretic, usually in the from of its preparations or alkaloids.

Adulterants.—(1) Cuprea bark obtained from *Remijia pedunculata* Triana and *R. Purdieana* Triana, plants growing in the U.S. of Colombia. This has a copper color and is more compact and heavy than Cinchona. It is characterized microscopically by the presence of numerous stone cells in cortex and phloem. (2) Loxa bark, from *Cinchona officinalis*, a native of

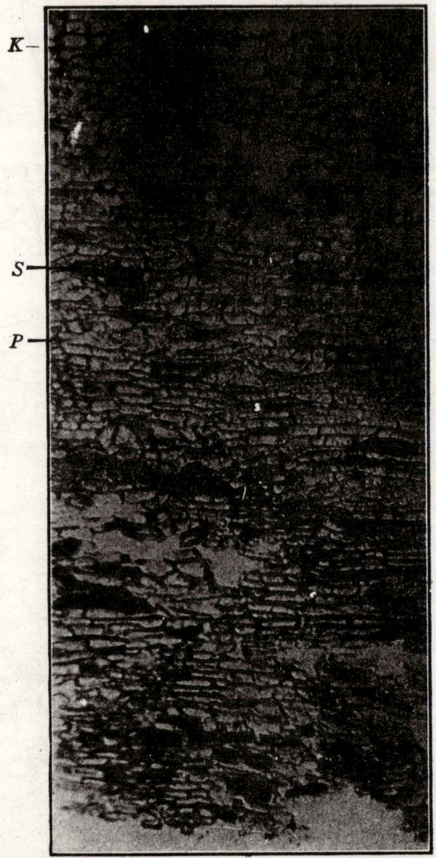

Fig. 259.—Transverse section Cuprea bark, a Cinchona adulterant. Cork (*K*); Parenchyma of cortex (*P*); stone cell (*S*).

Ecuador. This occurs in thin quills, fissured transversely, otherwise smooth and yields up to 4 per cent. of alkaloids. The medullary rays in this bark are quite narrow. Cuprea and Loxa barks contain quinine. (3) Barks of various species of *Cascarilla*, etc. which are devoid of cinchona alkaloids.

IPECACUANHA U. S. P. (IPECAC)

Synonyms.—Ipecac Root, Ipecacuanhæ radix, Poaya; *Fr.* Racine brésilienne; *Ger.* Brechwurzel, Ruhrwurzel.

Botanical Origin.—(1) *Cephaelis Ipecacuanha* (Brotero) A. Richard (*Uragoga Ipecacuanha* Baillon) and (2) *Cephaelis acuminata* Karsten (*Uragoga granatensis* Baillon).

Part Used.—The dried rhizome and roots.

Standard of Assay.—Not less than 1.75 per cent. of the ether-soluble alkaloids of Ipecac.

Limit of Impurities.—5 per cent. of its overground stems or 2 per cent. of other foreign organic matter.

Habitat.—(1) Brazil, (2) United States of Colombia, in forests.

Plants.—*Cephaelis Ipecacuanha* (*Evea Ipecacuanha* Standley), commonly known as Rio or Brazilian Ipecac, is a low, straggling shrub whose underground portion consists of a slender rhizome bearing annulated wiry roots and slender smooth roots. The rhizome arches upward and becomes continuous with a short, green, aerial stem bearing a few opposite, petiolate, stipulate, entire, obovate leaves. The flowers are small, white and capitate, occurring in the leaf axils, the corolla being infundibuliform. The fruit is a cluster of dark purple berries, each containing 2 plano-convex seeds.

Cephaelis acuminata somewhat resembles the Brazilian species but has a root with less pronounced annulations.

Production and Commerce.—Rio or Brazilian Ipecac grows in rich forest soil in Brazil and Bolivia. It is particularly abundant in the provinces of Matto-Grosso and Minas Geraes, Brazil. The roots together with portions of the rhizome, are gathered from January to late March by the natives, who then dry them in the sun and pack them in bales made of hide (serons). These bales are stored and later purchased by traders who ship them to Rio de Janeiro, Bahia, Pernambuco or Montevideo for export. Some Rio Ipecac is also grown in the Straits Settlement (Yohore or Indian Ipecac) but none of this reaches the United States.

Cartagena Ipecac grows in forests of United States of Colombia. It is exported to this country in bales from Cartagena and Savanilla, Colombia.

Description.—Rio or Brazilian Ipecac occurs as cylindrical pieces of roots of variable length mixed with nearly smooth, grayish-brown rhizomes, the latter up to about 3 mm. thick; root reddish-brown to blackish-brown, rarely grayish-brown, either closely annulated or smooth from 1 to 5 mm. in diameter, simple or branched, usually with transverse fissures, the latter often extending to the wood bark of annulated root about two-thirds the diameter of the root, bark of the smooth root, about one-ninth of the entire diameter; fracture of bark short, readily separable from the tough, yellowish-white wood; odor slight; taste bitter, nauseous and acrid. The rhizome, which is up to 10 cm. in length and 3 mm. in thickness, is finely longitudinally wrinkled and shows a few elliptical scars and a pith, the latter about one-sixth its diameter.

Cartagena Ipecac differs from Rio Ipecac macroscopically by the following points: It is thicker, being up to 7 mm. in diameter. Its color is gray or grayish-brown and its annulations are less numerous.

Histology.—Transverse sections of Ipecac show the following microscopical peculiarities passing from periphery toward the center:

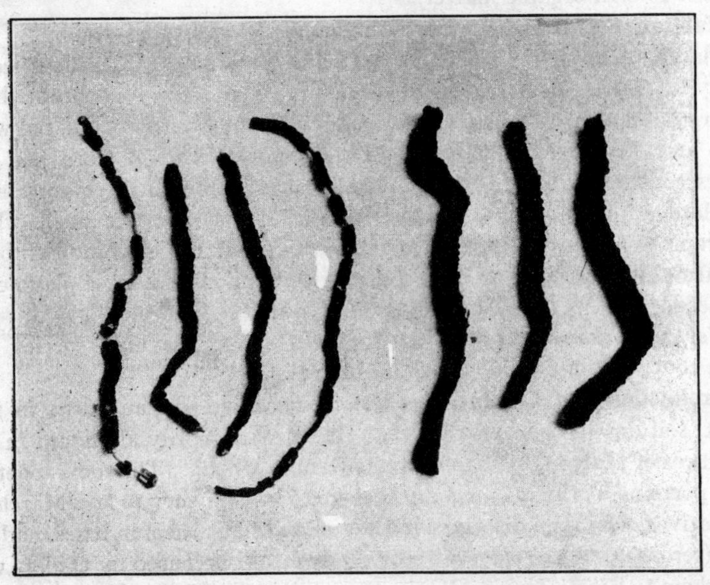

FIG. 260.—*A*, Rio Ipecac; *B*, Cartagena Ipecac, × ⅜. (*Photograph by Stoneback.*)

1. Cork of several layers of tabular cork cells.
2. Cork cambium of meristematic cells.
3. Cortex, a broad zone of irregularly rounded cells, most of which contain starch and active principles, a few, raphides of calcium oxalate.
4. Phloem, a narrow zone of more or less cone-shaped phloem patches composed of sieve tubes and phloem cells, the patches separated from each other by wedge-shaped strands of cortex.
5. Cambium of meristematic cells.
6. Xylem, taking up the remainder of the room in the sections and composed chiefly of porous tracheids with a few lignified wood fibers.

Coursing radially through the xylem are modified medullary-rays, the cells containing starch grains up to 10μ in diameter.

Longitudinal sections show the tracheids to be of two kinds, the one showing bordered pores, the other, slit-like simple pores.

Powdered Drug.—Light brown; fragments of thin-walled parenchyma loaded with starch; numerous simple or 2- to 7-compound starch grains, the individual grains spheroidal, plano-convex or angular in outline, up to 15μ (Rio Ipecac) or 20μ in diameter (Cartagena Ipecac); fragments of tracheids with bordered pore or simple pore markings; raphides of calcium oxalate up to 50μ in length; a few wood fibers and fragments of cork.

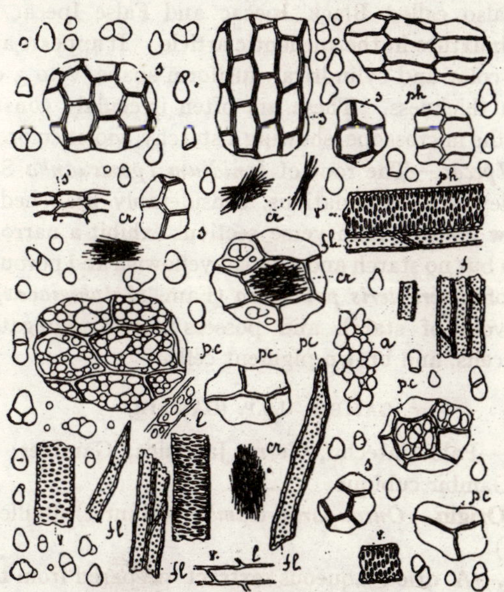

FIG. 261.—Powdered Undulated Ipecac (*Richardsonia scabra*). × 210. *a*, starch grains; *cr*, raphides of calcium oxalate; *fl*, pitted wood fibers; *l*, bast; *pc*, cortical parenchyma; *ph*, phelloderm; *s*, *s'*, cork in surface view and section; *v*, pitted tracheæ. (*From Sayre after Greenish and Collin.*)

When the powder contains stem admixture it shows in addition, elongated porous stone cells with lignified walls.

Constituents.—The alkaloids emetine ($C_{15}H_{22}NO_2$), cephaeline ($C_{14}H_{20}NO_2$), kryptonine and psychotrine; a glucoside termed ipecacuanhin, ipecacuanhic acid, starch, calcium oxalate, etc.

Uses.—Nauseating expectorant and emetic.

Adulterants and Substitutes: (1) *Ipecac Stems.*—These may be distinguished from the rhizome by the presence of opposite leaf scars in the terminal portion and by the presence of numerous chloroplasts.

(2) *Undulated Ipecac.*—The root of *Richardsonia scabra* St. Hilaire (Fam. *Rubiaceæ*) indigenous to Brazil occurs in tortuous pieces like Ipecac, but its upper portion is cylindrical, the crown showing several slender stem bases. It is less fissured and annulated than Ipecac, its wood is distinctly porous, due to the presence of pitted tracheæ, its bark frequently violet-colored and its starch grains attain a diameter of up to 40μ.

(3) *Greater Striated Ipecac.*—The root of *Psychotria emetica* L. (Fam. *Rubiaceæ*) resembles somewhat Cartagena Ipecac from which it may be distinguished in cross sections by its violet-colored bark and absence of starch.

(4) *Lesser Striated Ipecac.*—The root of an undetermined species of *Richardsonia*, also called Black Ipecac and False Ipecac, occasionally occurs as an admixture in the authentic article. It appears as short pieces of gray-brown color and cylindrical, fusiform shape, 2 to 3 cm. long and 2 to 3 mm. in thickness. These are often irregulaly constricted, cross sections under the microscope, showing a starchy, violet colored bark.

(5) *White Ipecac.*—The root of *Ionidium Ipecacuanha* St. Hil. (Fam. *Violaceæ*) is devoid of annulations, considerably branched, of grayish-white or yellow color. Transverse sections exhibit a narrow, dark bark with stone cells but no starch and a broad yellowish and porous wood.

(6) Roots of *Heteropteris pauciflora* (Fam. *Malphigiaceæ*) from Brazil which are devoid of starch and possess rosette aggregates of calcium oxalate, stone cells, and brown pigment cells.

GAMBIR U.S.P. (GAMBIR)

Synonyms.—Pale Catechu, Terra Japonica, Gambier; *Ger.* Gambir Catechu; *Fr.* Gambir cubique.

Botanical Origin.—*Ourouparia Gambir* (Hunter) Baillon. (*Uncaria Gambier* Roxb.).

Part Used.—A dried aqueous extract prepared from the leaves and twigs.

Purity Rubric.—Not less than 70 per cent. of water-soluble extractive and not less than 65 per cent. of alcohol-soluble extractive.

Habitat.—Malay Archipelago.

Plant.—A perennial, woody, climbing shrub having more or less angular stems somewhat thickened at the nodes, opposite, entire, oblong-ovate, petiolate, acuminate leaves, spherical axillary clusters of small pinkish flowers and capsular fruits. The seeds are very small, brownish and tailed at either end.

Production and Commerce.—The plant is cultivated chiefly in the East Indies. The extract is prepared mainly near Singapore from plants which are cultivated. The young leafy stems are cut up and boiled for about 6 hours in water, during which time they are continually bruised and stirred. The decoction is then strained, poured into copper pans, evaporated until it has reached a syrupy consistence and allowed to cool. During the cooling process, the extract is induced to crystallize by working a wooden stick up and down in the liquor until a mass of soft clay consistency is formed. This is usually carried to Singapore where it is cut into cubes and dried. It is then packed in wooden cases for export. Most of the world's supply of Gambir comes from Singapore.

Description.—In cubes about 25 mm. in diameter or irregularly shaped pieces, externally dull grayish-brown to reddish-brown; friable; internally light brown or dull earthy in color; inodorous; taste very astringent and bitterish.

If 1 Gm. of Gambir be macerated with 50 c.c. of water and filtered, the filtrate is pale yellowish-brown and gives an intense green color with diluted ferric chloride test solution and no precipitate with copper sulphate T.S.

Histology.—Scrapings of Gambir mounted in chloral hydrate solution show numerous acicular crystals (catechin) which gradually dissolve, thick-walled non-glandular hairs, leaf fragments, bacteria and starch grains of variable shape and up to 16μ in diameter.

Constituents.—From 25 to 50 per cent. of catechutannic acid, up to 33 per cent. of catechin; catechu red, etc.

Use.—Astringent.

COFFEA TOSTA N.F. (COFFEE)

Synonyms.—Roasted Coffee; *Fr.* Café; *Ger.* Kaffee.

Botanical Origin.—(1) *Coffea arabica* Linné and (2) *Coffea liberica* Bulliard.

Part Used.—The dried ripe seed, deprived of most of the seed coat and roasted until a dark brown color and a characteristic aroma are developed.

Purity Rubric.—Not less than 1 per cent. of caffeine, not less than 3 per cent. nor more than 5 per cent. of total ash and not less than 10 per cent. of fat.

Habitat.—Africa. (1) Abyssinia. (2) Liberia.

Plant.—Evergreen trees having opposite, oblong-ovate, coriaceous, glabrous and shining, acuminate leaves, axillary clusters of fragrant, white, tubular flowers and red or purple berry fruits about the size of cherries. Each flower consists of a 5-toothed calyx, a tubular, 5-lobed corolla, 5 stamens, a 2 celled ovary and a bifid style. The fruit consists of a 2-celled pericarp surrounding 2 plano-convex seeds, each with a longitudinal groove on its plane surface, both facing each other by their plane surfaces, each being surrounded by a thin membranous endocarp called "parchment."

Production and Commerce.—The coffee plants are extensively cultivated in Arabia, Java, Brazil, Venezuela, Ecuador, Peru, Colombia, Central America, West Indies, India and Hawaii. They are grown from seeds and yield mature fruits in 2 or three years but generally require 5 years before yielding a good crop. The fruits are gathered when fully mature and prepared for the market either by the dry or wet methods.

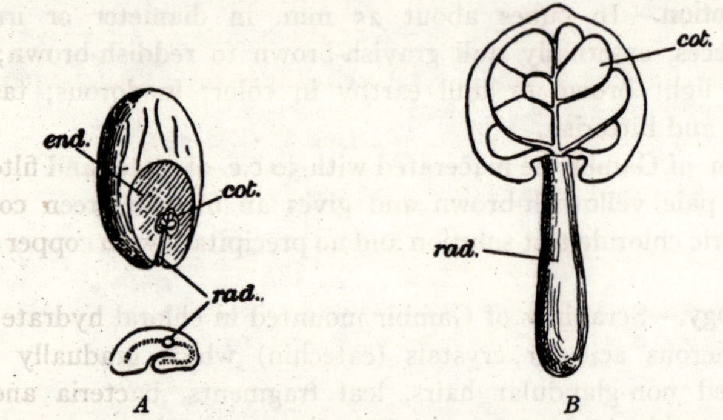

FIG. 262.—*A*, Diagram of coffee seed showing relative position of embryo, groove and endosperm. Cotyledons (*cot*) and radicle (*rad*) of embryo. *B*, Embryo of coffee seed showing one of the cotyledons (*cot*) and the radicle (*rad*). (Enlarged.) (*After Greenish.*)

The former consists of spreading the fruits out on a floor and exposing them to the drying action of the sun. The dried pulp and parchment are subsequently removed and the seeds liberated. This method is employed mainly in Arabia which produces Mocha coffee.

The wet method is the more modern and that now more generally employed.

It consists of placing the fruits in a tank of water. In this the ripe fruits sink and are drawn through pipes to a pulping machine where the fleshy portion is reduced to a pulp and the pulp and free seeds, enclosed in their parchment, conveyed to a second tank of water. Here they are stirred, the pulp being separated by washing and the seeds sinking to the bottom. The parchment coverings are removed by subsequently allowing them to slightly ferment, by trampling the seeds, stirring and washing. The seeds are then dried in the sun or by artificial heat. They constitute what is known as "raw coffee." In this condition the seeds are yellowish or dull green, each with papery spermoderm ("silver skin") in the longitudinal cleft on the flat side. The seeds are now graded for roasting by passing them through sieves having large, medium and small apertures. They are then garbled to remove split or otherwise defective seeds and foreign matter. The seeds are imported in bags usually in the raw or unroasted condition.

Most of the coffee imported into this country is roasted here. The process of roasting requires considerable skill and care, lest some of the aroma be lost. It is this process which causes the coffee seeds to swell up and become altered in their constituents. During this process the fragrant substance coffeol, which gives to coffee its flavor and aroma, is developed. During this process, also, a portion of the caffeine is liberated from the caffeotannic acid.

About eighty per cent. of all the coffee produced at the present time comes from Brazil. The United States consumes over one-half of the world's supply of coffee.

The following is a list of the most important commercial varieties of coffee, classified according to the countries or districts in which they are produced and from which they are exported.

Brazil.—Santos Rio, Mocha Seed Santos; Victoria.

Central America.—Mild grades.

Venezuela.—Caraccas; Porto Cabello (snappy acid, heavy style).

Maracaibo.—Light and heavy smooth types—Trujillo, Bocono, Tovar, Merida. Thick, syrupy type—Cucuta.

Colombia.—Bucramanga (resembles Sumatra and Java types); Bogata (heaviest grown); Tolima; Medellin—Mazizales; Cauca.

Mexico.—Cordova; Coatapec; Oaxaca; Tabasco (all strong fancy styles).

Costa Rica.—Heavy syrupy types.

Nicarauga.—Heavy syrupy types.

Guatemala.—Fancy rich style.

Honduras.—Fancy rich style.

Hayti.—Common to fair grades, wild grown.

Porto Rico.—Fanciest, aromatic, heavy types.

Arabia.
Abyssinia. } Mocha (sharp and aromatic).

Liberia.—Wild, coarse, powerful types.

East Indies.—Sumatra (finest grown); Padang; Interior; Macassar; Java.

Manila.—Light, aromatic, woody types.

Description.—Oval to ellipsoidal in outline, plane on one side, with a longitudinal groove showing traces of the papery seed coat, convex on the other, of variable size; dark brown; odor aromatic, characteristic; taste bitter.

Histology.—Coffee seeds may be prepared for sectioning by soaking over night in water. The remains of the spermoderm (seed coat) may be picked out of the groove with a fine pair of forceps and examined separately. The seeds present for examination 3 regions, viz: (1) spermoderm, (2) endosperm and (3) embryo.

The *spermoderm* consists of a layer of more or less obliterated parenchyma cells over which are scattered elongated, variously shaped, porous

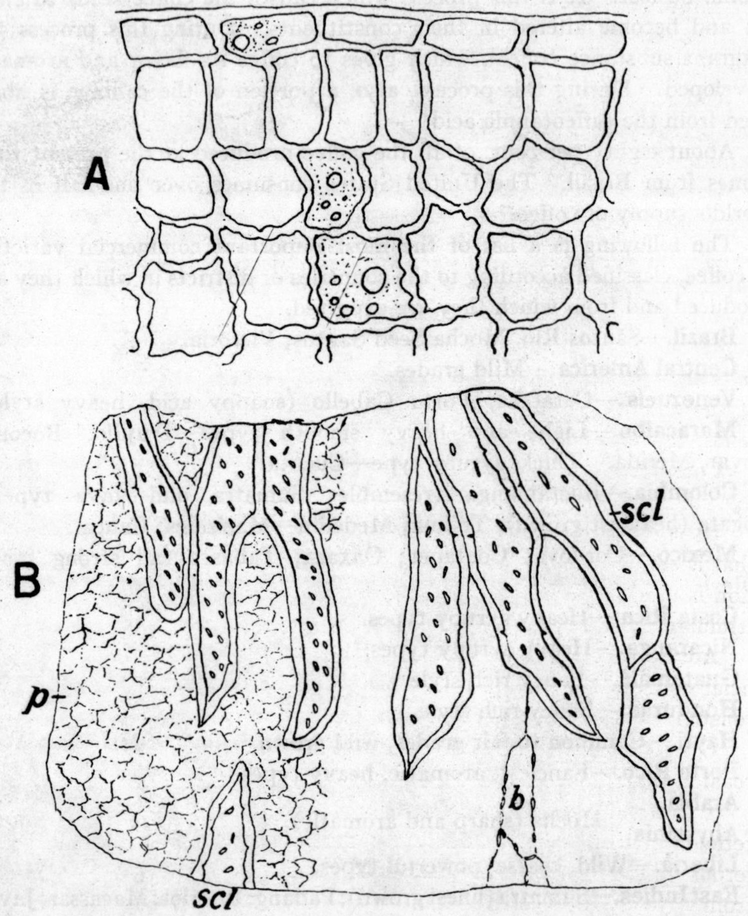

FIG. 263.—Coffee. *A*, Portion of outer endosperm of seed showing endosperm cells with reserve cellulose walls which, while nearly uniform in outer layer or two, become unevenly thickened and beaded farther inward. *B*, Portion of seed coat removed from the groove of a coffee seed. Parenchyma cells (*p*); sclerenchyma cells with oblique pores (*scl*); cells with minutely beaded walls (*b*). (Partly diagrammatic.)

stone cells from 100μ to over 1000μ in length and up to 135μ in breadth. These occur singly or in small groups, the latter showing intercellular-air-spaces between the component elements.

The *endosperm* takes up the greater area of the seed and consists of an outer layer of more or less square shaped cells with thick cuticle and a broad inner zone of larger cells having knotty walls of reserve cellulose about 10μ in thickness and containing oil globules and aleurone grains. A few minute starch grains may only occasionally be found in some of the cells.

The *embryo* consists of a blunt radicle 3 to 4 mm. in length and 2 small heart-shaped cotyledons, each pinnately 3-nerved.

Chloral hydrate solution, a mixture of equal parts of ammonia water and peroxide of hydrogen, are valuable clearing agents, when roasted coffee is under examination.

Ground Coffee.—This should be cleared with either of the aforementioned reagents before examination. Coarser particles may be picked out and sectioned after soaking in water or clearing solution, and paper fragments of the seed coat may be picked out with a forcep and mounted separately. The characteristic elements to be noted are the numerous fragments of seed coat with variously shaped, porous stone cells arranged singly or in small groups; the knotty-thickened walled cells of the endosperm (walls about 10μ in width) with aleurone and oil contents; few spiral tracheæ.

Constituents.—Coffeol, caffeine (1 to 2 per cent.), 10 to 13 per cent. of fixed oil, from 2 to 5 per cent. of tannin; proteins, glucose, dextrin, etc.

Uses.—Roasted coffee is widely used in the preparation of a decoction that is employed as a stimulating beverage. Medicinally, a strong decoction is used in the treatment of poisoning by alkaloids and as a cerebral stimulant. A source of caffeine.

Adulterants: Whole roasted coffee has been adulterated with artificial coffee seeds made by moulding and roasting dough and also with roasted masses of pea hulls, ground cereal and molasses.

Ground roasted coffee has been adulterated with the following ground roasted materials:

1. *Chicory root* (*Cichorium Intybus*) identified by its short, pitted and reticulate tracheæ with moderately elongated pores and numerous laticiferous vessels (usually less than 10μ broad). The tracheæ are averagely from 25 to 50μ in breadth.

2. *Taraxacum root*, identified by its pitted and reticulate tracheæ, up to 80μ in width, with elongated pores along with its laticiferous vessels.

3. *Cereals* and *Cereal Products*, identified by their characteristic hairs, cross cells and starch grains. See p. 94.

4. *Coffee hulls*, identified by a layer of elongated, curved, palisade cells with yellowish contents and whose walls take a red color with safranin, the contents remaining yellow.

5. *Leguminous seeds*, including peas, beans, chick peas, peanuts, carob beans, soja beans, coffee cassia, lupines, etc., characterized by fragments of leguminous palisade cells and starch grains.

6. *Acorn kernels*, characterized by distorted ellipsoidal or elongated starch grains, each with a prominent elongated hilum.

7. *Figs*, identified by fragments of mesocarp of receptacle containing abundant branching latex tubes up to 50μ in breadth, and rosette crystals of calcium oxalate, spiral and pitted vessels, by fragments of the epicarp with small thick-walled cells 20μ or less in diameter, arranged in radiate fashion around the circular bases of unicellular non-glandular hairs, that are frequently detached, and by the minute akenes which are usually imbedded in the roasted pulp.

8. *Ivory nut* (*Phytelephas macrocarpa*) characterized by its large thick-walled endosperm cells with porous walls of reserve cellulose from 35 to 50μ or more in thickness.

9. *Narcissus bulbs* (*Narcissus poeticus* and *N. pseudonarcissus*), which have elongated raphides of calcium oxalate that occur in long crystal cells and thin walled parenchyma containing swollen starch grains.

MITCHELLA N.F. (MITCHELLA)

Synonyms.—Squaw Vine, Partridge Berry, Checkerberry, Winter Clover, Squaw Berry, Twin Berry.

Botanical Origin.—*Mitchella repens* Linné.

Part Used.—The dried plant.

Purity Rubric.—Not more than 5 per cent. of foreign organic matter.

Habitat.—North America, from Nova Scotia to Minnesota south to the Gulf of Mexico.

Plant.—A low evergreen herb with slender, creeping, prostrate stems bearing opposite, shining, round-ovate, petioled leaves often with whitish veins and bright scarlet, 4-seeded berries usually occurring in pairs which remain on the plant over winter.

Commercial.—The commercial supplies of this drug are gathered in New Hampshire and the southern Appalachian district.

Description.—It occurs in loosely matted masses of branched, yellowish to brownish, filiform rhizomes bearing fine rootlets, stems and leaves and occasionally berries. The stems are quadrangular or flattened and bearing opposite leaves. The leaves are green, short petiolate, coriaceous, rounded-ovate, entire up to 2 cm. in length, with smooth, shining, dark-green upper surface, showing prominent midrib and veins and smooth pale green lower surface. The odor is faint and the taste, slightly bitter and astringent.

Powdered Drug.—Light grayish-green. Numerous fragments of chlorenchyma, some of the cells with a yellowish amorphous resinous content; fragments of epidermis with broadly elliptical stomata; numerous raphides of calcium oxalate up to 55μ in length, fragments of stem parenchyma often associated with fibrovascular tissue whose tracheæ exhibit spiral and reticulate markings; starch grains mostly simple, spheroidal or ellipsoidal and up to 10μ in diameter.

Constituents.—A saponin-like compound, resin, mucilage, wax, dextrin, calcium oxalate, etc.

Uses.—Diuretic, astringent and tonic.

CAPRIFOLIACEÆ (HONEYSUCKLE FAMILY)

Shrubs or rarely herbs. Leaves entire, opposite, exstipulate or with delicate, attenuate or filiform stipules. Inflorescence varying from a raceme of shortened cymes to a capitulum. Flowers varying from regular and small (*Sambucus*, *Viburnum*, etc.) to increasingly large, slightly irregular and ultimately very irregular, in some Honeysuckles and in a few *Weigelas* and allies; calyx pentamerous, superior; corolla superior, gamopetalous, limb pentafid, small in *Viburnum* and *Sambucus* to elongate, tubular or irregular infundibuliform in Loniceras; stamens five, inserted on tube of corolla and alternating with corolla segments; filaments equal or didynamous (in irregular flowers); ovary inferior, rarely five- to three-celled, usually three- or frequently two-celled; style terminal. Fruit a berry (*Viburnum and Snowberry*) from an inferior ovary, several celled, occasionally becoming one-celled with several to rarely one seed, or fruit a capsule (*Diervilla or Bush Honeysuckle and Weigela*). Seeds albuminous.

SAMBUCUS N.F. (SAMBUCUS)

Synonyms.—Elder Flowers, American Elder, Sweet Elder; *Ger.* Holunderblüthen; *Fr.* Fleurs de sureau.

Botanical Origin.—(1) *Sambucus canadensis* Linné and (2) *Sambucus nigra* Linné.

Part Used.—The air-dried flower.

Purity Rubric.—Not more than 2 per cent. of foreign organic matter.

Habitat.—(1) United States and lower Canada. (2) Europe.

Plants.—*Sambucus canadensis*, known as Common Elder or American Elder, is a shrub growing in moist soil, frequently on the border of meadows or swamps. Its stems attain a height of 4 m. and contain abundant white pith, the latter being employed for imbedding plant parts for sectioning purposes. Its leaves are imparipinnate with 5 to 11 oblong, glabrous leaflets, the lower ones being often 3-parted. The inflorescences are flat compound cymes. The flowers are small, white, each with 5 minute calyx lobes, an urn-shaped, 5-cleft gamopetalous corolla, 5 stamens

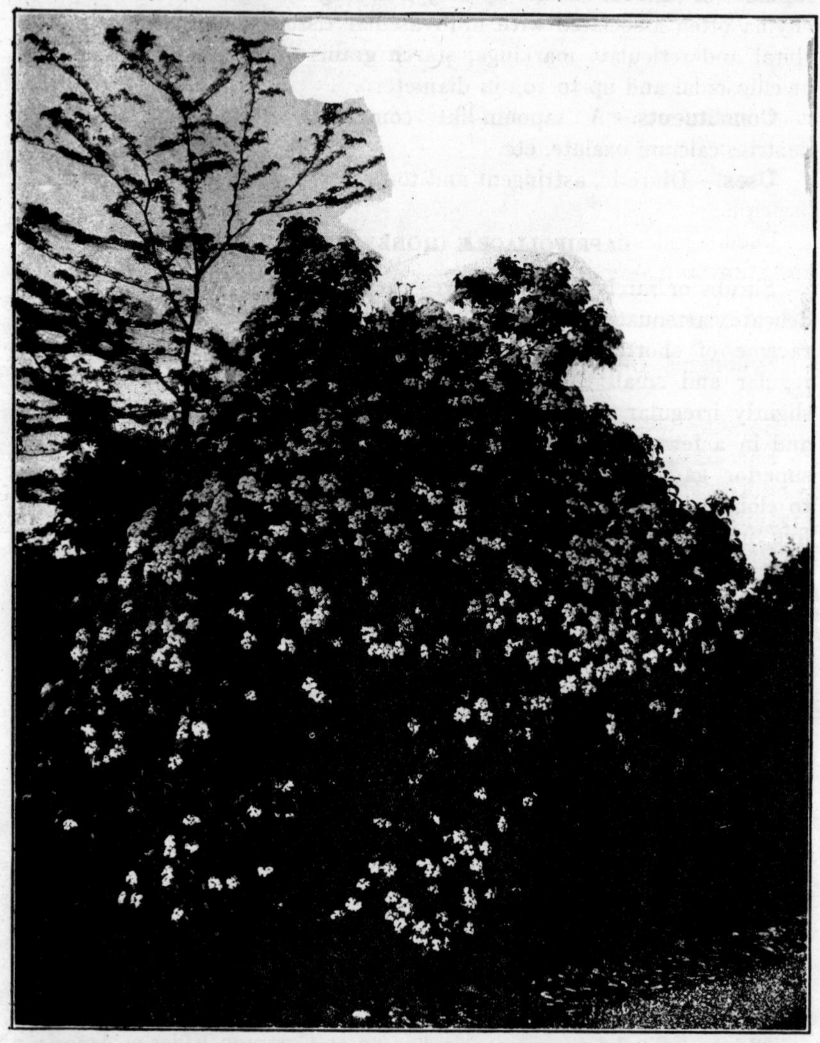

FIG. 264.—*Viburnum Lentago.* (*Courtesy of Arnold Arboretum.*)

and a tricarpellate pistil having 3 stigmas. The fruits are black-purple, edible, berry-like drupes.

Production and Commerce.—Elder flowers are gathered from wild plants in June and July, separated from the peduncles and pedicels, and carefully dried and preserved. Most of the drug is imported from Europe largely through Hamburg, Budapest and Trieste.

Description.—Flowers small and shriveled, 2 to 3 mm. broad; calyx superior, 5-lobed; corolla urn-shaped, 5-lobed, regular; stamens, 5, epipetalous, each possessing a slender filament and yellow, oblong anther; pollen ellipsoidal or tetrahedral and rounded, covered with finely punctate markings and showing 3 pores in the exosporium, odor faintly sweet and aromatic, taste slightly bitter.

Constituents.—Volatile oil, mucilage, gum, resin, tannin, bitter principle, etc.

Uses.—Elder flowers are employed in the form of a tea as a diaphoretic and stimulant.

VIBURNUM PRUNIFOLIUM N.F. (VIBURNUM PRUNIFOLIUM)

Synonyms.—Black Haw, Viburnum, Stag-bush; *Ger.* Schneeballrinde; *Fr.* Ecorce de boule de neige d'Amérique.

Botanical Origin.—*Viburnum prunifolium* L.

Part Used.—The dried root bark.

Purity Rubric.—Not more than 7 per cent. of wood or other foreign organic matter and not more than 3 per cent. of acid-insoluble ash.

Habitat.—United States from New York and Connecticut to Florida, west to Michigan and Texas.

Plant.—A shrub or small tree attaining a height of from 3 to 6 m., leaves opposite, petiolate, glabrous, ovate with serrate margins; flowers white and arranged in compound cymes; fruit an oval, black, sweet and edible drupe with a flat stone.

Production and Commerce.—Large quantities of Black Haw bark are gathered in North Carolina. While the root bark is alone official, the stem bark is also collected and sold to manufacturers.

Description.—In transversely curved pieces or quills, up to 6 cm. in length, 2 cm. in width and 1.5 mm. in thickness. Outer surface grayish-brown or brownish-red (when cork is missing) longitudinally wrinkled; inner surface reddish brown and striated; fracture weak, brittle and uneven; odor sourish; taste bitter and astringent.

Microscopical Characteristics.—Transverse sections of the bark show isolated groups of thick-walled, lignified stone cells in both cortex and phloem. Calcium oxalate crystals of the rosette and monoclinic types are found in numerous cells of both cortex and phloem regions. Rifts between parenchyma cells are also to be observed in the cortex and phloem. Tangential sections show that the medullary rays are 1–3 layers of cells broad. Crystal fibers containing rosette crystals of calcium oxalate may be observed in longitudinal sections.

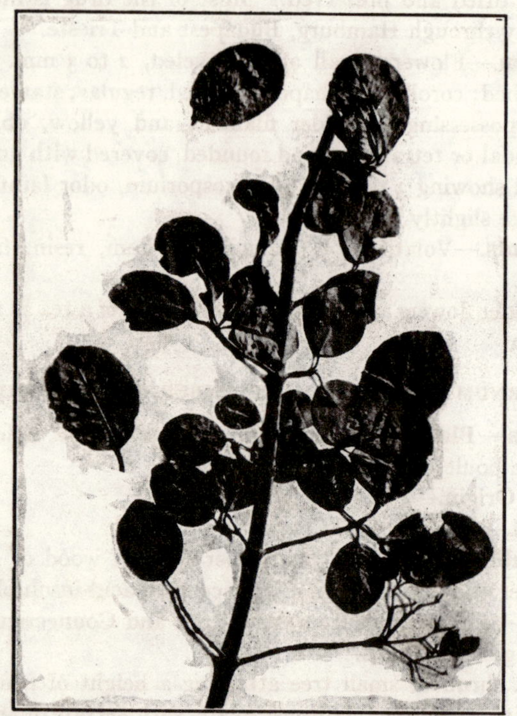

FIG. 265.—*Viburnum prunifolium.* Branch, leaves, inflorescence axis and fruits.

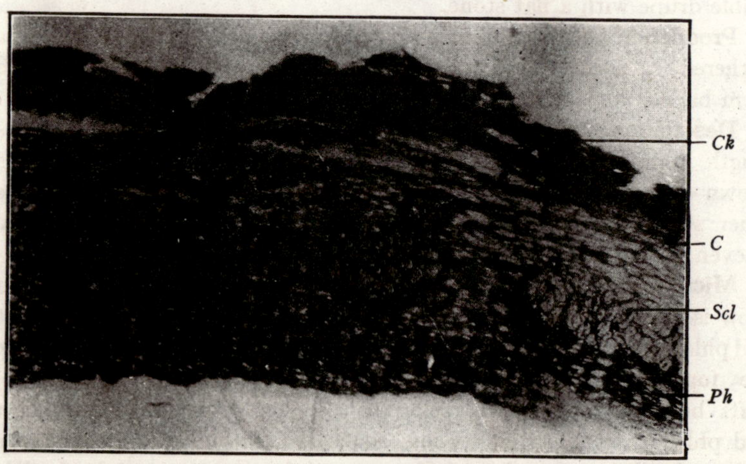

FIG. 266.—*Viburnum prunifolium.* Transverse section of bark showing cork (*Ck*); cortex (*C*); stone cells (*Scl*); phloem (*Ph*).

Powdered Drug.—Dark brown. Stone cells numerous, with thick, porous, lignified walls and from 40 to 150μ in length; numerous fragments of lignified cork; calcium oxalate in rosette aggregates or occasionally in monoclinic prisms up to 40μ in diameter; fragments of parenchyma, some of the cells containing starch grains up to 15μ in diameter, others brownish amorphous masses or oil globules; few sclerenchyma fibers.

Constituents.—Viburnin, an enzyme which splits viburnin into valeric acid and glucose, free valeric acid, resin, tannin, etc.

Uses.—Uterine tonic and sedative.

Substitutes and Adulterants.—The barks of other species of *Viburnum* notably *V. nudum* L. commonly known as Shonny Haw or Shawnee Haw and *V. Lentago* L. or Sheep Berry.

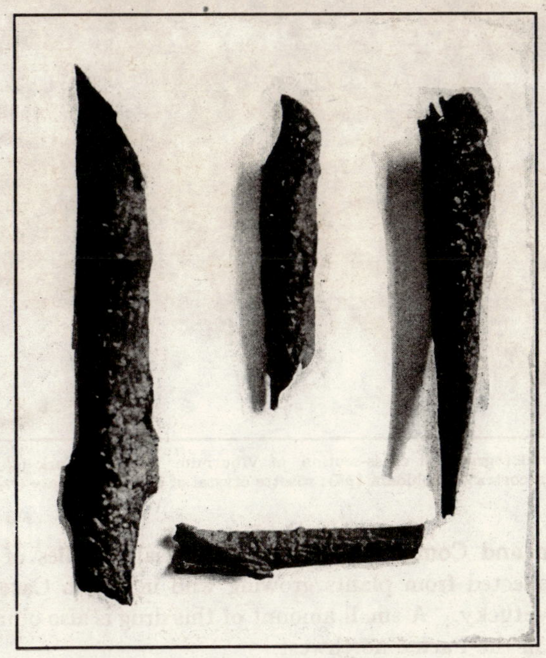

FIG. 267.—Bark of Viburnum Prunifolium, × ½.

VIBURNUM OPULUS N.F. (VIBURNUM OPULUS)

Synonyms.—High Bush Cranberry Bark, Cramp Bark, Wild Guelder Rose, Cranberry Tree Bush, White Dogwood, *Ger.* Wasserholderrinde; *Fr.* Ecorce d'Obier.

Botanical Origin.—*Viburnum Opulus* L. *var. americanum* (Miller) Aiton.

Part Used.—The dried bark.

Purity Rubric.—Not more than 5 per cent. of adhering wood or other foreign organic matter.

Habitat.—Southern Canada and Northern United States, growing wild in thickets along streams.

Plant.—A shrub attaining the height of 3.5 m. Leaves opposite, simple, palmately-veined and prominently 3-lobed, the lobes being toothed; petiole with 2 glands at its summit. Flowers white and arranged on peduncled cymes. Fruit an acid, light-red, globular drupe.

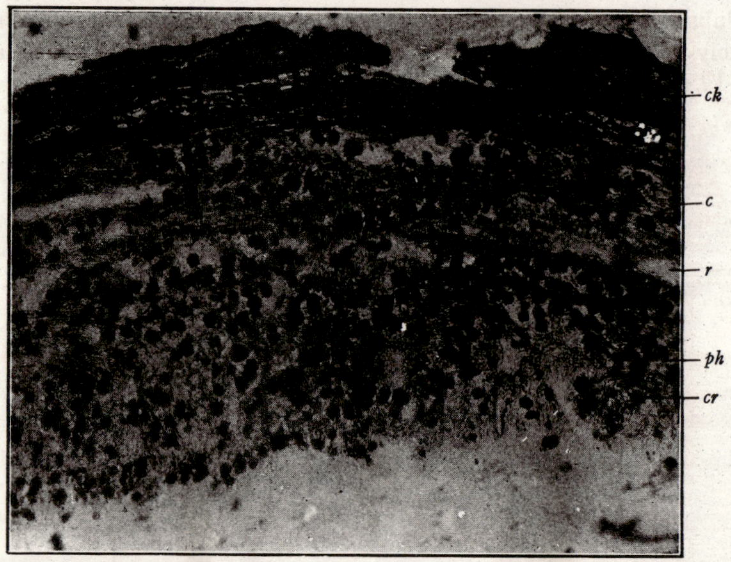

FIG. 268.—Photomicrograph of cross-section of Viburnum Opulus. Cork (*ck*); cortex (*c*); rift in cortex (*r*); phloem (*ph*); rosette crystal of calcium oxalate (*cr*).

Production and Commerce.—The commercial supplies of this bark are largely collected from plants growing wild in North Carolina, Tennessee and Kentucky. A small amount of this drug is also obtained from plants grown in the Pacific northwest.

Description.—Bark in strips, quills or chip-like fragments up to 3 mm. thick; outer surface of thinner pieces light-gray with crooked, longitudinal, purplish-brown stripes and small lenticels, the thicker pieces purplish-red to black, thin scaly or finely fissured, inner surface yellowish to rusty-brown; fracture short and weak; odor valerian like; taste astringent and bitter.

Microscopical Characteristics.—Passing from outer to inner surface The following peculiarities are evident.

1. Cork of 5 to 25 layers of suberous cells having almost colorless walls.
2. Cork cambium.
3. Cortex of about 10 layers of cortical parenchyma cells containing either starch grains, rosette crystals of CaO, a brownish-yellow amorphous substance or chloroplasts. Sclerenchyma fibers with lamellated walls are arranged either singly or in small groups of 2 to 10 in this region.

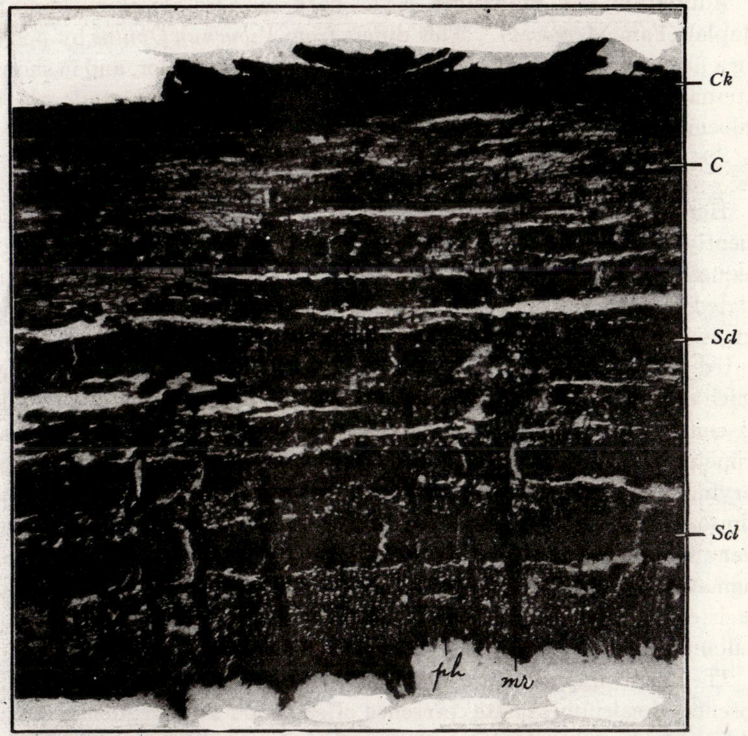

FIG. 269.—Transverse section of mountain maple bark (*Acer spicatum*). Cork (*Ck*); cortex (*C*); sclerenchyma fibers in groups (*Scl*); medullary-ray (*mr*); phloem patch (*ph*) between two medullary rays.

4. Phloem, a broad region composed of phloem patches separated by starch containing medullary rays, 1–2 cells wide. Most of the elements of the phloem patches are sieve tubes and phloem cells. Occasional sclerenchyma elements may occur in this region but are not seen in every section. The latter may contain either starch, rosettes of CaO or a reddish-brown amorphous substance. The starch grains are either simple or compound, the individual grains being 2–10μ in diameter.

Powdered Drug.—Grayish-brown. Fragments of cork having colorless cells, polygonal in surface view; parenchyma with rosette aggregates of CaO up to 40μ in diameter; fragments of parenchyma containing small starch grains up to 10μ in diameter or a brownish amorphous substance, occasional sclerenchyma fibers and reticulate or scalariform tracheæ from adhering wood, few stone cells.

Constituents.—Viburnin (glucoside), an enzyme which splits viburnin into valeric acid and glucose; resin, tannic acid, valeric acid, etc.

Uses.—Antispasmodic, uterine tonic and sedative.

Adulterant and Substitute.—The bark of *Acer spicatum* (Mountain Maple) (Fam. *Aceraceæ*). This differs from *Viburnun Opulus* by possessing a fibrous fracture, in being devoid of a valeric acid odor, and in showing internally tiers of lignified sclerenchyma fibers in cortex, pericycle and phloem, as well as scattered monoclinic prisms of calcium oxalate.

VALERIANACEÆ (VALERIAN FAMILY)

Herbaceous often low succulent plants with creeping rhizomes, frequently strongly scented and possessing stimulating properties. Leaves frequently dimorphic; the radical fascicled; the cauline opposite; petiole dilated, exstipulate. Inflorescence a raceme of dichesial or scorpioid cymes. Flowers more or less irregular; calyx absent as such but represented by a series of teeth that are incurved in the bud and flower and which expand later into a pappose crown and act in the fruit as a pappose disseminator; corolla pentamerous, gamopetalous, varying from rotate-synpetalous to irregular-tubular with petals diversely united, in color varying from greenish-white to white or pink (*Valeriana officinalis*) to crimson; stamens three, rarely two or one, epipetalous; pistil syncarpous; ovary inferior, 3-celled, only 1 cell being fertile; style filiform with three stigmatic surfaces. Fruit an akene from inferior ovary crowned by a persistent, expanded, pappose, calyx rudiment. Seeds anatropous, exalbuminous.

The most important histological features comprise the following: Absence of calcium oxalate; presence of secretion sacs frequently in subepidermal layer, containing volatile oil and possessing suberized walls; tracheæ with scalariform makings or simple pores.

VALERIANA U.S.P. (VALERIAN)

Synonyms.—Wild, Great Wild, Setwall, St. George's Herb, Cat's Valerian, Vandal Root, Garden Heliotrope; *Ger.* Baldrianwurzel; Fr. Racine de Valeriane.

Botanical Origin.—*Valeriana officinalis* Linné.

Part Used.—The dried rhizome and roots.

Purity Rubric.—Not more than 5 per cent. of foreign organic matter and not more than 10 per cent. of acid-insoluble ash.

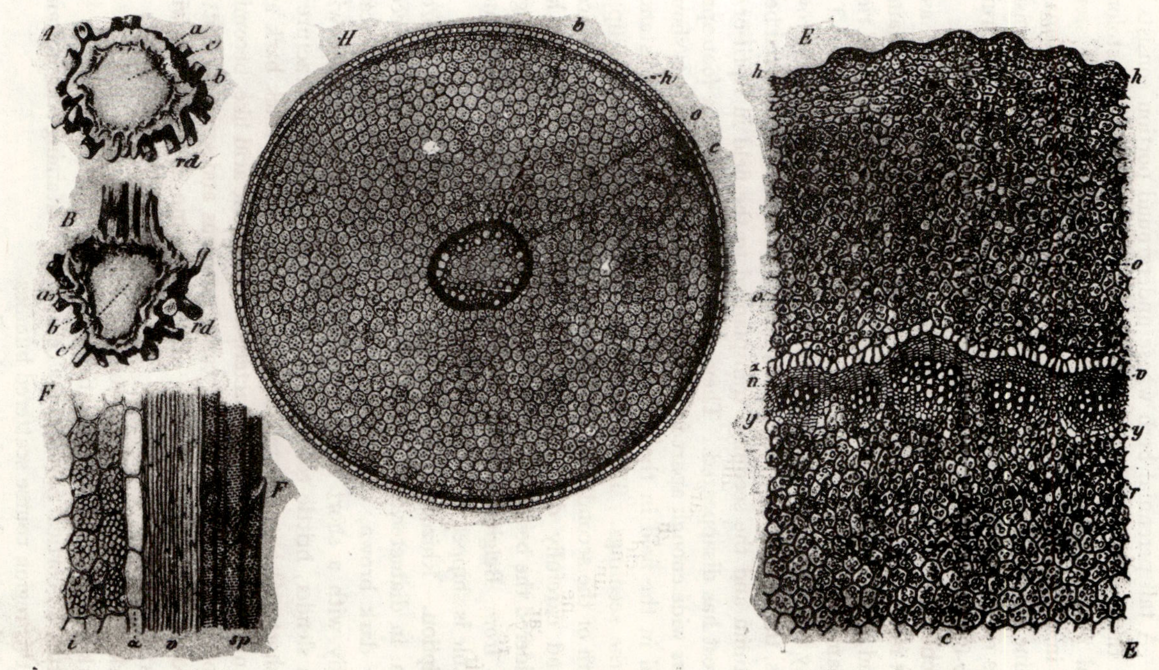

FIG. 270.—*Valeriana officinalis*. *A*, Transverse section of rhizome with lateral rootlet stumps (nat. size). *B*, Longitudinal section of rhizome showing leaf remnants above and lateral rootlet stumps (nat. size). *E*, Transverse section of stolon from rhizome, × 65. *F*, Radial-longitudinal section of a representative portion of stolon showing a few starch-parenchyma cells, endodermis, cambium, and pitted tracheæ of xylem. *H*, Transverse section of root, × 65. *a*, bark, *b*, wood, *c*, pith, *rd*, rootlet, *h*, epidermis, *i*, starch-parenchyma, *o*, cortex, *sp*, tracheæ, *x*, endodermis, *v*, cambium, on outer face of which is soft bast, *y*, xylem. (*After Berg.*)

Habitat.—Europe and Asia.

Plant.—A tall perennial herb whose underground portion consists of a vertical rhizome bearing numerous rootlets and one or more stolons. The aerial portion consists of a cylindrical, hollow, channelled stem, branched in the terminal region, bearing opposite, exstipulate, pinnatisect, cauline leaves with clasping petioles. The inflorescences consist of racemes of cymes whose flowers are small, white or pink. The fruits are oblong-ovate, 4-ridged, one-seeded akenes.

Production and Commerce.—*Valeriana officinalis* is cultivated as a drug plant in various localities of New England and New York but mainly in England, Belgium, Holland and Germany. It thrives best in rich, heavy, loamy soil which is abundantly supplied with moisture. The plants may be propagated from seeds or by dividing old roots. If grown from seeds, the seeds should be planted in cold frames or in protected beds in the autumn and the seedlings transplanted to the field in April or as soon as frost has disappeared. They should be set at least a foot apart and in rows wide enough apart for cultivation. Divided old roots should be planted in the field in the early autumn and set the same distances apart as the seedlings. The rhizomes and roots should be dug up in the autumn of the second year, the rhizomes cut into longitudinal slices, washed and carefully dried by artificial heat. English Valerian has been considered the best in the past. At the present most of the drug is imported from Belgium. Some has been arriving from Germany. Considerable is shipped through London.

Description.—Rhizome vertical, from 2 to 4 cm. in length and from 1 to 2 cm. in diameter, usually cut into 2 or more longitudinal pieces; externally dark brown, upper portion with stem bases and leaf scars, occasionally with a short horizontal stolon, the outer surface showing numerous slender, brittle rootlets and occasional root scars; fracture of rhizome short and horny; internally light-brown, with a thick bark and narrow central cylinder; odor characteristically valeric acid like, becoming stronger on ageing; taste sweetish, camphoraceous and somewhat bitter.

Histology.—Transverse sections of the **rhizome** show the following structures:

1. Cork, a narrow zone of suberous tissue.
2. Cork cambium of meristematic cells.
3. Cortex, of cortical parenchyma cells, most containing starch grains. Through this region course scattered bundles.
4. Endodermis, a layer of altered cells.
5. Fibrovascular bundles of the collateral type, somewhat twisted.
6. Medulla, a broad zone of starch-containing parenchyma.

Transverse section of the **rootlets** show the following peculiarities:

1. Epidermis, consisting of a single layer of papillose cells, a number showing outgrowths as root hairs. Cork replaces epidermis in older rootlets.

2. Hypodermis, a layer of subepidermal cells, some of which are modified as secretion sacs. These have suberized walls and usually contain small volatile oil globules, occasionally small prismatic crystals.

3. Cortical parenchyma of several layers of cells, most of which are filled with simple and compound starch grains; a few near the hypodermis may contain oil globules.

4. Endodermis, a single layer of thin-walled endodermal cells.

5. Pericambium, a layer or two of thin-walled cells.

6. Three to five fibrovascular bundles.

7. Pith.

Powdered Drug.—Brown; numerous starch grains, from 3 to 20μ in diameter, spherical, plano-convex, polygonal, 2- to 4-compound, each generally exhibiting a central cleft; fragments of pitted, scalariform and reticulate tracheæ as well as tracheæ with bordered pores; fragments of sclerenchyma fibers with thin lignified walls; fragments of cork and epidermis; fragments of parenchyma, some cells of which are modified as secretion sacs and contain globules of oil.

Constituents.—Volatile oil (up to 2 per cent.) containing bornyl isovalerianate, bornyl formate, bornyl acetate and bornyl butyrate, camphene, borneol and pinene; 2 alkaloids, chatinine and valerianine, a glucoside, resin, valeric acid, tannin, sugar, etc.

Use.—Valerian is used as a calmative in nervousness and hysteria and as a carminative.

Adulterants and Substitutes.—Rhizomes and roots of *Valeriana toluccana* and (2) *V. mexicana* from Mexico. Both of these contain a volatile oil and valeric acid. (3) Rhizomes and roots of *Valeriana Phu* from the Caucasus region. The rhizome is about twice as long as that of the official article and shows rootlets only on one side. This drug contains only about half as much volatile oil and valeric acid as true Valerian. (4) Rhizomes and roots of *Valeriana officinalis* var. *latifolia* Miq. or Japanese Valerian which yields up to 8 per cent. of volatile oil containing *l*-bornyl isovalerianate and acetate, kessyl acetate and terpenes. (5) Rhizomes and roots of *Veratrum* species.

CUCURBITACEÆ (GOURD FAMILY)

Herbaceous, very often annual (*Colocynth*, etc.), more rarely perennial (*Bryonia*, etc.), sometimes shrubby plants, the perennial and shrubby forms perennating by swollen roots, some of which are heavy and tuberous.

Stems very usually grooved and ridged, often provided with roughened and barbed hairs. Tendrils are frequently produced in the axils of leaves from tendril axillary buds (Pumpkin, Colocynth, Watermelon, Cucumber, Bryony, etc.). Leaves varying from entire, simple, usually deltoid to triangular through stages of trilobate, pentalobate, deeply palmatifid to palmatipartite to seldom approaching compound (Colocynth). Venation in nearly all cases palmate. Leaves thin, herbaceous, much expanded, often hairy. Vascular bundles of petioles, branches and stems, bicollateral. Inflorescence either of loose cymes or more frequently racemes or spikes or entire axillary inflorescence may become solitary-axillary. Flowers pentamerous, very rarely tetramerous, monœcious (*Bryonia alba*) or diœcious (*Bryonia dioica*); sepals five, gamosepalous, adnate to ovary; corolla of five, rarely four gamopetalous petals, varying in size and shape from small to large campanulate or broadly cup-shaped (Cucumber) and in color from greenish-yellow to greenish-white to pure yellow to yellowish-white to white; stamens typically five, epigynous, with anthers either joined by pairs or synantherous; carpels usually three; ovary inferior, one- to three-celled. Fruit a pepo (a berry from an inferior ovary with thick skin). Seeds flat and exalbuminous.

PEPO U.S.P. (PEPO)

Synonyms.—Pumpkin Seed, Squash Seed, Pompion; *Ger.* Kürbissamen; *Fr.* Semences de Potirons.

Botanical Origin.—Cultivated varieties of *Cucurbita Pepo* Linné.

Part Used.—The dried ripe seed.

Limit of Impurities.—5 per cent. of broken or defective seed or other foreign organic matter.

Habitat.—Tropical America.

Plants.—Annual, running, monoecious herbs with dark green, non-glossy, 3–5 lobed leaves and prickly stems and petioles. The flowers are large and yellow being arranged singly in the axils of leaves. With the gradual widening of the corolla toward the top, its lobes become upright and pointed. Calyx lobes are narrow. The gourd-fruit differs in size and shape in the many cultivated varieties, and the toughened, furrowed peduncle does not enlarge near it.

Production and Commerce.—The seeds are gathered from the fruits of varieties of *Cucurbita Pepo* grown in this country as field and pie pumpkins. They are dried in the sun or by artificial heat.

Description.—Broadly elliptical or ovate, flattened, from 15 to 23 mm. in length and 2 to 2.5 mm. in thickness; externally yellowish-white, smooth with a flat ridge and shallow groove parallel to and within 1 mm. of the margin; fracture short; spermoderm consisting of a white coriaceous outer layer and a green membranous inner layer; embryo white, oily, consisting of 2 plano-convex cotyledons and a short conical hypocotyl; odor indistinct; taste bland and oily.

Constituents.—Up to 30 per cent. of a reddish fixed oil conisting of a glyceride of linoleic acid, olein, palmatin and stearin; resin, protein, starch. etc.

Use.—Taenifuge.

COLOCYNTHIS U.S.P. (COLOCYNTH)

Synonyms.—Colocynth Pulp, Colocynth Apple, Bitter Apple; *Fr.* Coloquinte; *Ger.* Coloquinthenapfel.

Botanical Origin.—*Citrullus Colocynthis* (Linné) Schrader.

Part Used.—The dried pulp of the unripe but fully-grown fruit.

Purity Rubric.—Not more than 5 per cent. of seeds and 2 per cent. of epicarp. It yields not more than 2 per cent. of extractive with purified petroleum benzin and not more than 6 per cent. of acid-insoluble ash.

Habitat.—Asia and Africa.

Plant.—A monoecious, perennial vine with an angular hispid stem bearing long petioled, palmately cleft to parted leaves and short tendrils. The flowers are yellow and axillary. The fruit is a greenish-yellow, globular, 3-celled berry, becoming spuriously 1-celled on ripening.

Production and Commerce.—The Colocynth plant grows wild in Mediterranean countries and has been cultivated in India, Turkey, Spain, Cyprus, the Soudan, England and New Mexico. The berries are collected when turning yellow in autumn, and, after the epicarps are removed by peeling, are dried in the sun or by fire. The seeds constitute about 75 per cent. of the weight of the fruits. Colocynth occurs on the American market as pulp (*Colocynth Pulp*) and as whole fruits with the epicarp removed (*Colocynth Apples*). Most of the drug now being imported into this country comes from the Soudan. It is concentrated around Omdurman and Khartoum on the White Nile and is then shipped through Cairo to the United States. Smaller lots come from Aden, London, Marseilles and Hamburg. The pulp is usually packed in large bales, the "apples" in cases. From 5 to 30 per cent. of seeds have been found in recent importations of the pulp.

Description.—Berries, before the removal of the seeds, subspherical, from 4 to 7 cm. in diameter, frequently more or less crushed and in broken pieces, with occasional patches of the epicarp; yellowish-white; light and spongy; separable longitudinally, when entire, into 3 carpels, each containing near the outer surface compressed, ovoid, yellowish seeds; odor slight; taste intensely bitter.

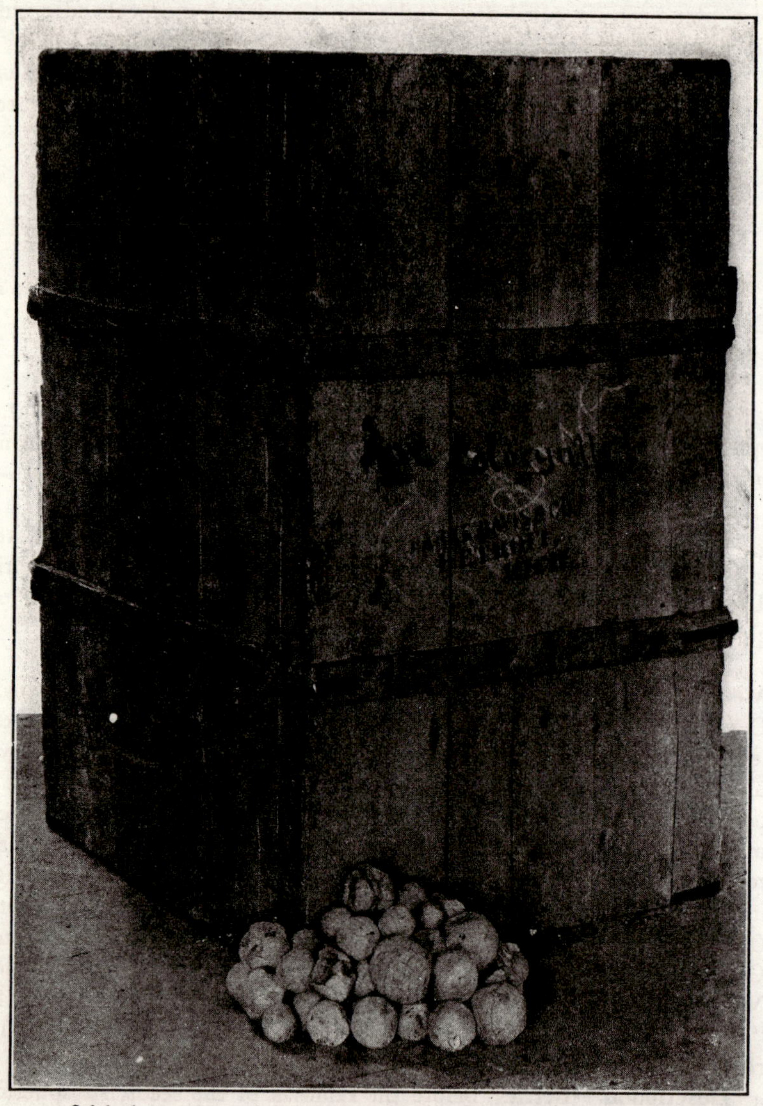

FIG. 271.—Original container of Colocynth fruits. (*After photograph by Parke, Davis and Company.*)

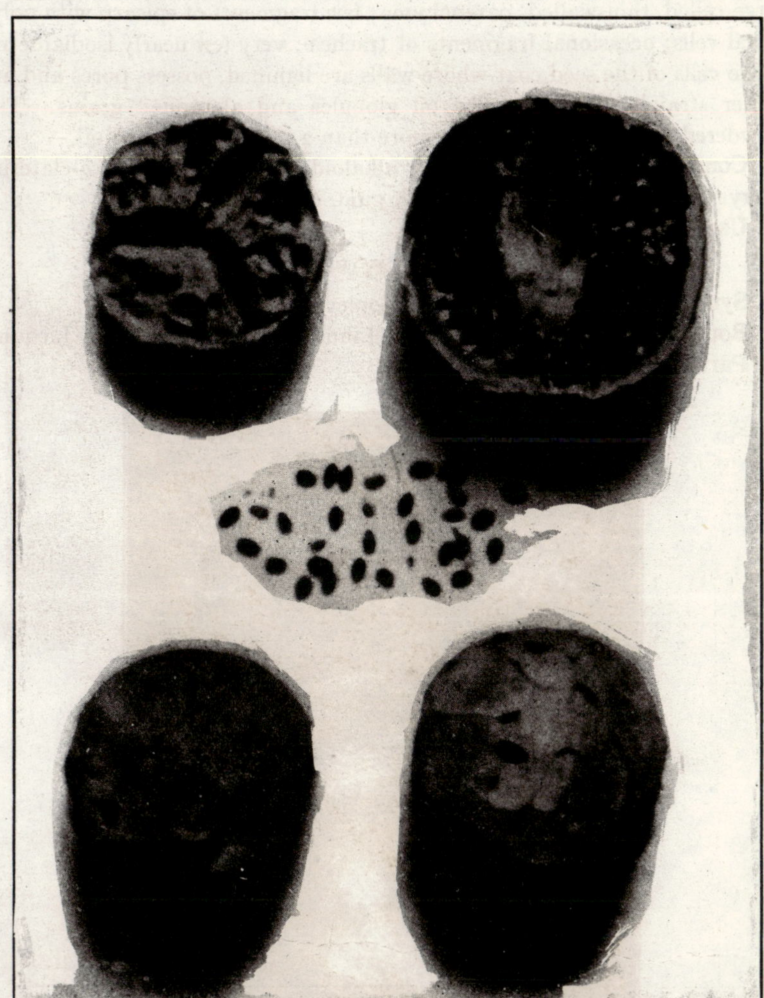

Fig. 272.—Colocynth apples. In lower part of figure are two fruits (berries) deprived of their epicarp. Upper figure to left shows the surface of a fruit cut crosswise. Note the three elliptical fissures with divided placentas between these bearing many seeds. Upper figure to right shows a longitudinally cut surface of fruit. Note groove, placenta and seeds. Seeds at center, × ⅔.

Powdered Drug.—Yellowish-white or buff; numerous fragments of large celled, thin-walled, parenchyma; few fragments of epicarp with polygonal cells; occasional fragments of tracheæ; very few nearly isodiametric stone cells of the seed coat whose walls are lignified, possess pores and are either straight or wavy; few oil globules and aleurone grains. The powdered drug should yield not more than 2 per cent. of fixed oil.

Constituents.—Resins and an alkaloid (both purgative), *a*-elaterin, a crystalline alcohol called citrullol, gum, etc.

Use.—Hydragogue cathartic.

BRYONIA N.F. (BRYONY)

Synonyms.—Bryony Root; *Fr.* Coulevree; *Ger.* Zaunrübe.

Botanical Origin.—*Bryonia alba* Linné and *Bryonia dioica* Jacquin.

Part Used.—The dried root.

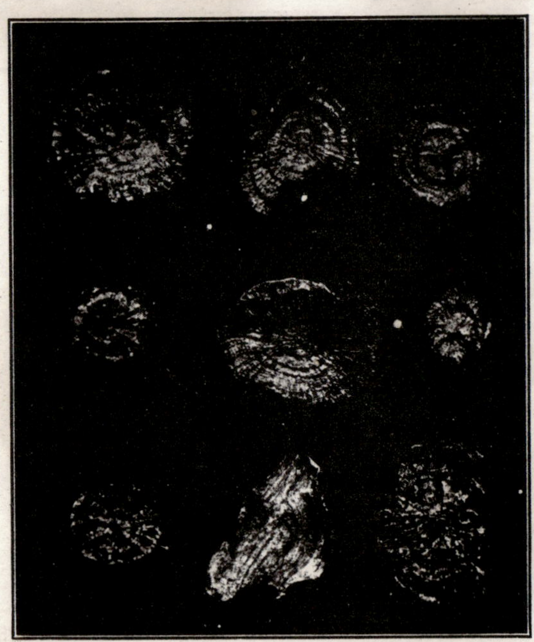

FIG. 273.—Bryonia, × ½.

Limit of Impurities.—2 per cent. of foreign organic matter.

Habitat.—Europe.

Plants.—Perennial climbing vines, monœcious (*B. alba*) or diœcious (*B. dioica*) bearing cordate, palmately 5-lobed leaves and small greenish-white to yellowish axillary flowers. The fruits are black (*B. alba*) or red (*B. dioica*) berries.

Production and Commerce.—The spindle shaped roots are dug up in late summer or early autumn, washed, cut into transverse slices and carefully dried. They are packed in sacks and shipped to Trieste and London whence they are exported to this country.

Description.—Usually in circular or elliptical slices from 1.5 to 10 cm. in breadth and from 3 to 15 mm. in thickness; the edges light gray or yellowish, rough and striate, the cut surface white or faintly yellow, showing a thin bark and broad wood, the latter exhibiting several concentric zones of bicollateral bundles; fracture short and mealy; whitish internally; odor characteristic but faint, taste bitter and nauseous.

Powdered Drug.—Pale yellow; fragments of parenchyma, numerous starch grains, both simple and 2- to 6-compound, the individual grains spheroidal, plano-convex and polygonal usually with a central hilum, and from 4 to 24μ in diameter frequently with a central cleft; fragments of broad tracheæ up to 250μ in width with reticulate and bordered pore markings; a few yellow cork fragments.

When sulphuric acid is added to the powder it becomes reddish-brown and then brownish-purple.

Constituents.—An amorphous alkaloid and a resin (both purgative) volatile oil, an alcohol termed bryonol, phytosterol glucoside, etc.

Uses.—Bryony is used as a hydragogue cathartic and diuretic, in pleurisy, dropsy, bronchitis, tonsilitis, etc.

CAMPANULACEÆ (BLUEBELL FAMILY)

Herbs of annual or more commonly perennial growth, rarely sub-shrubby or sub-woody in habit, frequently with laticiferous tubes containing a milky juice. Inulin occurs in place of starch in the species investigated. Cacium oxalate is absent. Stem upright or feeble and spreading. Leaves alternate, simple, exstipulate. Inflorescence primitively a racemose cyme condensing into a raceme, to a sub-capitulum and ultimately to a capitulum. Flowers regular, campanulate to campanulate-elongate to elongate and deeply cleft in petals; sepals five, only slightly synsepalous, epigynous; petals five, campanulate to campanulate-tubular to tubular-elongated to tubular and deeply cleft; corolla varying in color from greenish-yellow to yellowish-white to white or again, from yellowish-purple (rarely through yellowish-pink or red) to purple to pure blue; stamens five, epigynous, usually free from corolla; nectary epigynous; pistil usually tricarpellary; ovary as many celled as number of carpels and with central placenta; style single, elongate; stigmas as many as carpels. Fruit a capsule. Seeds albuminous. Glandular hairs are absent. The non-glandular hairs are unicellular.

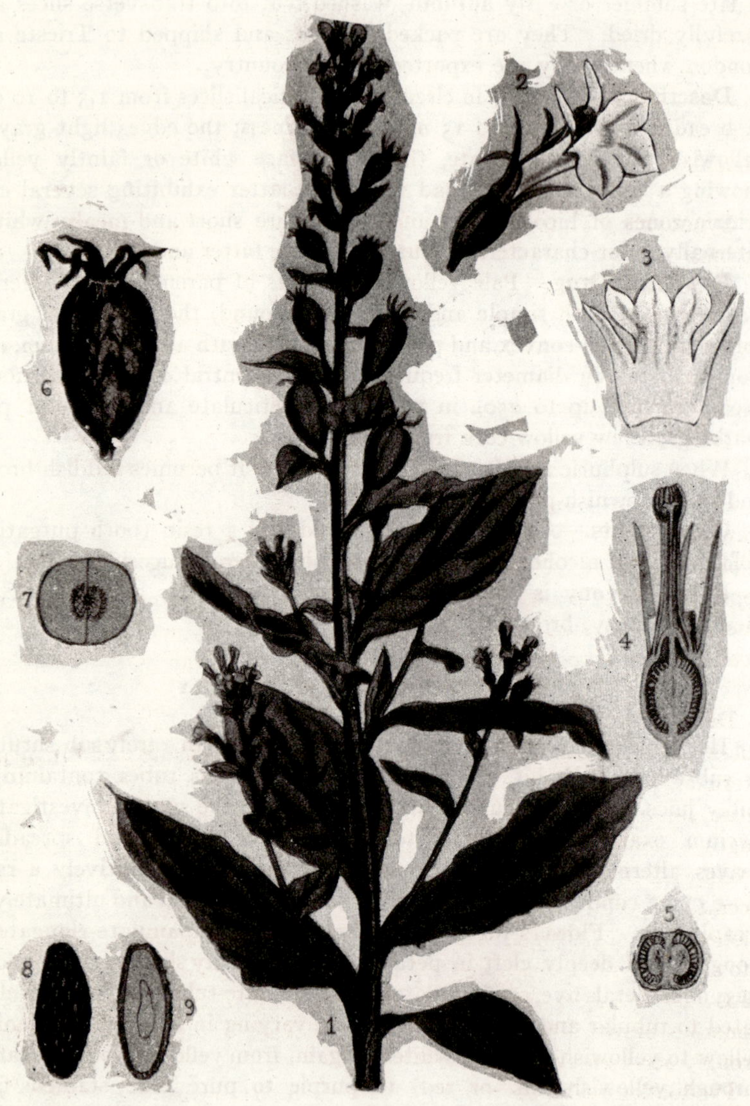

FIG. 274.—*Lobelia inflata*. 1. Upper part of plant. 2. Flower. 3. Corolla. 4. Vertical section of flower with corolla cut off. 5. Transverse section of ovary. 6. Ripe fruit. 7. Transverse section of fruit. 8. Seed. 9. Vertical section of same. (*After Bentley and Trimen.*)

Lobeliaceæ or Lobelia Family.—Herbs, with inulin and latex contents, the latter occurring in laticiferous vessels, which ramify through cortex, phloem, xylem and pith, corresponding with *Campanulaceæ* in their vegetative parts, but differing from that group by having irregular flowers (pale blue in *Lobelia inflata*), anthers always synantherous and pistil always bicarpellate with a two-celled ovary and bilobed or bilabiate stigma.

LOBELIA U.S.P. (LOBELIA)

Synonyms.—Indian Tobacco, Wild Tobacco, Bladder Podded Lobelia, Asthma or Emetic Weed; *Ger.* Lobelienkraut; *Fr.* Herbe de lobélie enflée,

Botanical Origin.—*Lobelia inflata* Linné.

Part Used.—The dried leaves and tops.

Purity Rubric.—Not more than 10 per cent. of stems or more than 2 per cent. of other foreign organic matter. It yields not more than 5 per cent. of acid-insoluble ash.

Habitat.—In open woods and meadows of United States and Canada East of the Mississippi.

Plant.—An annual herb with an erect, yellowish-green, pubescent, branched stem from .3 to .6 m. in height. The leaves are alternate, ovate or oblong with serrate denticulate margins, the lower short-petioled, the upper sessile. The inflorescences are terminal racemes of small, pale blue, short pedicelled flowers. The fruits are bladdery, ovoid or ellipsoidal, 2-celled capsules containing numerous small, oblong, coarsely reticulate, brown seeds.

Description.—Stems cylindrical, coarsely and irregularly furrowed, yellowish-green, occasionally purplish and with numerous hairs; leaves alternate, sessile or short petiolate, usually somewhat broken; when entire, laminæ pale green, pubescent, ovate or oblong, from 2 to 9 cm. in length, obtusely dentate or irregularly serrate-denticulate, each tooth with a yellowish-brown, glandular apex; flowers pale blue, in elongated loose racemes, calyx tube ovoid, with 5 teeth, corolla tubular, 5 parted, the upper 2-lobed portion cleft nearly to the base; stamens with anthers united above into a curved tube enclosing the bifid stigmas; capsules bladdery, ovoid or ellipsoidal, from 5 to 8 mm. in length, light-brown, inferior, and enclosing numerous brown, oblong and coarsely reticulate seeds; odor slight; taste strongly acrid and tobacco-like.

Production and Commerce.—The drug is obtained from both wild and cultivated plants. When cultivated, the seeds should be sown in the fall or spring in rows about 2 feet apart. The soil should be rich loam which has been made very fine before sowing. The seeds are best sown on the surface of the soil and the ground then made firm by placing a board over the row and walking upon it. Shallow cultivation is necessary.

About 1000 pounds of drug per acre can be harvested. Most of the drug is obtained from plants grown in Massachusetts, New York and Michigan. The leaves and flowering tops are collected after a portion of the capsules have become inflated and carefully dried in the shade.

Powdered Drug.—Dark green; fragments of stem with tracheæ showing annular or spiral thickenings or simple pores associated with narrow thin-walled wood fibers; fragments of leaf epidermis with elliptical stomata and usually 3 to 4 neighboring cells; numerous fragments of seed coat composed of more or less polygonal cells with thick yellowish-brown walls; non-glandular hairs, unicellular, short and pointed or elongated to elongated-conical with rounded distal end; spheroidal pollen grains up to 30μ in diameter.

Constituents.—The poisonous liquid, acrid alkaloid, lobeline; lobelic acid, lobelacrin, inflatin, resin, fixed oil, volatile oil (lobelianin), etc.

Uses.—Expectorant in asthma and bronchitis.

COMPOSITÆ (DAISY FAMILY)

Herbs, rarely shrubs or trees, of annual or perennial habit, and with watery or milky juice. Inulin is present in cell sap of parenchyma. Leaves alternate, rarely opposite, simple to compound, exstipulate. Inflorescence a capitulum or a raceme of capitula, each capitulum surrounded by an involucre or protective whorl of bracts, and composed of numerous florets that may be: (*a*) wholly regular, tubular and hermaphrodite (Thistle, Eupatorium, etc.); or (*b*) central florets as in (*a*), but marginals strap-shaped or ligulate and usually pistillate (Daisy, Dahlia, Chamomille, etc.); or (*c*) florets all ligulate and hermaphrodite (Dandelion, Chicory, Hawkweeds, Lettuce, etc.); or (*d*) florets in part or in whole bilabiate (Mutisia, etc.). Flowers small (florets), closely crowded, pentamerous, shaped as above, with ovary inferior and other floral parts superior. Sepals rudimentary, tooth-like (Sunflower), or reduced to a pappose or hairy rudiment above ovary that is functionless during flowering, but that expands in fruit as a hairy fruit disseminator (Dandelion, Thistle, etc.); or sepals wholly absorbed (Daisy). Petals synpetalous, tubular, ligulate or rarely bilabiate, greenish-yellow to white, or through pink-crimson and purple to blue (Chicory). Stamens five, epipetalous, filaments distinct, anthers united into an upright anther-box (so synantherous) into which pollen is shed before or during the opening of each floret. Carpels two, syncarpous, ovary inferior, one-celled with single ovule; style simple, at first short, later elongating and by collecting hairs sweeping pollen to top of anther box, then dividing into two stigmatic surfaces with stigmatic hairs for pollen reception. Fruit an indehiscent achene, often (Dandelion, Thistle) crowned by the pappose, calyx rudiment (pappus). Seed single, exalbuminous.

MATRICARIA N.F. (MATRICARIA)

Synonyms.—German Chamomile, Wild Chamomile; *Ger.* Kamillen; *Fr.* Fleurs de Chamomille commune.

Botanical Origin.—*Matricaria Chamomilla* Linné.

Part Used.—The dried flower head.

Purity Rubric.—Not more than 5 per cent. of stems or other foreign organic matter. It yields not more than 4 per cent. of acid-insoluble ash.

Habitat.—Europe and Western Asia.

Plant.—A branched annual herb attaining a height of about .6 m. bearing alternate, tripinnately-divided leaves below and bipinnately divided leaves above, both types having almost filiform lobes. The flower heads show a conical hollow receptacle surrounded by a flattened imbricated involucre, white ligulate florets and yellow tubular florets, the pappus being absent.

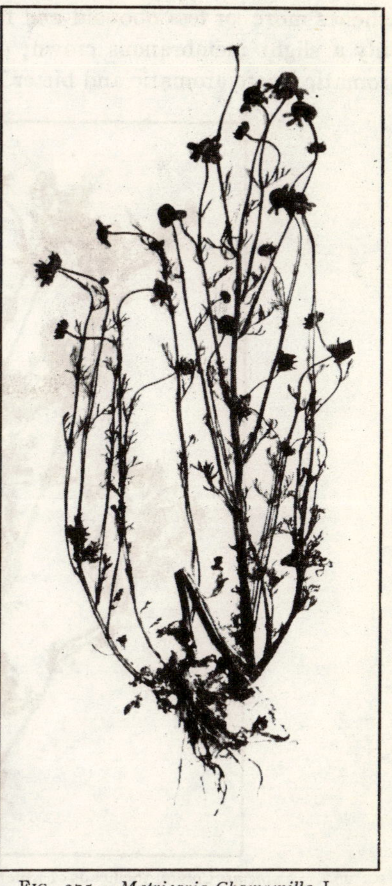

FIG. 275.—*Matricaria Chamomilla* L.

Production and Commerce.—The plant grows wild in this country and Europe but is also cultivated in gardens. It is propagated from seeds which may be sown broadcast in moderately heavy moist soil, rich in humus. The plants bloom in about 2 months after sowing the seed, so that it is possible in many sections to obtain 2 crops a year. The flower heads are gathered when plants are in full bloom, leaves and stems removed and dried on canvas sheets in the sun. They are then packed in cases or bales for the market. The present commercial supplies are largely obtained from Hungary and Germany. Siftings consisting of ray and disk florets are also imported, though not official.

Description.—Flower heads composed of a few white ligulate florets and numerous yellow tubular florets on conical, more or less hollow receptacles the latter being up to 10 mm. in breadth; tubular flowers perfect and without a pappus; ligulate flowers from 10 to 20, pistillate, corolla white, 3 toothed and 4 veined; involucre hemispherical, composed of from 20 to 30 imbricate, oblanceolate and pubescent scales; peduncles light green to brownish-green, longitudinally furrowed and more or less twisted; achenes more or less obovoid and faintly 3-to 5-ribbed; pappus none, or only a slight membranous crown; odor characteristically and fragrantly aromatic; taste aromatic and bitter.

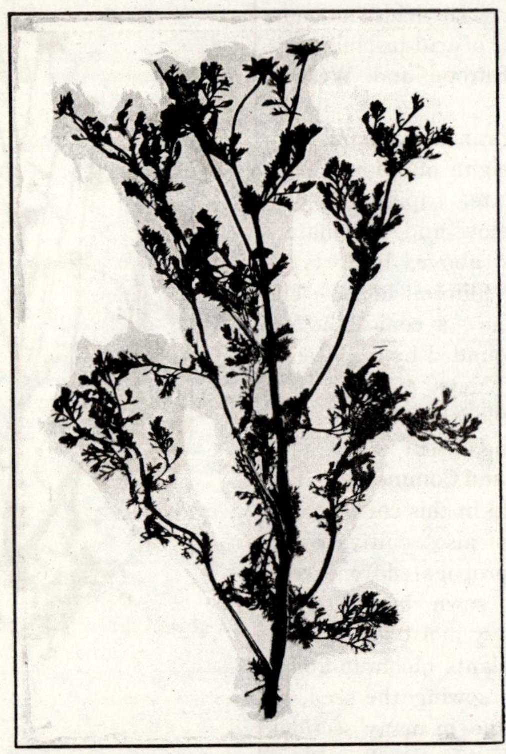

FIG. 276.—*Anthemis Cotula*, the heads of which have frequently been admixed with Matricaria.

Powdered Drug.—Greenish-yellow to yellowish-brown; epidermal cells of corolla with 8-celled glandular hairs; numerous spherical pollen grains up to 25μ in diameter with prominent conical projections of outer wall and 3 pores; papillose fragments of stigmas; fragments of collapsed parenchyma; fragments of fibrovascular bundles with spiral, annular and reticulate tracheæ and sclerenchyma fibers.

Constituents.—Volatile oil of a blue color due to azulene; anthemic acid, tannin, malic acid, etc.

Use.—Aromatic bitter.

Adulterants.—(1) The flower heads of *Anthemis Cotula* L., commonly known as Mayweed, Fetid Chamomile or Dog Fennel, an annual glabrous herb with a disagreeable fetid odor. It is widely distributed over lower Canada and United States, having been naturalized from Europe.

(2) The flower heads of wild plants of *Anthemis nobilis* L., a perennial, pubescent, procumbent herb indigenous to Europe but naturalized in most of the northeastern states.

DISTINCTIONS BETWEEN FLOWER HEADS OF MATRICARIA, ANTHEMIS COTULA AND ANTHEMIS NOBILIS.

Part	Matricaria	Anthemis Cotula	Anthemis nobilis (wild plant)
Receptacle	Hollow	Solid	Solid
Flower head	Ovoid becoming conical	Decidedly conical to oblong	Conical
Peduncle	Unicellular non-glandular hairs absent	Numerous unicellular non-glandular hairs	
Paleæ (scales on receptacle)	Absent	Present. Broad and membranous	Present. Broad and bristly acuminate
Ligulate florets	Pistillate, 3 toothed and 4 veined; 10–20 in one series	Neutral, mostly 3 toothed; 10–18 in one series	Pistillate, 3 toothed, 3–6 veined; 12–18 in one series.
Bracts	Entire, lanceolate	Fimbriated, obovate	Obtuse, pubescent, with scarious margins.
Achenes	Smooth, 3–5 ribbed	Rough, 10-ribbed	Oblong, obtusely 3-angled
Pappus	Absent or as toothed membrane	Absent	Absent

(3) Flower heads of *Santolina chamæcyparissus* L., or Garden Cypress have been detected by Clevenger and Ewing in a shipment of Matricaria from Spain. These differ from Matricaria in their absence of ligulate florets, in the recurving of the tubular florets and in their solid chaffy receptacle, the chaffy scales being very broad with rounded summits.

(4) Matricaria stems.

Allied Drug.—English or Roman Chamomile consists of the dried flower head of cultivated plants of *Anthemis nobilis* L. It occurs in hemispherical heads of a whitish or buff color (upon keeping) each with a solid conical receptacle bearing paleæ and numerous ligulate florets, the corollas of which possess 3 teeth and 4 veins, and subtended by an involucre of 3 rows of imbricate bracts with membranous margins. It contains up to 1 per cent. of a blue volatile oil, anthemic acid, etc. Aromatic bitter.

GRINDELIA N.F. (GRINDELIA)

Synonyms.—Gum Plant, Tar Weed; *Ger.* Grindelie; *Fr.* Grindelia.

Botanical Origin.—(1) *Grindelia camporum* Greene, (2) *Grindelia cuneifolia* Nuttall and (3) *Grindelia squarrosa* (Pursh) Dunal.

Part Used.—The dried leaves and flowering tops.

Limit of Impurities.—10 per cent. of stems over 2 mm. in diameter or 2 per cent. of other foreign organic matter.

Habitat.—Western North America.

Plants.—Perennial herbs with branched stems bearing alternate sessile or clasping, oblong to oblong-spatulate, serrate to dentate, pale green leaves and large heads composed of both ligulate and tubular,

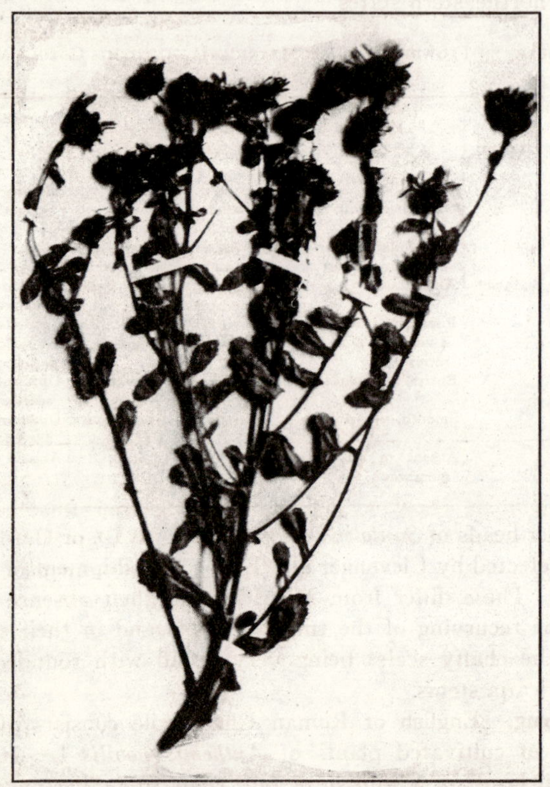

FIG. 277.—*Grindelia squarrosa.*

yellow flowers. The involucre of each flower head is hemispherical and consists of several series of slender bracts with recurved tips. The fruits are short, truncate, glabrous achenes. The pappus consists of from two to several awns which usually fall before the achene has completely matured.

Production and Commerce.—The leafy tops of the Grindelia plants are cut off in July and carefully dried in the sun. The present commercial supply of the drug chiefly comes from the south-western section of the United States.

TABLE OF COMPARISON BETWEEN OFFICIAL GRINDELIAS

Part	Grindelia camporum	Grindelia cuneifolia	Grindelia squarrosa
Stem	Cylindrical, pinkish to yellowish, with attached, alternate branches and small nodes	Cylindrical, pinkish to purplish-brown, with attached alternate branches and larger nodes	Cylindrical, grayish-green to yellowish, with alternate branches and larger nodes
Leaves	Sessile and clasping	Sessile and clasping	Sessile and clasping
Leaf outline	Oblong to oblong spatulate	Oblong to cuneate oblong	Oblong
Leaf apex	Acute	Acute	Obtuse
Leaf base	Subcordate	Subcordate	Subcordate
Leaf margin	Irregularly serrate	Entire below, serrate above, ciliate	Dentate
Upper surface	Pale green, shiny and resinous	Light green to greenish brown and pitted	Gray green or yellowish-green, resinous
Lower surface	Paler green, resinous	Pale green and devoid of resin.	Grayish-green, resinous
Length of leaf	Up to 6 cm.	Up to 9.8 cm.	Up to 5 cm.
Breadth of leaf	Up to 15 mm.	Up to 27 mm.	Up to 15 mm.
Involucral bracts	Linear lanceolate, imbricate, resinous with recurved tips	Linear lanceolate, imbricate, resinous with recurved tips	Linear lanceolate, resinous, imbricate with recurved tips
Ligulate florets	Orange brown, pistillate	Yellow, pistillate	Yellow, pistillate
Tubular florets	Yellow, perfect	Yellow, perfect	Yellow, perfect
Achenes	4-angled with biauriculate summit	4-angled, toothed, with biauriculate summit	4-angled, not toothed, truncate at summit
Odor	Balsamic	Balsamic	Balsamic
Taste	Aromatic and bitter	Aromatic and bitter	Aromatic and bitter

Powdered Drug.—Yellowish-brown. Numerous fragments of fibrovascular bundles showing lignified sclerenchyma fibers and annular, spiral and porous tracheæ; numerous fragments of pith parenchyma the cells of which contain a layer of protoplasm in which spheroidal granules are imbedded; spherical spinose pollen grains up to 35μ in diameter; fragments of mesophyll with adherent epidermis; fragments of glandular hairs, the multicellular heads of which show a rosette aggregate crystal of CaO up to 8μ in diameter in each cell.

Constituents.—Resins, grindeline (alkaloid), tannic acid, volatile oil, etc.

Uses.—Grindelia is used as a stimulating expectorant in bronchitis and often smoked with stramonium and other drugs in asthma. Its aqueous fluidextract is diluted with water and used locally for poison ivy dermatitis.

ABSINTHIUM (ABSINTHIUM)

Synonyms.—Wormwood, Absinth, Maderwort; Mingwort; *Fr.* Absinthe grande; *Ger.* Wermut, Alseikraut, Magenkraut, Bitterkraut.

Botanical Origin.—*Artemisia Absinthium* Linné.

Part Used.—The dried leaves and flowering tops.

Habitat.—Europe, Asia and Northern Africa.

Plant.—A shrubby, odorous, grayish-green, finely canescent herb with branched stem attaining a height of about 1 m. Its leaves are once, twice or thrice pinnately divided into many obovate or linear lobes, the lower, long petioled and the upper, short petioled or sessile. The inflorescence consists of racemose-paniculate heads, drooping on short pedicels. Each head is greenish-yellow, round ovoid and composed of tubular florets inserted on a pubescent receptacle which is subtended by a hemispherical involucre of imbricated bracts.

Production and Commerce.—The plant is extensively cultivated in various parts of Europe mainly for flavoring beer and for the manufacture of a liquor termed "absinthe." It is also cultivated in various sections of the United States and some of the commercial article is gathered in Michigan, Wisconsin and New York. The leaves and flowering tops are gathered in August and September, dried and stored in tin containers. The foreign commercial supplies to this country come largely from France and Italy.

Description.—Stems and leaves gray-green, silky hairy and glandular throughout; the largest leaves 10 to 12 cm. in length and of almost equal breadth, 2- to 3-pinnately lobed or divided, the ultimate segments oblong or obovate, obtuse, entire or slightly toothed; upper leaves becoming gradually shorter petioled, small and narrower, the uppermost only about 2 cm. long and resembling the ultimate segments of the larger lower ones; heads greenish-yellow, racemose-paniculate, from 3 to 4 mm. in breadth, globose-ovoid, with a hemispherical involucre of bracts, outer bracts linear-oblanceolate, obtuse; inner bracts broader and with membranous margins; receptacle pilose-hairy; florets all tubular; odor characteristically aromatic; taste very bitter.

Powdered Drug.—Brownish-green or yellowish-green; numerous whole or broken T-shaped non-glandular hairs from bracts, consisting of a short, 1- to 4-celled stalk and a single apical cell attached to near center and up to 800μ in length; long, unicellular, non-glandular hairs from florets; glandular hairs consisting when entire of a 1- to 2-celled stalk and a 4–8-celled head; fragments of epidermis with elliptical stomata; fragments of mesophyll; tracheæ with spiral markings or simple pores; few lignified sclerenchyma fibers; pollen grains spheroidal, up to 30μ in diameter; rosette aggregates of calcium oxalate about 10μ in diameter.

Constituents.—Volatile oil containing absinthol, a bitter glucoside termed absinthin, tannic acid, resin, etc.

Uses.—Aromatic bitter, diaphoretic and flavoring agent.

CALENDULA N.F. (CALENDULA)

Synonyms.—Marigold, Garden Marigold; *Ger.* Ringelblumen; *Fr.* Fleurs de tous les mois, Fleurs de souci.

Botanical Origin.—*Calendula officinalis* Linné.

Part Used.—The dried ligulate florets.

Purity Rubric.—Not more than 2 per cent. of foreign organic matter.

Habitat.—Mediterranean Basin and Southern Europe.

Plant.—An annual herb frequently found in gardens as an ornamental plant. Its stem is angular and hairy, grows to the height of .4 to .6 m. and bears oblanceolate to spatulate leaves with toothed margins. Its flower heads are terminal about 5 cm. in breadth. Each consists of yellow to orange ray and disk florets.

Production and Commerce.—Calendula is cultivated widely as a garden ornamental in this country and Europe. It thrives best in moderately rich garden soil. The seeds should be sown in drills about 1½ feet apart in the spring. As soon as the seedlings are sufficiently strong they should be thinned so as to stand about one foot apart. The plants bloom throughout the summer. The flower heads should be collected when fully expanded, the ligulate florets removed by hand and carefully dried. Some of the drug is produced in this country but most of it is imported from Spain, France and Italy.

Description.—Ligulate florets from 15 to 25 mm. in length, more or less shrivelled, yellow- or orange-colored, the limb 1- to 3-toothed, 4- or 5-veined, the short hairy tube occasionally enclosing the remnants of a filiform style and bifid stigma; odor slight; taste slightly bitter.

Histology.—Fragments of the corolla, mounted in water or chloral hydrate T. S., exhibit elongated epidermal cells with striated cuticle, the parenchyma cells beneath showing numerous, often yellow, oil globules. In the vicinity of the tube will be noted a few long non-glandular hairs, consisting of a double row of thin walled, more or less collapsed cells, with a one- to two-celled summit, and up to about 950μ in length. Coursing through the mesophyll will be noted strands of fibrovascular tissue, each possessing annular and spiral tracheæ. Spinose pollen grains, 3 pored, and up to 45μ in diameter will be noted adhering to the corolla.

Constituents.—Volatile oil, bitter principle, resin and calendulin (a tasteless gummy principle.)

Use.—Calendula is employed chiefly in the form of its tincture as a vulnerary.

Adulterants.—Ligulate florets of various species of the *Compositæ*.

ARNICA N.F. (ARNICA)

Synonyms.—Arnica Flowers, Wolf's Bane, Mountain Tobacco, Leopard's Bane; *Ger.* Arnikablüthen, Fallkraut; *Fr.* Fleurs d' Arnica.

Botanical Origin.—*Arnica montana* Linné.

Part Used.—The dried flower head.

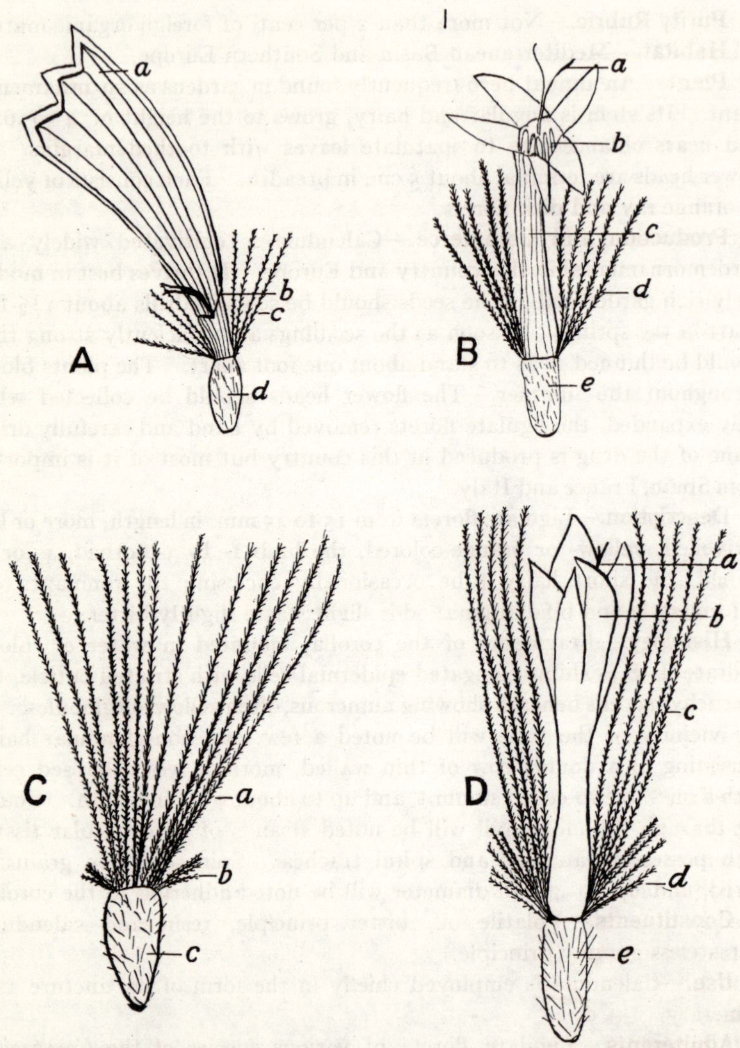

FIG. 278.—*A*, Ligulate floret of Arnica. Ligula of corolla (*a*); tubular portion of corolla p*b*); pappus (*c*); ovary (*d*). *B*, Tubular floret of Arnica. Stigma (*a*); stamens (*b*); corolla (*c*); pappus (*d*); ovary (*e*). *C*, Fruit of *Heterotheca inuloides*, an arnica adulterant. Inner, long pappus (*a*); outer, short pappus (*b*); akene (*c*). *D*, Tubular floret of *Heterotheca inuloides*. Style (*a*); corolla (*b*); inner long pappus (*c*); outer, short pappus (*d*); ovary (*e*).

Purity Rubric.—Not more than 3 per cent. of foreign organic matter.

Habitat.—In mountains and meadows of central Europe. Naturalized in northwest Asia and western North America.

Plant.—A perennial herb flourishing in the Alps and Pyrenees of Europe. Its underground portion consists of a rhizome and root system. Its aerial portion comprises a basal rosette of oblong-ovate leaves from the center of which arises a hairy, longitudinally striate stem bearing lanceolate, pubescent bright green leaves and both axillary and terminal stalked flower heads of sub-globular shape.

Production and Commerce.—Arnica is collected from plants growing wild in mountain meadows and upland moors of central Europe. Considerable of the drug which eventually reaches the United States is collected in Jugo-Slavia. Both rhizomes and flower heads are used in medicine. The flower heads are collected when fully expanded, deprived of their receptacles and involucres and dried. The commercial article is imported from Hamburg and Halle, Germany, and from Trieste and Nimes.

Description.—The drug occurs as tubular and ligulate florets, occasionally with receptacles and involucres present; bracts of involucre narrowly lanceolate, about 1 cm. in length, dark green and pubescent; receptacle solid, slightly convex, deeply pitted and densely hairy; ligulate florets bright-yellow, the ligula or limb up to 2 cm. in length, 3 toothed, 7 to 10 veined, pistillate tubular florets perfect, deep yellow; the achenes spindle shaped, from 5 to 7 mm. in length, dark brown, finely striate, glandular pubescent and surrounded by a long pappus composed of a single circle of barbellate bristles; odor agreeably aromatic; taste bitter and acrid.

Powdered Drug.—Yellowish-brown; numerous spherical spinose pollen grains up to 35μ in diameter; non-glandular hairs either unicellular or uniseriate, 4-to 6-celled or paired unicellular; glandular hairs either with a 4-celled stalk and a 1-celled head or a biseriate stalk of 10 cells and a 2-celled head or a 1-celled stalk and 1-celled head; fragments of barbed pappus consisting of a multicellular axis with one-celled branches.

Constituents.—Arnicin (bitter principle), volatile oil, resin, etc.

Use.—The tincture is used externally as a vulnerary.

Adulterants.—(1) The flower heads of *Inula britannica* L. which are characterized by the smaller ligulate florets with but 4 veins in each ligula, a smooth receptacle and a short achene having a length of about 1 mm. (2) Flower heads of *Heterotheca inuloides*. See Fig. 278 C, D.

PYRETHRI FLORES (PYRETHRUM FLOWERS)

Synonyms.—Insect Flowers; *Ger.* Bertramblüthen; *Fr.* Fleurs de pyrèthe.

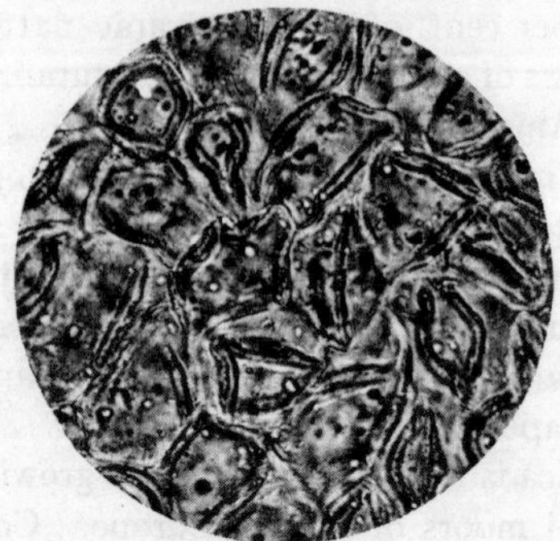

FIG. 279.—"Puckered" papillæ, ray floret, × 290.

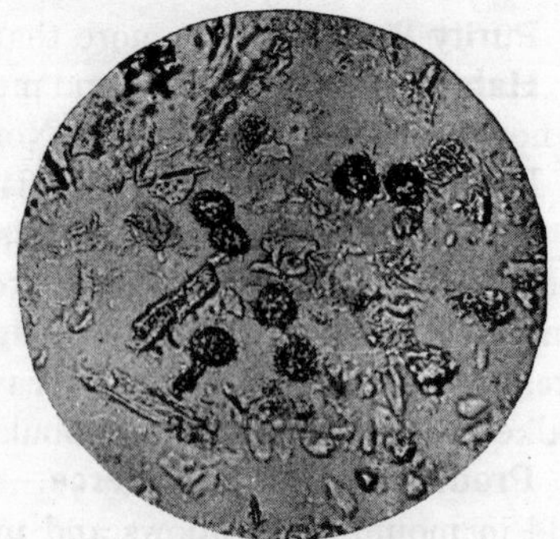

FIG. 280.—Pollen grains, × 140.

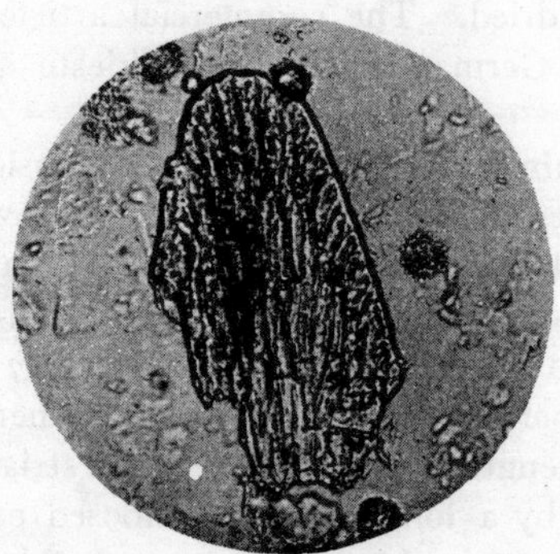

FIG. 281.—Tooth, disk floret, × 140.

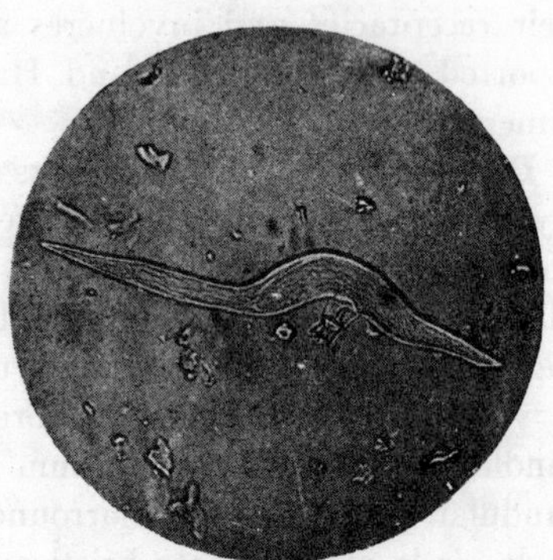

FIG. 282.—Stalked hair (magnified).

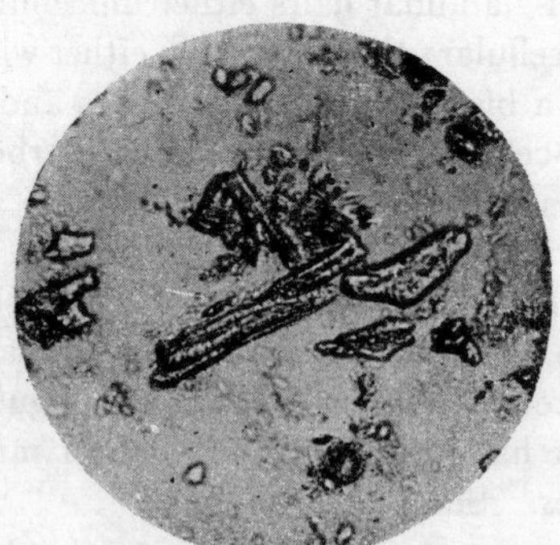

FIG. 283.—Stone cells, achene, × 134.

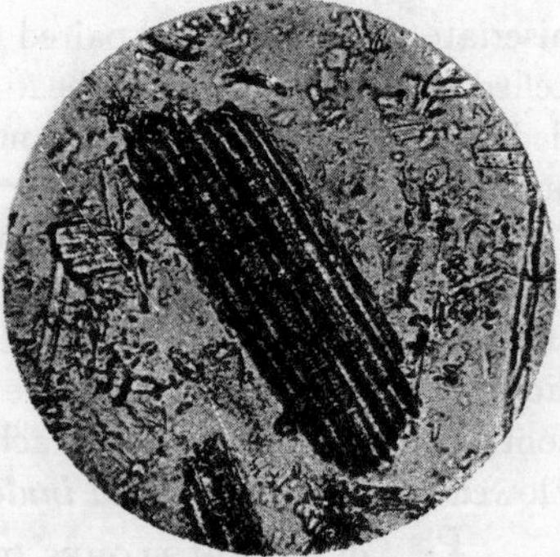

FIG. 284.—Stem tissues, × 84.

FIGS. 279–284.—Insect Powder (*Chrysanthemum cinerariæfolium*). (*Bull.* 824, U. S. *Dept. of Agriculture.*)

Botanical Origin.—(1) *Chrysanthemum cinerariæfolium* (Trev.) Bocc., (2) *Chrysanthemum roseum* Web. et Mohr and (3) *Chrysanthemum Marschalii* Aschers.

Part Used.—The dried flower heads.

Purity Rubric.—Insect flowers or Insect Powder should not contain more than 5 per cent. of insect flower stems (peduncles) and not more than

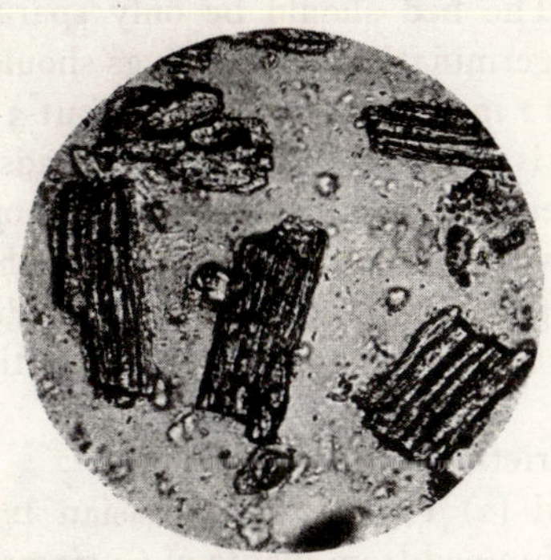

FIG 285.—Achene tissues, × 130.

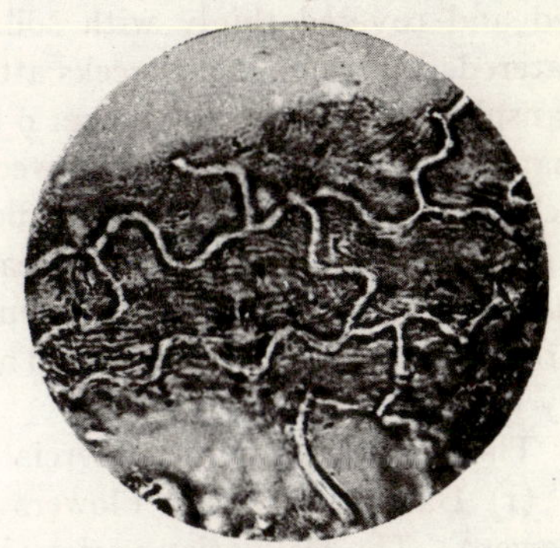

FIG. 286.—Sinuous cells, ray floret, × 254.

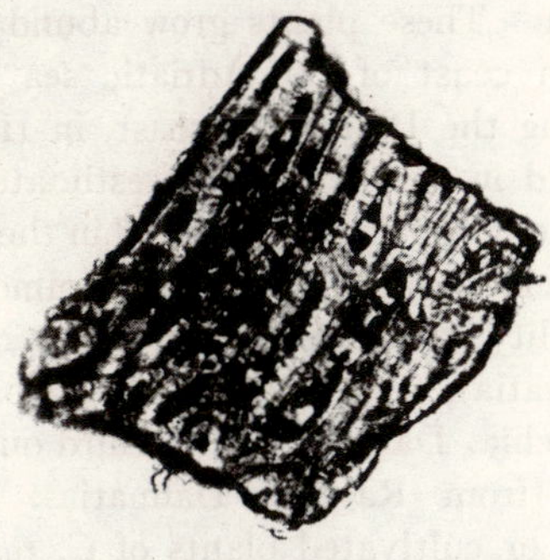

FIG. 287.—Achene tissue and crystals, × 204.

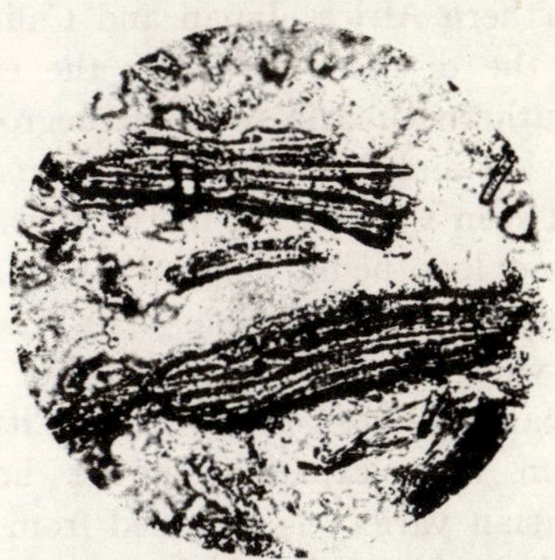

FIG. 288.—Bract tissues, × 120.

FIGS. 285–288.—Insect Powder (*Chrysanthemum cinerariæfolium.* (*Bull.* 824, *U. S. Dept. of Agriculture.*)

2 per cent. acid-insoluble ash, none of either of which has been purposely added.

Ash.—Not more than 2 per cent. ash insoluble in HCL.

Habitat.—(1) Dalmatia and Herzegovina. (2 and 3) Persia and Caucasus region.

Plants.—Perennial herbs with pinnatifid or divided leaves and hemispherical to top-shaped heads of yellow tubular and cream colored or reddish (*C. roseum*) ligulate flowers.

Production and Commerce.—The three species yielding Insect Flowers grow best in warm localities and in ordinary manured or fertilized field or garden soil which is well drained and not too clayey. A rocky soil and a southern exposure are desirable. They may be propagated either from seeds or by the division of old plants. When seeds are employed they should be mixed with sand and sown broadcast on the surface of the seed bed and covered thinly with soil. The bed should be only sparingly watered. In from 4 to 5 weeks after germination the seedlings should be transplanted to the field and set 9 to 12 inches apart in rows about 3 feet apart. Cultivation to remove weeds is essential. The flower heads are picked by hand or by means of a flower picker just as they begin to open, being plucked just beneath the head, spread out in a thin layer on sheets and dried in the shade or sun. During the drying process they should be turned at least twice a day. They should be preserved in air tight, dry containers.

There are two chief commercial varieties of these flowers, viz.:

(1) Dalmatian Insect Flowers and (2) Persian or Caucasian Insect Flowers. The Dalmatian variety is obtained from plants of *C. cinerariæfolium*, cultivated in Dalmatia, Herzegovina, Switzerland, Germany, northern Africa, Japan and California. These plants grow abundantly in the districts bordering the eastern coast of the Adriatic sea from Southern Croatia to Montenegro, along the Dalmatian coast, in Herzegovina and Albania. The annual yield in this territory is estimated at between 150 and 200 metric tons. The flower heads are dried in the sun, some lots being shipped entire, others powdered. Three commercial varieties are obtainable, viz.: First quality from unexpanded flower heads of wild plants (from Krivosije, Dalmatia), second quality from partly expanded flower heads (from Cittavecchia, Dalmatia), and third quality from fully expanded flower heads (from Ragusa, Dalmatia). The Persian variety is obtained from wild or cultivated plants of *C. roseum* and *C. Marschalii* which abound in the Caucasus regions and in northern Persia and Japan. At the present writing this variety is off the American market. Most of the Insect flowers used in United States are imported from Trieste, from Gravosa in Jugo Slovakia and from Osaka and Yokohama, Japan.

Description.—Flower heads nearly hemispherical (*C. cinerariæfolium*) or flattened top-shaped (*C.Marschallii* and *C. roseum*) up to about 12 mm. in diameter, consisting of a grayish-yellow rounded or conical receptacle subtended by a bell-shaped involucre consisting of an outer and inner series of imbricated scales and bearing up to 30 marginal, yellowish-white or straw-colored (Dalmatian) or purplish-red (Persian) pistillate, ligulate (ray) florets and a central broad disk of numerous, perfect, yellow, 5-

toothed tubular florets. The outer bracts of the involucre are keeled, lanceolate, light brown on their outer and straw colored on their inner surface (*C. cinerariæfolium*) or green to greenish-brown and reddish-brown along margins (*C. Marschallii* and *C. roseum*). The inner bracts are spatulate, somewhat longer than the outer bracts with pale scarious membranous margins (*C. cinerariæfolium*) or dark reddish-brown scarious margins (*C. roseum*) or dark red to black brown margins (*C. Marschallii*). The ligula (limb) of the ligulate florets terminates in 3 short obtuse teeth, the central one usually being smaller than the other two. The tubular florets are about 6 mm. and exhibit a 5-ribbed (*C. cinerariæfolium*) to 10 ribbed (*C. roseum* and *C. Marschallii*) ovary or achene, a toothed pappus and a 5-lobed yellow corolla enveloping a style which is surrounded by synantherous stamens and which terminates in 2 style arms bearing stigmatic surfaces.

Powdered Drug.—Yellowish brown; numerous T-shaped non-glandular hairs from bracts with 4 basal stalk cells (usually broken) and a horizontal, tapering, pointed and usually twisted or curved end cell; fragments of the outer epidermis of the outer bracts with somewhat polygonal to slightly wavy-walled epidermal cells and many broadly elliptical stomata which are usually surrounded by 3–4 neighboring cells; fragments of the inner epidermis of the corolla showing numerous striated papillae; fragments of outer epidermis of corolla with elongated, striated epidermal cells, and a few stomata that are surrounded by 4 to 5 neighboring cells; numerous fragments of the pistil and achene showing secretion reservoirs containing brownish resin contents, the latter colored yellowish-green changing to brownish-black with mineral acids; fragments of sclerenchyma tissue of somewhat rectangular shape from the achene showing short prisms or diamond-shaped crystals; fragments of the seed coat with elongated, thick-walled, porous stone cells and particularly abundant in powder ground from mature flower heads; spirally thickened cells from edge of pappus; fragments of ovary showing epidermis with club-shaped glandular hairs; fragments of teeth of the tubular florets with rows of longitudinally elongated cells becoming smaller toward the base, most of which contain a rosette aggregate of calcium oxalate; fragments of vascular bundles; a few monoclinic prisms; numerous round pollen grains from 27 to 29μ in diameter, the exine with 3 pores and numerous conical spines of different length.

A relatively larger percentage of pollen and relatively smaller percentage of stone cells is found in the powder ground from the unexpanded flower heads than in that ground from mature flower heads.

Constituents.—A mixture of acids and esters which appear to represent the insecticidal principles; resin, volatile oil, etc.

Use.—Insecticide.

Adulterants.—(1) The flower heads of *Chrysanthemum Leucanthemum* L. known commonly as the ox-eye daisy or common field daisy; (2) Flower heads of *Helichrysum arenarium* DC. or yellow immortelle; (3) entire peduncles of Insect Flowers.

Insect powder has been frequently adulterated with powdered Pyrethrum stems, turmeric, chromate of lead, yellow ocher and ground flower heads and stems of other *Compositæ*. Less frequently used past adulterants have been ground cereals, sawdust, almond shells, white hellebore, fustic, saffron, brick dust, barium chromate, potassium chromate, aloes, arsenic, borax, jalap, nux vomica, euphorbium, quassia, pepper, soap bark, senna leaflets, sumach berries, and starches.

The flower heads of the Daisy have been one of the most common adulterants of Insect Flowers. This plant grows in practically every region where Dalmatian Insect Flowers are gathered and is common in many sections of this country. Whole Daisy flowers may be detected by the presence of relatively shorter achenes than those of Insect Flowers, each of which possesses 10 whitish ribs alternating with black stripes and with knob-like projections on its broader end. Cross sections of these achenes show elongated, narrow, palisade cells in the outer region of each rib and secretion reservoirs, in the mesocarp, possessing a dark-red amorphous substance.

The most common recent adulterants for Insect Powder have been powdered insect flower stems or peduncles, powdered Daisy flowers and powdered turmeric.

Insect flower stems may be detected qualitatively, if present in considerable amounts, by the green color of the ether extract of the sample. Pure Insect flowers yield an intensely yellow ether extract, whereas that of pure stems yields one of a pronounced green color. Fragments of stem tissue may be detected in the powder by mounting it in phloroglucin and hydrochloric acid and examining microscopically, when long strands of tissues with frayed out ends and composed of collenchyma cells associated with pinkish- or reddish-stained tracheæ and sclerenchyma fibers will be evident.

No chemical method has yet been devised which will determine quantitatively even an approximate amount of the stem present in an adulterated sample. This is likewise true for Insect powder which has been adulterated with powdered Daisy flowers or Turmeric. It is possible, however, to determine the approximate percentage of these three sophisticants by certain methods of microscopic analysis. See page 659.

Powdered Daisy flowers can be definitely determined in Insect powder by the presence of dark red amorphous fragments of material from the secretion-reservoirs of the Daisy achene and by the closely arranged, narrow, thick-walled palisade cells of the outer portion of the ribs of this achene.

Powdered turmeric can be detected microscopically by the irregular deep yellow, altered, pasty masses of starch which become reddish-brown with KOH solution, blue with iodine T.S. and crimson with concentrated H_2SO_4. Unaltered turmeric starch grains, some with beaked ends as well as reticulate ducts represent corroborative evidence of the presence of this adulterant, although many samples of turmeric show no unaltered starch. See Curcuma.

SANTONICA (SANTONICA)

Synonyms.—Levant Wormseed; *Fr.* Semen Cinæ; *Ger.* Zittwersamen, Wurmsamen.

Botanical Origin.—*Artemisia Cina* (Berg.) Willkomm.

Part Used.—The dried unexpanded flower heads.

Ash.—8 per cent.

Habitat.—Turkestan.

Plant.—A small shrub the aerial portion of which consists of 6 to 8 stems bearing pinnately-dissected, grayish leaves and small, oblong-ovoid, obtuse, grayish-green flower heads.

Production and Commerce.—The greater bulk of the present world's supply of Santonica is obtained from plants growing in the desert of Kirghiz of Turkestan. The flower heads are collected in mid summer while unexpanded by stripping them from the stems, and rapidly dried. The commercial supplies are shipped here largely through London.

Description.—Oblong-ovoid, from 2 to 3.5 mm. in length and from 1 to 1.5 mm. in width, summit obtuse; consisting of an involucre of 14 to 20 glandular and imbricated bracts enclosing 3 to 5 tubular florets; apical marginal hairs absent from bracts; apices of corolla lobes devoid of trichomes and never more than slightly papillose; externally smooth, glossy, grayish-green to brownish-green; readily crumbling to powder upon crushing; odor aromatic, somewhat camphor-like; taste aromatic and bitter.

Constituents—Up to 3.5 per cent. of santonin (neutral principle); resin, volatile oil, artemisin, etc. Santonin, the chief active principle, rapidly disappears with the opening of the flower head. It is present in greatest abundance in flower heads collected just before expansion and rapidly dried. Santonin occurs in rhombic plates and responds positively to the furfural reaction.

Uses.—Anthelmentic and a source of santonin.

Adulterants.—(1) Santonin-less Santonica. This may be distinguished by the presence of apical marginal hairs upon the bracts of the flower heads and the presence of hairs on the leaves usually occurring in commercial samples. It is usually shipped from Persian Gulf ports. (2) Barbary Santonica from *Artemisia ramosa* and *Artemisia Sieberi.*

Substitutes.—The unexpanded flower heads of *Artemisia pauciflora* Weber and of *A. maritima var. Stechmanniana* Besser, both of which contain santonin. Santonin also occurs in the unexpanded flower heads of *Artemisia mexicana* Willd., *A. neo-Mexicana* Wooton and *A. Wrightii* Gray, growing in New Mexico and Mexico.

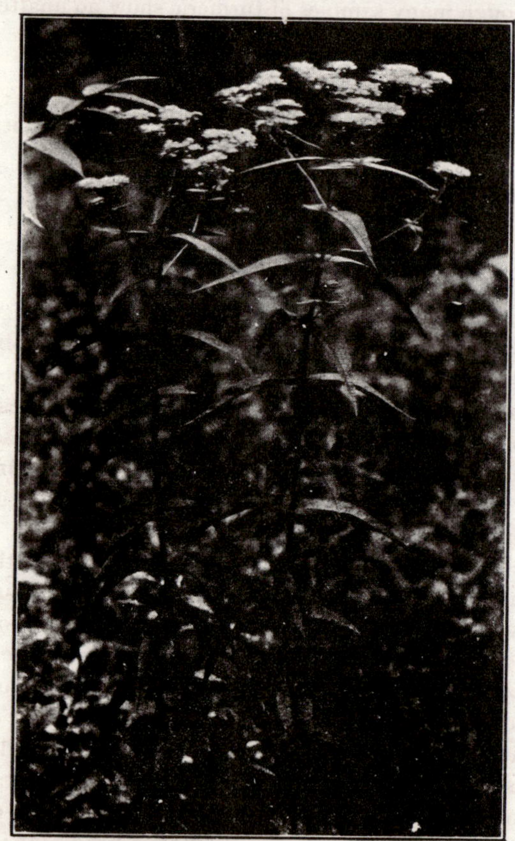

FIG. 289.—Boneset (*Eupatorium perfoliatum*). Note connate-perfoliate leaves and flower heads arranged in corymbs.

EUPATORIUM N.F. (EUPATORIUM).

Synonyms.—Boneset, Thoroughwort, Vegetable Antimony, Feverwort, Sweating Plant, Indian Sage; *Fr.* Herbe à fièvre; *Ger.* Durschwachsdost.

Botanical Origin—*Eupatorium perfoliatum* Linné.

Part Used.—The dried leaves and flowering tops.

Purity Rubric.—Not more than 10 per cent. of its stems and not more than 2 per cent. of foreign organic matter.

Habitat.—North America.

Plant.—A hardy perennial herb having an erect hairy stem from 0.5 to 1.5 m. in height which bears connate-perfoliate, bright green leaves and panicled corymbs of numerous small heads of white tubular florets.

Production and Commerce.—Boneset is a very common weed which spreads rapidly in fields and low grounds. In this country it is found

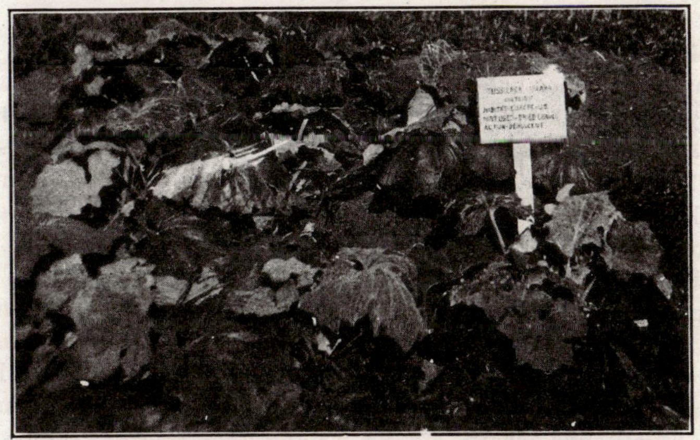

FIG. 290.—*Tussilago farfara* (coltsfoot). (*Photograph by Hogstad.*)

mostly east of the Mississippi. The drug is almost entirely obtained from wild plants which are cut down in late summer when in full bloom. The leaves and flowering tops are stripped from the stems by hand and carefully dried in the shade. The commercial supplies are obtained principally from central and southern United States.

Description.—Usually as more or less broken leaves and flowering tops; leaves connate-perfoliate, each consisting of 2 sessile lanceolate leaves, the bases of which are connate around the stem, up to 20 cm. in length and from 1.5 to 5 cm. in breadth, apex acute, margin crenate-serrate, venation rugose, upper surface rough and bright-green, lower surface yellowish-gray-green, tomentose and dotted with yellow resin; flower heads small, numerous, corymbed, with a campanulate involucre of linear lanceolate, imbricated hairy bracts and with 10 to 15 tubular, yellowish-white florets, each with a pappus consisting of a single row of bristles; odor characteristically but slightly aromatic; taste very bitter.

Constituents.—A bitter glucoside called eupatorin; resin, volatile oil, gallic acid, a glucosidal tannin, etc.

Use.—Boneset is chiefly used as a diaphoretic in systemic colds.

FARFARA N.F. (COLTSFOOT)

Synonyms.—Coltsfoot Leaves, Tussilago Leaves, Horse-, Bull's-, Fool's-, or Ass'-foot Leaves, British Tobacco, Herba Farfaræ, *Ger.* Huflattigblätter; *Fr.* Feuilles de tussilage.

Botanical Origin.—*Tussilago Farfara* Linné.

Part Used.—The dried leaf.

Purity Rubric.—Not more than 3 per cent. of foreign organic matter and not more than 4 per cent. of acid-insoluble ash.

Habitat.—Europe.

Plant.—A low perennial wooly herb whose underground portion consists of a horizontal rhizome and root system. Its aerial portion consists of a rosette of heart shaped to ovate-reniform, toothed, radical leaves and a scape bearing a single, terminal, yellow, flower head which is surrounded by reddish involucral bracts. The flowering scapes appear before the leaves in the spring.

Production and Commerce.—Coltsfoot grows in wet places and somewhat sandy soil in central and southern Europe and in the north eastern and north central part of the United States and lower Canada. The leaves are generally gathered in June and July and carefully dried. The commercial supply of the drug is obtained from Europe, largely through Trieste and Leghorn.

Description.—Leaves usually broken and folded together; when entire, petiole long and pubescent; lamina broadly ovate-reniform, nearly orbicular or cordate, from 8 to 18 cm. in length and up to 18 cm. in breadth, rounded or acute at the apex, deeply cordate at the base, angularly lobed and dentate with red-brown teeth along the margin, palmately 5- to 9-nerved; upper surface dull grayish-green, nearly glabrous; lower surface white-tomentose; odor indistinct, taste mucilaginous and bitter.

Constituents.—Traces of volatile oil and resin; tannin, etc.

Use.—Coltsfoot is used by the laity in the treatment of coughs.

SENECIO N.F. (SENECIO)

Synonyms.—Life Root, Golden Senecio, Ragwort.

Botanical Origin.—*Senecio aureus* Linné.

Part Used.—The dried plant.

Purity Rubric.—Not more than 10 per cent. of foreign organic matter.

Habitat.—In swampy grounds and moist thickets of eastern and central United States, south to Virginia and Arkansas.

Plant.—A perennial herb whose underground portion consists of a slender branching rhizome system from which arise erect stems bearing alternate lyrate to pinnatifid leaves, the uppermost ones being sessile and bractiform. The basal radical leaves are rounded ovate to oblong, deeply cordate at base, and form a rosette. The inflorescences consist of loose corymbs of bright yellow heads.

Production and Commerce.—The aerial portions of this plant are gathered from June to August when the plant is in flower and carefully dried. The commercial supplies of the drug come from central United States.

Description.—Usually in the form of a mixture of broken stems, leaves and flower heads; when entire, stems from 3 to 6 m. in length, when young white tomentose, when mature glabrous, and showing, if entire from base upward, a rosette of long petioled, rounded ovate, obtuse, cordate, crenate-dentate radical leaves and cauline leaves of transitional forms which pass from lyrate to sessile pinnatifid to amplexicaul, oblong and cleft and correspondingly smaller until quite bract like in uppermost region; flower heads in terminal loose corymbs, each up to 25 mm. in breadth and showing a flat naked receptacle surrounded by usually 2 series of lance-linear appressed bracts and bearing usually 10 bright yellow ligulate florets and numerous yellow, perfect, tubular florets, each with a white bristly pappus; odor aromatic; taste bitter, acrid and pungent.

Constituents.—Volatile oil, bitter principle, etc.

Uses.—Life Root is used as an emmenagogue.

TARAXACUM N.F. (TARAXACUM)

Synonyms.—Dandelion, Common Dandelion, Lion's Tooth, Puff- or Blow Ball; *Ger.* Löwenzahn, Pfaffenröhrchen; *Fr.* Dent de Lion, Couronne de moine.

Botanical Origin.—(*Taraxacum officinale* Weber) *Leontodon Taraxacum* L.

Part Used.—The dried rhizome and roots.

Purity Rubric.—Not more than 2 per cent. of foreign organic matter and not more than 4 per cent. of acid-insoluble ash.

Habitat.—Europe.

Plant.—A perennial herb naturalized in North America where it is common in grassy places, fields, meadows and along roadsides. It consists of an underground long, straight, tapering, fleshy brown root which is continued upward as a simple or branched rhizome. From this arises a rosette of bright-green runcinate leaves and later from the center of the rosette a hollow scape bearing on its summit a broad orange-yellow head of ligulate flowers. The fruit is a compressed, oblong-ovate achene, terminated by a slender stalk which is crowned by a silky, spreading pappus.

Production and Commerce.—Dandelion thrives in any good soil. The fruits are sown in the spring, being placed in rows from 1½ to 2 feet apart and covered by about ½ in of soil. The seedlings are later thinned to stand about a foot apart in each row. Cultivation is necessary to keep down weeds. The roots of wild plants are dug in the early spring before the vegetative processes begin or in the fall immediately after they cease. The roots of plants under cultivation are best dug in the fall of the

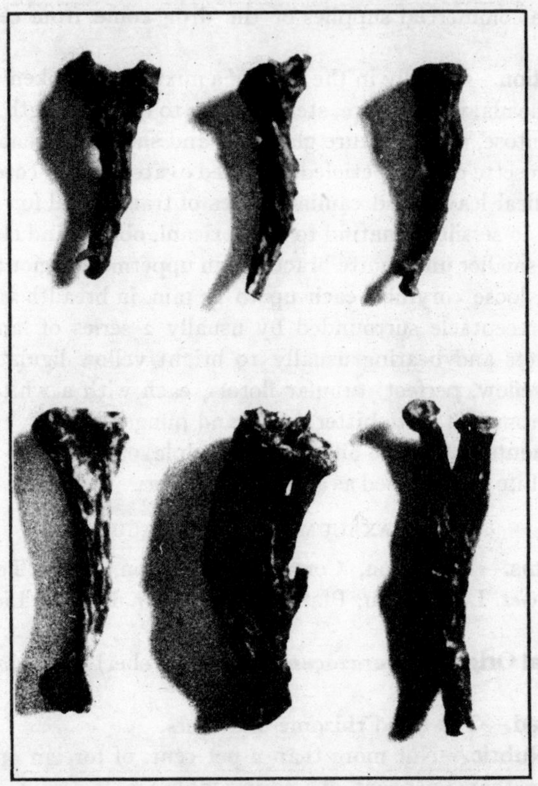

FIG. 291.—Taraxacum. Note the roots with multiple crowns. In the lower half of the figure, the characteristic depressed stem scars are evident, × ½.

second season after planting. They are then washed, the thicker roots sliced and all carefully dried and stored in closed containers to which a few drops of carbon tetrachloride are placed from time to time to prevent attacks by insects.

Most of the drug used in this country is collected from wild plants and is imported from London, Hamburg, Amsterdam and Budapest in burlap bags.

Description.—Cylindrical or somewhat flattened, gradually tapering, usually in broken segments up to 15 cm. in length and from 5 to 15 mm. in diameter; externally blackish-brown or dark-brown, longitudinally wrinkled with few root or rootlet scars; crown usually branched with numerous leaf-bases exhibiting annulate markings; fracture short and horny; internally bark light brown, containing concentrically arranged

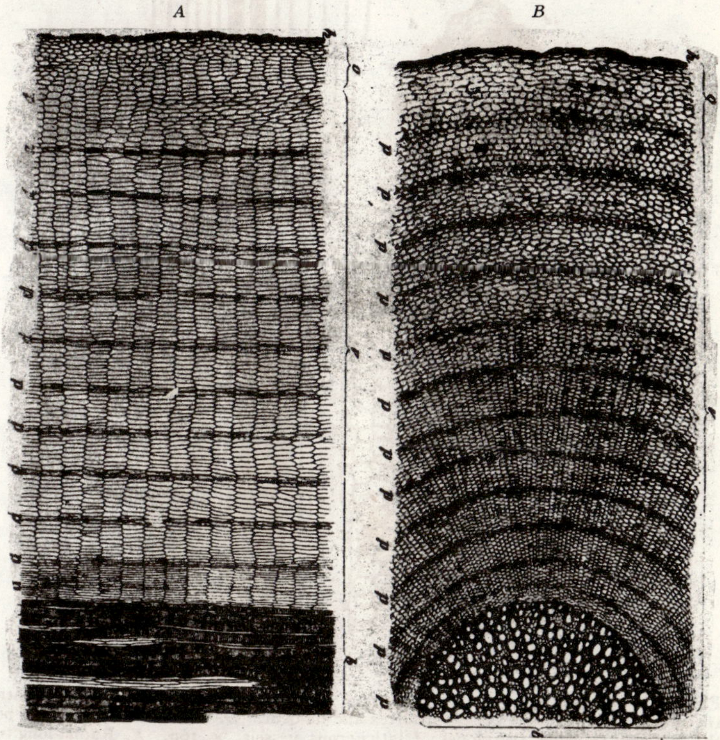

FIG. 292.—Taraxacum Root. *B*, Representative portion of transverse section and *A*, of longitudinal-radial section showing *h*, cork; *o*, cortex; *v*, phloem; *b*, xylem and *p*, laticiferous vessels, × 40. (*After Berg.*)

lighter and darker zones which represent parenchyma alternating with laticiferous vessels and sieve; wood light yellow and porous; odor slight; taste bitter.

Histology.—Transverse sections of macerated Dandelion root show the following peculiarities.

1. Cork, of several layers of cork cells with brownish contents.
2. Cork cambium.
3. Cortex of several layers of more or less tangentially elongated cells containing inulin.

4. Phloem, a broad zone of concentric layers of laticiferous vessels and sieve tubes alternating with parenchyma, the cells of which contain inulin.

5. Cambium, comprising several layers of small meristematic cells.

6. Xylem, filling the center of the root and composed of a matrix of

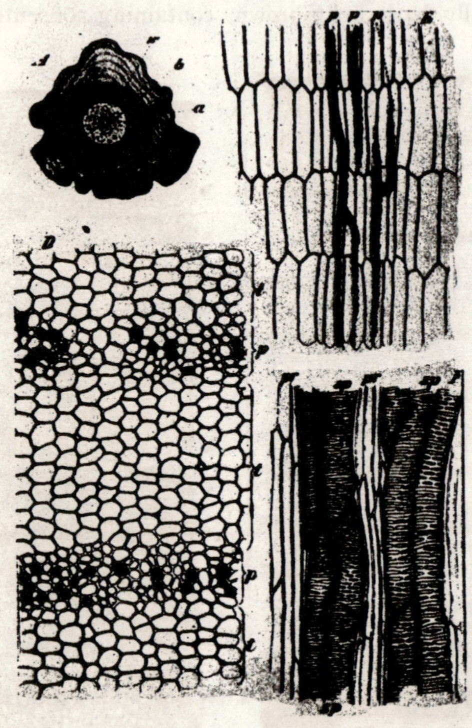

FIG. 293.—Taraxacum. *A*, Cross section of dried root (× 4) showing concentrically arranged lines of laticiferous vessels in cortex and phloem. *D*, Transverse section of a portion of the phloem showing two zones of laticiferous vessels, × 160. *E*, Radial-longitudinal section of a portion of the phloem showing a zone of laticiferous vessels, × 160. *F*, A portion of a radial-longitudinal section of the wood, × 160. *a*, bark; *b*, wood; *w*, cambium; *p*. laticiferous vessels; *l*, phloem parenchyma; *pr*, wood fibers; *sp*, reticulate tracheæ. (*After Berg.*)

non-lignified wood fibers and xylem cells in which are scattered numerous tracheæ.

The rhizomes differ mainly from the roots by showing a small pith in the center.

Tangential sections, cut through the phloem, and mounted in weak iodine, show a network of branching laticiferous vessels with brownish contents which anastomose with one another. Accompanying these latex carrying elements are sieve tubes. These and their callus plates may readily be made out by mounting a similar section in corallin soda solution, when the callus sieve plates take on a pink coloration.

Radial-longitudinal sections show that the tracheæ of the xylem are for the most part reticulate. The wood fibers accompanying them have simple and oblique pores.

Powdered Drug.—Light brown; numerous parenchyma cells containing irregular masses of inulin; fragments of sieve tubes and laticiferous vessels, the latter yellowish-brown; fragments of reticulated tracheæ associated with wood fibers having oblique and simple pores.

Constituents.—Taraxacin (bitter principle); taraxacerin, inulin, a sugar called lævulin, choline, resin, fat acids, 2 phytosterols, taraxasterol and homotaraxasterol, etc. Inulin is most abundant in autumn, sugar in spring.

Uses.—Taraxacum is chiefly used as a simple bitter and as a mild laxative in catarrhal jaundice.

Adulterants.—(1) Chicory, the rhizome and roots of *Cichorium Intybus* (*Compositæ*), which is frequently gathered by mistake along with Dandelion, since it frequently occurs in the same localities in which the latter abounds. Like Dandelion, it also contains laticiferous vessels but these are arranged with the sieve tubes in radiate fashion, as observed in transverse sections, the radiating phloem patches being separated by broad medullary-rays. (2) The roots of species of *Lactuca* (Lettuce) which show radial rows of tracheæ, usually one cell wide in the xylem patches, the latter separated from each other by medullary-rays, 2 to 3 cells in width.

LAPPA N.F. (LAPPA)

Synonyms.—Burdock Root, Beggar's Buttons, Hareburr; *Ger.* Klettenwurzel; *Fr.* Bardane.

Botanical Origin.—*Arctium Lappa* Linné and *Arctium minus* Bernhardi.

Part Used.—The dried root, collected from plants of the first year's growth.

Purity Rubric.—Not more than 5 per cent. of its leaf bases or more than 2 per cent. of other foreign organic matter.

Habitat.—Europe and Asia.

Plants.—*Arctium Lappa* or Great Burdock is a coarse biennial herb naturalized in this country and found as a common weed along roadsides and in waste places. The first year's aerial growth consists of a rosette of rough cordate-oblong leaves. During the second year a stem arises to the height of .6 to 1.8 m., becoming much branched and bearing alternate, petiolate, smaller ovate to cordate to cordate-oblong, irregularly toothed leaves and solitary or clustered capitula of purple tubular flowers.

Each head is 3 to 5 cm. broad and its receptacle is sourrounded by a glabrous involucre of imbricated, lanceolate to linear-attenuate bracts with hooked tips. The fruits consist of oblong, flattened and angular achenes.

Arctium minus or Common Burdock somewhat resembles the former species but its flower heads are only up to 3 cm. in breadth and possess shorter and more linear bracts.

Production and Commerce.—The root is collected from wild and cultivated first year plants in autumn, washed (the thicker roots longitudinally sliced to facilitate drying), and carefully dried. The plants are readily propagated from fruits sown in the fall or spring directly in the field.

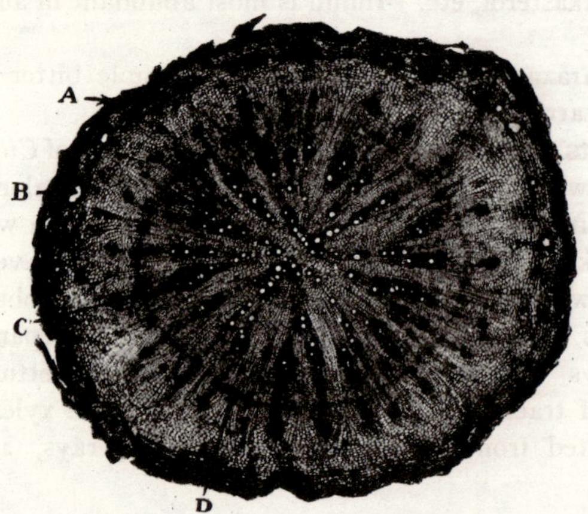

FIG. 294.—Lappa—cross-section of root. (10 diam.) (*A*) Cork; (*B*) resin cell; (*C*) xylem; (*D*) cambium. (*Sayre.*)

The commercial article is chiefly imported in bags from Belgium, Germany and France. The Belgian product appears to be the most esteemed at present.

Description.—Fusiform, of variable length, from 5 to 20 mm. in diameter near the crown; frequently split longitudinally or in broken segments; externally grayish-brown, longitudinally wrinkled, the crown annulate and frequently showing a woolly tuft of leaf remnants; fracture short and horny; a dark cambium separating the thick brown bark from the yellowish, porous and radiate wood; odor indistinct; taste mucilaginous, sweetish, then bitter.

Histology.—Transverse sections of young roots show the following structural characteristics:

1. *Cork*, composed of thin-walled, brownish, brick-shaped cork cells.
2. *Cork cambium*.

3. *Cortex*, a broad zone of parenchyma containing for the most part crystals or masses of inulin, when sections are mounted in alcohol. Other cells of this region contain a yellow resin.

4. *Phloem*, a narrow zone of slender patches of sieve tubes and phloem parenchyma, separated by broad phloem medullary rays.

5. *Cambium* composed of small, more or less collapsed, meristematic cells.

6. *Xylem*, filling up the center and composed of narrow, radiate xylem patches, separated by broad, wedge-shaped, xylem medullary-rays. Each xylem patch is composed of inulin-containing wood parenchyma and a few pitted tracheæ. Only occasional wood fibers with thin walls can be observed accompanying the tracheæ. (In old second year roots wood fibers are abundant.) The cells of the medullary-rays contain inulin.

Powdered Drug.—Light brown; numerous thin-walled cells of the cortex, wood parenchyma and medullary-rays containing glassy masses or sphaerocrystals of inulin; fragments of parenchyma containing yellow resin cells; fragments of pitted tracheæ; fragments of brownish cork tissue; only occasional slender sclerenchyma fibers.

Constituents.—Bitter principle, mucilage, inulin, fixed and volatile oils, tannin, sugar, etc.

Uses.—Burdock is used as a diaphoretic, diuretic and alterative.

PYRETHRUM (PYRETHRUM)

Synonyms.—Pellitory Root, Spanish Chamomile; *Fr.* Salivaire; *Ger.* Römische Bertramwurzel.

Botanical Origin.—*Anacylus Pyrethrum* (Linné) De Candolle.

Part Used.—The dried root.

Habitat.—Northern Africa.

Plant.—A perennial herb with long fusiform root. From this arises a rosette of pinnatifid radical leaves and numerous branched pubescent stems which are procumbent at the base, erect above. The stem leaves are sessile with linear lobes. The inflorescences consist of terminal heads of white, pistillate, ray flowers and yellow, tubular, disk flowers. The ligula of the ray flower is purple beneath. The fruits are obovate achenes each with a short pappus.

Production and Commerce.—The root is gathered in autumn from plants growing in Algeria, carefully dried and shipped direct or through France.

Description.—Roots sometimes entire, fusiform, frequently broken into segments up to 10 cm. in length and up to 22 mm. in diameter; externally dark brown, deeply longitudinally furrowed, beset with few or no hair-like rootlets, crown more or less annulate and frequently showing

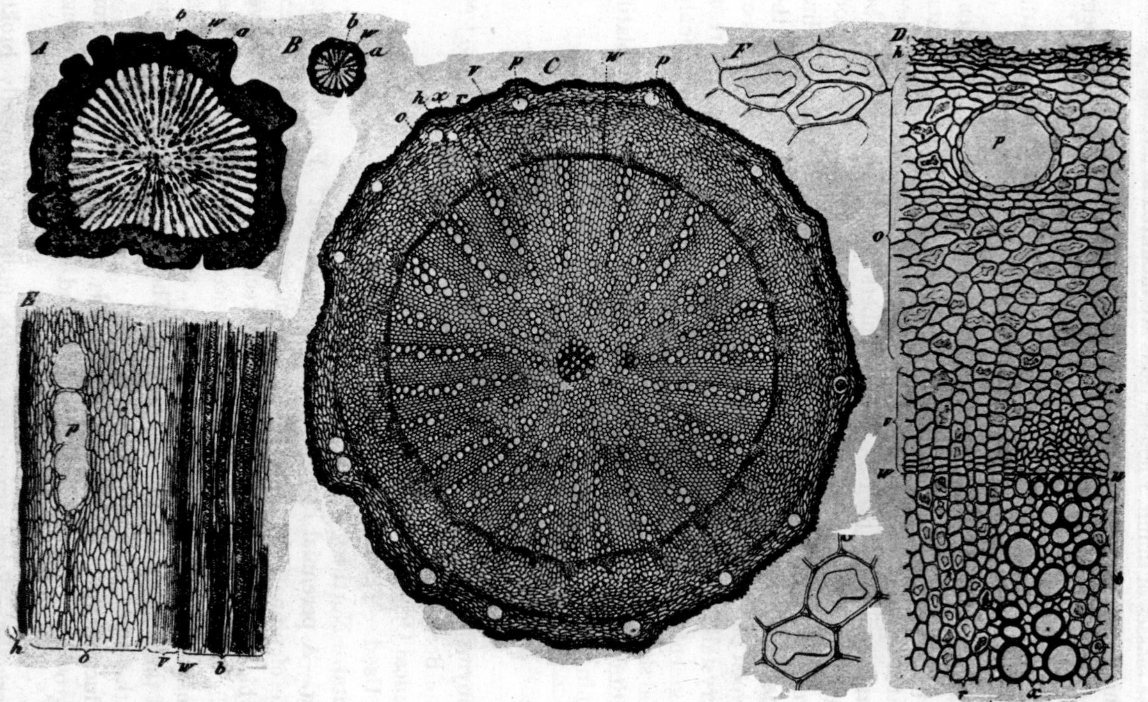

Fig. 295.—Pyrethrum. *A*, Transverse section of Italian Pellitory root (*Anacyclus Pyrethrum* DC.), × 3. *B*, Transverse section of German Pellitory root (*Anacyclus officinarum* Hayne), × 3. *C*. Transverse section of German Pellitory root, × 40. *D*, Segment of same from cork to within xylem, × 115. *E*, Segment of a radial-longitudinal section from cork to within outer region of xylem, × 65. *F* & *G*. Inulin-containing cells. *a*, bark; *b*, wood; *h*, cork; *o*, cortex; *p*, oleoresin reservoirs; *r*. medullary rays; *s*, soft bast; *v*, phloem; *w*, cambium; *x*, xylem. (*After Berg.*).

a tuft of long woolly hairs; fracture short; bark thick, dark brown with 1 or 2 circular rows of resin reservoirs; wood yellow, radiate and porous with resin reservoirs in the medullary-rays; odor distinct; taste at first sweetish, then pungent and persistently acrid, leaving a tingling sensation in the mouth and exciting a strong flow of saliva.

Powdered Drug.—Brown; numerous fragments of parenchyma cells containing inulin; yellow resin masses; fragments of brown cork tissue; reticulate, scalariform, and spiral tracheæ; more or less elongated stone cells with yellowish porous walls.

Constituents.—Pyrethrine (a pungent alkaloid), an acrid resin, volatile oil, inulin, etc.

Use.—Sialagogue and constituent of certain dentifrices.

INULA N.F. (INULA)

Synonyms.—Elecampane; *Fr.* Racine d'aunée; *Ger.* Alantwurzel.

Botanical Origin.—*Inula Helenium* Linné.

Part Used.—The dried rhizome and roots.

Limit of Impurities.—5 per cent. of its stem bases or 2 per cent. of other foreign organic matter.

Habitat.—Europe and Asia, along roadsides and in damp pasture land.

Plant.—A perennial herb growing to the height of 1.8 m., with a thick, solid, striated, hairy, branched stem bearing large, half clasping, alternate, cordate-oblong, unequally dentate-serrate leaves (lower radical leaves, petioled and elliptic-oblong) that are woolly beneath and large, golden-yellow, radiate heads of flowers. Each flower head is about 6 cm. wide and consists of a naked receptacle bearing yellow, pistillate, ligulate flowers along the margin and a disk of yellow, perfect, tubular flowers in the center, its exterior being covered by an imbricated involucre, the outer bracts of which are leaf-like. The fruit is a 4- to 5-ribbed achene.

Production and Commerce.—Elecampane is naturalized in the United States extending from Nova Scotia as far south as North Carolina and westward to Missouri. It has been cultivated to a small extent on drug farms for its rhizome and roots. It thrives best on a clay loam which has been deeply ploughed and kept moist. The plants are grown from seeds or from cuttings of old roots. If from the former, the seeds should be sown in seed beds early in the spring and the seedlings later transferred to the field, where they should be set 18 inches apart in rows with at least 3 feet between each row for cultivation. Root cuttings are planted in autumn in the same manner as the seedlings.

The rhizomes and roots should be dug up in August of the second year, washed, cut into longitudinal, transverse or oblique slices and dried in the shade. They should be preserved in air-tight containers to which carbon tetrachloride or chloroform is added from time to time to prevent insect attacks.

Most of the drug is imported in bales or bags from Trieste and Rotterdam.

Description.—Rhizome fleshy and fusiform, when entire, branching; usually cut into longitudinal or oblique or occasionally transverse pieces, to which may be attached one or more roots; of variable length and up to 4 cm. in diameter; externally grayish-brown to dark-brown, longitudinally wrinkled, with occasional buds or stem scars; inner or cut surface somewhat concave, the edges incurved with the overlapping bark, yellowish-brown to grayish-brown, longitudinally striate and more or less fibrous near the cambium zone; fracture short and horny; inner surface light brown and showing circular or elliptical markings; roots cylindrical and tapering, frequently twisted, up to 15 cm. in length and 1.6 cm. in diameter; odor characteristically aromatic; taste aromatic, then acrid and pungent.

Histology.—Transverse sections of rhizomes exhibit the following characteristics passing from periphery toward the center:

1. Cork, of several rows of thin-walled, brownish, tabular cells.
2. Cork cambium of meristematic cells.
3. Cortex, a zone of many layers of parenchyma cells containing inulin masses.
4. Pericycle, of several layers of parenchyma cells. In old rhizomes this region contains many discontinuous groups of sclerenchyma fibers.
5. Phloem, consisting of radially arranged phloem patches separated by broad medullary-rays. Circular oleoresin reservoirs are arranged in nearly radial rows and form interrupted circles in this region and cortex.
6. Cambium, of meristematic cells.
7. Xylem, in young rhizomes, consisting of radiate wedges separated by broad medullary-rays which contain oleoresin reservoirs. Each xylem patch consists of a matrix of inulin containing wood parenchyma, imbedded in which are a number of pitted and reticulate tracheæ associated occasionally with a few strongly lignified wood fibers. Xylem in old rhizomes shows narrow medullary rays and thick-walled, lignified wood fibers replacing wood parenchyma.
8. Pith, consisting of large-celled parenchyma containing inulin in smaller amounts than in the cortex. Intercellular-air-spaces in this zone are large.

Powdered Drug.—Light brown; consisting chiefly of fragments of parenchyma containing inulin and small, irregular, separated masses of inulin; fragments of highly colored oleoresin; occasional reddish-brown fragments of the walls of the oleoresin reservoirs; fragments of tracheæ with reticulate thickening or elliptical pores associated occasionally with wood fibers.

Constituents.—An active bitter principle termed **helenin**, **inulin**, acrid resin, volatile oil, inulenin, mucilage, etc.

Uses.—Elecampane is used as a constituent of **Warburg's Pills** and Warburg's Tincture, as an ingredient in veterinary pulmonic powders and numerous proprietary medicines. Its active constituent, **helenin**, is employed as an antiseptic in pulmonary diseases.

ECHINACEA N.F. (ECHINACEA)

Synonyms.—Cone Flower, Purple Cone Flower.

Botanical Origin.—*Brauneria pallida* (Nuttall) Britton and *Brauneria angustifolia* (DC.) Heller.

Part Used.—The dried rhizome and roots.

Purity Rubric.—Not more than 3 per cent. of foreign organic matter. It must be used after it has lost its characteristic odor and taste.

Habitat.—Central United States.

Plant.—*Brauneria pallida* is a perennial herb with stout stem arising to the height of 1 m. or less, bearing alternate, lanceolate, 3- to 5-nerved leaves below, naked above and terminating in a single, large, purplish, conical head of ligulate and tubular flowers. The ligulate flowers are slender and drooping with the 2-toothed limb. The fruit is a short 4-sided akene with a short-toothed pappus.

Production and Commerce.—Echinacea grows wild in the central states from Michigan and Kansas to Texas and Alabama and occurs sparingly in some of the eastern states. Plants propagated from seeds have been found to do well in moderately rich and well drained loam but the rhizomes do not attain a size suitable for marketing until three or four years from the time of sowing the seed. Whenever cultivated, the plants should be left in the seed-bed for two years before transplanting to the field. They should be set about 1½ feet apart in rows with sufficient space intervening between these for cultivation.

The rhizomes and roots are dug up in autumn, cleaned, and dried either by artificial heat or in the sun. The commercial supply of the drug comes from Kansas.

Description.—Usually as broken pieces of the rhizomes and roots of variable length and thickness. Rhizome vertical, usually twisted and crooked, slightly tapering, the summit showing a simple or multiple crown with one or more stem bases or V-shaped scars; rhizome and roots externally varying from grayish brown to purplish brown, longitudinally wrinkled, the rhizome slightly annulate in upper portion; fracture short-fibrous; internally exhibiting a very narrow bark and a broad wood zone composed of alternating wedge-shaped yellowish and blackish areas, the rhizome possessing a small central pith area; odor slightly aromatic; taste sweet and followed by a tingling sensation.

Histology.—Sections of the rhizome exhibit the following structural peculiarities:

1. Cork, composed of several rows of tabular cells with suberized walls.
2. Hypodermis, of several layers of tangentially elongated cells amongst which occur oleoresin reservoirs of schizogenous formation.

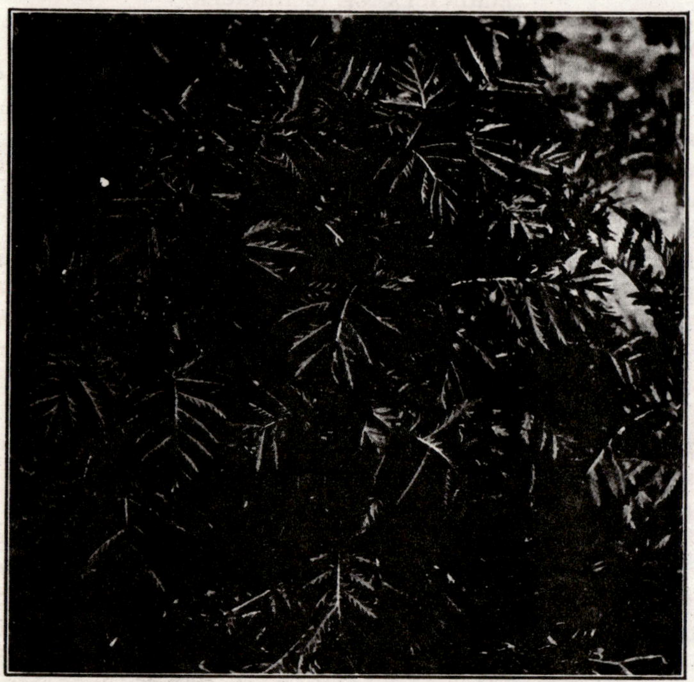

FIG. 296.—Tansy (*Tanacetum vulgare*). (*Photograph by Hogstad.*)

3. Cortex, of numerous layers of more or less polygonal to spheroidal inulin containing parenchyma, scattered amongst which are good sized secretion reservoirs with amber colored oleoresin and many somewhat elongated stone cells. In the intercellular spaces adjacent to the stone cells there is found a black, carbon-like substance termed *phytomelane*.
4. Pericycle, in which are imbedded strongly lignified, lamellated sclerenchyma fibers, arranged singly and in groups.
5. Fibrovascular bundles of the open collateral type, each consisting of a narrow cone-shaped phloem composed of soft bast, a prominent cambium and an elongated, wedge-shaped, radiate xylem composed of

radially arranged, often interrupted, rows of pitted, spiral and reticulate tracheæ imbedded in inulin-containing wood parenchyma. Broad medullary rays intervene between the bundles. These are composed for the most part of a matrix of inulin-containing parenchyma in which are scattered schizogenous oleoresin reservoirs and thick-walled, lamellated, distinctly porous stone cells, similar to those found in the cortex. In the intercellular-air-spaces adjacent to these occurs a black deposit of phytomelane.

6. Pith, composed of tissue similar to the cortex.

The root shows a somewhat similar histology but is devoid of pith.

Constituents.—Resins, inulin, saccharose, volatile oil, etc.

Uses.—Echinacea is employed in the treatment of ulcers, boils and septicæmia.

LACTUCARIUM (LACTUCARIUM).

Synonyms.—Wild Lettuce, Acrid Lettuce, Prickly Lettuce; *Fr.* Laitue vireuse; *Ger.* Giftlattichsaft.

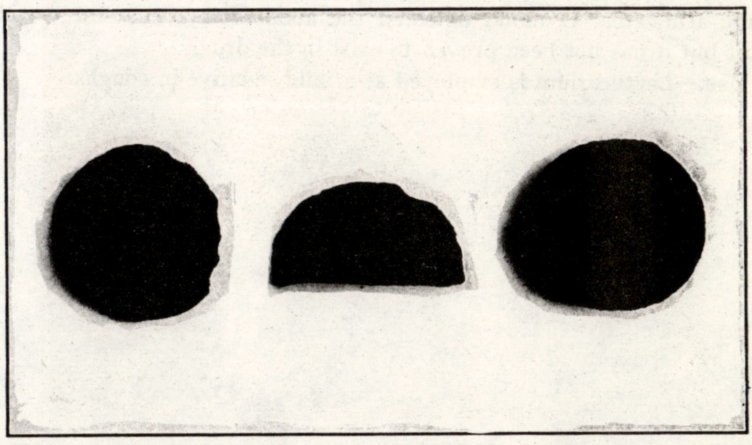

FIG. 297.—Lactucarium, × ⅝. (*Photograph by Stoneback.*)

Botanical Origin.—*Lactuca virosa* Linné.

Part Used.—The dried milk juice.

Habitat.—Europe and Western Asia.

Plant.—A biennial, latex-containing herb bearing a basal rosette of large, runcinate, radical leaves from the center of which arises an erect, prickly, pale green, often purple blotched stem, bearing alternate pale green, sessile, runcinate leaves which possess spines along the midrib of the lower surface. The inflorescence consists of panicles of pale yellow flowers.

Production and Commerce.—The plant grows wild in various sections of central and southern Europe and in New England. It has been cultivated for the milk juice in England, Scotland, France, Austria and Germany. The drug is collected mainly near Zell, Germany from May to September by collectors who cut off the tops of stems when a milk juice exudes. This is removed by the finger and transfered to china receptacles. Flesh slices of the stem are removed daily and an additional amount collected until the plants are exhausted. When sufficiently hardened in the receptacles, it is removed by gently heating the exterior of the cup and tapping, often cut into 2 or 4 pieces and allowed to become hard and dry. The commercial supplies are obtained chiefly from Germany.

Description.—In hemispherical cakes, or in halved or quartered hemispherical cakes, or rarely in irregular masses; externally dull reddish- or grayish-brown; fracture tough, waxy; internally light-brown, porous; odor somewhat opium-like; taste bitter.

Constituents.—The bitter principles, lactucin, lactucopicrin and lactucic acid; volatile oil, lactucerin, caoutchouc, citric acid, malic acid, oxalic acid, etc. Dymond detected the alkaloid, hyoscyamine, in the plant but it has not been proven to exist in the drug.

Use.—Lactucarium is employed as a mild sedative in coughs.

CHAPTER II

CRUDE DRUGS OF ANIMAL ORIGIN

CLASS INSECTA

The largest group of living animals, belonging to the Invertebrata Division of the Animal Kingdom. Their bodies are divisible into three distinct regions, viz., head, thorax and abdomen. Antennæ, eyes (simple and compound), and mouth parts consisting of maxillæ, mandibles, labium and hypopharynx (tongue) are found in the head. Wings either one or two pair on thorax together with three pairs of legs. Ten segments typical in abdomen. Respiration is by a system of branching tracheæ which extend from openings called spiracles on the exterior of the body. Examples. Grasshoppers, Dragon-flies, Bees, Moths, Beetles, Flies, etc.

ORDER HEMIPTERA

Insects having suctorial mouth parts, and direct metamorphosis (with the exception of the male members of the *Coccidæ*). Wings present and segments of the antennæ few.

SUBORDER HOMOPTERA

Characterized by four, sloping, membranous and similar wings. The head is very closely united to the thorax and the distal ends of the front legs touch the sides of the head.

FAMILY COCCIDÆ

This family comprises the scale insects and mealy bugs, which are injurious to cultivated plants.

The species differ greatly from other families of this order and also inter se. The males, unlike other Hemiptera, undergo a complete metamorphosis and possess only one pair of wings. The female has no mouth and is always devoid of wings. In addition, it is covered by means of scales, either in powder or in plates, which form a protective case or roof. Some members of this family yield shellac, wax, dye-stuffs, etc.

COCCUS U.S.P. (COCHINEAL)

Synonyms.—Cochineal Insect; Red Scale Insect; *Fr.* Cochenille; *Ger.* Coccionella.

Zoological Origin.—*Coccus cacti* Linné.

Part Used.—The dried female insect enclosing the young larvæ.

Habitat.—On species of the Cactus family found in Mexico, Central America, and Peru.

Production and Commerce.—The wingless female insects live on the stems of various members of the *Cactaceæ*, but are chiefly found on *Nopalea coccinellifera*, an abundant plant of the subtropics. They are placed on the branches by the natives and multiply very rapidly. The males alone have wings and, shortly after they copulate with the females, die. The fecundated females increase considerably in size and retain the larvæ in their bodies until they die. Up to 5 generations of these insects are produced yearly by breeders. The female insects are collected by brushing them from the branches after which they may be dried on trays for several hours in the sun or artificially in an oven at about 65°C., when the commercial variety known as "Silver Grain Cochineal" is obtained. The silvery color of the insects of this variety is due to the fact that their wax coating is not melted. If dried at a temperature higher than the melting point of their wax covering, *i.e.*, a temperature of more than 106°C., the commercial variety known as "Black Grain Cochineal" results. The "Granilla" variety consists of small, immature females and is deficient in coloring matter. Madres cochineal represents the first brood of the year and generally demands the highest price.

The insects have been introduced from Mexico and Central America to the Canary Islands, Algeria, Spain and the East and West Indies.

The commercial supplies used in this country come chiefly from Teneriffe, an island of the Canary group and from Mexico.

Description.—Insect, ovate in outline, convex on dorsal surface, concave on ventral surface, from 3.5 to 5 mm. in length, consisting of 9 to 12 segments; externally grayish, grayish-purple, grayish-black, or rosy-black; internally exhibiting numerous larvæ containing the red pigment, all of which are covered by the shell-like chitinous abdomen of the mother insect; the mature larvæ with 8-jointed antennæ, 3 pairs of legs, the lower having 6 to 8 segments, and a beak composed of 4 thread-like parts which pair off into 2 coils; odor characteristic; when tasted, slightly bitter and imparting a red color to the saliva.

The powdered drug is dark red and imparts a purple color to alkaline solutions and a reddish-yellow color to acids.

Adulterants.—The "Silver Grain" variety has been admixed with carbonate or sulphate of barium or lead as well as talcum. The "Black Grain" variety has been admixed with manganese dioxide, graphite and ivory black. These minerals may be detected by macerating in water and noting separation of an insoluble powder.

Constituents.—Carminic acid (coloring principle) fixed oil, wax, myristin, etc.

Use.—Coloring agent.

ORDER COLEOPTERA

Wings four, the front pair of which form the horny elytra which form a line at the middle of the back. The prothorax is large and the mouth has well-developed mandibles. Metamorphosis is indirect. Examples: Firefly, Tiger Beetle, Potato Beetle, Click Beetles, Blistering Beetles, etc.

FAMILY MELOIDEÆ

Five tarsal joints are present on each of the front and middle legs, but the last pair has only four with a pair of claws. Integument rather soft.

CANTHARIS U.S.P. (CANTHARIDES)

Synonyms.—Spanish Flies, Russian Flies, Blister Beetle; *Fr.* Cantharides; *Ger.* Spanische Fliegen.

Zoological Origin.—*Cantharis vesicatoria* De Geer.

Part Used.—The dried insects.

Standard of Assay.—Not less than 0.6 per cent. of cantharidin.

Habitat.—Europe and western Asia.

Production and Commerce.—The insects are found in southern and central Europe and western Asia on various shrubs and trees of the Olive and Honeysuckle families. They appear to be most frequent in Spain, southern Russia, Italy, Sicily, southern France and Hungary. They are collected mainly during the months of June and July by masked collectors who, during the early morning hours, while the beetles show little sign of activity, spread cloths beneath the shrubbery and trees harboring them and then beat the branches with poles. The beetles are shaken off, and gathered up in the cloth, are cast into suitable containers and killed by the vapors of ether, chloroform, ammonia or carbon disulphide. They are then carefully dried at a temperature not above 40°C. Cantharides with an ammoniacal odor should not be used. Not more than 10 per cent. of moisture should be present in the drug. The commercial supplies imported into the United States come from Spain and Russia in cases. The Russian article is shipped here through London and Hamburg.

Description.—Beetle oblong, up to 25 mm. in length and up to 8 mm. in breadth; of a brilliant green or bluish-green, metallic luster, changing in different regions, particularly beneath, to a golden green; head triangular, separated into two symmetrical halves by a faint median line; mouth parts mandibulate; antennæ filiform of 11 conical joints, the upper ones being black; neck recognizable; prothorax angulate; first and second pairs of legs with 5 tarsal joints, the third pair of legs with 4 tarsal joints and 2 distal claws; anterior pair of wings or elytra elongated, each with 2 parallel lines and finely wrinkled, covering over the folded posterior pair of wings which are brownish and membranous; odor strong and characteristic; taste pungent and acrid.

Powdered Drug.—Grayish brown, with shining green particles, showing in microscopical mounts fragments of striated muscles, long pointed unicellular hairs about 0.5 mm. in length, fragments of chitinous body wall, wings and frequently fragments of mites and their eggs.

Constituents.—From .5 to 1 per cent. cantharidin (vesicant principle), uric, formic and acetic acids, fixed oil, etc.

Uses.—Cantharides is chiefly used as a vesicant and counter irritant.

Substitute.—*Mylabris Cichorii* Fab. or Chinese Blistering Beetles from China and East Indies. These differ from Cantharis in having jet black

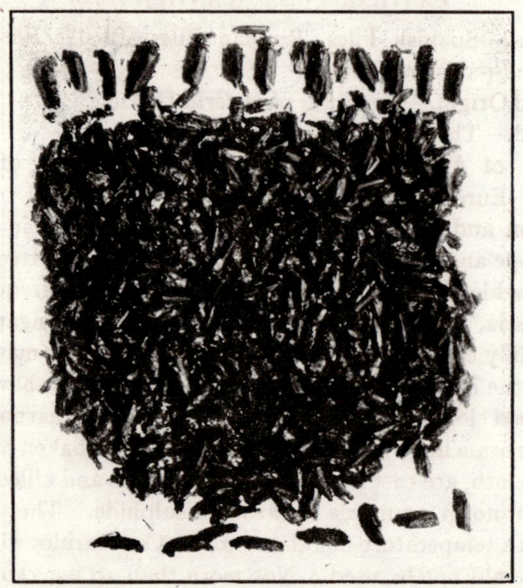

FIG. 298.—Spanish flies (*Cantharis vesicatoria*), × ⅜.

bodies, the elytra of which show 2 broad brownish-yellow or orange-yellow bands and in their anterior part 2 spots of the same color. They contain up to 1.2 per cent. of cantharidin. The present supplies of Mylabris to this country come in cases from Shanghai and Singapore.

ORDER HYMENOPTERA

Insects whose mouth parts are adapted for both chewing and sucking. The wings are four in number, alike, membranous with few irregular veins. The prothorax is small and united with other thorax segments. The ovipositor is modified to serve some special purpose such as sawing or boring. The metamorphosis is complete. Examples: Bees, Gall-flies, Wasps and Ants.

FAMILY APIDÆ

A large family of hymenopterous insects characterized by possessing short stout mouth parts and posterior tibiæ devoid of apical spurs. Examples: Honey Bee, Leaf Cutter and Carpenter Bee.

MEL U.S.P. (HONEY)

Synonyms.—Clarified Honey; *Fr.* Miel; *Ger.* Honig.

Zoological Origin.—*Apis mellifera* Linné.

Part Used.—A saccharine substance, gathered mostly from the nectaries of flowers and deposited in the honey-comb by the bee.

Habitat.—North America and Europe.

Animal.—This is the common honey bee much prized for its honey and wax. The species shows differentiation into three types of individuals, viz: the queen bee which is a sexually perfect female, the drones or males, and the worker which in reality is a sexually imperfect female. In respect to size, the queen is much larger than either drone or worker. Her sole duty is to lay eggs and thus reproduce the colony. The worker bees collect the honey, feed the young, and form the hive. All but the drones have a poison sac with a sharp sting attached. In nature, the honeybee is now found wild and lives in swarms consisting of thousands of individuals.

Production.—It is collected by draining the honey-comb, found in bee hives.

Description.—A thick, light yellowish or yellowish-brown syrupy liquid, translucent when fresh, but gradually becoming opaque and granular from crystallization of dextrose, crystalline; odor characteristic; taste sweet and faintly acrid. When diluted with twice its weight of water, it is only slightly turbid, not stringy and has a specific gravity of not less than 1.099. It is laevorotatory at 20°C.

When examined under the microscope it frequently shows the presence of the various types of pollen grains corresponding to those different plants which the bees have visited in gathering the honey.

Constituents.—Dextrose (which crystallizes), lævulose (which remains liquid), volatile oil, mucilage, proteids, coloring matter, a little wax and formic acid.

Use.—Honey is used as a nutritive, demulcent, mild laxative and as a vehicle for medicaments employed as gargles.

Adulterants.—(1) Syrup; (2) added invert sugar; (3) azo dyes and other foreign coloring substances.

CERA ALBA U.S.P. (WHITE WAX)

Synonyms.—White Bee's Wax; *Ger.* Weisses Wachs; *Fr.* Cire blanche.

Zoological Origin.—*Apis mellifera* Linné.

Part Used.—Bleached yellow wax.

Description.—A yellowish-white solid, occurring in circular cakes, melting between 62° and 65°C.; odor faint and characteristic; taste indistinct.

Production.—White wax is obtained by exposing thin sheets of yellow wax to moisture and sunlight.

Constituents.—Similar to yellow wax but containing little or no coloring matter.

Uses.—White wax is used pharmaceutically in the preparation of simple cerate and cold cream.

CERA FLAVA U.S.P. (YELLOW WAX)

Synonyms.—Beeswax, Yellow Bee's Wax; *Ger.* Gelbes Wachs; *Fr.* Cire jaune.

Zoological Origin.—*Apis mellifera* Linné.

Part Used.—A product obtained by melting and purifying the honey comb of the bee.

Description.—A yellow to brownish-yellow or grayish-brown solid occurring as variously molded cakes, brittle when cold and when broken exhibiting a dull granular fracture; specific gravity 0.950 to 0.960 at 25°C.; melting point between 62° and 65°C.; odor honey-like; taste faint but characteristic.

Constituents.—Hydrocarbons, myricyl palmitate, cerin, two alcohols, aromatic substance, coloring matter, etc.

Uses.—Yellow wax is used in the preparation of ointments, cerates and plasters.

Adulterants.—(1) Tallow, which lowers its specific gravity and softens it; (2) Rosin, which dissolves in 75 per cent. hot alcohol and can be subsequently precipitated by the addition of water; (3) Paraffine; (4) Starch.

CLASS PISCES

The first class of vertebrates or backbone animals including many forms which are adapted to life in the water. The majority of fishes have an internal skeleton consisting chiefly of bone and a protective exoskeleton of dermal scales. Their respiratory organs consist of gills which are covered by gill covers or opercula. There are 2 subclasses, the *Teleostomi* or bony fishes and the *Dipnoi* or lung fishes.

FAMILY GADIDÆ

A family of bony fishes (*Teleostomi*) comprising a number of valuable food fishes including the codfishes, haddocks, hakes and pollacks.

OLEUM MORRHUÆ U.S.P. (COD LIVER OIL)

Synonyms.—Oleum Jecoris Aselli, Cod Oil; *Ger*. Leberthran; *Fr*. Huile de Foie de Morue.

Zoological Origin.—*Gadus morrhua* Linné and other species of *Gadus*.

Part Used.—The fixed oil obtained from the fresh livers.

Habitat.—North Atlantic Ocean.

Production and Commerce.—The cod fish inhabits the cooler and deeper waters of the North Atlantic Ocean, visiting the coasts to spawn in the shallower waters during late winter and early spring. It is caught in vast numbers by trap nets, hand lines and set lines chiefly off the coasts of Newfoundland, Massachusetts, Norway and Great Britain, where the cod fisheries are an important industry. The livers are removed while the fish are still fresh either by hand gutting or mechanical splitters, care being exercised that the gall bladder is completely separated. They are then washed and the oil extracted either by the direct steam process, by subjecting livers to a gentle heat in iron pots, by cold expression or electrolysis.

In Newfoundland, the direct steam process is almost exclusively employed. In this process the livers, after being washed, are placed in a steam pan and live steam is passed into them until a white scum floats. The oil is then poured off and strained. This first fraction, known as "ordinary refined oil" is alone marketed for medicinal purposes. The residue is then steamed and the oil which separates to the top is decanted and strained. This second fraction is known as "common cod oil" and is not used medicinally. Cod liver oil is refined by chilling it in tin vessels at a low temperature (−5°C.) which causes the stearin or solid fat to separate, the liquid portion being decanted. It is sometimes assayed biologically for its vitamine-A content, the test animals employed being albino rats from a constant source. If so assayed, it should contain at least 50 units per gram.

The U.S.P. X requires that the vitamine-A potency of Cod Liver Oil be expressed in units per gram of oil. The unit represents the minimum daily amount of Cod Liver Oil which is required to cure induced symptoms of vitamine-A starvation in young albino rats and to cause a gain in weight from 10 to 20 Gm. within a period of 35 days under the conditions of growth and diet specified under this assay in the U.S.P. (See U.S.P. X, p. 469.) Cod liver oil should be standardized also for its vitamine-D content, for this vitamine represents the antirachitic element of the oil.

The Cod Liver Oil used in this country comes chiefly from Gloucester, Mass., Norway and Newfoundland.

Description.—A pale yellow, thin oil with a slightly fishy odor and taste, slightly soluble in alcohol and completely soluble in chloroform, ether, carbon disulphide and ethylacetate. Specific gravity: 0.918 to 0.927 at 25°C.

Constituents.—Vitamine-A (fat soluble), vitamine-D, traces of iodine and bromine organic compounds; jecolein, therapin, palmatin, biliary acids, cholesterin, the alkaloids aselline and morrhuine, etc. Vitamine-A represents the growth-promoting and antixerophthalmic element, whereas vitamine-D represents the antirachitic element of this oil.

Uses.—Cod Liver Oil is used as a nutritive and growth stimulating agent in rickets, malnutrition and tuberculosis.

Adulterants.—Seal oil and other fish oils.

CLASS AVES

Birds are warm blooded vertebrates which differ from all other vertebrates by possessing feathers. Their forelimbs are modified as wings and their young are hatched from eggs (oviparous).

FAMILY PHASIANIDÆ

Fowl-like birds of terrestrial or tree habit with a stout, convex beak, short, rounded wings and short, stout legs having toes adapted for scratching. To this family belong most of our game-birds including the chickens, quail, bob-whites, partridges, grouse and turkeys.

OVUM GALLINACEUM N.F. (FRESH EGG)

Synonyms.—Hen's Egg, Chicken's Egg; *Fr.* Œuf frais; *Ger.* Frisch Ei.

Zoological Origin.—*Gallus domesticus* Temminck.

Part Used.—The recently laid egg of the hen.

Habital.—Probably descended from the red jungle fowl, indigenous to India and other Asiatic countries.

Description.—Ovate and consisting of a thin calcareous shell enclosing a thin membrane which surrounds albuminous matter or egg white that in turn envelops the vitellus or egg yolk.

From this egg the shell or *Testa Ovi*, the white of egg, official as *Ovi Albumen Recens* N.F. and the egg yolk or yelk, official as *Ovi Vitellum Recens* N.F. are obtained.

Constituents.—Egg-shell is composed of from 90 to 97 per cent. of pure calcium carbonate, the remainder consisting of magnesium and calcium phosphates and organic matter.

Egg-white is composed of about 15 per cent. albumin and 85 per cent. of water with minute traces of sodium and potassium chlorides, fat and sugar.

Egg-yolk contains about 30 per cent. of fat, 16 per cent. vitellin, 52 per cent. water, 1.5 per cent. inorganic salts, traces of lactic acid and sugar, and coloring matter.

Uses.—The shell is occasionally used as an antacid. Egg-white is used as a nutrient and as an ingredient of Canada liniment and St. John Long's liniment. Egg-yolk is used as an emulsifying agent and in the preparation of Glycerite of egg-yolk and St. John Long's liniment.

CLASS MAMMALIA

The members of this class of vetebrates breathe by means of lungs, and are warm-blooded. Hair at some period in their life history is also present, and the young are nourished after birth by secretions from cutaneous glands. Examples: Rodents, Apes, Whales, Marsupials, Man, etc.

ORDER UNGULATA

Terrestrial and largely herb-feeding animals with more or less hair and with solid, tough, horny hoofs. The canine teeth are generally small or entirely absent, while the molars and premolars which are used in grinding are well developed and have broad crowns with roughened surface. There is no foramen over the inner condyle of the humerus, and the clavicle is absent.

FAMILY BOVIDÆ

Ruminants having hollow, unbranched horns, not shed each year, and which fit over bony projections on the skull. The stomach as a general rule is complex. Examples:—chamois, goats, musk-oxen, cows, gazelles, gnus, bison, sheep, oxen, etc.

PITUITARIUM U.S.P. (PITUITARY)

Synonyms.—Desiccated Pituitary Body, Hypophysis Sicca, Desiccated Hypophysis Cerebri.

Zoological Origin.—*Bos taurus* Linné, *Ovis aries* Linné and other domesticated animals which are used for food by man.

Part Used.—The posterior lobe of the pituitary body, cleaned, dried and powdered.

Habitat.—Domesticated.

Description.—A yellowish or grayish, amorphous powder, partially soluble in water and having a characteristic odor.

Constituent.—Pituitrin.

Uses.—Pituitary is used hypodermically to relieve uterine inertia and intestinal paralysis.

FEL BOVIS U.S.P. (OXGALL)

Synonym.—Ox Bile.

Zoological Origin.—*Bos taurus* Linné.

Part Used.—The fresh bile.

Description.—A dark green or brownish-green, somewhat viscid, neutral or faintly alkaline liquid, having a characteristic odor and a disagreeable, bitter taste. Its specific gravity ranges from 1.015 to 1.025 at 25°C.

Constituents.—Sodium and potassium glycocholates and taurocholates, bilirubin and biliverdin (bile pigments), cholesterin, choline, fat, urea, etc.

Use.—Cholagogue cathartic.

THYROIDEUM U.S.P. (THYROID)

Synonyms.—Thyroideum Siccum, Dried Thyroid Glands.

Zoological Origin.—*Bos taurus* Linne, *Ovis aries* Linné and other domesticated animals used by man as food.

Part Used.—The cleaned, dried and powdered thyroid gland, previously deprived of connective tissue and fat.

Purity Rubric.—It contains not less than 0.17 nor more than 0.23 per cent. of iodine in thyroid combination and must be free from iodine in inorganic or any other form of combination than that peculiar to the thyroid gland.

Description.—A yellowish, amorphous powder with a faint characteristic odor.

Constituent.—A proteid called iodothyrin or thyroxin (U.S.P.) which contains iodine and phosphorous.

Uses.—Thyroid and Thyroxin are used in myxœdema and cretinism.

SUPRARENALUM SICCUM (DRIED SUPRARENALS)

Synonyms.—Dried Adrenals, Desiccated Suprarenal Glands.

Zoological Origin.—Animals used for food by man.

Part Used.—The suprarenal or adrenal glands, cleaned, dried, freed from fat and powdered.

Description.—A light yellowish-brown powder, partly soluble in water, and with a slight characteristic odor.

Constituent.—Epinephrine (U.S.P.) or adrenalin which occurs in the medulla of the gland.

Uses.—Epinephrine and dried suprarenals are employed as vasoconstrictors in the treatment of bronchitis, in congestion and œdema of the lungs and in Addison's disease.

ORDER CARNIVORA

Chordates in which the young are nourished in the uterus of the mother for a time. Integument furry. Four or more digits developed on the fore and hind feet, all provided with claws. Clavicle absent or incomplete. The canine teeth are generally large, curved and pointed.

Molar and premolars compressed and the incisors are small and chisel-like. The stomach is not complex and the brain fairly large. Examples—Cats (*Felidæ*), Bears (*Ursidæ*), Otters (*Lutridæ*), Walruses (*Trichechidæ*). Cinets (*Viverridæ*) etc.

FAMILY VIVERRIDÆ

Small cat-like, carnivorous quadrupeds with, as a rule, short legs, a curly tail, a long body, and a sharp snout. The family is naturally divided into the aeluropod type or cat-footed, and the cynopod or dog-footed. Both types are instrumental in destroying vermin.

CIVETTA (CIVET)

Synonym.—Zibethum.

Zoological Origin.—1. *Viverra Civetta* Schreber and 2. *Viverra Zibetha* Schreber.

Part Used.—Unctuous secretion obtained from a pouch situated between the anus and genitalia of both male and female civets.

Habitat.—(1) Africa. (2) Southern Asia.

Production.—The secretion is removed at intervals and dried.

Description.—A yellowish to brownish, unctuous substance having a penetrating odor resembling musk; yellowish when fresh; taste bitter and acrid.

Constituents.—Volatile oil, resin, coloring matter, etc.

Use.—Civet is used chiefly by the perfume industry as a fixative.

FAMILY MOSCHIDÆ

Small, hornless deer with short tail and fairly high hind quarters. Canine teeth are well developed and, in the male, project from the upper jaw. The musk sac is located between the umbilicus and the preputial follicles.

MOSCHUS (MUSK)

Synonyms.—Tonquin Musk, Deer Musk; *Fr.* Musc; *Ger.* Bisam.

Zoological Origin.—*Moschus moschiferous* Linné.

Part Used.—The dried secretion from the musk sac.

Habitat.—In forests of the Himalaya mountains from India to Siberia.

Animal.—One of the members of the *Moschidæ*, inhabiting the highlands and plateaus of central Asia, especially Thibet. The male is about a yard in length and 20–22 inches in height, and its coat is brownish with white underparts. The musk sac is as large as a hen's egg and somewhat flattened on one side. It is lined by a convoluted, smooth membrane which secretes musk. In the case of the doe, the musk-sac is absent, and the deer is smaller than the male. The largest herds of musk-deer are found on the southern shores of the Koro-Nor.

Production and Commerce.—Musk is secreted in the hairy musk sac located between the umbilicus and the preputial follicles of the male musk deer. It is a brown, thick secretion, when first collected, and occurs in quantities up to 25 Gm. in the sac of the adult animal. It is collected, after trapping and killing the animal, by cutting off the sac and quickly drying by pressing against heated stones. Autumn and winter collected musk is considered the best. The chief markets for musk are Sungpan, Tachienlu and Yuchow. The sacs are packed in small rectangular cases

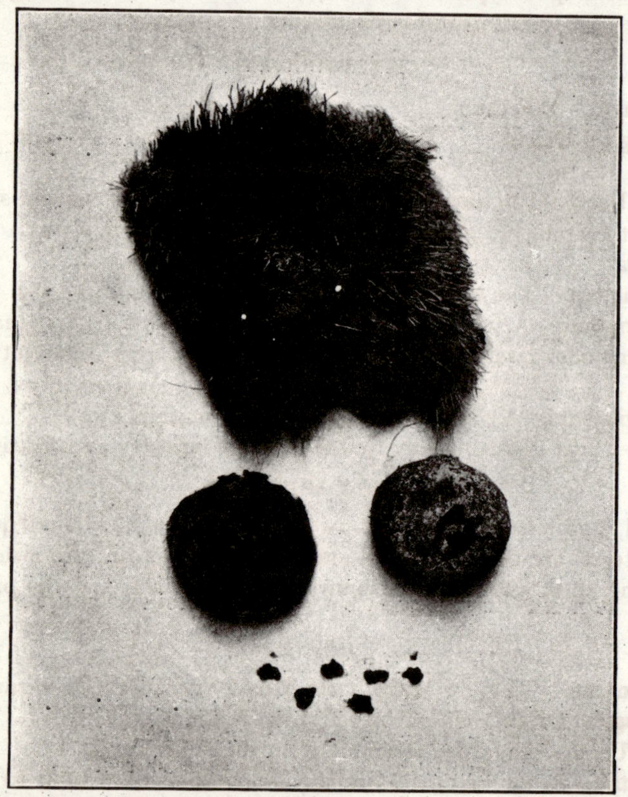

FIG. 299.—Moschus. Entire musk sac and contents, × ½. (*Photograph by Stoneback.*)

lined with tin foil and shipped via Shanghai or Calcutta to purchasers in Europe and the United States. China is the chief exporter of musk.

Description.—In small, irregular, oily and glistening granules, not more than 2 mm. in thickness, blackish or brownish, becoming grayish on aging; odor peculiar, penetrating, powerful and persistent; taste somewhat bitter. Not less than 50 per cent. of musk should be water-soluble.

If a few granules of musk be added to a small quantity of chloroform in a watch crystal, the grains float on the surface; upon stirring with a glass rod the solution remains nearly colorless, and as it evaporates a small quantity of a whitish oily substance separates around the particles.

Constituents.—Volatile oil, resin, cholesterin, protein, fat, calcium and ammonium compounds, etc.

Uses.—Musk is employed chiefly in the manufacture of perfumery. It has been used as an antispasmodic.

Adulterants.—1. Starch, detected by mounting crushed granules on a slide, adding iodine and examining under a microscope and noting bluish stained granules. (2) Artificial musk, a synthetic, consisting of trinitro—isobutyl—methyl—benzol. This is a brownish mass having a musk odor which rapidly disappears on exposure. (3) Peas. (4) Barley. (5) Acorns; (6) Fried liver. (7) Powdered beef.

ORDER CETACEA

Aquatic mammals of fish-like form which for the greater part live in salt water. Posterior limbs and hairs are generally absent, although in some members (*whales*) rudiments of posterior limbs occur beneath the skin. The anterior limbs are paddle-like flippers. To this order belong the toothed or sperm whales which yield spermaceti, the toothless or baleen whales which yield whalebone and oil, the porpoises and the dolphins.

CETACEUM U.S.P. (SPERMACETI)

Synonyms.—Sperm Whale, Cachalot; *Ger.* Wallrath; *Fr.* Cétine.

Zoological Origin.—*Physeter macrocephalus* Linné.

Part Used.—A fatty substance obtained from the head of the sperm whale.

Habitat.—Pacific and Indian Oceans.

Animal.—A huge, toothed whale averaging 70 to 80 feet in length with a massive head, truncated in front and about one-third the length of the body. On the upper surface of its skull occurs a large cavity containing fatty tissue from which spermaceti is obtained. The flippers are short and antero-lateral. On the dorsal surface there occurs a rudimentary dorsal fin as a low projection.

Production.—A short time after the animal is killed, the fat cavity is opened and the oil collected in buckets. This, upon hardening, forms a yellowish mass which is placed in bags, drained and pressed to remove olein, purified by melting in hot water and skimming, boiled with weak alkaline solution, washed with water and allowed to harden.

Description.—A pearl-white, waxy, rather translucent mass having a somewhat scaly-crystalline fracture, faint odor and bland taste. It fuses at about 45°C. It is soluble in fixed and volatile oils, chloroform and ether. On exposure to air it becomes yellow and rancid.

Constituents.—Cetyl palmitate and small percentages of other fatty substances.

Use.—As a base for cerates and ointments.

BIBLIOGRAPHY

United States Pharmacopœia x.
National Formulary v.
United States Dispensatory.
A. Vogl: "Pharmakognosie."
A. E. Vogl: "Anatomischer Atlas zur Pharmakognosie."
Albert Weigand: "Lehrbuch der Pharmakognosie."
G. C. Wittstein: "Pharmakognosie des Pflanzenreichs."
F. A. Fluckiger: "Pharmakognosie des Pflanzenreichs."
F. A. Fluckiger and Daniel Hanbury: "Pharmacographia."
Joseph Moeller: "Pharmakognostischer Atlas."
Joseph Moeller: "Lehrbuch der Pharmakognosie."
Joseph Moeller: "Mikroskopie der Nahrungs und Genussmittel."
E.Gilg: "Lehrbuch der Pharmakognosie."
Tschirch and Oesterle: "Anatomischer Atlas."
A. Tschirch: "Handbuch der Pharmakognosie."
H. Zörnig: "Arzneidrogen."
H. Behrens: "Anleitung zur Microchemischen Analyse."
Hans Molisch: "Grundriss einer Histochemie der Pflanzlichen Genussmittel."
Otto Tunmann: "Pflanzenmikrochemie."
A. Engler und K. Prantl: "Die Naturlichen Pflanzenfamilien."
Eugene Collin: "Traite de Toxocologie Végétale."
T. F. Hanausek and A. Winton: "Microscopy of Technical Products."
Winton and Moeller: "Microscopy of Vegetable Foods."
Henry G. Greenish: "A Text Book of Materia Medica." (4th Ed.)
Henry G. Greenish: "Microscopical Examination of Foods and Drugs. (3rd. Ed.)
Henry G. Greenish and Eugene Collin: "Anatomical Atlas of Vegetable Powders."
Strasburger, Jost, Schenck and Karsten: "A Text-book of Botany."
John M. Maisch: "Organic Materia Medica."
Charles F. Millspaugh: "American Medicinal Plants."
E. S. Bastin: "College Botany." (Revised by W. B. Day.)
Smith E. Jeliffe: "Introduction to Pharmacognosy."
Henry Kraemer: "Scientific and Applied Pharmacognosy."
Otto A. Wall: "Pharmacognosy."
D. M. R. Culbreth: "Materia Medica and Pharmacology."
L. E. Sayre: "Organic Materia Medica and Pharmacognosy." (4th Ed.)
William Mansfield: "Histology of Medicinal Plants."
Albert Schneider: "Microanalysis of Powdered Vegetable Drugs."
H. Solereder: "Systematic Anatomy of the Dicotyledons." (Vols. 1 and 2.)
Small: "Flora of the Southern States."
Bentley and Trimen: "Medicinal Plants." (Vol. I to IV.)
Britton and Brown: "An Illustrated Flora of the Northern United States, Canada and British Possessions." (2nd Ed.)
Gray: "New Manual of Botany." (7 Ed.) (Revised by B. L. Robinson and M. L. Fernald).
Heber W. Youngken: "Pharmaceutical Botany." (4th. Ed.)
Bailey: "Standard Cyclopedia of Horticulture."
T. A. Henry: "Plant Alkaloids." (2nd Ed.)
J. U. Lloyd: "Origin and History of all the Pharmacopeial Vegetable Drugs, etc."
Hegner: "College Zoology."

PARKER and HASWELL: "Textbook of Zoology."
WILLIAM MANSFIELD: "Squibb's Atlas of the Official Drugs."
Index Kewensis.
Botanical Abstracts.
Commerce Reports.
Bulletins of the United States Department of Agriculture.
National Geographic Magazine.
Journals of the American Pharmaceutical Association.
Year Books of the American Pharmaceutical Association.
American Journal of Pharmacy.
Pharmaceutical Journal, London.
British Pharmaceutical Codex, 1923.
Druggists Circular.
Pharmaceutical Era.

CHAPTER III

MICROANALYTICAL METHODS

Microanalysis may be defined as that method of laboratory procedure which involves the use, in analytical work, of a microscope, simple, compound, petrographical or any other type. Microanalytical methods, which are largely qualitative, make it possible to identify plant and animal materials by certain diagnostic histological characters and to confirm the identification of material by certain physical constants. Quantitative microanalytical methods are also of considerable value.

The early microanalyst's field of activity was restricted to the identification of plant ingredients. For that reason he needed chiefly a strong foundation in botanical subjects, particularly those relating to plant anatomy and histological structures. The microscopy of vegetable foods and drugs, therefore, became his largest field of activity. This has broadened to include animal materials. More recently microchemical technique and the application of optical-crystallographic methods to the identification of small quantities of crystalline material have become part of the microanalyst's work.

For the microscopical identification of plant or animal ingredients in powdered material, the microanalyst must be prepared to detect differences in structure readily and to evaluate their importance properly. The eye must be trained to recognize diagnostic structures that serve to differentiate powdered stem materials from flower powder and roots from stems, the presence or absence of characteristic crystalline material, variation in the shape and size of characteristic plant hairs, abundance and shape of sclerenchyma elements, the characteristic structure of bone and meat fragments, and the reaction of various cell structures to microchemical reagents.

A microscopical study of plant and animal structures furnishes the basis upon which to build the fund of specialized information obtained by practical experience. As the field of study enlarges, the microanalyst rapidly accumulates a large working acquaintance with many substances in the powdered condition, a first-hand knowledge of which enables him at once to determine the presence or absence of a certain ingredient in a mixture.

The critical microscopical study of any powdered material implies a thorough study by the analyst of the various parts of the ingredients which he has been called upon to identify. For instance, in the case of a product consisting of powdered flower and stem materials, it is reasonable to suppose that the microanalyst has first studied the various parts of the flower, including the stem material, in the whole as well as in the powdered condition. Freehand sections of the various parts are useful in showing the proper relationship of the different structures. It is quite as advantageous, however, to separate the parts of the flower, for example, and examine them in the powdered condition. In this manner the different structures are broken up into sections and fragments of sections, quite unlike any found in freehand sections made with a razor. A microscopical study of these powdered parts from any particular ingredient makes it possible to recognize them in a finely ground commercial product. This procedure, varied to meet special conditions, is valuable in the initial study of any product.

Mixing the unknown sample is a prequisite of a microscopical examination. This is best done by spreading the sample upon a sheet of clean white paper and mixing the powder with a spatula or rolling it back and forth. After thorough mixing, a composite portion is drawn from various parts of the sample. It is desirable to make the first examination in water, to make certain that foreign starches are absent. A drop of iodine in potassium iodide solution may be drawn under the cover glass for subsequent confirmation of the presence of starchy material. For further examination a small portion of the powder should be mounted in chloral hydrate solution and gently warmed. This solution serves to dissolve any starch that may be present, and clears the tissues generally.

A nest of sieves, ranging from 30-mesh to 100-mesh, and a dissecting microscope, are also valuable aids in general microanalytical work. Sifting a powdered sample through a sieve often makes it possible to pick out larger fragments, which may be identified by their general appearance or sectioned for more detailed study. The coarse material left on the sieve can be advantageously studied with a dissecting microscope provided with a transparent glass stage and lenses giving a magnification of approximately 8 and 16.

Quantitative Microanalysis.—Although surprisingly accurate and trustworthy results may be obtained by the quantitative microanalysis of certain classes of products, this branch of microanalytical work has its limitations and its use may at times be difficult. Experience is necessary for the successful manipulation of these methods. Carefully prepared standard reference samples containing known amounts of the suspected ingredient and as nearly identical as possible (slightly finer if anything) in fineness of powder with the product under examination are essential. A thorough mixing of the standard reference samples is also an important precaution. Various workers have used different methods of attack. Some have used diluents, while others have used certain specific diagnostic tissue elements as criteria. Every problem in quantitative microanalysis must be considered on its own merits rather than on general conclusions applicable in all cases.

Method for Determination of Percentage of Powdered Daisy Flowers in Insect Powder

The equipment essential for carrying out this method consists of a compound microscope equipped with ocular and objective and giving a magnification of 90 to 120 diameters, an analytical balance, ruled microscopic slides similar to that shown in Fig. 300, disecting needle, small camel's hair brush, 7/8 inch square cover glasses, and fine mesh sieves.

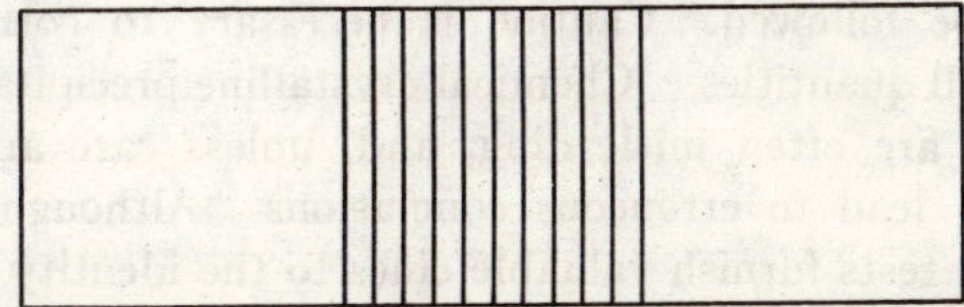

FIG. 300.—Ruled microscopic slide, useful in making certain quantitative microscopical counts.

Standard reference samples are first prepared by grinding together known amounts of Daisy (*Chrysanthemum Leucanthemum*) flower heads and Pyrethri Flores. The resulting powder should be reduced to the same degree of fineness as that of the sample to be determined. Both should be thoroughly mixed and passed through number 60 to 80 meshed sieves before further procedure.

Weigh out at least two lots of 2 mg. each of the reference sample. Transfer each to the ruled microscopic slides by means of a camel's hair pencil, add sufficient chloral hydrate solution and apply cover glass. It is important that all of the material on each slide be distributed as evenly as possibly beneath cover glass and none outside of cover glass.

Calculate the number of characteristic deep red amorphous masses of the Daisy achene in each mount by moving the slide slowly in the direction parallel to the rulings and by counting particles between each two ruled lines until the entire mount is covered. Determine average for 2 mg.

Weigh out at least two lots of 2 mg. each of the sample to be determined, transfer to ruled microscopic slides and proceed with the same technique as for the reference samples. Calculate the average as above. Compare counts which will give the necessary ratio for determining the percentage of Daisy flowers present.

Thus, if the average for 2 mg. of a reference sample containing 50 per cent. Daisy flowers was 60 and the average for the 2 mg. sample of the material under investigation was 30, then;

$$30 : (60 \times 2) 120 :: x : 100$$
$$120\,x = 3000$$
$$x = 25 \text{ per cent.}$$

This same method may be employed with but slight modifications in the determination of Insect Flower stems and Turmeric admixture. In determining the percentage of Insect Flower stems the mounts are made in Phloroglucin and Hydrochloric acid reagent and the fragments of fibrovascular tissues counted, whereas Turmeric mounts are made in water and the irregular masses of altered starch are counted.

Microchemical Tests.—Microchemical tests are invaluable in microanalytical work and often serve to rapidly and accurately identify small quantities of material. Many textbooks on microchemistry describe the methods to be followed. Caution is necessary to correctly interpret results on small quantities. Chemical crystalline precipitates of a certain definite habit are often misleading, and, unless care and judgment is exercised may lead to erroneous conclusions. Although the results of microchemical tests furnish valuable clues to the identity of a substance, unfortunately, they tell only half the story. For instance, they may show the presence of two metals in an admixture, but they can give no indication as to the combination of the metals with any acid radicals that might be identified. Such tests are purely qualitative and somewhat limited.

Optical-crystallographic Methods.—Small quantities of crystalline material, which cannot be wasted in making many qualitative tests, must often be identified. An examination of this material mounted in a suitable oily liquid soon establishes its identity. A microscope equipped with nicol prisms is necessary for this examination and a 4-millimeter, an 8-millimeter, and a 16-millimeter objective are usually the only lenses required. The other accessories furnished with a petrographic microscope are useful but not absolutely necessary in establishing the identity of crystalline material. The procedure followed in identifying a crystalline substance is the same as that used by petrographers in the identification of rock fragments. The most important optical constants which serve to identify a product with certainty are the refractive indices. These are determined by immersing the crystalline material in oily liquids of known refractive index. The value of the index of refraction of each liquid is first determined by means of a refractometer. For most identification purposes, the quidlis used differ in index only by two units in the second decimal place, that is, 1.48, 1.50, or by three units, that is, 1.485, 1.490. The refractive indices of a crystalline substance vary in number, depending upon the system in which the substance crystallizes. In crystals of the triclinic, monoclinic, and orthorhombic systems, three indices can be determined, the smallest being designated α, the intermediate β, and the largest γ. In those belonging to the hexagonal, tetragonal, and trigonal systems, two indices can be determined, ω and ϵ. Crystals belonging to the cubic system give but one index, indicated as n.

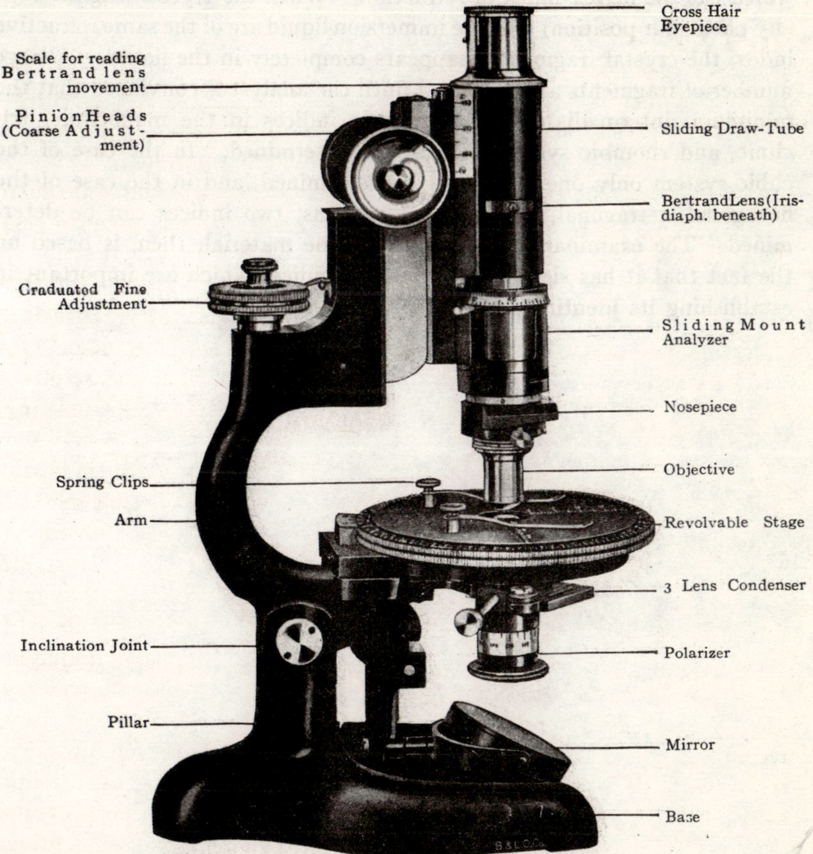

FIG. 301.—Petrographic microscope.

The determination of the refractive indices of the substance is based on matching the refractive index of a crystalline fragment oriented in a certain position against that of the oily liquid which has been predetermined on a refractometer. The fragment of material, immersed in the liquid on a slide, is examined under the microscope with the polarizer (lower nicol) in place. Attention is then paid to the direction in which the band of light surrounding the fragment moves when the microscope tube is raised. If it passes into the crystal the refractive index in the crystallographic direction lying parallel to the plane of the nicol is higher than that of the crystal. In other words, when the microscope tube is raised, the band of light passes toward the medium (either liquid or crystal) which has the higher index of refraction. When the crystal fragment (in any particular position) and the immersion liquid are of the same refractive index, the crystal fragment disappears completely in the liquid. A large number of fragments are examined until the analyst is convinced that the minimum, intermediate, and maximum indices in the monoclinic, triclinic, and rhombic systems have been determined. In the case of the cubic system only one index can be determined, and in the case of the hexagonal, tetragonal, and trigonal systems, two indices can be determined. The examination of any crystalline material, then, is based on the fact that it has significant refractive indices which are important in establishing its identity.

BIBLIOGRAPHY

WALLIS, T. E.: "Analytical Microscopy." 1924.

WALLIS, T. E.: "The use of lycopodium in quantitative microscopy." Pharm. Jour., 103: 75–76, 1919.

LEFFMANN, HENRY: "Some applications of the microscope in research." Jour. Franklin Institute, 193: 81–88, 1922.

KEENAN, GEO. L.. "The Value of Microanalytical Methods and Examples of Their Application." Jour. Amer. Pharm. Assoc., 14: 112–113, Feb., 1925.

CLARK, CHAS. H.: "Practical Methods in Microscopy. (5th Ed.)" 1924.

GREENISH, HENRY G.: "Microscopical Methods with Special Reference to the Examination of Drugs." The Analyst, July, 1916, pp. 195–203.

BARNARD, J. E.: "The limitations of microscopy." Jour. Royal Microscopical Soc., Jan., 1919, pp. 1–13.

WRIGHT, P. E.: "The Petrographic Microscope." Jour. Optical Soc. of America, 1: 15–21, Jan., 1917.

WRIGHT, F. E.: "The Petrographic Microscope in Analysis." Jour. Amer. Chem. Soc., 38: 1647–1658, Sept., 1916.

JOHANNSEN, A.: "Manual of Petrographic Methods." (2nd Ed.) 1918.

PREGL, FRITZ: "Quantitative Organic Microanalysis." Trans. by Ernest Fyleman. 1924.

EMICH, F.: "Mikrochemisches Praktikum." Munich, 1924.

BEHRENS, H. & KLEY, P. D. C.: "Mikrochemische analyse." Leipzig, 3d. ed. 1915.

CHAMOT, E. M.: "Elementary Chemical Microscopy." (2nd. Ed.) 1921.

BEHRENS, H.: "A Manual of Microchemical Analysis." 1894.

WRIGHT, F. E.: "The Methods of Petrographic-Microscopic Research." Bul. 158, Carnegie Inst., Washington, 1911.

GAGE, S. H.: "The Microscope." (14th Ed.)

WINTON, A. L.: "The Microscopy of Vegetable Foods." (2nd. Ed.) 1916.

KEENAN, GEO. L. & LYONS, MARY A.: "The Microscopical Examination of Flour." Bul. 839, U.S. Dept. Agriculture, Aug., 1922.

HANAUSEK, T. F. & WINTON, A. L.: "The Microscopy of Technical Products." 1907.

KEENAN, GEO. L.: "The Application of Optical Methods to the Examination of Insecticides and Fungicides." Jour. Amer. Pharm. Assoc., 10: 331–336, May, 1921.

KEENAN, GEO. L.: The Microscopical Identification of Some Sodium and Potassium Salts." Jour. Amer. Pharm. Assoc., 13: 122–125, Feb., 1924.

HINRICHS, C. G.: "Microchemical Analysis." 1904.

STEPHENSON, CHAS. H.: "Some Microchemical Tests for Alkaloids." 1921.

FRY, WILLIAM H.: "Tables for the Microscopic Identification of Inorganic Salts." Bul. No. 1108, U.S. Dept. of Agriculture, Nov. 6, 1922.

WHERRY, EDGAR T.: "The Application of Optical Methods of Identification to Alkaloids and Other Organic Compounds." Bul. No. 679, U.S. Dept. of Agriculture, May 20, 1918.

WALLIS, T. E., "The use of Synthesis in Quantitative Microscopy," Pharm. Jour. 109: 192-6, 1922.

WHEATLEY, [illegible], "The Limitations of Microscopy," Jour. Royal Microscopical Soc., Jan., 1926, pp. 1-13.

HOFFMAN, C. G., "Microchemical Analysis," 1909.

INDEX